PHARMACOLOGY

A SAUNDERS TEXT

PHARMACOLOGY

GEORGE M. BRENNER, Ph.D.

Professor of Pharmacology
and
Chairman, Department of Pharmacology and Physiology
Oklahoma State University, Center for Health Sciences
Tulsa, Oklahoma

SAUNDERS
An Imprint of Elsevier

SAUNDERS
An Imprint of Elsevier

The Curtis Center
Independence Square West
Philadelphia, Pennsylvania 19106

Library of Congress Cataloging-in-Publication Data

Brenner, George M.
Pharmacology/George M. Brenner—1st ed.

p.   cm.   (Saunders text and review series)

ISBN 0–7216–7757–6

I. Title. II. Series.
  [DNLM: 1. Pharmacology.   2. Drug Therapy.   3. Pharmaceutical
  Preparations. QV 4 B838p 2000]

RM300 B74 2000

615′1—dc21   99–051716

ISBN 0–7216–7757–6

Pharmacology

Permissions may be sought directly from Elsevier's Health Sciences Rights
Department in Philadelphia, USA: phone: (+)215-238-7869, fax: (+)215-238-2239,
email: healthpermissions@elsevier.com. You may also complete your request on-line via
the Elsevier Science homepage (http://www.elsevier.com), by selecting 'Customer Support'
and then 'Obtaining Permissions'.

Printed in the United States of America.

Last digit is the print number: 9   8   7   6   5

PREFACE

Medical pharmacology is primarily concerned with the mechanisms by which drugs alter the functions of living cells to relieve the symptoms and pathophysiologic manifestations of disease. It is an applied science that utilizes clinical data and basic science material from numerous fields, including biochemistry, microbiology, physiology, and pathology, to explain how drugs affect the human body. For this reason, the study of pharmacology provides an opportunity for students to review basic science concepts and apply these concepts to clinical problems.

Students in the health professions are often overwhelmed by the vast amount of pharmacologic information that is available today. Many traditional textbooks contain more information than an individual can possibly learn, and the most important points are often lost in a maze of details. Other books have the opposite problem and fail to cover important concepts and clinical applications. This book is the outgrowth of teaching pharmacology to medical, nursing, and pharmacy students for over 25 years. It provides the essential information and concepts that students need to be successful in their courses, but it omits details that are primarily of interest to research scientists or clinical specialists.

Because of the large number of drugs that are available today, the text emphasizes the general properties of drug categories and prototypical drugs. Throughout the book, the pharmacologic information is organized in the same format. A drug classification box is included at the beginning of the chapter to familiarize students with categories, subcategories, and examples of individual drugs to be discussed in the chapter. Within the chapter, discussion focuses on mechanisms of action, drug effects, and clinical uses for each drug category. Pharmacologic and clinical terms are clearly defined so that readers do not need to look up this information in other sources. Numerous illustrations are used to depict drug mechanisms and other conceptual information, while well-organized tables are included to highlight differences in the specific properties of drugs within a therapeutic category. At the end of each chapter, a summary of important points is provided to reinforce the pharmacologic concepts and clinical applications that are crucial for students to remember.

The text is divided into seven sections, the first of which covers basic principles of pharmacology. Five of the remaining sections are concerned with drugs that act on various organ systems, and the last section provides data on antimicrobial and cancer chemotherapy. Most of the chapters deal with drugs that are used to treat one or two particular types of disease. For example, in Section IV (Central Nervous System Pharmacology), Chapter 20 describes antiepileptic drugs for seizure disorders, and

Chapter 22 discusses psychotherapeutic drugs for depression and schizophrenia. The sections in the book are organized in the same sequence used in many pharmacology courses for students of medicine and related disciplines. While *Pharmacology* is primarily intended for use by students taking their first pharmacology course, it will also be useful for those who are preparing to take medical board examinations.

This book would not have been possible without the encouragement and advice of mentors, colleagues, and editorial personnel. I am particularly grateful to Dr. David John and Dr. Edward Goljan, the friends and colleagues who inspired me to undertake this task and whose personal experiences as textbook authors were invaluable to me. I am indebted to my editor at W.B. Saunders, Bill Schmitt, for his interest and support. A special word of appreciation is extended to Sharon Maddox for her continuous advice, encouragement, and editorial work on the manuscript. I am also indebted to Kristin Mount for preparing the excellent illustrations in the book. Finally, I would like to thank my wife and family for their understanding and patience throughout this endeavor.

GEORGE M. BRENNER

CONTENTS

SECTION III

CARDIOVASCULAR, RENAL, AND HEMATOLOGIC PHARMACOLOGY

SECTION IV

CENTRAL NERVOUS SYSTEM PHARMACOLOGY

SECTION V

PHARMACOLOGY OF THE RESPIRATORY, GASTROINTESTINAL, AND OTHER ORGAN SYSTEMS

SECTION VI

ENDOCRINE PHARMACOLOGY

SECTION VII

CHEMOTHERAPY

SECTION I

PRINCIPLES OF

PHARMACOLOGY

CHAPTER ONE

INTRODUCTION

TO PHARMACOLOGY

PHARMACOLOGY AND RELATED SCIENCES

History and Role of Pharmacology

Although people have attempted to treat diseases with substances derived from plants, animals, and minerals for over 4000 years, the science of pharmacology is less than 150 years old. Historically, the selection and use of drugs were based on superstition or on experience (empiricism). Knowledge of the physiologic mechanisms by which drugs produce their therapeutic effects has largely been acquired during the past century, ushering in the era of rational pharmacotherapeutics.

In the first or earliest phase of drug usage, noxious plant and animal preparations were administered to the diseased patient to rid the body of the evil spirits believed to cause illness. The Greek word *pharmakon,* from which the term *pharmacology* is derived, originally meant a magic charm for treating disease. Later, *pharmakon* came to mean a remedy or drug.

In the second phase of drug usage, people learned by experience which substances were actually beneficial in relieving particular disease symptoms. The first effective drugs were probably simple external preparations such as cool mud or a soothing leaf, and the earliest known prescriptions from 2100 BCE included salves containing thyme. Over many centuries, people learned the therapeutic value of natural products through trial and error. By 1500 BCE, Egyptian prescriptions called for castor oil, opium, and other drugs still in use today. Dioscorides, a Greek army surgeon of the first century CE, described over 600 medicinal plants that he collected and studied as he traveled with the Roman armies. During the Middle Ages, Islamic physicians (such as Avicenna) and Christian monks cultivated and studied the use of herbal medicines.

The third phase of drug usage, the rational or scientific phase, gradually evolved with important advances in chemistry and physiology that gave rise to the new science of pharmacology. At the same time, a more rational understanding of disease mechanisms provided a scientific basis for employing drugs whose physiologic actions and effects were understood. Some of the critical events leading to the development of pharmacology and pharmacotherapeutics are listed in Table 1–1.

The advent of pharmacology was particularly dependent on the isolation of pure drug compounds from natural sources and on the development of experimental physiology methods to study these compounds. The isolation of morphine from opium in 1804 was rapidly followed by the extraction of many other drugs from plant sources, providing a diverse array of pure drugs for pharmacologic experimentation. Advances in physiology allowed pioneers such as François Magendie and Claude Bernard to conduct some of the earliest pharmacologic investigations, including studies that localized the site of action of curare to the neuromuscular junction. The first medical school pharmacology laboratory was started by Rudolf Büchheim in Estonia. Büchheim and one of his students, Oswald Schmiedeberg, trained many other pharmacologists, including John Jacob Abel, who began the first pharmacology departments in the USA.

The goal of pharmacology is to understand the mechanisms by which drugs interact with biologic systems so as to enable the rational use of effective agents in the diagnosis and treatment of disease. The success of pharmacology in this task has led to an explosion of new drug development, particularly in the past 50 years. Twentieth-century developments include the isolation and use of insulin for diabetes, the discovery of antimicrobial and antineoplastic drugs, and the advent of modern psychopharmacology. Recent advances in molecular biology, genetics, and drug design suggest that new drug development and pharmacologic innovations will provide even greater advances in the treatment of medical disorders in the future.

Pharmacology and Its Subdivisions

Pharmacology is the biomedical science concerned with the interaction of chemical substances with living cells, tissues, and organisms. It is particularly concerned with the mechanisms by which drugs counteract the manifestations of disease and by which drugs affect fertility. Pharmacology is not primarily concerned with the synthesis or isolation of drugs or with the preparation of pharmaceutical

TABLE 1–1.   Important Persons and Events in the History of Pharmacology

Person and Life Span	Event
Paracelsus (1493–1541)	Refuted the tenets of humoralism. Advocated the use of a specific chemical to treat a particular disease (such as the use of mercury to treat syphilis).
John Wepfer (1620–1695)	Published studies on the toxicity of drugs and poisons in animals.
Felice Fontana (1730–1805)	Studied the toxicity of crude drug preparations.
Frederick Sertürner (1783–1841)	Isolated morphine from opium in 1804, becoming the first scientist to isolate the active ingredient of a natural drug.
François Magendie (1783–1855)	Proposed that the sites of action of drugs could be localized to specific organs in the body.
Claude Bernard (1813–1878)	Localized the site of action of curare to the neuromuscular junction in 1856.
Rudolf Büchheim (1820–1879)	Established the first medical school laboratory to be used exclusively for pharmacologic studies. Proposed that drugs exert their effects via their physiochemical interaction with cell constituents.
Oswald Schmiedeberg (1838–1921)	Was a student of Büchheim and later trained many pharmacologists, including John Jacob Abel. Defined pharmacology as the science concerned with effects of chemicals on living organisms.
Paul Ehrlich (1854–1915)	Demonstrated that drugs can destroy microbes. Developed antimicrobial chemotherapy.
John Jacob Abel (1857–1938)	Was the first pharmacology professor in the USA. Started pharmacology society and journals.

products. The sciences that deal with these subjects are described below.

Pharmacology has been divided into two subdivisions, **pharmacokinetics** and **pharmacodynamics.** The relationship between these subdivisions is shown in Fig. 1–1. Pharmacokinetics is concerned with the processes that determine the concentration of drugs in body fluids and tissues over time, including **drug absorption, distribution, biotransformation,** and **excretion.** Pharmacodynamics is the study of the actions of drugs on target organs. It is particularly concerned with the **biochemical mechanisms** by which drugs produce their physiologic effects and with the **dose-response relationship,** defined as the relationship between the concentration of a drug in a tissue and the magnitude of the tissue's response to that drug. Most drugs produce their effects by binding to macromolecular **receptors** in target tissues, a process that activates a cascade of events known as **signal transduction.** Pharmacokinetics and pharmacodynamics are discussed in greater detail in Chapters 2 and 3.

Toxicology

Toxicology is the science of poisons and toxicity. It focuses on the harmful effects of drugs and other chemicals and on the mechanisms by which toxic agents produce pathologic changes, disease, and death. Like pharmacology, toxicology is concerned with the relationship between the dose of an agent and the resulting tissue concentration and biologic effects that the agent produces. For this reason, some authorities consider toxicology to be a subdivision of pharmacology.

Pharmacotherapeutics

Pharmacotherapeutics is the medical science concerned with the use of drugs in the treatment of disease. Pharmacology provides a rational basis for pharmacotherapeutics by explaining the mechanisms and effects of drugs on the body and the relationship between dose and drug response. Human studies known as **clinical trials** are then used to determine the efficacy and safety of drug therapy in

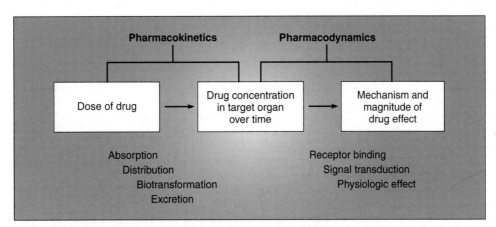

FIGURE 1–1. Relationship between pharmacokinetics and pharmacodynamics.

human subjects. The purpose, design, and evaluation of human drug studies are discussed in Chapter 4.

Pharmacy and Related Sciences

Pharmacy is the science and profession concerned with the preparation, storage, dispensing, and proper utilization of drug products. Related sciences include pharmacognosy, medicinal chemistry, and pharmaceutical chemistry. **Pharmacognosy** is concerned with the isolation and characterization of drugs from natural sources, including plants, microbes, animal tissues, and minerals. **Medicinal chemistry** is a branch of organic chemistry that specializes in the design and chemical synthesis of drugs. **Pharmaceutical chemistry, or pharmaceutics,** is concerned with the formulation and chemical properties of pharmaceutical products, such as tablets, liquid solutions and suspensions, and aerosols.

DRUG SOURCES AND PREPARATIONS

A **drug** can be defined as a natural product, chemical substance, or pharmaceutical preparation intended for administration to a human or animal for the purpose of diagnosing or treating a disease. The word *drug* is derived from the French *drogue,* which traditionally meant dried herbs and which was originally used in the context of the sale and marketing of herbs, rather than the medicinal use of these substances. **Medication** and **medicament** are terms often used synonymously with the word *drug.*

Natural Sources of Drugs

Drugs have been obtained from **plants, microbes, animal tissues,** and **minerals.** Among the various types of drugs derived from plants are **alkaloids,** which are nitrogenous substances that give an alkaline reaction in aqueous solution. Examples of alkaloids include morphine, cocaine, atropine, and quinine. **Antibiotics** have been isolated from numerous microorganisms, including *Penicillium* and *Streptomyces* species. **Hormones** are the most common type of drug obtained from animals, while minerals have yielded a small number of useful therapeutic agents, including the lithium compounds used in psychotherapy.

Synthetic Drugs

The rise of modern chemistry in the 19th century enabled scientists to synthesize new compounds and to modify naturally occurring drugs. Aspirin, barbiturates, and local anesthetics such as procaine were among the first drugs to be synthesized in the laboratory. Semisynthetic derivatives of naturally occurring compounds, such as morphine, have enabled the development of drugs with improved pharmacokinetic and pharmacodynamic properties.

In some cases, scientists have discovered new drug compounds either by accident or by actively screening various agents for their potential pharma-

cologic activity. With some classes of drugs, however, scientists have been able to discern a **structure-activity relationship** (a relationship between the chemical structure and the pharmacologic activity), and this information has guided the synthesis of new compounds. Recently, chemists have developed new drugs with the aid of computer programs that model the receptor of a particular drug and facilitate the design of drug structures that best fit the three-dimensional conformation of the receptor. This approach has been used, for example, to design agents that inhibit angiotensin synthesis and agents that inhibit the maturation of the human immunodeficiency virus.

Drug Preparations

Drug preparations include crude drug preparations obtained from natural sources, pure drug compounds isolated from natural sources or synthesized in the laboratory, and pharmaceutical preparations of drugs intended for administration to patients. The relationship between these types of drug preparations is illustrated in Fig. 1–2.

Crude Drug Preparations

Some crude drug preparations are made by drying or pulverizing a plant or animal tissue. Others are made by extracting substances from a natural product with the aid of hot water or a solvent such as alcohol. Three familiar examples of crude drug preparations are coffee, tea, and opium (the dried

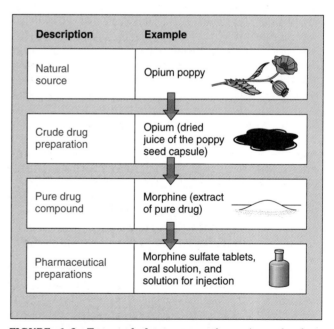

Description	Example
Natural source	Opium poppy
Crude drug preparation	Opium (dried juice of the poppy seed capsule)
Pure drug compound	Morphine (extract of pure drug)
Pharmaceutical preparations	Morphine sulfate tablets, oral solution, and solution for injection

FIGURE 1–2. Types of drug preparations. A crude drug preparation retains most or all of the active and inactive compounds contained in the natural source from which it was derived. After a pure drug compound (for example, morphine) is extracted from a crude drug preparation (in this case, opium), it is possible to manufacture pharmaceutical preparations that are suitable for administration of a particular dose to the patient.

juice of the poppy seed capsule). Many herbal medicines are available today in the form of crude drug preparations containing the same active and inactive ingredients that are found in the original source.

Pure Drug Compounds

It is difficult to identify and quantify the pharmacologic effects of crude drug preparations because these products contain multiple ingredients, the amounts of which vary from batch to batch. Hence, the development of methods to isolate pure drug compounds from natural sources was an important step in the growth of pharmacology and rational therapeutics. Frederick Sertürner, a German apothecary, isolated the first pure drug from a natural source when he extracted and purified morphine from opium in 1804 and named it after Morpheus, the Greek god of dreams. The subsequent isolation of many other drugs from natural sources provided pharmacologists with a number of pure compounds for study and characterization. One of the greatest medical achievements of the early 20th century was the isolation of insulin from the pancreas. This achievement by Frederick Banting and Charles Best led to the development of insulin preparations for treating diabetes mellitus.

Pharmaceutical Preparations

Pharmaceutical preparations or dosage forms are drug products suitable for administration of a specific dose of a drug to a patient by a particular route of administration. Most of these preparations are made from pure drug compounds, but a few are made from crude drug preparations.

Tablets and Capsules. Tablets and capsules are the most common preparations for oral administration because they are suitable for mass production, are stable, are convenient to use, and can be formulated to release the drug immediately after ingestion or to release it over a period of hours.

In the manufacture of tablets, a machine with a punch and die mechanism is used to compress a mixture of powdered drug and inert ingredients into a relatively hard disk. The **inert ingredients** include specific components that provide bulk, prevent sticking to the punch and die, prevent disintegration in the bottle, and facilitate disintegration of the tablet when it reaches gastrointestinal fluids. These ingredients are called **fillers, lubricants, adhesives,** and **disintegrants,** respectively.

A tablet must disintegrate after it is ingested, and then the drug must dissolve in gastrointestinal fluids before it can be absorbed into the circulation. Variations in the rate and extent of tablet disintegration and drug dissolution may give rise to differences in the oral bioavailability of drugs from different tablet formulations.

Tablets may be coated with various types of coatings. **Enteric coatings** consist of polymers that will not disintegrate in gastric acid but will break

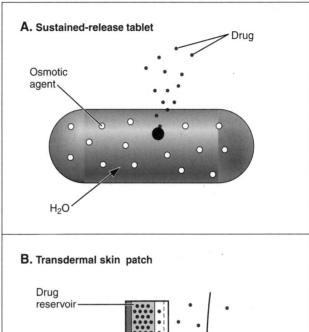

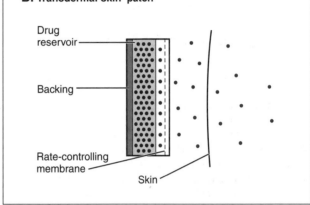

FIGURE 1–3. Mechanisms of sustained-release drug products. (A) In the sustained-release tablet, water is attracted by an osmotic agent in the tablet, and this forces the drug out through a small orifice. (B) In the transdermal skin patch, the drug diffuses through a rate-controlling membrane and is absorbed through the skin into the circulation.

down in the more alkaline intestines. Enteric coatings are used to protect drugs that would otherwise be destroyed by gastric acid.

Sustained-release products, or **extended-release products,** release the drug from the preparation over many hours. The two methods that are used to extend the release of the drug are **controlled diffusion** and **controlled dissolution.** Diffusion of the drug from the drug product may be regulated by means of a rate-controlling membrane. Dissolution is controlled by means of inert polymers that gradually break down in body fluids. These polymers may be part of the tablet matrix, or they may be used as coatings over small pellets of drug enclosed in a capsule. In either case, the drug is gradually released into the gastrointestinal tract as the polymers dissolve.

Some products utilize **osmotic pressure** to provide a sustained release of a drug. These products contains an osmotic agent that attracts gastrointestinal fluid at a constant rate. The attracted fluid then forces the drug out of the tablet through a small laser-drilled orifice (Fig. 1–3A).

Capsules are hard or soft gelatin shells enclosing a powdered or liquid medication. **Hard capsules** are used to enclose powdered drugs, whereas **soft capsules** enclose a drug in solution. The gelatin shell quickly dissolves in gastrointestinal fluids to release the drug for absorption into the circulation.

Solutions and Suspensions. Drug solutions and particle suspensions are the most common liquid pharmaceutical preparations and may be formulated for oral, parenteral, or other routes of administration. Solutions and suspensions provide a convenient method for administering drugs to pediatric and other patients who cannot easily swallow solid dosage forms. They are less convenient than solid dosage forms, however, because the liquid must be measured each time a dose is given.

Solutions and suspensions for oral administration are often sweetened and flavored to increase palatability. Sweetened aqueous solutions are called **syrups,** whereas sweetened aqueous-alcoholic solutions are known as **elixirs.** Alcohol is included in elixirs as a solvent for drugs that are not sufficiently soluble in water alone.

Sterile solutions and suspensions are available for parenteral administration with a needle and syringe or with an intravenous infusion device. Many drugs are formulated as sterile powders for reconstitution with sterile liquids at the time the drug is to be injected, because the drug is not stable for long periods of time in solution. Sterile ophthalmic solutions and suspensions are suitable for administration with a dropper into the conjunctival sac.

Skin Patches. Skin patches are drug preparations in which the drug is slowly released from the patch for absorption through the skin into the circulation. Most skin patches use a rate-controlling membrane to regulate the diffusion of the drug from the patch (see Fig. 1–3B). Such devices are most suitable for drugs that are effective at a relatively low dosage and have sufficient lipid solubility to enable skin penetration.

Aerosols. Aerosols are a type of drug preparation administered by inhalation through the nose or mouth. They are particularly useful for treating respiratory disorders because they deliver the drug directly to the site of action and may thereby minimize the risk of systemic side effects. Some aerosol devices contain the drug dispersed in a pressurized gas and are designed to deliver a precise dosage each time they are activated by the patient. **Nasal sprays,** another type of aerosol preparation, can be used either to deliver drugs that have a localized effect on the nasal mucosa or to deliver drugs that are absorbed through the mucosa and exert an effect on another organ. For example, butorphanol, an opioid analgesic, is available as a nasal spray for the treatment of pain.

Ointments, Creams, Lotions, and Suppositories. Ointments and creams are semisolid preparations intended for topical application of a drug to the skin or mucous membranes. These products contain an active drug that is incorporated into a vehicle such as polyethylene glycol or petrolatum, which enables the drug to adhere to the tissue for a sufficient length of time to exert its effect. Lotions are liquid preparations that are often formulated as oil-in-water emulsions and find use in treating dermatologic conditions. Suppositories are products in which the drug is incorporated into a solid base that melts or dissolves at body temperature. Suppositories are usually intended for rectal, vaginal, or urethral administration and may provide either localized or systemic drug therapy.

ROUTES OF DRUG ADMINISTRATION

Some routes of drug administration, such as the four enteral and parenteral routes compared in Table 1–2, are intended to elicit systemic effects and are commonly called systemic routes. Other routes of administration, such as the inhalational route, may elicit either localized effects or systemic effects, depending on the drug being administered.

Enteral Administration

The enteral routes of administration are those in which the drug is absorbed from the gastrointestinal tract. These include sublingual, buccal, oral, and rectal routes.

In **sublingual administration,** a drug product is placed under the tongue. In **buccal administration,**

TABLE 1–2. Advantages and Disadvantages of Four Common Routes of Drug Administration

Route	Advantages	Disadvantages
Oral	Is convenient, relatively safe, and economical.	Cannot be used for drugs that are inactivated by gastric acid, for drugs that have a large first-pass effect, or for drugs that irritate the gut.
Intramuscular	Is suitable for suspensions and oily vehicles. Absorption is rapid from solutions and is slow and sustained from suspensions.	May be painful. Can cause bleeding if the patient is receiving an anticoagulant.
Subcutaneous	Is suitable for suspensions and pellets. Absorption is similar to the intramuscular route but is usually somewhat slower.	Cannot be used for drugs that irritate cutaneous tissues or for drugs that must be given in large volumes.
Intravenous	Bypasses absorption to give an immediate effect. Allows for rapid titration of dosage. Has 100% bioavailability.	Poses more risks for toxicity and tends to be more expensive than other routes.

the drug is placed between the cheek and the gums. Sublingual and buccal administration enable the rapid absorption of certain drugs and are not affected by first-pass drug metabolism in the liver. Drugs for sublingual and buccal administration must be given in a relatively low dosage and must have good solubility in water and lipid membranes. Larger doses might be irritating to the tissue and would likely be washed away by saliva before the drug would be absorbed. Two examples of drugs available for sublingual and buccal administration are nitroglycerin for treating ischemic heart disease and hyoscyamine for treating bowel cramps.

In medical orders and prescriptions, **oral administration** is often designated as *per os* (PO) and refers to drug administration by mouth. The medication is swallowed, and the drug is absorbed from the stomach and small intestines. Because the oral route of administration is convenient and relatively safe and economical, it is the most commonly used route. It does have some disadvantages, however. Absorption of orally administered drugs may be quite variable because of the interaction of drugs with food and gastric acid, the varying rates of gastric emptying and intestinal transit, and the varying rates of tablet disintegration and dissolution. Moreover, some drugs are inactivated by the liver following their absorption from the gut, and oral administration is not suitable for use by patients who are sedated, comatose, or suffering from nausea and vomiting.

Rectal administration of drugs in suppository form may result in either a localized effect or a systemic effect. Suppositories are useful when patients cannot take medications by mouth, such as in the treatment of nausea and vomiting. They may also be administered for localized conditions such as hemorrhoids. Drugs absorbed from the rectum undergo relatively little first-pass metabolism in the liver.

Parenteral Administration

Parenteral administration refers to drug administration with a needle and syringe or with an intravenous infusion device. The most commonly used parenteral routes are the intravenous, intramuscular, and subcutaneous routes.

Intravenous administration bypasses the process of drug absorption and provides the greatest reliability and control over the dose of drug reaching the general circulation. It is often preferred for administration of drugs that have short half-lives and drugs whose dosage must be carefully titrated to the physiologic response, such as agents used to treat hypotension, shock, and acute heart failure. The intravenous route is widely used to administer antibiotics and antineoplastic drugs to critically ill patients, as well as to treat various types of medical emergencies. The intravenous route is potentially the most dangerous, because rapid administration of drugs by this route may cause serious toxicity.

Intramuscular administration and **subcutaneous administration** are suitable for treatment with drug solutions and particle suspensions. Solutions are absorbed more rapidly than particle suspensions, so suspensions are often employed to extend the duration of action of a drug over many hours or days. Most drugs are absorbed more rapidly after intramuscular than after subcutaneous administration because of the greater circulation of blood to the muscle.

Intrathecal administration refers to injection of a drug through the theca of the spinal cord and into the subarachnoid space. In cases of meningitis, the intrathecal route is useful in administering antibiotics that do not cross the blood-brain barrier.

Other less commonly used parenteral routes include **intra-articular administration** of drugs used to treat arthritis.

Transdermal Administration

Transdermal administration refers to the application of drugs to the skin for absorption into the circulation. Application may be via a skin patch or, less commonly, via an ointment. Transdermal administration bypasses first-pass hepatic inactivation and is a reliable route of administration for drugs that are effective when given in a relatively low dosage and that are highly soluble in lipid membranes. Two examples of transdermal preparations are estradiol transdermal patches and nitroglycerin ointment.

Inhalational Administration

Inhalational administration may be used to produce either a localized or a systemic drug effect. A localized effect on the respiratory tract is obtained with drugs used to treat asthma or rhinitis, whereas a systemic effect is observed when a general anesthetic, such as halothane, is inhaled.

Topical Administration

Topical administration refers to the application of drugs to the surface of the body to produce a localized effect. It is often used for treating disorders of the skin, eyes, nose, mouth, throat, rectum, and vagina.

DRUG NAMES

A drug often has several names, including a chemical name, a nonproprietary name, and a proprietary name.

The **chemical name** specifies the chemical structure of the drug and uses standard chemical nomenclature. Some chemical names, such as acetylsalicylic acid, are relatively short. Others are relatively long because of the size and complexity of the drug molecule. For most drugs, the chemical name is primarily of interest to the chemist.

The **nonproprietary name,** or **generic name,** is the type of drug name most suitable for use by health care professionals. In the USA, the preferred nonproprietary names are the **United States Adopted Names (USAN)** designations. These designations are often derived from the chemical names of drugs and provide some indication of the class to which a particular drug belongs. For example, oxacillin can be easily recognized as a type of penicillin. The designations are selected by the USAN Council, which is a nomenclature committee representing the medical and pharmacy professions and the United States Pharmacopeia (see Chapter 4), with advisory input from the Food and Drug Administration. The USAN is often the same as the **International Nonproprietary Name** (INN) and the **British Approved Name** (BAN). However, international names for drugs may vary with the language in which they are used.

The **proprietary name, trade name,** or **brand name** for a drug is a registered trademark belonging to a particular drug manufacturer and used to designate a drug product marketed by that manufacturer. Many drugs are marketed under two or more trade names, especially those drugs which are contained in combination drug products. Drugs may also be marketed under their USAN. For these reasons, it is often less confusing and more precise to use the USAN rather than a trade name for a drug. The proprietary name may provide some indication of the drug's pharmacologic or therapeutic effect. For example, Diuril is a proprietary name for a diuretic, Calan is a name for a calcium antagonist, and Maxair is a product used to treat asthma.

Summary of Important Points

- The development of pharmacology was made possible by important advances in chemistry and physiology that enabled scientists to isolate and synthesize pure chemical compounds (drugs) and to design methods for identifying and quantifying the physiologic actions of the compounds.
- Pharmacology has two subdivisions. Pharmacodynamics is concerned with the mechanisms of drug action and the dose-response relationship, whereas pharmacokinetics is concerned with the relationship between the drug dose and the plasma drug concentration over time.
- The sources of drugs are natural products (including plants, microbes, animal tissues, and minerals) and chemical synthesis. Drugs may exist as crude drug preparations, pure drug compounds, or pharmaceutical preparations used to administer a specific dose to a patient.
- The primary routes of administration are enteral (for example, oral ingestion), parenteral (for example, intravenous, intramuscular, and subcutaneous injection), transdermal, inhalational, and topical. Most routes produce systemic effects. Topical administration produces a localized effect at the site of administration.
- All drugs (pure compounds) have a nonproprietary name (a generic name, such as a USAN designation) as well as a chemical name. Some drugs also have one or more proprietary names (trade names or brand names) under which they are marketed by their manufacturer.

Selected Readings

Cowan, D. L., and W. H. Helfand. Pharmacy: An Illustrated History. New York, Harry N. Abrams, Inc., 1990.

Fleeger, C. A., ed. USP Dictionary of USAN and International Drug Names. Rockville, Md., United States Pharmacopeia, 1997.

Lyons, A. S., and R. J. Petracelli. Medicine: An Illustrated History. New York, Harry N. Abrams, Inc., 1978.

Tyler, V. E. The Honest Herbal, 3rd ed. New York, Pharmaceutical Products Press, 1993.

CHAPTER TWO

PHARMACOKINETICS

OVERVIEW

Pharmacokinetics is concerned with the relationship between the **dose** of a particular drug and the **concentration** of that drug in body fluids and tissues over time, as determined by the rates of **drug absorption, drug distribution,** and **drug elimination.** Drug elimination includes the **biotransformation** (metabolism) of a drug to one or more drug metabolites as well as the **excretion** of the drug from the body. The relationship between these processes is shown in Fig. 2–1.

To derive and use expressions for pharmacokinetic parameters, the first step is to establish a mathematical model that accurately relates the plasma drug concentration to the rates of drug absorption, distribution, and elimination. The **one-compartment model** is the simplest model of drug disposition, but the **two-compartment model** provides a more accurate representation of the pharmacokinetic behavior of many drugs (Fig. 2–2). In the two-compartment model, drugs are absorbed into the central compartment (the blood), distributed from the central compartment to the peripheral compartment (the tissues), and eliminated from the central compartment. Rate constants can be determined for each process and used to derive expressions for other pharmacokinetic parameters, such as the elimination half-life of a drug. In this chapter, each process of drug disposition will be considered in greater detail.

DRUG ABSORPTION

Except for topically administered drugs that are absorbed directly into the target tissue, drug absorption refers to the passage of a drug from its site of administration into the circulation. Absorption requires the passage of drugs across one or more layers of cells. In the gut, lungs, and skin, drugs must first be absorbed through a layer of epithelial cells that have tight junctions (Fig. 2–3). Drugs that are injected into the subcutaneous tissue and muscle bypass the epithelial barrier and are more easily absorbed through spaces between capillary endothelial cells. For this reason, drugs face a greater barrier to absorption after oral administration than after parenteral administration.

Processes of Absorption

Most drugs are absorbed by **passive diffusion** across a biologic barrier and into the circulation. The rate of absorption is proportional to the drug concentration gradient across the barrier and the surface area available for absorption at that site. Drugs may be absorbed passively through cells either by lipid diffusion or by aqueous diffusion. **Lipid diffusion** is a process in which the drug dissolves in the lipid components of the cell membranes. This process is facilitated by a high degree of lipid solubility. **Aqueous diffusion** occurs by passage through the aqueous pores in cell membranes. Because aqueous diffusion is restricted to drugs with molecular weights lower than 200, most drugs are too large to be absorbed by this process.

A few drugs are absorbed by **active transport** or by **facilitated diffusion.** For example, some cephalosporin antibiotics are partly absorbed by the transporter for dipeptides, which is located in intestinal epithelial cells. Investigators have suggested that drug absorption could be enhanced by designing drugs that would utilize such transporters for absorption.

Effect of pH on Absorption of Weak Acids and Bases

Many drugs are weak acids and bases that exist in both ionized and nonionized forms in the body. Only the nonionized form of these drugs is sufficiently soluble in membrane lipids so as to be readily transferred across cell membranes (Box 2–1). The ratio of the two forms at a particular site influences the rate of drug absorption, distribution, or elimination.

The protonated form of a weak acid is nonionized, whereas the protonated form of a weak base is ionized. The ratio of the protonated form to the nonprotonated form of these drugs can be calculated using the **Henderson-Hasselbalch equation** (see Box 2–1). At a pH equal to the pK_a, equal amounts of the protonated and nonprotonated forms are present. If the pH is less than the pK_a, the protonated form predominates. If the pH is greater than the pK_a, the nonprotonated form predominates.

In the stomach, with a pH of 1, weak acids and bases are highly protonated. At this site, the nonionized form of weak acids (pK_a = 3–5) and the ionized form of weak bases (pK_a = 8–10) will predominate. Hence, weak acids are more readily absorbed from the stomach than are weak bases. In the intestines, with a pH of 6–7, weak bases are also mostly ionized, but much less so than in the stomach, and weak bases are absorbed more readily from the intestines than

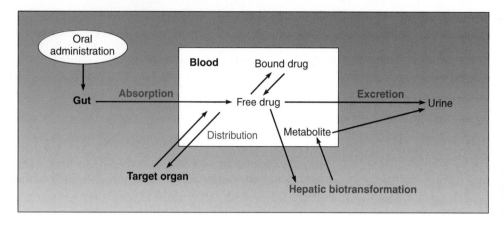

FIGURE 2-1. The absorption, distribution, hepatic biotransformation, and excretion of a typical drug after its oral administration.

FIGURE 2-2. Two models of the processes of drug absorption, distribution, and elimination. K_a, K_d, and K_e are the rate constants, representing the fractional completion of each process per unit of time. **(A)** In the one-compartment model, the drug concentration at any time (C) is the amount of drug in the body at that time (D) divided by the volume of the compartment (V). Thus, D is a function of the dose administered and the rates of absorption and elimination represented by K_a and K_e, respectively. **(B)** In the two-compartment model, the drug concentration in the central compartment (the blood) is a function of the dose administered and the rates of drug absorption, distribution to the peripheral compartment (the tissues), and elimination from the central compartment.

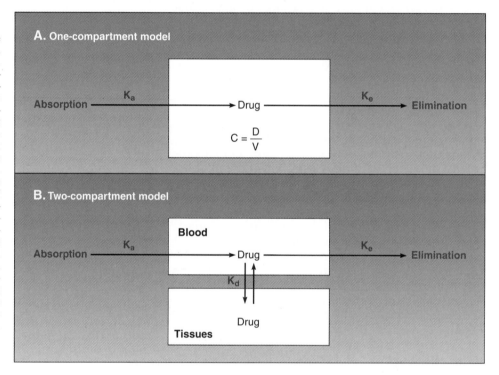

FIGURE 2-3. Drug absorption after oral, subcutaneous, or intramuscular administration.

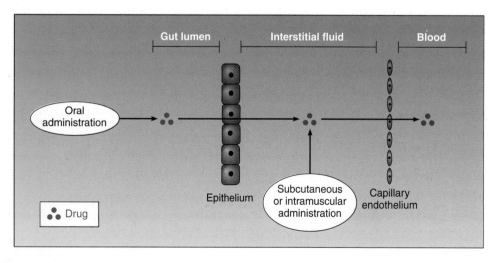

from the stomach. Weak acids may also be absorbed more readily from the intestines than from the stomach, despite their greater ionization in the intestines, because the intestines have a greater surface area than the stomach for absorption of the nonionized form of a drug, and this outweighs the influence of greater ionization in the intestines.

DRUG DISTRIBUTION

Drugs are distributed to organs and tissues via the circulation, from which they may diffuse into interstitial fluid and cells. Most drugs are not uniformly distributed throughout the total body water, and some drugs are restricted to the extracellular fluid or plasma compartment. Drugs with sufficient lipid solubility can diffuse into cells, and some drugs are concentrated in cells by the phenomenon of ion trapping, which is described below. Drugs may also be actively transported into cells. For example, some drugs are actively transported into hepatic cells, where they may undergo enzymatic biotransformation. In the intestines, carrier-mediated drug transport in the blood-to-lumen direction leads to a net secretion of anticancer drugs into the intestinal tract,

---

BOX 2–1. Effect of pH on the Absorption of a Weak Acid and a Weak Base

Weak acids (HA) donate a proton (H⁺) to form anions (A⁻), whereas **weak bases** (B) accept a proton to form cations (HB⁺).

$$HA \rightleftharpoons H^+ + A^-$$

For weak acids, the protonated form is nonionized.

$$B + H^+ \rightleftharpoons HB^+$$

For weak bases, the protonated form is ionized.

Only the **nonionized form** of a drug can readily penetrate cell membranes.

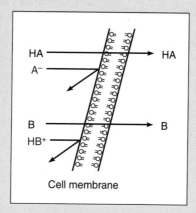

Cell membrane

The **pK$_a$** of a weak acid or weak base is the **pH** at which there are equal amounts of the protonated form and the nonprotonated form. The **Henderson-Hasselbalch equation** can be used to determine the ratio of the two forms:

$$\log \frac{[\text{Protonated form}]}{[\text{Nonprotonated form}]} = pK_a - pH$$

For **salicylic acid,** which is a weak acid with a pK$_a$ of 3, log [HA]/[A⁻] is 3 minus the pH. At a pH of 2, then, log [HA]/[A⁻] = 3 − 2 = 1. Therefore, [HA]/[A⁻] = 10/1.

Protonated   Nonprotonated

Continued

For **amphetamine,** which is a weak base with a pK_a of 10, log $[HB^+]/[B]$ is 10 minus the pH. At a pH of 8, then, log $[HB^+]/[B] = 10 - 8 = 2$. Therefore, $[HB^+]/[B] = 100/1$.

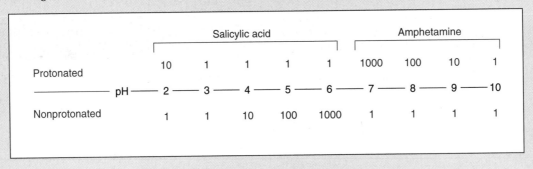

The following are the ratios of the protonated form to the nonprotonated form at different pH levels:

	Salicylic acid					Amphetamine			
Protonated	10	1	1	1	1	1000	100	10	1
pH	2	3	4	5	6	7	8	9	10
Nonprotonated	1	1	10	100	1000	1	1	1	1

thereby serving as a secretory detoxifying mechanism.

Volume of Distribution

The volume of distribution (V_d) can be defined as the volume of fluid in which a drug would need to be dissolved in order to have the same concentration in that volume as it does in plasma. The V_d does not represent the volume in a particular physiologic body compartment; instead, as shown in Fig. 2–4, it is a virtual volume (apparent volume) that represents the relationship between the dose of a drug and the resulting plasma concentration of the drug.

Calculation

The V_d is calculated by dividing the dose of a drug (usually, the dose given intravenously) by the plasma drug concentration immediately after distribution. As shown in Fig. 2–4C, this drug concentration can be determined by extrapolating the plasma drug concentration back to time zero. The plasma drug concentration at time zero (Cp_0) represents the plasma concentration of a drug that would be obtained if it were instantaneously dissolved in its V_d. This equation can be rearranged to determine the dose of a drug that is required to establish a specified plasma drug concentration (see below).

Interpretation

Although the V_d does not correspond to a physiologic body fluid compartment, it does provide an indication of the physiologic distribution of a drug. A low V_d that approximates plasma volume or extracellular fluid volume usually indicates that the drug's distribution is restricted to a particular compartment (the plasma or extracellular fluid). When the V_d of a drug is equivalent to total body water (as occurs, for example, with ethanol ingestion) this usually indicates that the drug has reached the intracellular fluid as well. Many drugs have a V_d that is much larger than total body water. A large V_d usually indicates that the drug is concentrated intracellularly, with a resulting low concentration in the plasma.

Many weak bases have an extremely large V_d because of the phenomenon of **ion trapping.** Weak bases are less ionized within plasma than they are within cells, and this is because of the difference in pH. After a weak base diffuses into a cell, a larger fraction is ionized in the more acidic intracellular fluid. This restricts its diffusion across cell membranes into the interstitial fluid and results in a large V_d.

Rate of Distribution

When drugs are administered orally, distribution occurs simultaneously with absorption, and the rate of distribution cannot be determined from the plasma drug concentration curve. After rapid intravenous drug administration, the plasma drug concentration falls rapidly at first, as the drug is distributed from the central compartment to the peripheral compartment (see Fig. 2–4C), and the

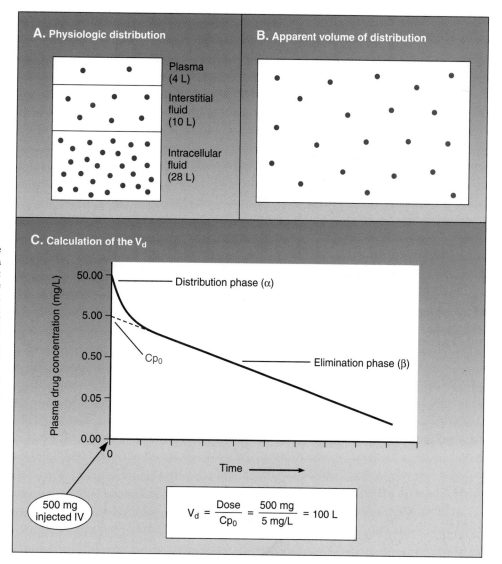

FIGURE 2–4. Calculating the volume of distribution (V_d) of a drug. Unlike the physiologic distribution of a drug **(A)**, the calculated V_d of a drug is an apparent (virtual) volume that can be defined as the volume of fluid in which a drug would need to be dissolved in order to have the same concentration in that volume as it does in the plasma **(B)**. The graph **(C)** provides an example of how the V_d is calculated. In this example, a dose of 500 mg was injected intravenously (IV) at time zero, and plasma drug concentrations were measured over time. The terminal elimination curve (β) was extrapolated back to time zero to determine that the plasma drug concentration at time zero (Cp_0) was 5 mg/L. Then the V_d was calculated by dividing the dose by the Cp_0. In this case, the result was 100 L.

rate of distribution can be determined from this portion of the curve.

Factors Affecting Distribution
Organ Blood Flow

The rate at which a drug is distributed to various organs after a drug dose is administered depends largely on the proportion of cardiac output received by the organs. Drugs are rapidly distributed to highly perfused tissues, such as brain, heart, liver, and kidney, and this enables a rapid onset of action of drugs affecting these tissues. Drugs are distributed more slowly to less highly perfused tissues, such as skeletal muscle, and even more slowly to those with the lowest blood flow, such as skin and adipose tissue.

Plasma Protein Binding

Almost all drugs are reversibly bound to plasma proteins, primarily albumin. The extent of binding depends on the affinity of a particular drug for protein-binding sites and ranges from less than 10% to as high as 99% of the plasma concentration. As the free (unbound) drug diffuses into interstitial fluid and cells, drug molecules dissociate from albumin to maintain the equilibrium between free drug and bound drug.

Plasma protein binding is saturable, and a drug may be displaced from binding sites by other drugs that have a higher affinity for such sites. This causes a temporary increase in the free concentration of the displaced drug and may lead to an increased tissue concentration and pharmacologic effect. However, this effect is usually short-lived because the increased free drug concentration will accelerate drug biotransformation and excretion.

Molecular Size

Molecular size is a factor affecting the distribution of extremely large molecules, such as heparin. Heparin is largely confined to the plasma, although it does undergo some biotransformation in the liver.

Lipid Solubility

Lipid solubility is a major factor affecting the extent of drug distribution, particularly to the brain, where the blood-brain barrier restricts the penetration of polar and ionized molecules. The barrier is formed by tight junctions between the capillary endothelial cells and also by the presence of glial cells that surround the capillaries and retard the penetration of polar molecules into brain neurons.

DRUG BIOTRANSFORMATION

Drug biotransformation and excretion are the two processes responsible for the decline of the plasma drug concentration over time during the terminal elimination phase (β). Drug biotransformation, which is often called **drug metabolism,** is the enzyme-catalyzed conversion of drugs to their metabolites. Most drug biotransformation takes place in the liver, but there are drug-metabolizing enzymes in many other tissues, including the gut, kidneys, brain, lungs, and skin.

Role of Drug Biotransformation

The primary biologic purpose of biotransformation enzymes is to inactivate and detoxify drugs and other foreign compounds (xenobiotics) that may cause harm to the body. Drug metabolites are usually more water-soluble than the parent molecule and are therefore more readily excreted by the kidneys. However, there is no particular relationship between biotransformation and pharmacologic activity. Some drug metabolites are active, while others are inactive. As a general rule, most conjugated drug metabolites are inactive, but there are a few exceptions.

Formation of Active Metabolites

Many pharmacologically active drugs are biotransformed to active metabolites. Some agents, known as **prodrugs,** are administered as inactive compounds and are subsequently biotransformed to active metabolites. This type of agent is usually developed because the prodrug is better absorbed than its active metabolite. For example, dipivefrin is a prodrug that is converted to its active metabolite, epinephrine, by corneal enzymes after topical ocular administration. Orally administered prodrugs are converted to their active metabolite by hepatic

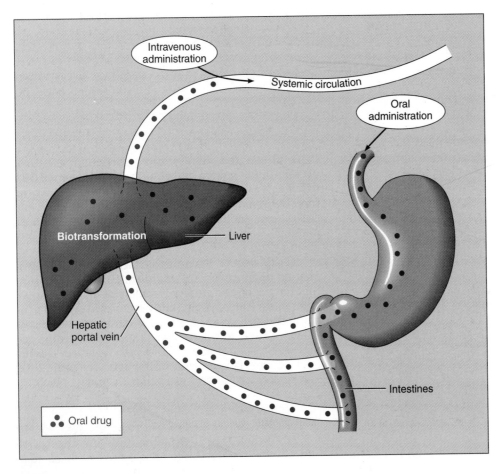

FIGURE 2–5. First-pass drug biotransformation. Drugs that are absorbed from the gut may be biotransformed by enzymes in the gut wall and liver before reaching the systemic circulation. This process lowers their degree of bioavailability.

enzymes, often during their first pass through the liver.

First-Pass Biotransformation

Drugs that are absorbed from the gut reach the liver via the hepatic portal vein before entering the systemic circulation (Fig. 2–5). Many drugs are extensively converted to inactive metabolites during their first pass through the liver and have low bioavailability after oral administration (see below). This phenomenon is called the first-pass effect. Drugs administered by the sublingual or rectal route undergo less first-pass metabolism and may have a higher degree of bioavailability than do drugs administered by the oral route.

Phases of Drug Biotransformation

Drug biotransformation can be divided into two phases, each comprising unique biotransformation reactions. In many cases, phase I reactions create or unmask a chemical group required for a phase II reaction. In some cases, however, drugs bypass phase I biotransformation and go directly to phase II. While phase I metabolites often have pharmacologic activity, most phase II metabolites do not.

Phase I Biotransformation

Phase I biotransformation includes oxidative, hydrolytic, and reductive reactions (Fig. 2–6).

Oxidative Reactions. Oxidative reactions are the most common type of phase I biotransformation. They are catalyzed by enzymes that are isolated in the microsomal fraction of liver homogenates (the fraction derived from the endoplasmic reticulum) and by cytoplasmic enzymes.

The **microsomal cytochrome P450 monooxygenase system** is a family of enzymes that catalyzes the biotransformation of drugs with a wide range of chemical structures. The microsomal **monooxygenase reaction** requires the following: cytochrome P450 (a hemoprotein); a flavoprotein that is reduced by nicotinamide adenine dinucleotide phosphate (NADPH) and is called NADPH–cytochrome P450 reductase; and membrane lipids in which the system is embedded. In the drug-oxidizing reaction, one atom of oxygen is used to form a hydroxylated metabolite of a drug, as shown in Fig. 2–7, while the other atom of oxygen forms water when combined with electrons contributed by NADPH. The hydroxylated metabolite may be the end product of the reaction or may serve as an intermediate leading to the formation of another metabolite.

The most common chemical reactions catalyzed by cytochrome P450 enzymes are aliphatic hydroxylation, aromatic hydroxylation, N-dealkylation, and O-dealkylation.

Various **cytochrome P450 isoforms** have been identified, and their role in metabolizing specific drugs is currently being elucidated. Each isoform catalyzes a different, but overlapping, spectrum of oxidative reactions. The majority of drug biotransformations are catalyzed by three P450 families, called CYP1, CYP2, and CYP3. The members of each of these families have more than 40% identical protein sequences. Each family is divided into subfamilies, the members of which have more than 55% identical protein sequences. The CYP3A subfamily catalyzes over half of all microsomal drug oxidations.

Many drugs alter drug biotransformation by inhibiting or inducing cytochrome P450 enzymes, and **drug interactions** may occur when these drugs are administered concurrently with other drugs that are metabolized by cytochrome P450 (see Chapter 4). Two examples of **inducers of cytochrome P450** are phenobarbital and rifampin. The inducers stimulate the transcription of genes encoding cytochrome P450 enzymes, and this results in increased messenger RNA and protein synthesis. There is evidence that P450 enzyme inducers combine with a nuclear receptor to initiate P450 gene transcription, and other gene regulatory elements have been identified.

A few drugs are metabolized by **cytoplasmic enzymes.** For example, ethanol is oxidized by alcohol dehydrogenase, and caffeine and theophylline are biotransformed by xanthine oxidase. Other cytoplasmic oxidases include monoamine oxidase.

Hydrolytic Reactions. Esters and amides are hydrolyzed by a variety of enzymes. These include the cholinesterases and other plasma esterases that inactivate choline esters, local anesthetics, and drugs such as esmolol (an agent that blocks β-adrenergic receptors).

Reductive Reactions. Reductive reactions are less common than are oxidative and hydrolytic reactions. Chloramphenicol and a few other drugs are partly metabolized by a hepatic nitroreductase, and this process appears to involve cytochrome P450. Nitroglycerin undergoes reductive hydrolysis catalyzed by glutathione–organic nitrate reductase.

Phase II Biotransformation

In phase II biotransformation, drug molecules undergo **conjugation reactions** with an endogenous substance such as acetate, glucuronate, sulfate, or glycine (Fig. 2–8). Conjugation enzymes are present in the liver and other tissues and serve to conjugate various drugs with the endogenous substance to form water-soluble metabolites that are more easily excreted. Except for microsomal glucuronosyltransferases, these enzymes are located in the cytoplasm. Most conjugated drug metabolites are pharmacologically inactive.

Acetylation. Acetylation is accomplished by N-acetyltransferase enzymes that utilize acetyl coenzyme A (acetyl CoA) as a source of the acetate.

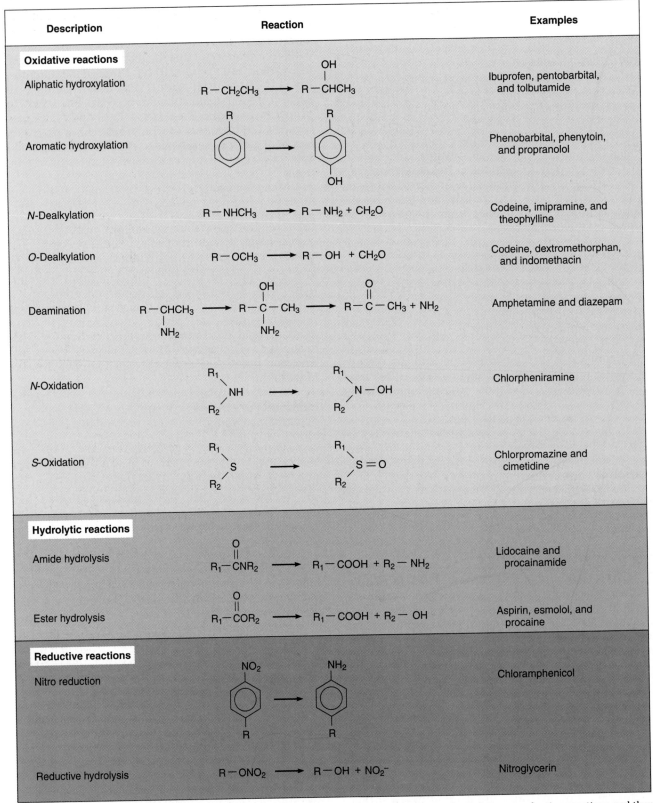

Description	Reaction	Examples

Oxidative reactions

Aliphatic hydroxylation — $R-CH_2CH_3 \longrightarrow R-CHCH_3$ (OH) — Ibuprofen, pentobarbital, and tolbutamide

Aromatic hydroxylation — Phenobarbital, phenytoin, and propranolol

N-Dealkylation — $R-NHCH_3 \longrightarrow R-NH_2 + CH_2O$ — Codeine, imipramine, and theophylline

O-Dealkylation — $R-OCH_3 \longrightarrow R-OH + CH_2O$ — Codeine, dextromethorphan, and indomethacin

Deamination — $R-CHCH_3\,(NH_2) \longrightarrow R-C(OH)-CH_3\,(NH_2) \longrightarrow R-C(=O)-CH_3 + NH_2$ — Amphetamine and diazepam

N-Oxidation — $R_1 R_2 NH \longrightarrow R_1 R_2 N-OH$ — Chlorpheniramine

S-Oxidation — $R_1 R_2 S \longrightarrow R_1 R_2 S=O$ — Chlorpromazine and cimetidine

Hydrolytic reactions

Amide hydrolysis — $R_1-CNR_2\,(=O) \longrightarrow R_1-COOH + R_2-NH_2$ — Lidocaine and procainamide

Ester hydrolysis — $R_1-COR_2\,(=O) \longrightarrow R_1-COOH + R_2-OH$ — Aspirin, esmolol, and procaine

Reductive reactions

Nitro reduction — $NO_2 \longrightarrow NH_2$ — Chloramphenicol

Reductive hydrolysis — $R-ONO_2 \longrightarrow R-OH + NO_2^-$ — Nitroglycerin

FIGURE 2–6. Phase I drug biotransformation. Many drugs are biotransformed by oxidative, hydrolytic, or reductive reactions and then undergo conjugation with endogenous substances. A few drugs bypass phase I reactions and directly enter phase II biotransformation.

Glucuronide Formation. Glucuronide formation is the most common conjugation reaction and utilizes glucuronosyltransferases to conjugate a glucuronate molecule with a drug.

Sulfation. Sulfotransferases catalyze the conjugation of several drugs, including minoxidil and triamterene, whose sulfate metabolites are pharmacologically active.

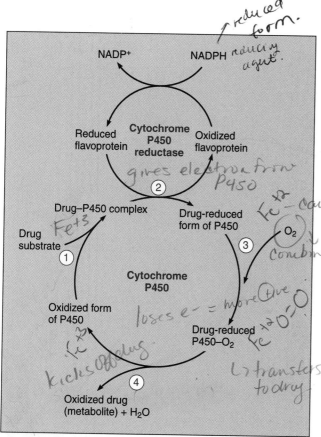

FIGURE 2–7. The cytochrome P450 reductase mechanism for drug oxidation. There are four steps in the cytochrome P450 reaction: First, the drug substrate binds to the oxidized form of P450 (namely, Fe^{3+}). Second, the drug–P450 complex is reduced by cytochrome P450 reductase, using electrons donated by the reduced form of nicotinamide adenine dinucleotide phosphate (NADPH). Third, the drug-reduced form of P450 (namely, Fe^{2+}) interacts with oxygen. Fourth, the oxidized drug (metabolite) and water are produced.

Genetic Variations in Drug Biotransformation
Variations in Acetylation of Drugs

Individuals may exhibit slow or fast acetylation of some drugs, such as isoniazid and hydralazine, because of genetically determined differences in the activity of acetyltransferases located in the gut and liver. The genetic variations are attributed to different isozymes. Slow acetylation is an autosomal recessive trait, and persons with the slow phenotype are homozygous for the slow allele (r/r). In contrast, persons with the fast phenotype are heterozygous (R/r) or homozygous dominant (R/R). The distribution of these phenotypes varies from population to population. The fast acetylation phenotype predominates in the Japanese population; the slow acetylation phenotype predominates in some Middle Eastern populations; and about half of the US population exhibits each phenotype.

Variations in Oxidation of Cytochrome P450

Variations in oxidation of some drugs have been attributed to genetic differences in cytochrome P450 enzymes. Because there are numerous P450 isoforms

with overlapping substrate specificity, the implications for pharmacotherapy are complex. Genetic variations in a CYP2D6 4-hydroxylase that metabolizes a marker drug called debrisoquine have been elucidated, and populations of "extensive metabolizers" and "poor metabolizers" have also been identified. Persons who lack CYP2D6 have been found to obtain little or no pain relief from codeine, because they cannot convert it to its active metabolite, morphine. The genetics of P450 isoforms continue to be investigated.

Other Variations in Drug Metabolism

About 1 in 3000 individuals exhibits a familial atypical cholinesterase that will not metabolize succinylcholine, a neuromuscular blocking agent, at a normal rate. Affected individuals are subject to prolonged apnea after receiving the usual dose of the drug. For this reason, patients should be screened for atypical cholinesterase before receiving succinylcholine.

Genetically determined variations in the rate of metabolism of other drugs, such as warfarin, have been observed, but most of these variations are relatively rare.

DRUG EXCRETION
Renal Drug Excretion

Most drugs are excreted in the urine, either as the parent compound or as drug metabolites. Drugs are handled by the kidneys in the same manner as physiologic substances and undergo the processes of glomerular filtration, active tubular secretion, and passive tubular reabsorption. The amount of drug excreted is the sum of the amounts filtered and secreted minus the amount reabsorbed. The relationship between these processes, the rate of drug excretion, and renal clearance is shown in Box 2–2.

Glomerular Filtration

Glomerular filtration is the first step in renal drug excretion. In this process, the free drug enters the renal tubule as a dissolved solute in the plasma filtrate (see Box 2–2). If a drug has a large fraction bound to plasma proteins, it will have a low rate of glomerular filtration.

Active Tubular Secretion

Some drugs, particularly weak acids and bases, undergo active tubular secretion by transport systems located primarily in proximal tubular cells. This process is competitively inhibited by other drugs of the same chemical class. For example, the secretion of penicillins and other weak acids is inhibited by probenecid.

Active tubular secretion is not affected by plasma protein binding. This is because when the free drug is actively transported across the renal tubule, this fraction of drug is replaced by a fraction that

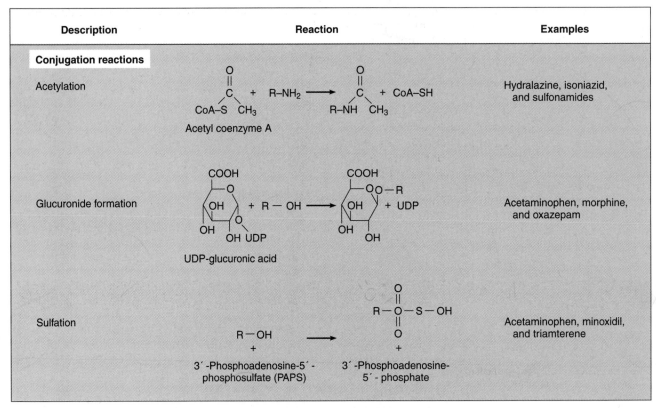

Description	Reaction	Examples

Conjugation reactions

Acetylation — Acetyl coenzyme A — Hydralazine, isoniazid, and sulfonamides

Glucuronide formation — UDP-glucuronic acid — Acetaminophen, morphine, and oxazepam

Sulfation — 3´-Phosphoadenosine-5´-phosphosulfate (PAPS) → 3´-Phosphoadenosine-5´-phosphate — Acetaminophen, minoxidil, and triamterene

FIGURE 2–8. Phase II drug biotransformation. UDP = uridine diphosphate.

dissociates from plasma proteins in order to maintain the equilibrium of free drug and bound drug.

Passive Tubular Reabsorption

The extent to which a drug undergoes passive reabsorption across renal tubular cells and into the circulation depends on the **lipid solubility** of the drug. Drug biotransformation facilitates drug elimination by forming polar drug metabolites that are not as readily reabsorbed as the less polar parent molecules.

Most nonelectrolytes, including ethanol, are passively reabsorbed across tubular cells. Ionized weak acids and bases are not reabsorbed across renal tubular cells, and they are more rapidly excreted in the urine than are nonionized drugs that undergo passive reabsorption. The proportion of ionized and nonionized drugs is affected by **renal tubular pH,** which may be manipulated in order to increase the excretion of a drug after a drug overdose (Box 2–3).

Biliary Excretion and Enterohepatic Cycling

Many drugs are excreted in the bile as the parent compound or a drug metabolite. Biliary excretion favors compounds with molecular weights that are higher than 300.

Numerous conjugated drug metabolites, including the glucuronate and sulfate derivatives of steroids, are excreted in the bile. After the bile empties into the intestines, a fraction of the drug may be reabsorbed into the circulation and eventually return to the liver. This phenomenon is called enterohepatic cycling (Fig. 2–9). Conjugated drugs may be hydrolyzed to the free drug by intestinal bacteria, and this facilitates the drug's reabsorption, since conjugated metabolites are more polar and less lipid-soluble than are the parent compounds. Antibiotics that kill the intestinal bacteria may reduce the enterohepatic circulation of estrogens and thereby cause a reduction in their plasma concentration and therapeutic effect. This type of drug interaction between antibiotics and orally administered steroids is sometimes responsible for the failure of oral contraceptives to prevent pregnancy.

Other Routes of Excretion

The **sweat** and **saliva** represent minor routes of excretion for some drugs. In pharmacokinetic studies, saliva measurements serve as a useful addition or alternative to plasma measurements, because the saliva concentration of a drug reflects the intracellular concentration of the drug in target tissues. For some drugs, the saliva concentration and plasma concentration are almost equal. For other drugs, one is much greater than the other. Among the factors that influence saliva concentrations are whether a drug has an active transport system and whether a drug is subject to ion trapping.

PHARMACOKINETIC CALCULATIONS

Most drugs exhibit **first-order kinetics,** in which the rate of drug elimination is proportional to the plasma drug concentration. A few drugs, such as ethanol, exhibit **zero-order kinetics,** in which the rate of drug elimination is constant and is independent of the plasma drug concentration. The **kinetic order** refers to the exponent of the drug concentration (0 or 1) in the expression shown in Fig. 2–10.

Pharmacokinetics concerns the relationship between the dose of a particular drug and the concentration of that drug in body fluids and tissues over time. For drugs that exhibit first-order kinetics, the plasma drug concentration can be estimated from a drug's dose and its clearance. Because the plasma drug concentration is often correlated with the magnitude of a drug's effect, it is possible to use pharmacokinetic calculations to determine and ad-

just drug dosages to achieve a desired therapeutic effect.

First-Order Kinetics

The following principles pertain to first-order kinetics: a drug's rate of elimination is equal to the plasma drug concentration multiplied by the drug clearance; the elimination rate declines as the plasma concentration declines (see Fig. 2–10A); and the half-life and clearance of the drug remain constant as long as renal and hepatic function do not change.

Elimination Half-Life

The elimination half-life is the time required to eliminate half of the amount of a drug in the body or

---

BOX 2–2. The Renal Excretion and Clearance of a Weak Acid, Penicillin G

Description and Chemical Structure

Penicillin G (benzylpenicillin) is an example of a weak acid. It has a **pK_a** of 2.8 and is primarily excreted via renal tubular secretion. About 60% of penicillin G is bound to plasma proteins. The pharmacokinetic calculations below are based on a urine **pH** of 5.8, a **plasma drug concentration** of 3 µg/mL, a **glomerular filtration rate** of 100 mL/min, and a **measured drug excretion rate** of 1200 µg/min. Because 40% of penicillin G is free (unbound), the **free drug plasma concentration** is 0.4×3 µg/mL = 1.2 µg/mL.

Renal Excretion

The discussion and accompanying figure illustrate the relationship between the rates of glomerular filtration, active tubular secretion, passive tubular reabsorption, and excretion.

(1) Filtration. The **drug filtration rate** is calculated by multiplying the glomerular filtration rate by the free drug plasma concentration: 100 mL/min × 1.2 µg/mL = 120 µg/min.

(2) Secretion. The **drug secretion rate** is calculated by subtracting the drug filtration rate from the drug excretion rate: 1200 µg/min – 120 µg/min = 1080 µg/min. This amount indicates that 90% of the drug's excretion occurs by the process of tubular secretion.

(3) Reabsorption. The ratio of the nonionized form to the ionized form of the drug in the urine is equal to the antilog of the pK_a minus the pH: antilog of 2.8 – 5.8 = antilog of –3 = 1:1000. Since most of the drug is ionized in the urine, the **drug reabsorption rate** is probably <1 µg/min.

(4) Excretion. The drug excretion rate was initially given as 1200 µg/min. It was determined by measuring the drug concentration in urine and multiplying it by the urine flow rate. Note that the drug excretion rate is equal to the drug filtration rate (120 µg/min) plus the drug secretion rate (1080 µg/min) minus the drug reabsorption rate (<1 µg/min).

Renal Clearance

The renal clearance is calculated by dividing the excretion rate (1200 µg/min) by the plasma drug concentration (3 µg/mL). The result is 400 mL/min, which is equal to 24 L/h.

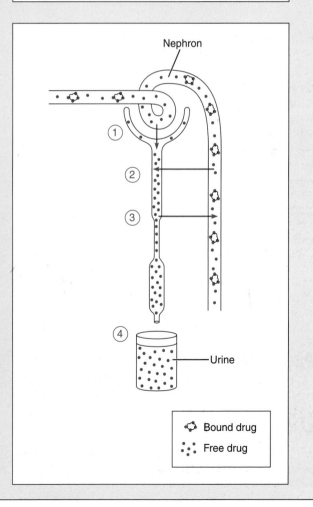

BOX 2–3.   Urine Acidification and Alkalinization in the Treatment of Drug Overdose

If a drug or other compound is a weak acid or base, its degree of ionization and rate of renal excretion will depend on its pK_a and on the pH of the renal tubular fluid. The rate of excretion of a **weak acid** can be accelerated by **alkalinizing the urine,** whereas the rate of excretion of a **weak base** can be accelerated by **acidifying the urine.** These procedures have been used to enhance the excretion of drugs and poisons, but they are not without risk to the patient, and their benefits have been established for only a few drugs.

To make manipulation of the urine pH worthwhile, a drug must be excreted to a large degree by the kidneys. The short-acting barbiturates, such as secobarbital, are eliminated almost entirely via biotransformation to inactive metabolites, so modification of the urine pH has little effect on their excretion. In contrast, phenobarbital is excreted to a large degree by the kidneys, so urine alkalinization is useful in treating an overdose of this drug. Urine acidification to enhance the elimination of weak bases, such as amphetamine, has been largely abandoned because it does not significantly increase the elimination of these drugs and poses a serious risk of metabolic acidosis.

In cases involving an overdose of aspirin or other salicylate, alkalinization of the urine produces the dual benefits of increasing drug excretion and counteracting the metabolic acidosis that occurs with serious aspirin toxicity. For patients suffering from phenobarbital overdose or from poisoning due to the herbicide 2,4-dichlorophenoxyacetic acid (2,4-D), alkalinization of the urine is also helpful and is accomplished by administering sodium bicarbonate intravenously every 3–4 hours to increase the urinary pH to 7–8.

the drug's half-life will change when either of these factors is altered. Disease, age, and other physiologic variables may alter drug clearance or volume of distribution and thereby change the half-life (see Chapter 4).

Drug Clearance

Clearance is defined as the volume of body fluid from which a substance is removed per unit of time.

Total Clearance.   The total clearance is the sum of the renal clearance, the hepatic clearance, and any other clearance (such as respiratory clearance). Total clearance can be calculated by multiplying a drug's apparent volume of distribution by the elimination rate constant (see Fig. 2–11). This relationship indicates that a drug's clearance represents that fraction of the volume of distribution from which a drug is eliminated per unit of time. The clearance does not change as the plasma drug concentration declines, but the amount of drug in the clearance volume decreases as the plasma concentration decreases.

Renal Clearance.   Renal clearance can be calculated as the renal excretion rate divided by the plasma drug concentration (see Box 2–2). Drugs that are eliminated primarily by glomerular filtration, with little tubular secretion or reabsorption, will have a renal clearance that is approximately equal to the creatinine clearance, which is normally about 100 mL/min in an adult. If the renal drug clearance is higher than the creatinine clearance, this indicates that the drug is a substance that undergoes tubular secretion. If the renal drug clearance is lower than the creatinine clearance, this suggests that the drug is highly bound to plasma proteins or that it undergoes passive reabsorption from the renal tubules.

Hepatic Clearance.   Hepatic clearance is more difficult to determine than renal clearance. This is

to reduce the plasma drug concentration by 50%. It can be calculated from the elimination rate constant, but it is usually determined from the plasma drug concentration curve (Fig. 2–11). The half-life may also be expressed in terms of the drug's clearance and volume of distribution, indicating that

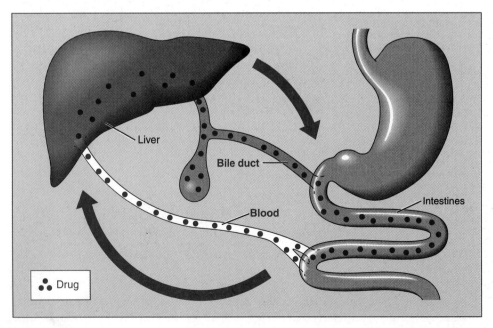

FIGURE 2–9. Enterohepatic cycling. Drugs and drug metabolites with molecular weights higher than 300 may be excreted via the bile, stored in the gallbladder, delivered to the intestines by the bile duct, and then reabsorbed into the circulation. This process reduces the elimination of drugs and prolongs their half-life and duration of action in the body.

Elimination.

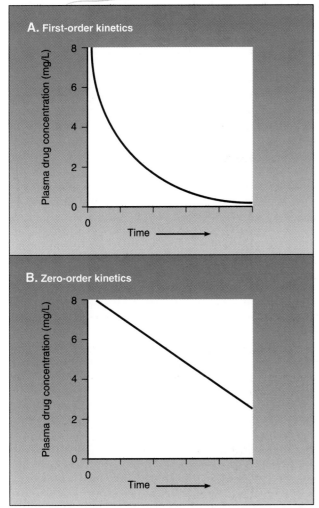

FIGURE 2–10. **The kinetic order of drugs.** In first-order kinetics **(A),** the rate of drug elimination is proportional to the plasma drug concentration. In zero-order kinetics **(B),** the rate of drug elimination is constant. The kinetic order of a drug is derived from the exponent, n, in the following expression:

$$\Delta[\text{Drug}]/\Delta t = [\text{Drug}]^n\, k$$

where Δ represents change, [Drug] represents the plasma drug concentration, and t is time. If n is 1, then $\Delta[\text{Drug}]/\Delta t$ is proportional to [Drug]. If n is 0, then $\Delta[\text{Drug}]/\Delta t$ is constant (k), since $[\text{Drug}]^0$ equals 1.

because hepatic drug elimination includes the biotransformation and biliary excretion of parent compounds. For this reason, hepatic clearance is usually determined by multiplying hepatic blood flow by the arteriovenous drug concentration difference.

Zero-Order Kinetics

The following principles pertain to zero-order kinetics: the rate of drug elimination is constant (see Fig. 2–10B); the drug's elimination half-life is proportional to the plasma drug concentration; the clearance is inversely proportional to the drug concentration; and a small increase in dosage can produce a disproportionate increase in the plasma drug concentration.

In many cases, the reason that the rate of drug elimination is constant is that the elimination process becomes saturated. This occurs, for example, at most plasma concentrations of ethanol. In some cases, drugs exhibit zero-order elimination when high doses are administered—as occurs, for example, with

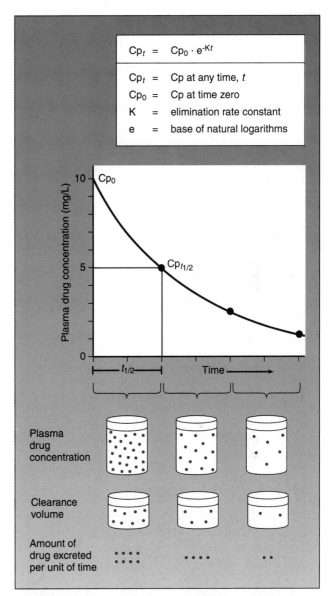

FIGURE 2–11. **Drug half-life and clearance.** The elimination half-life $(t_{1/2})$ is the time required to reduce the plasma drug concentration (Cp) by 50%. The formula is as follows:

$$t_{1/2} = 0.693/K_e$$

where 0.693 is the natural logarithm of 2, and K_e is the elimination rate constant. The half-life is often determined from the plasma drug concentration curve shown here. The clearance (Cl) is the volume of fluid from which a drug is eliminated per unit of time. It can be calculated as the product of the volume of distribution (V_d) and K_e. If $0.693/t_{1/2}$ is substituted for K_e, the equation is as follows:

$$\text{Cl} = 0.693\, V_d/t_{1/2}$$

Thus, a drug's clearance is directly proportional to its volume of distribution and is inversely proportional to its half-life.

aspirin and the anticonvulsant phenytoin—or when a hepatic or renal disease has impaired the drug elimination processes.

SINGLE-DOSE KINETICS
Plasma Drug Concentration Curve

The plasma drug concentration curve, which plots the concentration over time, provides useful information about drug absorption, distribution, and elimination. After a single dose of drug is administered, the plasma concentration increases as the drug is absorbed, reaches a peak as absorption is completed, and then declines as the drug is eliminated (Fig. 2–12A). Except in the case of a rapid intravenous

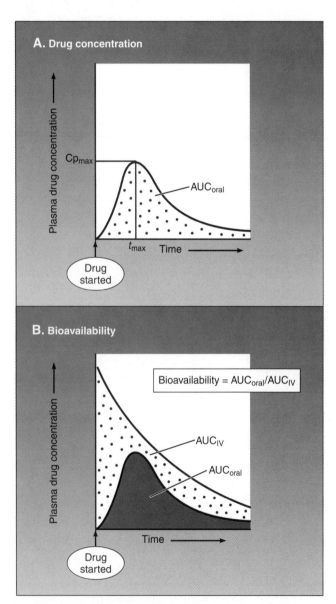

FIGURE 2–12. Plasma drug concentration and drug bioavailability. The plasma drug concentration curve for a single dose of a drug given orally **(A)** shows the maximum plasma concentration (Cp_{max}), the time at which the maximum plasma concentration occurred (t_{max}), and the area under the curve (AUC). To determine bioavailability **(B)**, the AUC of the orally administered drug (AUC_{oral}) can be divided by the AUC of the intravenously administered drug (AUC_{IV}).

injection, the process of drug distribution occurs simultaneously with drug absorption and cannot be easily discerned.

Bioavailability

In the plasma drug concentration curve, the rate and extent of drug absorption after oral administration are indicated by the maximum plasma drug concentration (Cp_{max}), the time at which the maximum concentration occurs (t_{max}), and the area under the curve (AUC). These measures are useful for comparing the bioavailability of different pharmaceutical formulations or of drugs given by different routes of administration.

Bioavailability is defined as the fraction of the administered dose of a drug that reaches the systemic circulation in an active form. As shown in Fig. 2–12B, the oral bioavailability of a particular drug is usually determined by dividing the AUC of an orally administered dose of the drug (AUC_{oral}) by the AUC of an intravenously administered dose of the same drug (AUC_{IV}). The assumption is that the intravenously administered drug has 100% bioavailability.

The bioavailability of orally administered drugs is of particular concern because it can be reduced by so many pharmaceutical and biologic factors. Pharmaceutical factors include the rate and extent of tablet disintegration and drug dissolution. Biologic factors include the effects of food, which may sequester or inactivate a drug; the effects of gastric acid, which may inactivate a drug; and the effects of gut and liver enzymes, which may biotransform a drug during its absorption and first pass through the liver.

The bioavailability of drugs administered intramuscularly or via other routes may be determined in the same manner as the bioavailability of drugs administered orally.

CONTINUOUS- AND MULTIPLE-DOSE KINETICS
Drug Accumulation and the Steady-State Principle

When a drug that exhibits first-order pharmacokinetics is administered to a patient continuously or intermittently, the drug will accumulate until it reaches a plateau or steady-state plasma drug concentration.

The basis for this accumulation to a steady state is shown in Fig. 2–13. When the drug is first administered, the rate of administration is much greater than the rate of elimination, because the plasma concentration is so low. As the drug continues to be administered, the rate of drug elimination gradually increases, whereas the rate of administration remains constant. Eventually, as the plasma concentration rises sufficiently, the rate of drug elimination equals the rate of drug administration. At this point, the steady-state condition is achieved.

Time Required to Reach the Steady-State Condition

Drug accumulation to a steady state is a first-order process and therefore obeys the rule that half

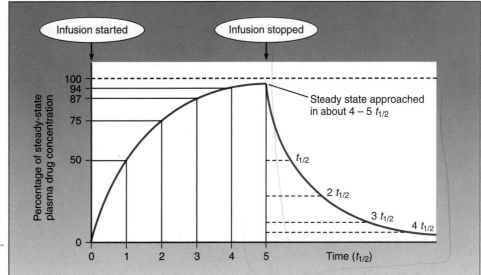

FIGURE 2–13. Drug accumulation to the steady state. The time required to reach the steady state depends on the half-life ($t_{1/2}$); it does not depend on the dose or dose interval. The steady-state drug concentration depends on the drug dose administered per unit of time and on the drug's clearance or half-life.

of the process is completed in a defined time. Since the time to reach the steady state is dependent on the time it takes for the rate of drug elimination to equal the rate of drug administration, the time to reach the steady state is a function of the elimination half-life of the drug. Any first-order process requires about 4–5 half-lives to reach completion, and the time to reach the steady-state drug concentration is about 4–5 drug half-lives. Note that the time required to reach the steady state is independent of the drug dose and is also independent of the rate or frequency of drug administration.

Steady-State Drug Concentration

The steady-state drug concentration depends on the drug dose administered per unit of time and on the half-life of the drug. If the dose is doubled, the steady-state concentration is also doubled. Likewise, if the half-life is doubled, the steady-state concentration is doubled.

Fig. 2–14 illustrates typical plasma concentration curves after drugs are administered continuously or intermittently. A drug administered intermittently will accumulate to a steady state at the same rate as a drug given by continuous infusion, but the plasma drug concentration will fluctuate as each dose is absorbed and eliminated. The average steady-state plasma drug concentration with intermittent intravenous administration will be the same as if the equivalent dose were administered by continuous infusion. With intermittent oral administration, the fractional bioavailability will also influence the steady-state plasma concentration.

Dosage Calculations
Loading Dose

The purpose of the loading dose, or **priming dose,** is to rapidly establish a therapeutic plasma drug concentration. The loading dose can be calcu-

lated by multiplying the volume of distribution by the desired plasma drug concentration (Box 2–4). The loading dose is usually larger than the maintenance dose and is generally administered as a single dose, but it may be divided into several parts that are given over a number of hours. The divided loading dose may be used with drugs that are more toxic, such as the digitalis glycosides.

Maintenance Dose

The purpose of a maintenance dose is to establish or maintain a desired steady-state plasma drug concentration. For drugs given intermittently, the maintenance dose is one of a series of doses administered at regular intervals. The amount of drug to be given is based on the principle that at the steady state, the rate of drug administration equals the rate of drug elimination. To determine the rate of drug elimination, the drug clearance is multiplied by the average steady-state plasma drug concentration. The maintenance dose is then calculated as the rate of drug elimination multiplied by the dosage intervals. If the drug is administered orally, its fractional bioavailability must be included in the equation.

Summary of Important Points

- Most drugs are absorbed by passive diffusion across or between cells. The rate of passive diffusion of a drug across cell membranes is proportional to the drug's lipid solubility. Only the nonionized form of weak acids and bases is lipid-soluble.
- The ratio of the ionized form to the nonionized form of a weak acid or base can be determined from the pK_a of the drug and the pH of the body fluid in which the drug is dissolved.
- The distribution of a drug is influenced by organ blood flow and by the plasma protein binding, molecular size, and lipid solubility of the drug.

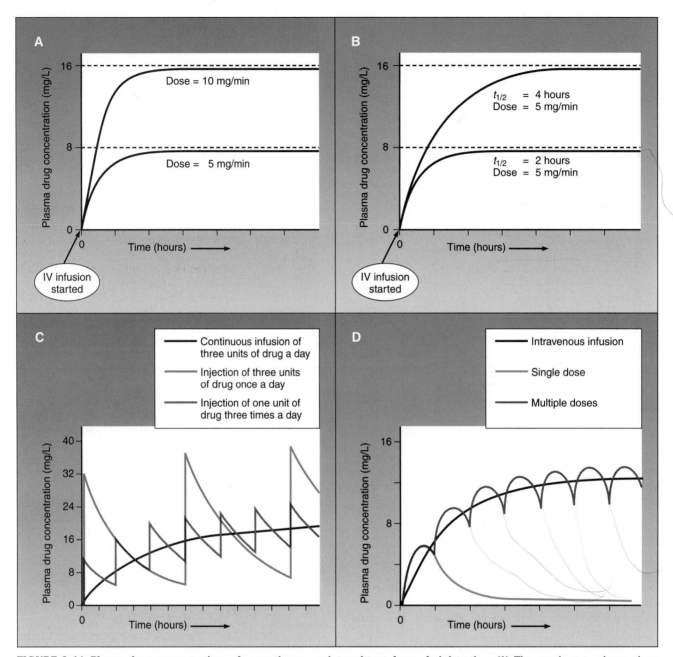

FIGURE 2–14. Plasma drug concentrations after continuous or intermittent drug administration. (A) The steady-state plasma drug concentration is proportional to the dose administered per unit of time. **(B)** The steady-state plasma drug concentration is directly proportional to the half-life (and is inversely related to clearance). **(C)** The average steady-state concentration is the same for intermittent infusion as it is for continuous infusion. However, with intermittent drug administration, the plasma concentrations fluctuate between doses, and the size of fluctuations increases as the dosage interval increases. **(D)** Plasma drug concentrations after intermittent oral administration are affected by the rates of drug absorption, distribution, and elimination. If only one dose is given, the peak in plasma drug concentration is followed by a continuous decline in the curve.

Only drugs with high lipid solubility can penetrate the blood-brain barrier.

- The volume of distribution is the volume of fluid in which a drug would need to be dissolved in order to have the same concentration in that volume as it does in plasma. It is calculated by dividing the drug dose by the plasma drug concentration at time zero.

- Many drugs are biotransformed before excretion. Drug metabolites may be pharmacologically active or inactive. Phase I reactions include oxidative, reductive, and hydrolytic reactions, whereas phase II reactions conjugate a drug with an endogenous substance. The cytochrome P450 enzymes located in the endoplasmic reticulum of liver cells are the most important oxidative biotransformation enzymes.

- Most drugs are excreted in the urine, either as the parent compound or as drug metabolites, and undergo the processes of glomerular filtration, active tubular secretion, and passive tubular reabsorption. The renal clearance of a drug can be calculated by dividing the renal excretion rate by the plasma drug concentration.

- Most drugs exhibit first-order kinetics, in which the rate of drug elimination is proportional to the

---

BOX 2–4. Drug Dosage Calculations

Loading Dose

The loading dose, or priming dose, of a drug is determined by multiplying the **volume of distribution** (V_d) of the drug by the **desired plasma drug concentration** (desired Cp). The clinician usually finds this information in the medical literature. For theophylline, for example, the estimated V_d for an adult weighing 70 kg is 35 L, and the desired Cp is 15 mg/L. The calculation is as follows:

$$\begin{aligned} \text{Loading dose} &= V_d \times Cp \\ &= 35\ L \times 15\ mg/L \\ &= 525\ mg \end{aligned}$$

As discussed in Chapter 4, the patient's age, body weight, and other characteristics affect the V_d and therefore should be considered in determining the appropriate loading dose for a particular patient.

Maintenance Dose

Calculations of the maintenance dose must take into consideration the **intended frequency of drug administration.** With intermittent administration, the fluctuations in Cp increase as the dosage interval increases. A twofold fluctuation in Cp will occur when the dosage interval is equal to the drug's half-life. This is because the Cp will fall 50% between doses. For many drugs, the half-life is a convenient and acceptable dosage interval.

The maintenance dose is designed to establish or maintain a **desired steady-state Cp.** The amount of drug to be given is based on the principle that at the steady state, the rate of drug administration equals the rate of drug elimination. The rate of elimination is equal to the clearance multiplied by the steady-state drug concentration. For example, if the steady-state gentamicin concentration is 2 mg/L and the clearance for gentamicin is 100 mL/ min (0.1 L/min), then the elimination rate is 0.1 L/min × 2 mg/L = 0.2 mg/min. If the drug is to be administered every 8 hours, then the dosage would be calculated as follows:

$$\begin{aligned} \text{Maintenance dose} &= \text{Hourly rate} \\ &\quad \times \text{dosage interval} \\ &\quad \text{in hours} \\ &= 0.2\ mg/min \\ &\quad \times 60\ \text{minutes in an hour} \\ &\quad \times 8\ \text{hours} \\ &= 96\ mg\ \text{every 8 hours} \end{aligned}$$

If a drug is to be administered orally, the calculated dose must be divided by the fractional bioavailability to determine the administered dose.

Dosage Adjustment Using Pharmacokinetic Values

First, choose the target Cp and administer the initial dose on the basis of the standard published values (general population values) for clearance or V_d. Second, measure the patient's plasma drug levels and calculate the patient's V_d and clearance. Third, revise the dosage based on the patient's V_d and clearance.

---

plasma drug concentration at any given time. If drug elimination mechanisms (biotransformation and excretion) become saturated, a drug may exhibit zero-order kinetics, in which the rate of drug elimination is constant.

- In first-order kinetics, a drug's half-life and clearance are constant as long as physiologic elimination processes are constant. The half-life is the time required for the plasma drug concentration to decrease by 50%. The clearance is the volume of plasma from which a drug is eliminated per unit of time.

- The oral bioavailability of a drug is the fraction of the administered dose that reaches the circulation in an active form. It is determined by dividing the area under the plasma drug concentration curve after oral administration (AUC_{oral}) by the area after intravenous administration (AUC_{IV}). Factors that reduce bioavailability include incomplete tablet disintegration and first-pass and gastric inactivation of a drug.

- With continuous or intermittent drug administration at a constant rate per unit of time, the plasma drug concentration increases until it reaches the steady-state condition, in which the rate of drug elimination is equal to the rate of drug administration.

- The steady-state drug concentration can be calculated as the dose per unit of time divided by the clearance, and this equation can be rearranged to determine the dose per unit of time required to establish a specified steady-state drug concentration.

- A loading dose is a single or divided dose given to rapidly establish a therapeutic plasma drug concentration. The dose can be calculated by multiplying the volume of distribution by the desired plasma drug concentration.

Selected Readings

Kinirons, M. T., and P. Crome. Clinical pharmacokinetic considerations in the elderly: an update. Clin Pharmacokinet 33:302–312, 1997.

Levine, R. R. Pharmacology: Drug Actions and Reactions, 5th ed. New York, Parthenon, 1996.

Loebstein, R., A. Lalkin, and G. Koren. Pharmacokinetic changes during pregnancy and their clinical relevance. Clin Pharmacokinet 33:328–343, 1997.

McCormack, J. P., and B. Carleton. A simpler approach to pharmacokinetic dosage adjustment. Pharmacotherapy 17:1349–1351, 1997.

Melmon, K. L., et al., eds. Clinical Pharmacology: Basic Principles in Therapeutics, 3rd ed. New York, McGraw-Hill, 1992.

Pratt, W. B., and P. Taylor. Principles of Drug Action: The Basis of Pharmacology, 3rd ed. New York, Churchill Livingstone, 1990.

Rescigno, A. Fundamental concepts in pharmacokinetics. Pharmacol Res 35:363–390, 1997.

Rowland, M., and T. N. Tozer. Clinical Pharmacokinetics: Concepts and Applications, 3rd ed. Philadelphia, Lea and Febiger, 1995.

CHAPTER THREE

PHARMACODYNAMICS

OVERVIEW

Pharmacodynamics is concerned with the mechanisms by which drugs produce their biochemical and physiologic effects. It is also concerned with the dose-response relationship, which is the relationship between drug concentration (dose) and the magnitude of drug effect. Pharmacodynamics provides a scientific basis for the selection and use of drugs to counteract specific pathophysiologic mechanisms in particular diseases.

MECHANISMS OF DRUG ACTION
Nature of Drug Receptors

Most drugs produce their effects by interacting with specific cell molecules known as receptors (Table 3–1). Among the few drugs that produce their effects without interacting with receptors are drugs that neutralize gastric acid and drugs that exert an osmotic effect in tissue.

Many drugs bind to **hormone and neurotransmitter receptors** located in the plasma membrane of target cells. These receptors are transmembrane proteins that have a ligand (drug or neurotransmitter) binding site on the external surface of the membrane and have an effector site on the internal surface. The effector site is involved in signal transduction, a process that triggers a physiologic effect and is described below.

Some drugs bind to specific **enzymes** and inhibit their function, either by competing with the enzyme substrate for the active site **(competitive inhibition)** or by changing the enzyme's conformation and thereby reducing its catalytic activity **(noncompetitive inhibition).** Other drugs bind to **membrane transport proteins,** such as ion channels and transporters for ions and neurotransmitters, and inhibit their function. A few drugs interact with **membrane lipids** or **nucleic acids.** For example, some of the antineoplastic drugs bind to DNA and prevent its replication and transcription.

Drug-Receptor Interactions
Receptor Binding and Affinity

In order to initiate a cellular response, a drug must first bind to a receptor. In most cases, drugs bind to their receptor by forming hydrogen, ionic, or hydrophobic (Van der Waals) bonds with a receptor site (Fig. 3–1). These weak bonds are reversible and enable the drug to dissociate from the receptor as the tissue concentration of the drug declines. The binding of drugs to receptors often exhibits stereospecificity, so that only one of the stereoisomers will form a three-point attachment with the receptor. In a few cases, drugs form relatively permanent covalent bonds with a specific receptor. This occurs, for example, with antineoplastic drugs that bind to DNA and with drugs that irreversibly inhibit the enzyme cholinesterase.

The tendency of a drug to combine with its receptor is called affinity and is a measure of the strength of the drug-receptor bonding. According to the law of mass action, the number of receptors [R] occupied by a drug depends on the drug concentration [D] and the drug-receptor association and dissociation rate constants (k_1 and k_2):

$$[D] + [R] \underset{k_2}{\overset{k_1}{\rightleftharpoons}} [D\text{-}R] \longrightarrow \text{Effect}$$

The ratio of k_2 to k_1 is known as the K_D and represents the drug concentration required to saturate 50% of the receptors. The lower the K_D, the greater is the drug's affinity for the receptor. Most drugs have a K_D in the micromolar to nanomolar (10^{-6} to 10^{-9} molar) range of drug concentrations. As discussed below, receptor affinity is the primary determinant of drug potency.

Signal Transduction

Signal transduction is the process by which receptor binding initiates a cascade of biochemical events that ultimately leads to a physiologic effect.

Membrane receptors are often coupled with a G protein, an ion channel, or an enzyme (Table 3–2). The receptors coupled with G proteins constitute a superfamily of receptors for a large number of physiologic ligands and drugs, including receptors for acetylcholine, epinephrine, histamine, opioids, and serotonin. Fig. 3–2 illustrates signal transduction for a receptor that is coupled with G proteins.

The G proteins are guanine nucleotide–binding proteins that have three subunits known as α, β, and γ. The α subunit serves as the site of guanosine triphosphate (GTP) hydrolysis, a process catalyzed by GTPase. There are several types of α subunit, each of which determines a specific cellular response. For example, the α_s (stimulating) subunit stimulates

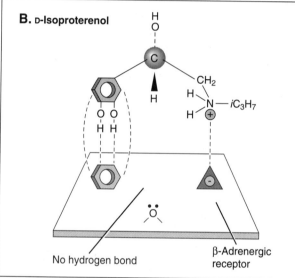

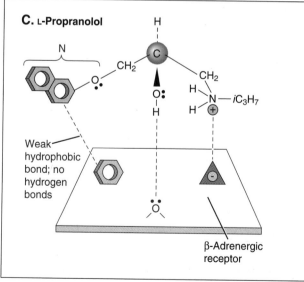

FIGURE 3–1. Drug binding to receptors. (A) L-Isoproterenol, a β-adrenergic receptor agonist, forms hydrogen, ionic, and hydrophobic (Van der Waals) bonds with three sites on the β-adrenergic receptor. **(B)** D-Isoproterenol binds to two sites on the β-adrenergic

TABLE 3–1. Types of Drug Receptors

Receptors for hormones and neurotransmitters
Adrenergic receptors
Histamine receptors
5-Hydroxytryptamine (serotonin) receptors
Insulin receptors
Muscarinic receptors
Nicotinic receptors
Opioid receptors
Steroid receptors

Enzymes
Carbonic anhydrase
Cholinesterase
Cyclooxygenase
DNA polymerase
DNA topoisomerase
Human immunodeficiency virus (HIV) protease
Monoamine oxidase
Na^+,K^+-adenosine triphosphatase
Xanthine oxidase

Membrane transport proteins
Ion channels
Ion transporters
Transporters for neurotransmitters

Other macromolecules
Membrane lipids
Nucleic acids

adenylyl cyclase and thereby increases the production of cyclic adenosine monophosphate (cyclic AMP, or cAMP). The α_i (inhibitory) subunit inhibits adenylyl cyclase and decreases the production of cyclic AMP. Another G protein activates phospholipase C and leads to the formation of inositol triphosphate (IP_3) and diacylglycerol (DAG) from membrane phospholipids. Several other α subunits have been identified.

Cyclic AMP, IP_3, DAG, and other second messengers activate or inhibit unique cellular enzymes in each target cell. Cyclic AMP activates a number of tissue-specific protein kinases. These kinases regulate muscle contraction, ion channel activity, and the activity of enzymes such as glycogen phosphorylase. IP_3 and DAG evoke the release of calcium from intracellular storage sites and thereby augment calcium-induced processes such as muscle contraction and glandular secretion.

Intrinsic Activity

The ability of a drug to initiate a cellular effect is called intrinsic activity. Drugs that have both receptor affinity and intrinsic activity are called **agonists,** whereas drugs that have receptor affinity but lack intrinsic activity are called **antagonists.** With a few

receptor but is unable to bind with the third site. **(C)** L-Propranolol, a β-adrenergic receptor antagonist, binds to two sites on the receptor in the same way that L-isoproterenol does. The naphthyloxy group (N) forms weak bonds with the third receptor site, but these are not sufficiently strong for the drug to have intrinsic (agonist) activity. iC_3H_7 = isopropyl.

TABLE 3–2. Examples of Drug Receptors and Signal Transduction Mechanisms*

Family and Type of Receptor	Mechanism of Signal Transduction	Drug Ligands
G protein–coupled receptors		
α_1-Adrenergic receptors	Activation of phospholipase	Phenylephrine (Ag)
α_2-Adrenergic receptors	Inhibition of adenylyl cyclase	Clonidine (Ag)
β-Adrenergic receptors	Stimulation of adenylyl cyclase	Isoproterenol (Ag) and propranolol (Ant)
Muscarinic receptors	Activation of phospholipase	Atropine (Ant)
Ligand-gated ion channels		
GABA$_A$ receptors	Chloride flux	Benzodiazepines (Ag) and flumazenil (Ant)
Nicotinic ACh receptors	Sodium flux	Carbachol (Ag) and tubocurarine (Ant)
Membrane-bound enzymes		
Atrial natriuretic factor receptors	Activation of guanylyl cyclase	Nitroglycerin
Insulin receptors	Activation of tyrosine kinase	Insulin
Nuclear receptors		
Steroid receptors	Activation of gene transcription	Adrenal and gonadal steroids
Thyroid hormone receptors	Activation of gene transcription	Thyroxin

*Ag = agonist; Ant = antagonist; GABA = gamma-aminobutyric acid; and ACh= acetylcholine.

classes of drugs, such as the β-adrenergic receptor agonists and antagonists, the specific structures responsible for affinity and intrinsic activity have been identified. Both agonists and antagonists have the structural components sufficient for receptor affinity, but only agonists have the structure required for intrinsic activity (see Fig. 3–1).

There are three types of agonists. **Full agonists** have the ability to produce the maximal response obtainable in a tissue. **Partial agonists** can only produce a submaximal response. In the presence of a full agonist, a partial agonist will act like an antagonist because it will prevent the full agonist from binding to the receptor and exerting a maximal response.

Inverse agonists, which are also called **negative antagonists,** are involved in a special type of drug-receptor interaction. The effect of inverse agonists is based on the concept that signal transduction proceeds at a basal rate in the absence of any ligand binding to the receptor (Fig. 3–3). A full agonist increases the rate of signal transduction when it binds to the receptor, whereas an inverse agonist decreases the rate of signal transduction. Antagonists can prevent the action of agonists and inverse agonists by occupying receptor-binding sites. Only a few inverse agonists have been identified, and drugs that bind to the benzodiazepine receptor located in the central nervous system are examples.

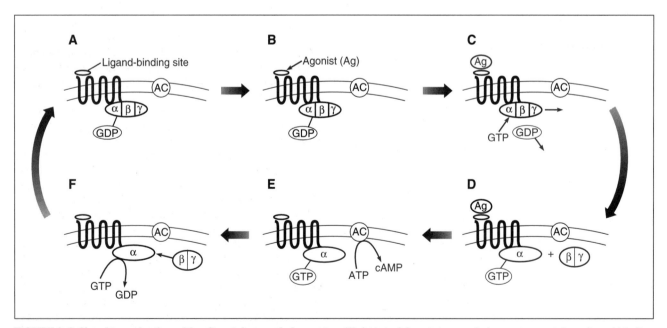

FIGURE 3–2. Signal transduction with a G protein–coupled receptor. (A) A typical G protein–coupled receptor contains a ligand-binding site on the external surface of the plasma membrane and a G protein–binding site on the internal surface. In the inactive state, guanosine diphosphate (GDP) is bound to the α subunit of the G protein. **(B) and (C)** When the agonist (Ag) binds to the receptor, guanosine triphosphate (GTP) binds to the G protein and causes the dissociation of GDP. **(D)** Activation of the α subunit by GTP causes the dissociation of the β and γ subunits. **(E)** The α subunit is then able to activate adenylyl cyclase (AC) and thereby stimulate the conversion of adenosine triphosphate (ATP) to cyclic adenosine monophosphate (cyclic AMP, or cAMP). **(F)** GTP hydrolysis, catalyzed by α subunit GTPase, leads to reassociation of the β and γ subunits.

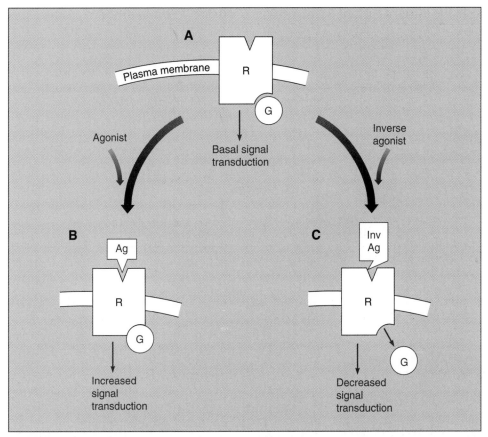

FIGURE 3–3. Mechanism of action of an inverse agonist (negative antagonist) on a G protein receptor. (A) In the basal state, a low level of signal transduction occurs in the absence of ligand binding. **(B)** An agonist (Ag) facilitates the binding of G protein (G) to the receptor (R) by stabilizing the G protein–receptor complex, and this increases the level of signal transduction. **(C)** An inverse agonist (Inv Ag) destabilizes the G protein–receptor complex and causes the signal transduction to dip below the basal level.

Receptor Classification

Drug receptors have been classified according to drug specificity, tissue location, and molecular structure. For example, adrenergic receptors were initially divided into two types (α and β), based on their affinity for and reaction to norepinephrine, epinephrine, and other agents in different tissues. Subsequently, the distinction between the types was confirmed by the development of selective antagonists that blocked either α-adrenergic or β-adrenergic receptors. Later, the two types of receptors were divided into subtypes, based on more subtle differences in agonist potency, tissue distribution, and effects. More recently, many receptors have been cloned and their amino acid sequence determined, so as to provide a molecular basis for receptor classification.

Receptor Regulation and Drug Tolerance

Receptors may undergo dynamic changes with respect to their density (number per cell) and their affinity for drugs and other ligands. The continuous or repeated exposure to agonists can reduce the number of receptors via a process called **down-regulation.** In contrast, continuous or repeated exposure to antagonists can increase the number of receptors via **up-regulation.** The magnitude of these

effects is usually proportional to the drug concentration and duration of drug administration. Altered receptor density may be mediated by altered synthesis of receptor protein as well as by **internalization,** a process in which the receptor-binding sites move into the cell and are no longer exposed to the drug on the cell surface.

Receptor down-regulation is often responsible for **pharmacodynamic tolerance,** a type of drug tolerance in which increasing doses of a drug are required to produce a given magnitude of effect. The rapid development of pharmacodynamic tolerance is called **tachyphylaxis.** Pharmacodynamic tolerance is distinct from **pharmacokinetic tolerance** in that the latter is caused by accelerated drug elimination.

Disease states may alter the number and function of receptors and thereby affect the response to drugs. For example, myasthenia gravis is an autoimmune disorder in which antibodies destroy some of the nicotinic receptors in skeletal muscle, leading to impaired neurotransmission and muscle weakness. This condition is treated by administration of nicotinic receptor agonists (see Chapter 6).

DOSE-RESPONSE RELATIONSHIPS

In pharmacodynamic studies, different doses of a drug can be tested in a group of subjects or on isolated organs, tissues, or cells. The relationship between the concentration of a drug at the receptor site and the magnitude of the response is called the dose-response relationship. Depending on the purpose of the studies, this relationship may be described in terms of a graded (arithmetic) response or a quantal (all-or-none) response.

Graded Dose-Response Relationships

In graded dose-response relationships, the response elicited with each dose of a drug is described in terms of a percentage of the **maximal response** and is plotted against the **log dose** of the drug (Fig. 3–4).

Graded-dose response curves illustrate the relationship between drug dose, receptor occupancy, and the magnitude of the resulting physiologic effect. For a given drug, the maximal response is produced when all of the functional receptors are occupied, and the half-maximal response is produced when 50% of the functional receptors are occupied. In some cases, only a small percentage of the total number of

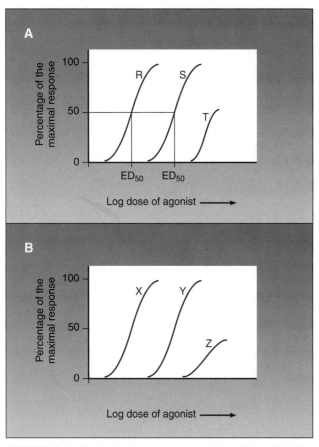

FIGURE 3–4. Graded dose-response relationships. (A) The dose-response curves of three agonists (R, S, and T) are compared. Drugs R and S are full agonists. Both have maximal efficacy, but R is more potent than S. Drug T is a partial agonist and is therefore incapable of producing the same magnitude of effect as a full agonist. T is also less potent than R and S. The ED_{50} is the median effective dose. **(B)** The effects that antagonists have on an agonist's dose-response curve are compared. X = agonist alone; Y = agonist in the presence of a competitive antagonist; and Z = agonist in the presence of a noncompetitive antagonist.

receptors must be occupied in order to produce the maximal response. This is because only some of the receptors are considered "functional," while the rest are considered to be "spare" receptors.

Potency is the dose required to produce a defined magnitude of drug effect. It is usually expressed in terms of the **median effective dose** (ED_{50}), which is the dose that produces 50% of the maximal response. The potency of a drug varies inversely with a drug's ED_{50}, so that a drug whose ED_{50} is 4 mg is 10 times more potent than a drug whose ED_{50} is 40 mg. Potency is determined by the affinity of a drug for its receptor, because drugs with greater affinity require a lower dose to occupy 50% of the functional receptors.

The maximal response produced by a drug is known as its **efficacy.** A **full agonist** has maximal efficacy, whereas a **partial agonist** has less than maximal efficacy and is incapable of producing the same magnitude of effect as a full agonist, even at the very highest doses (see Fig. 3–4A). As discussed earlier, when a partial agonist is administered with an agonist, the partial agonist may act as an antagonist by preventing the agonist from binding to the receptor and thereby reducing its effect.

The effect that an **antagonist** has on the dose-response curve of an agonist will depend on whether the antagonist is competitive or noncompetitive (see Fig. 3–4B). A **competitive antagonist** binds reversibly to a receptor, and its effects are surmountable if the dose of the agonist is increased sufficiently. A competitive antagonist shifts the agonist's dose-response curve to the right, but it does not reduce the maximal response. Although a **noncompetitive antagonist** also shifts the agonist's dose-response curve to the right, it binds to the receptor in a way that reduces the ability of the agonist to elicit a response. The amount of reduction is in proportion to the dose of the antagonist. The effects of a noncompetitive antagonist cannot be surmounted.

Quantal Dose-Response Relationships

In quantal dose-response relationships, the response elicited with each dose of a drug is described in terms of the cumulative percentage of subjects exhibiting a defined **all-or-none effect** and is plotted against the **log dose** of the drug (Fig. 3–5). An example of an all-or-none effect is sleep when a sedative is given. With the quantal dose-response relationship, the median effective dose (ED_{50}) is the dose that produces the defined effect in 50% of the subjects.

Quantal relationships may be defined for both toxic and therapeutic drug effects, so as to allow calculation of the **therapeutic index** (TI) and the **certain safety factor** (CSF) of a drug. The TI and CSF are based on the difference between the toxic dose and the therapeutic dose in a population of subjects. The TI is defined as the ratio between the median lethal dose (LD_{50}) and the median effective dose (ED_{50}). It provides a general indication of the margin

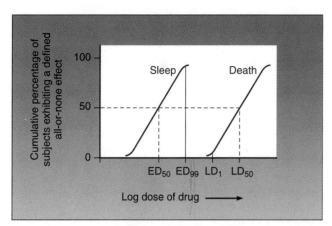

FIGURE 3–5. Quantal dose-response relationships. The dose-response curves for a therapeutic effect (sleep) and a toxic effect (death) of a drug are compared. LD is the lethal dose, and ED is the effective dose. The ratio of the LD_{50} to the ED_{50} is the therapeutic index. The ratio of the LD_1 to the ED_{99} is the certain safety factor.

of safety of a drug, but the CSF is a more realistic estimate of drug safety. The CSF is defined as the ratio between the dose that is lethal in 1% of subjects (LD_1) and the dose that produces a therapeutic effect in 99% of subjects (ED_{99}). When phenobarbital was tested in animals, for example, it was found to have a TI of 10 and a CSF of 2. Since the dose that will kill 1% of animals is twice the dose that is required to produce the therapeutic effect in 99% of animals, the drug has a good margin of safety.

Summary of Important Points

- Most drugs form reversible, stereospecific bonds with macromolecular receptors located in target cells.
- The tendency of a drug to bind to a receptor is called affinity and is directly related to potency. The affinity of a drug is often expressed as the K_D, which is the drug concentration required to saturate 50% of the functional receptors.
- The ability of a drug to initiate a response is called intrinsic activity. Agonists have both affinity and intrinsic activity, whereas antagonists have only receptor affinity.
- Graded dose-response curves show the relationship between the dose and the magnitude of the drug effect in a group of subjects or in a particular tissue, organ, or type of cell. The median effective dose (ED_{50}) produces 50% of the maximal response.
- A competitive antagonist and a noncompetitive antagonist will both cause a rightward shift in the dose-response curve of an agonist, but only a noncompetitive antagonist will reduce the maximal response of the agonist.
- Quantal dose-response curves show the relationship between the dose and the cumulative percentage of subjects exhibiting an all-or-none effect. The ratio of the median lethal dose (toxic dose) to the median effective dose (therapeutic dose) is called the therapeutic index and is an indication of the margin of safety of a drug.

Selected Readings

Chahdi, A. Drugs interacting with G protein alpha subunits: selectivity and perspectives. Fundam Clin Pharmacol 12:121–132, 1998.
Clark, W. P., and R. A. Bond. The elusive nature of intrinsic efficacy. Trends Pharmacol Sci 19:270–276, 1998.
Costa, T., et al. Drug efficacy at guanine nucleotide–binding regulatory protein-linked receptors: thermodynamic interpretation of negative antagonism and of receptor activity in the absence of ligand. Mol Pharmacol 41:549–560, 1992.
Levy, G. Predicting effective drug concentrations for individual patients: determinants of pharmacodynamic variability. Clin Pharmacokinet 34:323–333, 1998.
Pratt, W. B., and P. Taylor. Principles of Drug Action: The Basis of Pharmacology, 3rd ed. New York, Churchill Livingstone, 1990.
Smith, H. J. Introduction to the Principles of Drug Design and Action, 3rd ed. Newark, N. J., Harwood Academic Publishers, 1998.

CHAPTER FOUR

DRUG DEVELOPMENT AND SAFETY

OVERVIEW

Drugs have the potential to produce harmful and beneficial effects when they are administered to humans or animals. As the Renaissance physician Paracelsus argued, "All substances are poisons: there is none which is not a poison. The right dose differentiates a poison from a remedy" (quoted in Klaassen 1996, p. 4). Indeed, investigators have not yet discovered a drug that does not have the potential to cause toxicity. This chapter begins with a description of drug development and the processes for evaluating drug safety and efficacy and then provides information on the various types of adverse effects and interactions that are caused by drugs.

DRUG DEVELOPMENT

Drug development in most countries has many features in common, beginning with the discovery and characterization of a new drug and proceeding through the clinical investigations that ultimately lead to regulatory approval for marketing the drug. Steps in the process of drug development in the USA are depicted in Fig. 4–1.

Discovery and Characterization

New drug compounds are either synthesized or isolated from a natural product in a chemical laboratory. Synthetic drugs may be patterned after other drugs with known pharmacologic activity, or their structure may be designed to bind a particular receptor and be based on computer modeling of the drug and receptor. Because the likely activity of some new compounds is relatively uncertain, they must be submitted to a battery of screening tests to determine their effects. There are cases in which a particular pharmacologic activity of a drug was discovered accidentally after the drug was administered to patients for other purposes. For example, the antihypertensive effect of clonidine was discovered when a physician administered a small dose to an office secretary to treat nasal congestion (the anticipated clinical use of the drug) and found that the secretary experienced a profound hypotensive episode. This led to the drug's subsequent development and use in treating hypertension.

Experimental Studies

Before a new drug is administered to humans, its pharmacologic effects are thoroughly investigated in studies involving animals. The studies are designed to ascertain whether the new drug has any harmful or beneficial effects on vital organ function, including cardiovascular, renal, and respiratory function; to elucidate the drug's mechanisms and therapeutic effects on target organs; and to determine the drug's pharmacokinetic properties, thereby providing some indication of how the drug would be handled by the human body.

Federal regulations require that extensive toxicity studies in animals be conducted to predict the risks that will be associated with administering the drug to healthy human subjects and patients. The value of the experimental studies is based on the proven correlation between a drug's toxicity in animals and its toxicity in humans. As outlined in Table 4–1, the studies involve short-term and long-term administration of the drug and are designed to determine the risk of **acute, subacute, and chronic toxicity,** as well as the risk of **teratogenesis, mutagenesis,** and **carcinogenesis.** After animals are treated with the new drug, their behavior is assessed; their blood samples are analyzed for indications of tissue damage, metabolic abnormalities, and immunologic effects; their tissues are removed and examined for gross and microscopic pathologic changes; and their offspring are also studied for adverse effects.

Studies in animals do not usually reveal all of the adverse effects that will be found in human subjects, either because of the low incidence of particular effects or because of differences in susceptibility among species. This means that some toxic reactions will not be detected until the drug is administered to humans. Because the studies of long-term effects in animals may require many years for completion, it is usually possible to begin human studies while animal studies are being completed if the acute and subacute toxicity studies have not revealed any serious problems in animals.

The Investigational New Drug (IND) Application

The **Food and Drug Administration** (FDA) must approve an application for an investigational new drug (IND) before the drug can be distributed for the purpose of conducting studies in human subjects. The IND application includes a complete description of the drug, the results of all experimental studies completed to date, a description of the design and methods of the proposed clinical studies, and de-

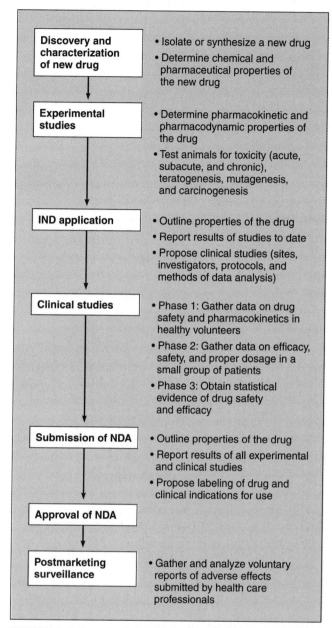

| Discovery and characterization of new drug | • Isolate or synthesize a new drug
• Determine chemical and pharmaceutical properties of the new drug |

| Experimental studies | • Determine pharmacokinetic and pharmacodynamic properties of the drug
• Test animals for toxicity (acute, subacute, and chronic), teratogenesis, mutagenesis, and carcinogenesis |

| IND application | • Outline properties of the drug
• Report results of studies to date
• Propose clinical studies (sites, investigators, protocols, and methods of data analysis) |

| Clinical studies | • Phase 1: Gather data on drug safety and pharmacokinetics in healthy volunteers
• Phase 2: Gather data on efficacy, safety, and proper dosage in a small group of patients
• Phase 3: Obtain statistical evidence of drug safety and efficacy |

| Submission of NDA | • Outline properties of the drug
• Report results of all experimental and clinical studies
• Propose labeling of drug and clinical indications for use |

| Approval of NDA | |

| Postmarketing surveillance | • Gather and analyze voluntary reports of adverse effects submitted by health care professionals |

FIGURE 4–1. Steps in the process of drug development in the USA. IND = investigational new drug; and NDA = new drug application.

tailed information pertaining to the qualifications of the investigators.

Clinical Studies

Phase 1 studies seek to determine the pharmacokinetic properties and safety of an IND in healthy human subjects. In the past, most of the subjects were men. Today, women are being included in phase 1 studies to determine if gender has any influence on the properties of the IND. The subjects typically undergo physical examination, imaging studies, and chemical and pharmacokinetic analyses of samples of blood and other body fluids. The pharmacokinetic analyses provide a basis for estimating doses to be employed in the next phase of studies, and the other examinations seek to determine if the drug is safe for use in humans.

Phase 2 studies are the first studies to be performed in human subjects who have the particular disease for which the IND is to be used. These studies use a small number of patients to obtain a preliminary assessment of the drug's efficacy and safety in diseased individuals and to establish a dosage range for further clinical studies.

Phase 3 studies are conducted to compare the safety and efficacy of the IND with that of another substance or treatment approach. Phase 3 studies employ a larger group of subjects, often consisting of hundreds or even thousands of patients, and usually involve multiple clinical sites and investigators. Phase 3 studies are rigorously designed to prevent investigator bias and are often double-blind and placebo-controlled. A **double-blind study** is one in which neither the investigator nor the patient knows if the patient is receiving the IND or another substance. With some diseases, it is unethical to administer a placebo because of the proven benefits of standard drug therapy. In such cases, the IND is compared with the standard drug. Phase 3 trials often involve **crossover studies,** in which the patients receive one medication or placebo for a period of time and then are switched, after a washout period, to the other medication or placebo.

In many cases, the data are analyzed statistically at various points to determine whether the IND is sufficiently effective or toxic to justify terminating a clinical study. For example, if a statistically significant therapeutic effect can be demonstrated after 6 months in the group of patients who are receiving the IND, it is unethical to continue giving a placebo to the other group, the members of which could also benefit from receiving the IND. A clinical study is also stopped if an IND has been found to cause a significant increase in the rate of mortality or serious toxicity.

The New Drug Application (NDA) and Its Approval

After phase 3 studies are completed and analyzed, the drug developer may submit a new drug application (NDA) to the FDA to request approval to market the drug. This application includes the results of all experimental and clinical studies, as well as the proposed labeling and clinical indications for the drug. The NDA typically constitutes an enormous amount of written material.

The FDA usually takes a number of months to review the NDA before deciding whether to permit the drug to be marketed.

Postmarketing Surveillance

If a drug is approved for marketing, its safety in the general patient population is monitored by an informal procedure known as postmarketing surveillance. The FDA seeks voluntary reporting of adverse

TABLE 4–1. Drug Toxicity Studies in Animals

Type of Study	Method	Observations
Acute toxicity	Administer a single dose of the drug in two species via two routes.	Behavioral changes, LD_{50},* and mortality.
Subacute toxicity	Administer the drug for 90 days in two species via a route intended for humans.	Behavioral and physiologic changes, blood chemistry levels, and pathologic findings in tissue samples.
Chronic toxicity	Administer the drug for 6–24 months, depending on the type of drug.	Behavioral and physiologic changes, blood chemistry levels, and pathologic findings in tissue samples.
Teratogenesis	Administer the drug to pregnant rats and rabbits during organogenesis.	Anatomic defects and behavioral changes in offspring.
Mutagenesis	Perform the Ames test in bacteria. Examine cultured mammalian cells for chromosomal defects.	Evidence of chromosome breaks, gene mutations, chromatid exchange, trisomy, or other defects.
Carcinogenesis	Administer the drug to rats and mice for their entire lifetime.	Higher than normal rate of malignant neoplasms.

*The LD_{50} (the medial lethal dose) is the dose that kills half of the animals in a 14-day period after the dose is administered.

drug reactions from all health care professionals through its MedWatch program, and standard forms for this purpose are disseminated widely in professional publications. Postmarketing surveillance is particularly important for detecting drug reactions that are rare in the population and are therefore unlikely to be found during clinical trials.

FEDERAL DRUG LAWS AND REGULATIONS IN THE USA

There are two major types of legislation pertaining specifically to drugs. One type concerns **drug safety and efficacy** and regulates the processes by which drugs are evaluated, labeled, and marketed. The other type focuses on the **prevention of drug abuse.** In both cases, the laws and regulations reflect society's concern with minimizing the harm that may result from drug use while permitting the therapeutic use of safe and beneficial agents.

Drug Safety and Efficacy
Pure Food and Drug Act

The Pure Food and Drug Act of 1906 was the first federal legislation concerning drug product safety and efficacy in the USA. The act was passed in response to the sale of patent medicines that often contained toxic, habit-forming, or other nonbeneficial ingredients. The legislation required accurate labeling of the ingredients in drug products and sought to prevent the adulteration of products through the substitution of inactive or toxic ingredients for the labeled ingredients. Because the courts refused to allow the use of this act to prevent fraudulent advertising, the legislation was only partially successful in eliminating unsafe drug products.

Food, Drug, and Cosmetic Act

The Food, Drug, and Cosmetic Act of 1938 came in response to a tragic incident in which over 100 people died after ingesting an elixir that contained sulfanilamide and ethylene glycol. The legislation, which is still in force today, made major strides by requiring evidence of drug safety before a drug product could be marketed, by establishing the FDA to enforce this requirement, and by giving legal authority to the drug product standards contained in the **United States Pharmacopeia** (USP).

First compiled in 1820, the USP has been updated and published at regular intervals by a private organization that is called the **United States Pharmacopeial Convention** and is composed of representatives of medical and pharmacy colleges and societies from each state. The USP contains information on the chemical analysis of drugs and indicates how much variance in drug content is allowable for each drug product. For example, the USP states that aspirin tablets must contain not less than 90% and not more than 110% of the labeled amount of $C_9H_8O_4$ (aspirin). In addition, the USP outlines standards for tablet disintegration and many other aspects of drug product composition and analysis.

Amendments to the Food, Drug, and Cosmetic Act

The Food, Drug, and Cosmetic Act has been amended many times.

The **Durham-Humphrey Amendment** was passed in 1952 and created a legal distinction between nonprescription and prescription drugs. According to this amendment, **prescription drugs** must bear the following notice: "Caution: federal law prohibits dispensing without prescription." Agents that are classified as prescription drugs include new drugs, habit-forming drugs, and drugs that are unsafe for use without the supervision of a physician or another designated health care professional. The FDA has the authority to reclassify drugs that have been found to be safe enough to be used without professional supervision. For example, topical cortisone products, some antifungal drugs for treating candidiasis, and some antihistamines and decongestants were originally classified as prescription drugs but are now classified as nonprescription drugs.

The **Kefauver-Harris Amendments** were passed in 1962, largely in response to reports of severe malformations in the offspring of women who took thalidomide during pregnancy. In fact, thalidomide had not been marketed in the USA, because a female scientist at the FDA, Frances Kelsey, had held up the drug's approval. Nevertheless, because the members of Congress believed that drug development should be regulated more strictly, they passed amendments that required the demonstration of both safety and efficacy in studies involving animals and humans before a drug product could be marketed. Although the processes of new drug development and testing have not changed substantially since this amendment was passed, the FDA review of new drugs has been streamlined in recent years.

The **Orphan Drug Amendments** were passed in 1983 to provide tax benefits and other incentives for drug manufacturers to test and produce drugs that are used in the treatment of rare diseases and are therefore unlikely to generate large profits. The act appears to have been successful, as several hundred orphan drugs are now available. Examples are drugs used for the treatment of urea cycle enzyme deficiencies, Gaucher's disease, homocystinuria, and other rare metabolic disorders.

The **Drug Price Competition and Patent Restoration Act** of 1984 extended the patent life of drug products (which at that time was 17 years) by the amount of time required for regulatory review of a new drug application. It also accelerated the approval of **generic drug products** by allowing investigators to submit an abbreviated new drug application (ANDA) in which the generic product is shown to be therapeutically equivalent to an approved brand name product. Therapeutic equivalence is demonstrated on the basis of a single-dose oral bioavailability study that compares the generic drug with the brand name drug. If the variance is within a specified range (usually ±20%), the generic drug may be approved for marketing. The cost of such a study is relatively small compared with the millions of dollars required for the development of a completely new drug.

In 1992, **accelerated drug approval** was authorized for **new drugs to treat life-threatening conditions** such as acquired immunodeficiency syndrome (AIDS) and cancer. Under the new regulations, patients with these conditions can be treated with an investigational drug before clinical trials have been completed.

Drug Abuse Prevention
Harrison Narcotics Act

The Harrison Narcotics Act of 1914 was the first major drug abuse legislation in the USA. It was prompted by the growing problem of heroin abuse, which followed the synthesis of this potent and rapid-acting derivative of morphine. The act sought to control narcotics through the use of tax stamps on legal drug products (a practice similar to the use of tax stamps on alcoholic beverages today) and was enforced by the US Treasury Department. The Harrison Narcotics Act had a profound and controversial effect on the treatment of drug dependence in that it prohibited physicians from administering drugs to addicts as part of their treatment program.

Comprehensive Drug Abuse Prevention and Control Act

During the 1960s, the prevalence of drug abuse increased, especially among adolescents and young adults, who were using a wide range of drugs that included prescription sedatives and stimulants as well as illicit substances such as lysergic acid diethylamide (LSD), marijuana, and other hallucinogens. Believing that the drug abuse problem required a new approach, members of Congress passed the Comprehensive Drug Abuse Prevention and Control Act of 1970. This law is often called the **Controlled Substances Act** (CSA).

The CSA classified abused drugs into five schedules, based on their potential for abuse and their clinical usage. **Schedule I drugs** have a high abuse potential and no legitimate medical use, and their distribution and possession are prohibited. **Schedule II drugs** have a high abuse potential but a legitimate medical use, and their distribution is highly controlled through requirements for inventories and records and through restrictions on prescriptions. **Schedule III, IV, and V drugs** have lower abuse potential and fewer restrictions on distribution. The CSA requires that all distributors, practitioners, and medical institutions using controlled drugs register with the Drug Enforcement Agency, which is responsible for enforcing the act.

ADVERSE EFFECTS OF DRUGS

Adverse effects, or **side effects,** can be classified with respect to their mechanisms of action and predictability. Those due to excessive pharmacologic activity are the most predictable and are often the easiest to prevent or counteract. Organ toxicity caused by other mechanisms is often unpredictable, because its occurrence depends on the drug susceptibility of the individual patient, the drug dosage, and numerous other factors. Hypersensitivity reactions are responsible for a large number of adverse organ system effects. These reactions occur frequently with some drugs but only rarely with others.

Excessive Pharmacologic Effects

Drugs often produce adverse effects by the same mechanism that is responsible for their therapeutic effect on the target organ. For example, atropine may cause dry mouth and urinary retention by the same mechanism that reduces gastric acid secretion in the treatment of peptic ulcer—namely, by muscarinic receptor blockade. This type of adverse effect may be managed by reducing the drug dosage or by substituting a drug that is more selective for the target organ.

Hypersensitivity Reactions

Hypersensitivity reactions, or **drug allergies,** are responsible for a large number of organ toxicities that range in severity from a mild skin rash to major organ system failure. An allergic reaction occurs when the drug, acting as a hapten, combines with an endogenous protein to form an antigen that induces antibody synthesis. The antigen and antibody subsequently interact with body tissues to produce a wide variety of adverse effects.

In the **Gell and Coombs classification system,** allergic reactions are divided into four general types, each of which can be produced by drugs. **Type I reactions** are immediate hypersensitivity reactions that are mediated by immunoglobulin E (IgE) antibodies. Examples of these reactions are urticaria (hives), atopic dermatitis, and anaphylactic shock. **Type II reactions** are cytolytic reactions that involve complement and are mediated by immunoglobulins G and M (IgG and IgM). Examples are hemolytic anemia, thrombocytopenia, and drug-induced lupus erythematosus. **Type III reactions** are mediated by immune complexes. The deposition of antigen-antibody complexes in vascular endothelium leads to inflammation, lymphadenopathy, and fever (serum sickness). An example is the severe skin rash seen in patients with a life-threatening form of drug-induced immune vasculitis that is known as Stevens-Johnson syndrome. **Type IV reactions** are delayed hypersensitivity reactions that are mediated by sensitized lymphocytes. An example is the ampicillin-induced skin rash that occurs in patients with viral mononucleosis.

Adverse Effects on Organs

In some cases, the adverse effects and therapeutic effects of a drug are caused by different mechanisms. For example, in patients taking aspirin, an adverse reaction such as tinnitus or hyperventilation that leads to respiratory alkalosis is caused by neurotoxic effects that do not appear to be mediated by the drug's primary mechanism of action, which is inhibition of prostaglandin synthesis. A variety of drugs (Table 4–2) produce toxicity of the liver, kidneys, or other vital organs, and this toxicity may not be readily apparent until significant organ damage has occurred. Patients receiving these drugs should be monitored with appropriate laboratory tests. For example, hepatotoxicity may be detected by monitoring serum aminotransferase (transaminase) levels, while hematopoietic toxicity may be detected by periodically performing blood cell counts.

Hematopoietic Toxicity

Bone marrow toxicity, one of the most frequent types of drug-induced toxicity, may present as **agranulocytosis, anemia, thrombocytopenia,** or a combination of these **(pancytopenia).** The effects are often reversible when the drug is withdrawn, but they may have serious consequences before toxicity can be detected. For example, patients who develop agranulocytosis may succumb to a fatal infection before the problem is recognized.

Many drugs cause hematopoietic toxicity by triggering hypersensitivity reactions directed against the progenitor cells in the bone marrow or their derivatives. Chloramphenicol, however, produces a reversible form of anemia by blocking the action of the enzyme ferrochelatase and thereby preventing the incorporation of iron into heme.

The most serious form of hematopoietic toxicity is **aplastic anemia,** which may be associated with several types of blood cell deficiencies and may lead to pancytopenia. Aplastic anemia is probably due to a hypersensitivity reaction and is often irreversible, although it has recently been treated by administration of hematopoietic growth factors (see Chapter 17).

TABLE 4–2. Drug-Induced Organ Toxicities

Organ Toxicity	Examples of Adverse Effects	Examples of Inducers
Cardiotoxicity	Cardiomyopathy. Inflammatory fibrosis.	Daunorubicin, doxorubicin, and idarubicin. Methysergide.
Hematopoietic toxicity	Agranulocytosis.*	Captopril, chlorpromazine, chlorpropamide, clozapine, and propylthiouracil.
	Aplastic anemia.* Hemolytic anemia.* Thrombocytopenia.*	Chloramphenicol and phenylbutazone. Captopril, levodopa, and methyldopa. Quinidine, rifampin, and sulfonamides.
Hepatotoxicity	Cholestatic jaundice.* Hepatitis.*	Erythromycin estolate and phenothiazines. Amiodarone, captopril, isoniazid, phenytoin, and sulfonamides.
Nephrotoxicity	Acute tubular necrosis. Interstitial nephritis.*	Aminoglycoside antibiotics, amphotericin B, and vancomycin. Nonsteroidal anti-inflammatory drugs (NSAIDs) and penicillins (especially methicillin).
Ototoxicity	Vestibular and cochlear disorders.	Aminoglycoside antibiotics, furosemide, and vancomycin.
Pulmonary toxicity	Inflammatory fibrosis. Pulmonary fibrosis.	Methysergide. Amiodarone, bleomycin, busulfan, and nitrofurantoin.
Skin toxicity	All forms of skin rash.*	Antibiotics, diuretics, phenytoin, sulfonamides, and sulfonylureas.

*Immunologic mechanisms known or suspected.

Hepatotoxicity

A large number of drugs produce liver toxicity, either via an immunologic mechanism or via their direct effect on the hepatocytes. Liver toxicity can be classified as cholestatic or hepatocellular. **Cholestatic hepatotoxicity** is often caused by a hypersensitivity mechanism producing inflammation and stasis of the biliary system. **Hepatocellular toxicity** is sometimes caused by a toxic drug metabolite. For example, acetaminophen and isoniazid have toxic metabolites that may cause hepatitis. With many hepatotoxic drugs, elevated serum aminotransferase levels may provide an early indication of liver damage. When the levels become highly elevated, the drug should be discontinued.

Nephrotoxicity

Renal toxicity is caused by various drugs, including several groups of antibiotics. The forms of renal toxicity can be classified according to site and mechanism and include **interstitial nephritis, renal tubular necrosis,** and **crystalluria** (the precipitation of insoluble drug in the renal tubules). Nephrotoxicity often reduces drug clearance, thereby elevating plasma drug concentrations and leading to greater toxicity. With some drugs that routinely cause renal toxicity, such as cisplatin, the kidneys can be protected by means of forced diuresis, in which the drug is administered with large quantities of intravenous fluid so as to lower the drug concentration in the renal tubules.

Bladder toxicity is less common than renal toxicity, but it may occur as an adverse effect of a few drugs. One example is cyclophosphamide, an antineoplastic drug whose metabolite causes **hemorrhagic cystitis.** This disorder can be prevented by administering mesna, a sulfhydryl-releasing agent that conjugates the toxic metabolite in the urine.

Other Organ Toxicities

Pulmonary toxicity occurs through a variety of mechanisms. Some drugs cause **respiratory depression** via their effects on the brain stem respiratory centers. Drugs such as bleomycin and amiodarone produce **pulmonary fibrosis,** so patients who are being treated with these agents should have periodic chest x-rays and blood gas measurements to detect early signs of fibrosis.

Relatively few drugs produce **cardiotoxicity.** Anthracycline anticancer drugs, such as doxorubicin, produce adverse cardiac effects that resemble congestive heart failure.

Skin rashes of all varieties, including macular, papular, maculopapular, and urticarial rashes, may be produced by drug hypersensitivity reactions. A mild skin rash may disappear with continued drug administration. Nevertheless, because rashes may lead to more serious skin or organ toxicity, they should be monitored carefully.

Idiosyncratic Reactions

Idiosyncratic reactions are unexpected drug reactions caused by a genetically determined susceptibility. For example, patients who have glucose-6-phosphate dehydrogenase deficiency may develop hemolytic anemia when they are exposed to an oxidizing drug such as primaquine or to a sulfonamide.

DRUG INTERACTIONS

A drug interaction is defined as a change in the pharmacologic effect of a drug that results when it is given concurrently with another drug or with food. Drug interactions may be caused by changes in the pharmaceutical, pharmacodynamic, or pharmacokinetic properties of the affected drug (Table 4–3).

Pharmaceutical Interactions

Pharmaceutical interactions, often called **drug incompatibilities,** are usually due to a chemical reaction between drugs prior to their administration or absorption. Pharmaceutical interactions occur most frequently when drug solutions are combined before they are given intravenously. For example, if a penicillin solution and an aminoglycoside solution are mixed, they will form an insoluble precipitate, because penicillins are negatively charged and aminoglycosides are positively charged. Many other

TABLE 4–3.   Types and Mechanisms of Drug Interactions

Type	Mechanism
Drug interactions with food	Altered drug absorption.
Pharmaceutical interactions (drug incompatibilities)	Chemical reaction between drugs prior to their administration or absorption.
Pharmacodynamic interactions	Additive, synergistic, or antagonistic effects on a microbe or tumor cells.
	Additive, synergistic, or antagonistic effects on a tissue or organ system.
Pharmacokinetic interactions	
Altered drug absorption	Altered gut motility or secretion.
	Binding or chelation of drugs.
	Competition for active transport.
Altered drug distribution	Displacement from plasma protein binding sites.
	Displacement from tissue binding sites.
Altered drug biotransformation	Altered hepatic blood flow.
	Enzyme induction.
	Enzyme inhibition.
Altered drug excretion	Altered biliary excretion or enterohepatic cycling.
	Altered urine pH.
	Drug-induced renal impairment.
	Inhibition of active tubular secretion.

drugs are incompatible and should not be combined before they are administered.

Pharmacodynamic Interactions

Pharmacodynamic interactions occur when two or more drugs have additive, synergistic, or antagonistic effects on a tissue, organ system, microbe, or tumor cells. An **additive effect** is equal to the sum of the individual drug effects, whereas a **synergistic effect** is greater than the sum of the individual drug effects. Some pharmacodynamic interactions occur when two or more drugs act on the same receptor, and others occur when the drugs affect the same physiologic function through actions on different receptors. For example, epinephrine and histamine affect the same function but have **antagonistic effects.** Epinephrine activates adrenergic receptors to cause bronchial smooth muscle relaxation, whereas histamine activates histamine receptors to produce bronchial muscle contraction.

Pharmacokinetic Interactions

In pharmacokinetic interactions, a drug alters the absorption, distribution, biotransformation, or excretion of another drug or drugs. Mechanisms and examples of pharmacokinetic interactions are provided in Tables 4–3 and 4–4.

Altered Drug Absorption

There are several mechanisms by which a drug may affect the absorption and bioavailability of another drug. One mechanism involves binding to another drug in the gut and preventing its absorption. Cholestyramine, for example, binds to digoxin and prevents its absorption. Another mechanism involves altering gastric or intestinal motility so as to affect the absorption of another drug. Drugs tend to be absorbed more rapidly from the intestines than from the stomach. Therefore, a drug that slows gastric emptying often delays the absorption of another drug. A drug that increases intestinal motility may reduce the time available for the absorption of another drug, thereby causing its incomplete absorption.

Altered Drug Distribution

Many drugs displace other drugs from plasma proteins and thereby increase the plasma concentra-

TABLE 4–4. Management of Clinically Significant Pharmacokinetic Drug Interactions

Examples of Inducers or Inhibitors	Examples of Affected Drugs	Management
Inducers of drug biotransformation		
Barbiturates, carbamazepine, and rifampin	Warfarin.	Increase warfarin dosage as indicated by prothrombin time (international normalized ratio).
Carbamazepine	Theophylline.	Monitor plasma theophylline concentration and adjust dosage as needed.
Rifampin	Phenytoin.	Monitor plasma phenytoin concentration and adjust dosage as needed.
Inhibitors of drug absorption		
Aluminum, calcium, and iron	Tetracycline.	Give tetracycline 1 hour before or 2 hours after giving the other agent.
Cholestyramine	Digoxin and warfarin.	Give digoxin or warfarin 1 hour before or 2 hours after giving cholestyramine.
Inhibitors of drug biotransformation		
Cimetidine	Benzodiazepines, lidocaine, phenytoin, theophylline, and warfarin.	Instead of giving cimetidine, substitute a histamine blocker that does not inhibit drug metabolism.
Disulfiram	Ethanol.	Make sure the patient understands that disulfiram is used therapeutically to promote abstinence from alcohol (ethanol).
Erythromycin	Carbamazepine and theophylline.	Lower the dose of the affected drug during erythromycin therapy.
Erythromycin, itraconazole, and keto-conazole	Astemizole, cisapride, and terfenadine.	Avoid concurrent therapy and thereby avoid potential QT interval prolongation and fatal cardiac arrhythmias.
Monoamine oxidase inhibitors	Levodopa and sympathomimetic drugs.	Avoid concurrent therapy if possible; otherwise, give a subnormal dose of the affected drug.
Inhibitors of drug clearance		
Diltiazem, quinidine, and verapamil	Digoxin.	Give a subnormal dose of digoxin and monitor the plasma drug concentration.
Probenecid	Cephalosporins and penicillin.	Advise the patient that the combination of drugs is intended to increase the plasma concentration of the antibiotic.
Thiazide diuretics	Lithium.	Give a subnormal dose of lithium and monitor the plasma drug concentration.

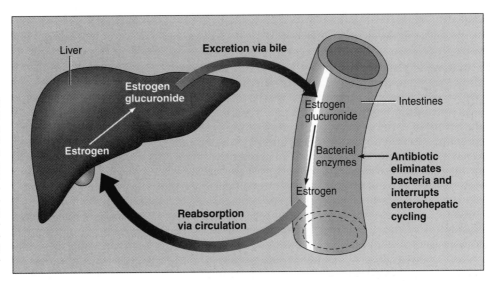

FIGURE 4–2. Interaction of antibiotics with estrogens found in oral contraceptives. Estrogen is conjugated with glucuronate and sulfate in the liver, and the conjugates are excreted via the bile into the intestines. Intestinal bacteria hydrolyze the conjugates, and estrogen is reabsorbed into the circulation. The enterohepatic cycling is interrupted if concurrently administered antibiotics destroy the intestinal bacteria. Contraceptive failure may result.

tion of the free (unbound) drug, but the magnitude and duration of this effect are usually small. As the free drug concentration increases, so does the drug's rate of elimination, and any change in the drug's effect on target tissues is usually short-lived.

The enterohepatic cycling of some drugs is dependent on intestinal bacteria that hydrolyze drug conjugates excreted by the bile and thereby enable the more lipid-soluble parent compound to be reabsorbed into the circulation (Fig. 4–2). Antibiotics administered concurrently with these drugs may kill the bacteria and reduce the enterohepatic cycling and plasma drug concentrations. When antibiotics are taken concurrently with oral contraceptives containing estrogen, for example, they may reduce the plasma concentration of estrogen and cause contraceptive failure.

Altered Drug Biotransformation

In some cases, biotransformation is affected by drugs that alter hepatic blood flow. In many cases, it is affected by drug interactions that either induce or inhibit drug-metabolizing enzymes (see Table 4–4).

Inducers of cytochrome P450 enzymes include barbiturates, carbamazepine, and rifampin. The rate of induction depends on the dose and frequency of administration, but it usually peaks after several days of continuing drug administration. Enzyme induction increases the clearance and reduces the half-life of drugs biotransformed by the enzyme. When the inducing drug is discontinued, the synthesis of P450 enzymes gradually returns to the pretreatment level.

Inhibitors of cytochrome P450 enzymes include cimetidine, erythromycin, and itraconazole. Significant interactions occur when these drugs reduce the clearance and increase the plasma concentration of other drugs. For example, itraconazole inhibits the biotransformation of cisapride and terfenadine. Elevated concentrations of either of these drugs may

prolong the QT interval and thereby precipitate serious cardiac arrhythmias.

Altered Drug Excretion

Drugs can alter the renal or biliary excretion of other drugs by several mechanisms. A few drugs, such as carbonic anhydrase inhibitors, alter the renal pH. This in turn can change the ratio of another drug's ionized form to its nonionized form and affect its renal excretion. Probenecid competes with other organic acids, such as penicillin, for the active transport system in renal tubules. Quinidine and verapamil decrease the biliary clearance of digoxin and thereby increase serum digoxin levels. Potentially nephrotoxic drugs, such as the aminoglycoside antibiotics, may impair the renal excretion of other drugs via their effect on renal function.

Clinical Significance of Drug Interactions

The clinical significance of drug interactions varies widely. In some cases, toxicity is severe and can only be prevented by avoiding the concurrent administration of drugs. In other cases, toxicity can be avoided by proper dosage adjustment and other measures (see Table 4–4). For example, when quinidine and digoxin are administered concurrently, a subnormal dose of digoxin should be used to prevent adverse effects. Fortunately, most drug interactions are of minor significance, and the interacting drugs can usually be administered concurrently without affecting their efficacy or the patient's safety. Drug interactions are more likely to occur if the affected drug has a low therapeutic index or is being used to treat a critically ill patient.

FACTORS AFFECTING DRUG SAFETY AND EFFICACY

Age, disease, pregnancy, and lactation are important biologic variables that can alter the response to drugs in particular patients.

Age

Factors affecting drug disposition in different age populations are summarized in Table 4–5.

In neonates and especially in premature infants, the capacity to metabolize and excrete drugs is often greatly reduced because of low levels of drug biotransformation enzymes. Oxidative reactions and glucuronate conjugation occur at a lower rate in neonates than in adults, whereas sulfate conjugation is well developed in neonates. Consequently, some drugs that are metabolized primarily by glucuronate conjugation in adults (drugs such as acetaminophen) are metabolized chiefly by sulfate conjugation in neonates. Nevertheless, the overall rate of biotransformation of most drugs is lower in neonates and infants than it is in adults.

In comparison with children and young adults, elderly adults tend to have a reduced capacity to metabolize drugs. Biotransformation via oxidative reactions usually declines more than biotransformation via drug conjugation. Therefore, in elderly patients, it may be safer to use drugs that are conjugated. For example, benzodiazepines that are metabolized by conjugation (such as lorazepam and temazepam) are believed to be safer for treatment of the elderly than are benzodiazepines that undergo oxidative biotransformation (such as diazepam and flurazepam).

Renal function is lower in neonates and elderly adults than it is in young adults, and this affects the renal excretion of many drugs. For example, the half-lives of aminoglycoside antibiotics are greatly prolonged in neonates. Glomerular filtration declines 35% between the ages of 20 and 90 years, with a corresponding reduction in the renal elimination of many drugs.

Because the very young and the very old tend to have increased sensitivity to drugs, the dosage per kilogram of body weight should be reduced when most drugs are used in the treatment of these populations.

Disease

Hepatic and renal disease may reduce the capacity of the liver and kidneys to biotransform and excrete drugs, thereby reducing drug clearance and necessitating a dosage reduction to avoid toxicity. Heart failure and other conditions that reduce hepatic blood flow may also reduce drug biotransformation. Oxidative drug metabolism is usually impaired in patients with hepatic disease, whereas conjugation processes may be little affected.

Guidelines for dosage adjustment in patients with hepatic or renal disease have been developed and can be found in many clinical references and textbooks. Dosage adjustments are made by reducing the dose, increasing the interval between doses, or both. Adjustments for individual patients are usually based on laboratory measurements of renal or hepatic function and on plasma drug concentration.

Pregnancy and Lactation

Drugs taken by a woman during pregnancy or lactation can cause adverse effects in the fetus or infant.

The risk of drug-induced developmental abnormalities known as **teratogenic effects** is the greatest during the period of organogenesis from the 4th to the 10th week of gestation. After the 10th week, the major risk is to the development of the brain and spinal cord. An estimated 1–5% of fetal malformations are attributed to drugs. Although only a few drugs have been proven to cause teratogenic effects (Table 4–6), the safety of many other drugs has not yet been determined.

The FDA has divided drugs into five categories, based on their safety in pregnant women. Drugs in categories A and B are relatively safe. For drugs in category C, risk to the fetus cannot be ruled out. Drugs in category D show positive evidence of risk to the fetus, and drugs in category X are contraindicated during pregnancy. Drugs of choice for pregnant

TABLE 4–5. Factors Affecting Drug Disposition in Different Age Populations

Process of Drug Disposition	Population		
	Neonates and Infants	Children	Elderly Adults
Absorption	Altered absorption of some drugs.	No major changes, but first-pass inactivation may be increased.	No major changes.
Distribution	Incomplete blood-brain barrier; higher volumes of distribution for water-soluble drugs.	No major changes.	Higher volumes of distribution for fat-soluble drugs.
Biotransformation	Lower rate of oxidative reactions and glucuronate conjugation.	Biotransformation rate for some drugs higher than in adults.	Reduced oxidative metabolism; relatively unchanged conjugation metabolism.
Excretion	Reduced capacity to excrete drugs.	No major changes.	Reduced capacity to excrete drugs.

TABLE 4–6. Examples of Teratogenic Drugs and Their Effects on the Fetus or Newborn Infant*

Drug	Adverse Effects
Alkylating agents and antimetabolites (anticancer drugs)	Cardiac defects; cleft palate; growth retardation; malformation of ears, eyes, fingers, nose, or skull; and other anomalies.
Carbamazepine	Abnormal facial features; neural tube defects, such as spina bifida; reduced head size; and other anomalies.
Coumarin anticoagulants	Fetal warfarin syndrome (characterized by chondrodysplasia punctata, malformation of ears and eyes, mental retardation, nasal hypoplasia, optic atrophy, skeletal deformities, and other anomalies).
Diethylstilbestrol (DES)	Effects in female offspring: clear cell vaginal or cervical adenocarcinoma; irregular menses; and reproductive abnormalities, including decreased rate of pregnancy and increased rate of preterm deliveries. Effects in male offspring: cryptorchidism, epididymal cysts, and hypogonadism.
Ethanol	Fetal alcohol syndrome (characterized by growth retardation, hyperactivity, mental retardation, microcephaly and facial abnormalities, poor coordination, and other anomalies).
Phenytoin	Fetal hydantoin syndrome (characterized by cardiac defects; malformation of ears, lips, palate, mouth, and nasal bridge; mental retardation; microcephaly; ptosis; strabismus; and other anomalies).
Retinoids (systemic)	Spontaneous abortions. Hydrocephaly; malformation of ears, face, heart, limbs, and liver; microcephaly; and other anomalies.
Tetracycline	Hypoplasia of tooth enamel and staining of teeth.
Thalidomide	Deafness, heart defects, limb abnormalities (amelia or phocomelia), renal abnormalities, and other anomalies.
Valproate	Cardiac defects, central nervous system defects, lumbosacral spina bifida, and microcephaly.

Other substances known to be teratogenic: lead, lithium, methyl mercury, penicillamine, polychlorinated biphenyls, and trimethadione. Other drugs that should be avoided during the second and third trimester of pregnancy: angiotensin-converting enzyme inhibitors, chloramphenicol, indomethacin, prostaglandins, sulfonamides, and sulfonylureas. Other drugs that should be used with great caution during pregnancy: antithyroid drugs, aspirin, barbiturates, benzodiazepines, corticosteroids, heparin, opioids, and phenothiazines.

women are listed in clinical references and textbooks and are selected on the basis of their safety to the fetus as well as their therapeutic efficacy.

Some drugs can be taken by lactating women without posing a risk to their breast-fed infants. Other drugs place the infant at risk for toxicity. As a general rule, breast-feeding should be avoided if a drug taken by the mother would cause the infant's plasma drug concentration to be greater than 50% of the mother's plasma drug concentration. Clinical references pro-

vide guidelines on the use of specific drugs by lactating women.

Summary of Important Points

- The process of drug development includes chemical and pharmacologic characterization, experimental studies to test for toxicity in animals, and clinical studies to determine efficacy and safety in humans.
- Drug development is regulated by the Food and Drug Administration (FDA). An investigational new drug (IND) application must be completed before clinical studies can be started, and a new drug application (NDA) must be submitted and approved before the drug can be marketed.
- Phase 1 studies provide data about drug safety and pharmacokinetics in healthy subjects; phase 2 studies provide data about the proper dosage and potential efficacy in a small group of patients; and phase 3 studies provide statistical evidence of efficacy and safety in a controlled clinical trial.
- The Food, Drug, and Cosmetic Act established the FDA to regulate the development, manufacturing, distribution, and usage of drugs. Amendments have established the prescription class of drugs, stricter requirements for human drug testing, incentives for developing orphan drugs for rare diseases, and abbreviated procedures for marketing generic drug products.
- The Comprehensive Drug Abuse Prevention and Control Act, also called the Controlled Substances Act (CSA), classifies potentially abused drugs in five categories (Schedules I through V), requires registration of legitimate drug distributors and health care professionals, and limits the prescription and distribution of controlled substances.
- The adverse effects of drugs may be due to excessive pharmacologic effects, hypersensitivity reactions, or other mechanisms responsible for organ toxicities. The bone marrow, liver, kidney, and skin are frequent sites of drug toxicity.
- Drug interactions occur when one drug alters the pharmacologic properties of another drug. Most interactions are due to pharmacokinetic effects, particularly inhibition or induction of drug biotransformation.
- Age, disease, pregnancy, and lactation are factors that must be considered in drug selection and dosage. The very young and the very old tend to have an increased sensitivity to therapeutic agents, usually because of a reduced capacity to eliminate drugs. Target organs may also be more sensitive to drugs in these populations.

Selected Readings

Bennett, W. M. Guide to drug dosage in renal failure (Appendix D). *In* Speight, T. M., and N. H. Holford, eds., Avery's Drug Treatment, 4th ed. Auckland, Adis International, 1997.

Charifson, P. S. Practical Application of Computer-Aided Drug Design. New York, Marcel Dekker, 1997.

Hammerlein, A., H. Derendorf, and D. T. Lowenthal. Pharmacokinetic and pharmacodynamic changes in the elderly: clinical implications. Clin Pharmacokinet 35:49–64, 1998.

Hansten, P. D. Hansten and Horn's Drug Interactions Analysis and Management. Vancouver, Wash., Applied Therapeutics, 1997.

Hebert, M. F. Guide to drug dosage in hepatic disease (Appendix F). *In* Speight, T. M., and N. H. Holford, eds., Avery's Drug Treatment, 4th ed. Auckland, Adis International, 1997.

Klaassen, C. D. Casarett and Doull's Toxicology: The Basic Science of Poisons, 5th ed. New York, McGraw-Hill, 1996.

Kuhlmann, J. Drug research: from the idea to the product. Int J Clin Pharmacol Ther 35:541–552, 1997.

Quinn, D. I., and R. O. Day. Clinically important drug interactions. *In* Speight, T. M., and N. H. Holford, eds., Avery's Drug Treatment, 4th ed. Auckland, Adis International, 1997.

AUTONOMIC AND

NEUROMUSCULAR

PHARMACOLOGY

CHAPTER FIVE

INTRODUCTION TO AUTONOMIC AND NEUROMUSCULAR PHARMACOLOGY

OVERVIEW OF NEUROPHARMACOLOGY

The nervous system consists of the central and peripheral nervous systems. The **central nervous system** includes the brain and spinal cord, whereas the **peripheral nervous system** includes the autonomic nervous system and the somatic nervous system.

Drugs alter nervous system function primarily by affecting **neurotransmitters** or their **receptors.** In some cases, drugs affect the synthesis, storage, release, inactivation, or neuronal reuptake of neurotransmitters. In other cases, they activate or block neurotransmitter receptors. Some drugs are relatively specific for a particular neurotransmitter or receptor, while other drugs affect several neurotransmitters. The spectrum of effects produced by a drug depends on the distribution of the affected neurotransmitters in the central and peripheral nervous systems. The actions of some drugs are localized to either the central or the peripheral nervous system, while the actions of other drugs (such as cocaine and amphetamine) affect both central and peripheral functions.

This chapter reviews the anatomy and physiology of the peripheral nervous system and provides an overview of the mechanisms by which drugs affect nervous system function. Drugs that act primarily on the central nervous system are discussed in the chapters of Section IV.

ANATOMY AND PHYSIOLOGY OF THE PERIPHERAL NERVOUS SYSTEM

The **autonomic nervous system** involuntarily regulates the activity of smooth muscles, exocrine glands, cardiac tissue, and certain metabolic activities, while the **somatic nervous system** activates skeletal muscle contraction, thereby enabling voluntary body movements. Both the autonomic and somatic nervous systems are part of the peripheral nervous system, and both are controlled by the central nervous system. The autonomic nervous system is regulated by brain stem centers responsible for cardiovascular, respiratory, and other visceral functions. The somatic nervous system is activated by corticospinal tracts, which originate in the motor cortex, and by spinal reflexes.

Autonomic Nervous System

The autonomic nervous system consists of sympathetic and parasympathetic divisions. In the **sympathetic nervous system,** nerves arise from the thoracic and lumbar spinal cord and have a short preganglionic fiber and a long postganglionic fiber. Most of the ganglia are located in the paravertebral chain adjacent to the spinal cord, but a few prevertebral ganglia (the celiac, splanchnic, and mesenteric ganglia) are located more distally to the spinal cord. The **parasympathetic nervous system** includes portions of cranial nerves III, VII, IX, and X (the oculomotor, facial, glossopharyngeal, and vagus nerves, respectively) and some of the nerves originating from the sacral spinal cord. The parasympathetic nerves have long preganglionic fibers and short postganglionic fibers, with the ganglia often located in the innervated organs.

The origins, neurotransmitters, and receptors of the sympathetic and parasympathetic systems are shown in Fig. 5–1. The sympathetic nervous system tends to discharge as a unit, producing a diffuse activation of target organs. Preganglionic sympathetic neurons synapse with a large number of postganglionic neurons, and this contributes to widespread activation of the organs during sympathetic stimulation. In addition, the release of epinephrine and norepinephrine from the adrenal medulla into the circulation enables the activation of target tissues throughout the body, including some tissues that are not directly innervated by sympathetic nerves. In contrast to the sympathetic system, the parasympathetic system is capable of discretely activating specific target tissues. For example, it is possible for parasympathetic nerves to slow the heart rate without simultaneously stimulating gastrointestinal or bladder function. This is partly because there is a low ratio of postganglionic fibers to preganglionic fibers in the parasympathetic system.

As shown in Fig. 5–2, the sympathetic and parasympathetic nervous systems often have opposing effects on organ function. Activation of the

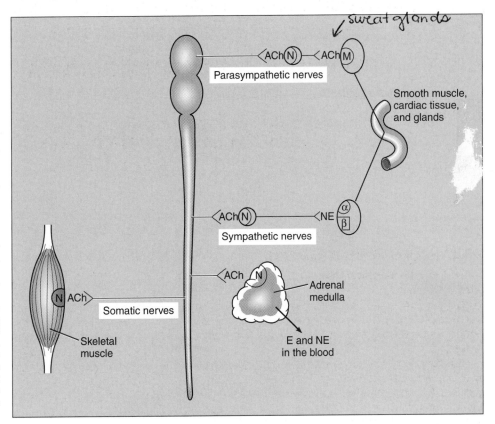

FIGURE 5–1. Neurotransmission in the autonomic and somatic nervous systems. The parasympathetic nervous system consists of cranial and sacral nerves with long preganglionic and short postganglionic fibers. The sympathetic nervous system consists of thoracic and lumbar nerves with short preganglionic and long postganglionic fibers. The sympathetic system includes the adrenal medulla, which releases catecholamines into the blood. The somatic nervous system consists of motor neurons to the skeletal muscle. ACh = acetylcholine; E = epinephrine; NE = norepinephrine; M = muscarinic receptors; N = nicotinic receptors; α = α-adrenergic receptors; and β = β-adrenergic receptors.

sympathetic system produces the **"fight or flight" response,** which enables a person to respond to threatening situations. During this response, cardiovascular stimulation provides skeletal muscles with the oxygen and energy substrates required to support vigorous physical activity. Increases in glycogenolysis and lipolysis also help provide the required energy fuels. The parasympathetic system is sometimes called the **"rest and digest" system,** because it slows the heart rate and promotes more vegetative functions, such as digestion, defecation, and micturition. Many parasympathetic effects (including pupillary constriction, bronchoconstriction, and stimulation of gut and bladder motility) are caused by smooth muscle contraction.

Somatic Nervous System

The somatic nervous system consists of the motor neurons to the skeletal muscle. These neurons are comprised of a single nerve fiber that releases acetylcholine at the neuromuscular junction.

Enteric Nervous System

The enteric nervous system (ENS) is sometimes called the third division of the autonomic nervous system. The ENS consists of a network of autonomic nerves that are located in the gut wall and regulate gastrointestinal motility and secretion. The ENS includes the submucosal, myenteric, and subserosal plexuses and receives innervation from the sympathetic and parasympathetic nervous systems. The ENS has afferent fibers and efferent fibers, and it integrates input received from autonomic nerves with localized reflexes, so as to synchronize the waves of peristalsis (the propulsive contractions of gut muscle). Parasympathetic stimulation activates the ENS, whereas sympathetic stimulation inhibits the ENS. The ENS can function independently of autonomic innervation following autonomic denervation.

NEUROTRANSMITTERS AND RECEPTORS
Neurotransmitters

The primary neurotransmitters found in the autonomic and somatic nervous systems are **acetylcholine** and **norepinephrine** (see Fig. 5–1). Acetylcholine is the transmitter at all autonomic ganglia, at parasympathetic neuroeffector junctions, and at somatic neuromuscular junctions. It is also the transmitter at a few sympathetic neuroeffector junctions, including the junctions of nerves in sweat glands and vasodilator fibers in skeletal muscle. The presence of acetylcholine in several types of autonomic and somatic synapses contributes to the lack of specificity of drugs acting on cholinergic neurotransmission.

Although norepinephrine is the primary neurotransmitter at most sympathetic postganglionic neuroeffector junctions, **epinephrine** is the principal catecholamine released from the adrenal medulla in

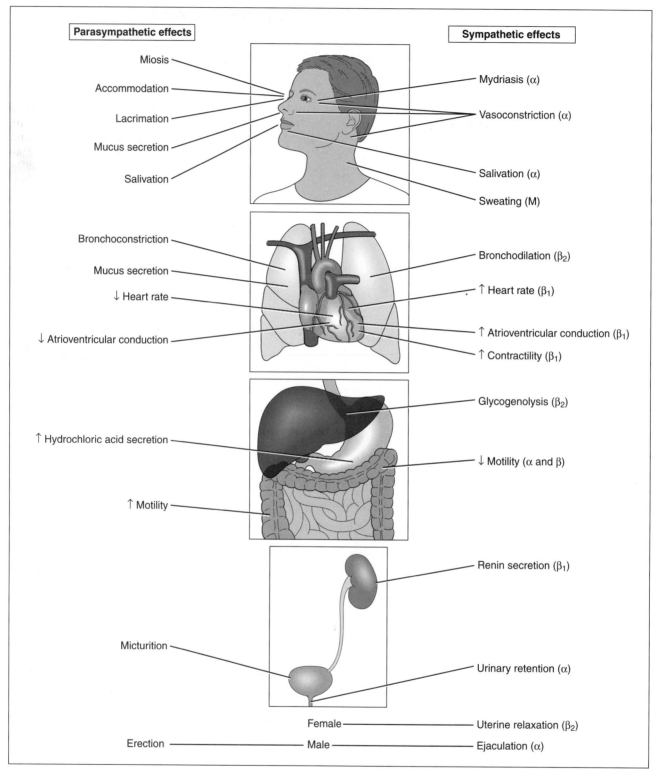

Parasympathetic effects

Miosis
Accommodation
Lacrimation
Mucus secretion
Salivation

Bronchoconstriction
Mucus secretion
↓ Heart rate
↓ Atrioventricular conduction

↑ Hydrochloric acid secretion

↑ Motility

Micturition

Erection ——————————— Male

Sympathetic effects

Mydriasis (α)
Vasoconstriction (α)
Salivation (α)
Sweating (M)

Bronchodilation (β_2)
↑ Heart rate (β_1)
↑ Atrioventricular conduction (β_1)
↑ Contractility (β_1)

Glycogenolysis (β_2)

↓ Motility (α and β)

Renin secretion (β_1)

Urinary retention (α)

Female ——————— Uterine relaxation (β_2)
Ejaculation (α)

FIGURE 5–2. Autonomic nervous system effects on organs. All parasympathetic effects are mediated by muscarinic receptors. Sympathetic effects are mediated by α-adrenergic receptors (α), β-adrenergic receptors (β), or ~~muscarinic~~ *nicotinic* receptors (~~M~~ N).

response to activation of the sympathetic nervous system.

A number of other neurotransmitters have been identified in autonomic nerves called nonadrenergic-noncholinergic (NANC) neurons. These neurons are primarily found in the ENS of the gastrointestinal tract, as well as in the genitourinary tract and certain blood vessels. The transmitters released by NANC neurons include **neuropeptide Y, vasoactive intestinal polypeptide** (VIP), **enkephalin, substance P, serotonin** (5-hydroxytryptamine), **adenosine triphosphate** (ATP), and **nitric oxide.** In some tissues, ATP released by so-called purinergic nerves is converted to **adenosine,** which may then activate adenosine receptors in a number of tissues (see Chapter 27). Nitric oxide is an important NANC neurotransmitter that produces vasodilation in many vascular beds and is also found in the ENS.

Receptors for Acetylcholine, Norepinephrine, and Epinephrine

The receptors for acetylcholine are called **cholinergic receptors** and have been divided into two types, based on their selective activation by one of two plant alkaloids. **Muscarinic receptors** are cholinergic receptors that are activated by muscarine and are primarily located at parasympathetic neuroeffector junctions. **Nicotinic receptors** are cholinergic receptors that are activated by nicotine and are found in all autonomic ganglia and at somatic neuromuscular junctions. When they are activated, muscarinic receptors mediate smooth muscle contraction (except sphincter contraction), cardiac slowing, and gland secretion. Activation of nicotinic receptors in autonomic ganglia excites neurotransmission, whereas activation of these receptors in skeletal muscle mediates muscle contraction.

The receptors for norepinephrine and epinephrine at sympathetic neuroeffector junctions are called **adrenergic receptors.** The term *adrenergic* is derived from adrenaline, another name for epinephrine. There are two types of adrenergic receptors, called α-**adrenergic receptors** and β-**adrenergic receptors,** and these are distinguished on the basis of their selective activation and blockade by adrenergic agonists and antagonists. The α-adrenergic receptors mediate smooth muscle contraction, whereas the β-adrenergic receptors mediate smooth muscle relaxation and cardiac stimulation. As discussed in Chapters 8 and 10, investigators have recently attributed some of the effects of α-adrenergic receptor agonists to activation of a new type of receptor called the **imidazoline receptor.**

NEUROTRANSMISSION AND SITES OF DRUG ACTION

Cholinergic and adrenergic neurotransmission have many basic similarities. In both cases, the neurotransmitter is synthesized in nerve terminals, stored in membrane-bound vesicles, and released into the synapse in response to nerve stimulation. After the neurotransmitter activates postjunctional receptors to initiate a physiologic effect, neurotransmitter action is terminated either by metabolism or neuronal reuptake. Various cholinergic and adrenergic drugs exert their effects at specific steps in the process.

Examples and sites of action for drugs that affect cholinergic and adrenergic neurotransmission are shown in Fig. 5–3, and the mechanisms of action are listed in Table 5–1.

Cholinergic Neurotransmission

Acetylcholine is synthesized from choline and acetate in the neuronal cytoplasm by choline acetyltransferase, and then it is stored in vesicles. When a cholinergic nerve is stimulated, the action potential induces calcium influx into the neuron, and calcium mediates release of the neurotransmitter by a process called exocytosis. During exocytosis, the vesicle membrane and plasma membrane fuse, and the neurotransmitter is released into the synapse through an opening in the fused membranes. After acetylcholine activates postsynaptic cholinergic receptors, it is rapidly hydrolyzed by the enzyme cholinesterase to form choline and acetate. Choline is recycled through the process of reuptake by the presynaptic neuron. This process is mediated by a membrane protein that transports choline into the neuron. Acetylcholine may also activate presynaptic autoreceptors, and this inhibits further release of the neurotransmitter by the neuron.

Drugs Affecting Cholinergic Neurotransmission

Fig. 5–3A shows the sites of various agents that affect cholinergic neurotransmission.

Hemicholinium blocks choline transport into the neuron and thereby inhibits the synthesis of acetylcholine, whereas **vesamicol** prevents the vesicular storage of acetylcholine. Neither of these drugs has any current medical use.

Several toxins affect the release of acetylcholine. One example, **black widow spider venom,** has been found to stimulate the release of acetylcholine. Another example, **botulinum toxin,** is produced by *Clostridium botulinum* and has been used to treat localized spasms of the ocular and facial muscles. In this application, botulinum toxin is injected directly into the muscle, where it blocks the exocytotic release of acetylcholine and inhibits neuromuscular transmission.

After acetylcholine is released, it may activate postsynaptic muscarinic or nicotinic receptors. Many drugs, including choline esters such as **bethanechol** and plant alkaloids such as **pilocarpine,** mimic the effect of acetylcholine at these same receptors. These drugs are called **direct-acting cholinergic receptor agonists** because they directly bind and activate cholinergic receptors.

Another group of drugs, the **cholinesterase inhibitors,** prevent the breakdown of acetylcholine and thereby increase the synaptic concentration of acetylcholine. Because this action leads to an increase in the activation of cholinergic receptors by acetylcholine, these drugs are called **indirect-acting cholinergic receptor agonists** (see Chapter 6).

The most important group of drugs that inhibit cholinergic neurotransmission consists of **cholinergic receptor antagonists.** The group is divided into two subgroups. The first consists of **muscarinic receptor antagonists** and includes drugs such as atropine, while the second consists of **nicotinic receptor antagonists** and includes **ganglionic blocking agents**

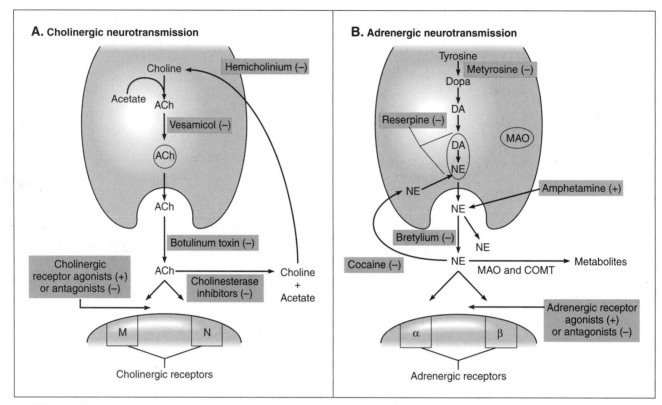

FIGURE 5–3. **Cholinergic and adrenergic neurotransmission and sites of drug action.** **(A)** Acetylcholine (ACh) is synthesized from choline and acetate, stored in neuronal vesicles, and released into the synapse by nerve stimulation. Hemicholinium blocks choline uptake by the neuron and inhibits ACh synthesis. Vesamicol blocks ACh storage, and botulinum toxin blocks ACh release. ACh breakdown is inhibited by cholinesterase inhibitors. Postjunctional cholinergic receptors are activated or blocked by cholinergic receptor agonists or antagonists, respectively. **(B)** Norepinephrine (NE) is synthesized from tyrosine in a three-step reaction: tyrosine to dopa (dihydroxyphenylalanine), dopa to dopamine (DA), and dopamine to NE. The conversion of tyrosine to dopa is inhibited by metyrosine. The vesicular storage of DA and NE is blocked by reserpine, and the release of NE in response to nerve stimulation is blocked by bretylium. After activating postsynaptic receptors, NE is sequestered by neuronal reuptake, a process blocked by cocaine. Amphetamine increases the release of NE into the synapse. Postsynaptic adrenergic receptors are activated or blocked by adrenergic receptor agonists or antagonists, respectively. M = muscarinic receptors; N = nicotinic receptors; α = α-adrenergic receptors; β = β-adrenergic receptors; MAO = monoamine oxidase; COMT = catechol-*O*-methyltransferase; (−) = inhibits; and (+) = stimulates.

(such as trimethaphan) and **neuromuscular blocking drugs** (such as tubocurarine).

Adrenergic Neurotransmission

Norepinephrine is synthesized via the following steps: tyrosine → dopa → dopamine → norepinephrine.

First, the amino acid tyrosine is converted to dopa (dihydroxyphenylalanine) by tyrosine hydroxylase, the rate-limiting enzyme in the pathway. Dopa is then converted to dopamine by L-aromatic amino acid decarboxylase (dopa decarboxylase). At this point, dopamine is accumulated by neuronal storage vesicles. Inside the vesicles, dopamine is converted to norepinephrine by dopamine-β-hydroxylase.

TABLE 5–1. Examples of Drugs Affecting Autonomic Neurotransmission

Mechanism of Action	Drugs Affecting Cholinergic Neurotransmission	Drugs Affecting Adrenergic Neurotransmission
Inhibit synthesis of neurotransmitter	Hemicholinium.*	Metyrosine.
Prevent vesicular storage of neurotransmitter	Vesamicol.*	Reserpine.
Inhibit release of neurotransmitter	Botulinum toxin.	Bretylium and guanethidine.
Stimulate release of neurotransmitter	Black widow spider venom.*	Amphetamine.
Inhibit reuptake of neurotransmitter	—	Antidepressants and cocaine.
Inhibit metabolism of neurotransmitter	Cholinesterase inhibitors.	Monoamine oxidase inhibitors.
Activate postsynaptic receptors	Acetylcholine, bethanechol, and pilocarpine.	Albuterol, dobutamine, and epinephrine.
Block postsynaptic receptors	Atropine and tubocurarine (block muscarinic and nicotinic receptors, respectively).	Phentolamine and propranolol (block α-adrenergic and β-adrenergic receptors, respectively).

*These agents have no current medical use.

Like acetylcholine, norepinephrine is released into the synapse by calcium-mediated exocytosis in response to nerve stimulation. Once in the synapse, norepinephrine activates postjunctional α-adrenergic and β-adrenergic receptors. It also activates prejunctional autoreceptors that exert negative feedback and inhibit norepinephrine release.

Norepinephrine is removed from the synapse primarily by neuronal reuptake via a transport protein located in the presynaptic neuronal membrane. Once inside the neuron, norepinephrine is sequestered in storage vesicles. It is recycled by adrenergic neurons in a manner similar to that used by cholinergic neurons to recycle choline.

The enzymes catechol-*O*-methyltransferase (COMT) and monoamine oxidase (MAO) primarily serve to inactivate norepinephrine that is not sequestered by presynaptic neurons. These enzymes are found in many tissues, including the liver and gut. MAO is also located inside neuronal mitochondria and degrades cytoplasmic norepinephrine that is not accumulated by storage vesicles.

BOX 5–1. The Use of Direct-Acting and Indirect-Acting Adrenergic Receptor Agonists in the Diagnosis of Horner's Syndrome

Case Introduction: L. B., a 26-year-old woman, recently sustained injuries that required physical therapy and the use of analgesics and a nonsteroidal anti-inflammatory drug to alleviate pain and reduce immobility in her left shoulder and neck. Today, she returned to the clinic because her left eye is sore, her left eyelid is drooping, and she noticed during exercise that she did not sweat on the left side of her forehead. A physical examination reveals conjunctival hyperemia and ptosis of the left eyelid. The patient's left pupil is 2 mm in diameter and does not dilate when she is placed in a dark room. Her right pupil is 3 mm in diameter and dilates normally in the dark. Ophthalmologic testing is scheduled.

In this case, the physician suspects Horner's syndrome, a disorder caused by damage to the sympathetic innervation of the head, usually secondary to unilateral cervical trauma or the presence of a tumor. Whether the lesion is in a preganglionic or postganglionic site can be determined by testing with drugs that mimic sympathetic nervous system stimulation of the pupil dilator muscle in the iris.

Case Continuation: L. B. reports for ophthalmologic testing of her pupillary response to topical ocular administration of a direct-acting adrenergic receptor agonist (phenylephrine) and an indirect-acting adrenergic receptor agonist (hydroxyamphetamine). Her right pupil dilates normally in response to administration of either drug. Her left pupil is unresponsive to hydroxyamphetamine, but it dilates maximally after administration of a low concentration of phenylephrine.

Drugs may either directly or indirectly activate adrenergic receptors in tissues innervated by the sympathetic nervous system. Direct-acting agonists activate postjunctional receptors. Indirect-acting agonists increase the concentration of norepinephrine in the synapse, either by increasing norepinephrine release (as occurs with amphetamine) or by blocking norepinephrine reuptake (as occurs with cocaine). Indirect-acting agonists require the presence of a functional postganglionic neuron to produce their effects. In Horner's syndrome, the manner in which the pupils respond to direct-acting and indirect-acting adrenergic receptor agonists can help determine the site of the lesion:

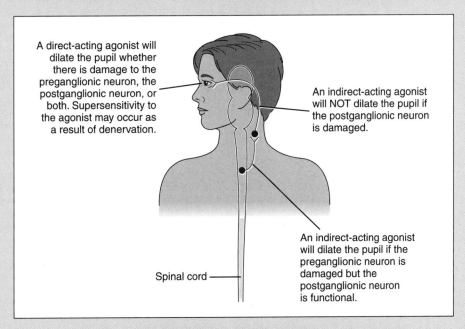

A direct-acting agonist will dilate the pupil whether there is damage to the preganglionic neuron, the postganglionic neuron, or both. Supersensitivity to the agonist may occur as a result of denervation.

An indirect-acting agonist will NOT dilate the pupil if the postganglionic neuron is damaged.

An indirect-acting agonist will dilate the pupil if the preganglionic neuron is damaged but the postganglionic neuron is functional.

Spinal cord

Case Conclusion: Based on the results of testing with phenylephrine and hydroxyamphetamine, the physician concludes that the patient's injury affected the postganglionic sympathetic innervation of the eye, and appropriate treatment is instituted.

Drugs Affecting Adrenergic Neurotransmission

Fig. 5–3B shows the sites of various agents that affect adrenergic neurotransmission.

The synthesis of norepinephrine is inhibited by **metyrosine,** a drug that is a competitive inhibitor of tyrosine hydroxylase. The storage of norepinephrine in neuronal vesicles is blocked by **reserpine,** a drug that inhibits the transporter for amines located in the vesicular membrane. The release of norepinephrine in response to nerve stimulation is inhibited by **bretylium** and **guanethidine.** As discussed in Chapters 10 and 14, these and other drugs that inhibit the synthesis, storage, or release of norepinephrine are called **neuronal blocking agents.**

Some endogenous substances and synthetic compounds directly activate α-adrenergic or β-adrenergic receptors and are therefore called **direct-acting adrenergic receptor agonists.** Examples include **albuterol, dobutamine,** and **epinephrine.** Other drugs indirectly increase the activation of adrenergic receptors, either by increasing norepinephrine release or by blocking norepinephrine reuptake and thereby increasing the synaptic concentration of the neurotransmitter. These drugs are called **indirect-acting adrenergic receptor agonists,** and examples include **amphetamine** and **cocaine.** As described in Box 5–1, indirect-acting agonists require the presence of a functional postganglionic neuron to exert their effects.

Another group of drugs act by inhibiting the breakdown of norepinephrine by COMT or MAO. As discussed in Chapters 21 and 22, these **catechol-*O*-methyltransferase inhibitors** and **monoamine oxidase inhibitors** primarily exert their effects on the central nervous system.

Drugs that inhibit sympathetic stimulation of target organs include the neuronal blocking agents (described above) and the **adrenergic receptor antagonists.** Examples of the latter are **phentolamine,** which selectively blocks α-adrenergic receptors; **propranolol,** which selectively blocks β-adrenergic receptors; and **labetalol,** which blocks both receptor types.

Drugs Modulating the Baroreceptor Reflex

In addition to exerting their primary pharmacologic actions, a number of adrenergic receptor agonists and antagonists modulate the baroreceptor reflex (Fig. 5–4).

When a drug or a physiologic action increases blood pressure, this activates stretch receptors (mechanoreceptors) located in the aortic arch and in the carotid sinus at the bifurcation of the carotid artery. Receptor activation initiates impulses that travel via afferent nerves to the brain stem vasomotor center. Stimulation of the vagal motor nucleus (via nerves from the solitary tract nucleus) leads to an increase in vagal (parasympathetic) outflow, a decrease in heart rate, and a decrease in the sympathetic nerve outflow from the vasomotor center. The effect on the heart rate is called **reflex bradycardia.**

If a drug lowers the blood pressure sufficiently, it may reduce the baroreceptor tone and thereby produce an acceleration of the heart rate and activation of sympathetic vasoconstriction. In this case, the effect on the heart rate is called **reflex tachycardia.**

Summary of Important Points

- The sympathetic and parasympathetic divisions of the autonomic nervous system have opposing effects in many tissues. Drugs that activate one

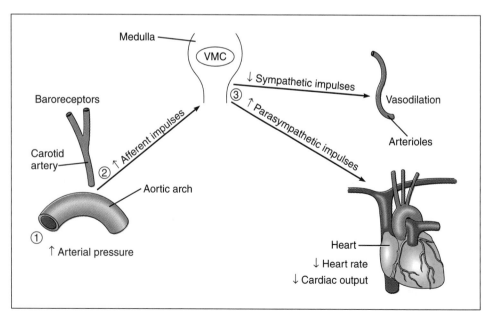

FIGURE 5–4. The baroreceptor reflex. (1) Increased arterial pressure activates stretch receptors in the aortic arch and carotid sinus. (2) Receptor activation initiates afferent impulses to the brain stem vasomotor center (VMC). (3) Via solitary tract fibers, the VMC activates the vagal motor nucleus, which increases vagal (parasympathetic) outflow and slows the heart. At the same time, the VMC reduces stimulation of spinal intermediolateral neurons that activate sympathetic preganglionic fibers, and this decreases sympathetic stimulation of the heart and blood vessels. By this mechanism, drugs that increase blood pressure produce reflex bradycardia. Drugs that reduce blood pressure attenuate this response and cause reflex tachycardia.

division often have the same effects as drugs that inhibit the other division.

- Acetylcholine is the primary neurotransmitter at parasympathetic and somatic neuroeffector junctions, and norepinephrine is the transmitter at most sympathetic junctions. In the autonomic nervous system, there are a number of nonadrenergic-noncholinergic neurotransmitters, including peptides, nitric oxide, and serotonin.
- Most autonomic drugs activate or block receptors for acetylcholine or norepinephrine in smooth muscle, cardiac tissue, and glands. Activation of muscarinic and α-adrenergic receptors produces smooth muscle contraction, whereas activation of β-adrenergic receptors produces smooth muscle relaxation and mediates cardiac stimulation.
- Some drugs have effects on neurotransmitter synthesis, storage, release, or metabolism. These are called indirect-acting drugs.
- Indirect-acting agonists increase the concentration of a neurotransmitter at synapses, either by inhibiting transmitter inactivation (cholinesterase inhibitors), increasing transmitter release (amphetamine and tyramine), or blocking transmitter reuptake (cocaine).
- Indirect-acting agonists require the presence of a functional postganglionic neuron to exert their effects.

Selected Readings

Boeckxstaens, G. E., and P. A. Pelckmans. Nitric oxide and the nonadrenergic noncholinergic neurotransmission. Comp Biochem Physiol Physiol 118:925–937, 1997.

Bousquet, P. Commentary: imidazoline receptors. Neurochem Int 30:3–7, 1997.

Chapple, C., and R. Chess-Williams. Latest developments in the field of neurotransmitters. Eur Urol 34(supplement 1):45–47, 1998.

Goldstein, D. S. Catecholamine receptors and signal transduction: overview. Adv Pharmacol 42:379–390, 1998.

Langer, S. Z., Twenty-five years since the discovery of presynaptic receptors: present knowledge and future perspectives. Trends Pharmacol Sci 18:95–99, 1997.

Sleight, P. The importance of the autonomic nervous system in health and disease. Aust N Z J Med 27:467–473, 1997.

Vanhatalo, S., and S. Soinila. The concept of chemical neurotransmission: variations on the theme. Ann Med 30:151–158, 1998.

CHAPTER SIX

CHOLINERGIC RECEPTOR AGONISTS

CLASSIFICATION OF CHOLINERGIC RECEPTOR AGONISTS

DIRECT-ACTING CHOLINERGIC RECEPTOR AGONISTS
  Choline esters
  - Acetylcholine
  - Bethanechol
  - Carbachol

  Plant alkaloids
  - Muscarine
  - Nicotine
  - Pilocarpine

INDIRECT-ACTING CHOLINERGIC RECEPTOR AGONISTS
  Drugs that inhibit cholinesterase
  Reversible cholinesterase inhibitors
  - Donepezil
  - Edrophonium
  - Neostigmine
  - Physostigmine
  - Pyridostigmine
  - Tacrine

  Irreversible cholinesterase inhibitors
  - Echothiophate
  - Isoflurophate
  - Malathion

  Drugs that increase acetylcholine release
  - Cisapride
  - Metoclopramide

OTHER CHOLINERGIC RECEPTOR AGONISTS
  - Sildenafil

OVERVIEW OF CHOLINERGIC PHARMACOLOGY

Cholinergic Receptors

Cholinergic receptors (cholinoceptors) are divided into two types, **muscarinic receptors** and **nicotinic receptors,** based on their selective activation by the alkaloids muscarine and nicotine.

Muscarinic Receptors

Muscarinic receptors are found in smooth muscle, cardiac tissue, and glands at parasympathetic neuroeffector junctions. They are also found in the central nervous system, on presynaptic sympathetic and parasympathetic nerves, and at autonomic ganglia. Activation of muscarinic receptors on presynap-tic autonomic nerves inhibits further neurotransmitter release. The presence of muscarinic receptors on sympathetic nerve terminals provides for interaction between the parasympathetic and sympathetic nervous systems: the release of acetylcholine from parasympathetic nerves inhibits the release of norepinephrine from sympathetic nerves.

Muscarinic receptors are divided into five subtypes, M_1 through M_5, based on their selective activation or inhibition by experimental compounds and on their selective binding by radioactive compounds. The principal subtypes found in most tissues are M_1, M_2, and M_3 receptors (Table 6–1).

The cholinergic receptor agonists that are currently available for clinical use do not selectively activate subtypes of muscarinic receptors, but an M_1 selective antagonist, pirenzepine, has been developed (see Chapter 7).

Nicotinic Receptors

Nicotinic receptors are found at all autonomic ganglia, at somatic neuromuscular junctions, and in the central nervous system. At autonomic ganglia, activation of nicotinic receptors produces neuronal excitation leading to the release of neurotransmitters at postganglionic neuroeffector junctions. At junctions of skeletal muscle and nerves, activation of nicotinic receptors depolarizes the motor end plate and leads to the release of calcium from the sarcoplasmic reticulum and to the contraction of muscles.

Signal Transduction

Muscarinic receptor stimulation leads to the activation of guanine nucleotide–binding proteins (G proteins), which increase or decrease the formation of other second messengers (see Chapter 3). Activation of M_1 and M_3 receptors stimulates the formation of inositol triphosphate (IP_3) and diacylglycerol (DAG) in most smooth muscles, whereas activation of M_2 receptors increases potassium efflux or decreases cyclic adenosine monophosphate (cyclic AMP, or cAMP).

In the circulation, activation of M_3 receptors in vascular endothelial cells stimulates the conversion of arginine to nitric oxide, a reaction catalyzed by nitric oxide synthase. Nitric oxide then diffuses to vascular smooth muscle cells, where it stimulates G protein–coupled receptors that activate guanylyl

TABLE 6-1. Properties of Cholinergic Receptors

Type of Receptor	Principal Locations	Mechanism of Signal Transduction	Effects
Muscarinic			
M_1 ("neural")	Autonomic ganglia, presynaptic nerve terminals, and central nervous system.	Increased inositol triphosphate (IP_3) and diacylglycerol (DAG).	Modulation of neurotransmission.
M_2 ("cardiac")	Cardiac tissue (sinoatrial and atrioventricular nodes).	Increased potassium efflux or decreased cyclic adenosine monophosphate (cAMP).	Slowing of heart rate and conduction.
M_3 ("glandular")	Smooth muscle and glands.	Increased IP_3 and DAG.	Contraction of smooth muscles and stimulation of glandular secretions.
	Vascular smooth muscle.	Increased cyclic guanosine monophosphate (cGMP) due to nitric oxide stimulation.	Vasodilation.
Nicotinic			
N_M (in muscles)	Somatic neuromuscular junctions.	Increased sodium influx.	Contraction of muscles.
N_N (in neurons)	Autonomic ganglia.	Increased sodium influx.	Excitation of postganglionic neurons.

cyclase and increase the formation of cyclic guanosine monophosphate (cyclic GMP, or cGMP). Cyclic GMP causes smooth muscle relaxation, which in turn leads to vasodilation. This mechanism is responsible for stimulation of penile erection by sacral parasympathetic nerves.

Nicotinic receptors are ligand-gated sodium channels whose activation leads to sodium influx, membrane depolarization, and excitation of autonomic postganglionic neurons and skeletal muscle.

Classification of Cholinergic Receptor Agonists

The cholinergic receptor agonists can be classified as direct-acting or indirect-acting. The **direct-acting agonists** bind and activate cholinergic receptors, whereas the **indirect-acting agonists** increase the synaptic concentration of acetylcholine. Although most of the indirect-acting agents inhibit cholinesterase and the breakdown of acetylcholine, some of them increase the release of acetylcholine from nerve terminals.

DIRECT-ACTING CHOLINERGIC RECEPTOR AGONISTS

The direct-acting agonists include the **choline esters** and the **plant alkaloids.** These drugs all bind and activate cholinergic receptors, but they differ with respect to their affinity for muscarinic and nicotinic receptors and their susceptibility to hydrolysis by cholinesterase (Table 6–2).

Choline Esters

The choline esters include acetylcholine and synthetic acetylcholine analogues, such as bethanechol and carbachol. Their structures are shown in Fig. 6–1A.

Drug Properties

The choline esters are positively charged quaternary ammonium compounds that are poorly absorbed from the gastrointestinal tract and are not distributed to the central nervous system. Acetylcholine and carbachol activate both muscarinic and nicotinic receptors, whereas bethanechol activates only muscarinic receptors. Because of their lack of specificity for muscarinic receptor subtypes, the muscarinic receptor agonists cause a wide range of effects on many organ systems.

Ocular Effects. Muscarinic receptor agonists increase lacrimal gland secretion and stimulate contraction of the iris sphincter muscle and the ciliary muscles. Contraction of the iris sphincter muscle produces pupillary constriction (miosis), whereas contraction of the ciliary muscles enables accommodation of the lens to focus on close objects (Fig. 6–2).

Respiratory Tract Effects. Stimulation of muscarinic receptors increases bronchial muscle contraction and causes an increase in the secretion of mucus throughout the respiratory tract. Because muscarinic receptor agonists may cause bronchoconstriction, they should be avoided or used with extreme caution in patients with asthma and other forms of obstructive lung disease.

Cardiac Effects. Muscarinic receptor agonists decrease impulse formation in the sinoatrial node by reducing the rate of diastolic depolarization. As a result, they slow the heart rate. In addition, they slow conduction of the cardiac action potential through the atrioventricular node, and this leads to an increased PR interval on the electrocardiogram.

Gastrointestinal and Urinary Tract Effects. When muscarinic receptor agonists are taken, they stimulate salivary, gastric, and other secretions in the gastrointestinal tract. They also increase contraction of gastrointestinal smooth muscle (except sphincters) by stimulating the enteric nervous system located in the gut wall. This, in turn, increases

TABLE 6–2. Properties and Clinical Uses of Direct-Acting Cholinergic Receptor Agonists

Drug	Receptor Specificity	Hydrolyzed by Cholinesterase	Route of Administration	Clinical Use
Choline esters				
Acetylcholine	Muscarinic and nicotinic.	Yes.	Intraocular.	Miosis during ophthalmic surgery.
			Intracoronary.	Coronary angiography.
Bethanechol	Muscarinic.	No.	Oral or subcutaneous.	Postoperative or postpartum urinary retention.
Carbachol	Muscarinic and nicotinic.	No.	Topical ocular.	Glaucoma.
			Intraocular.	Miosis during ophthalmic surgery.
Plant alkaloids				
Muscarine	Muscarinic.	No.	None.	None.
Nicotine	Nicotinic.	No.	Oral or transdermal.	Smoking cessation programs.
Pilocarpine	Greater affinity for muscarinic than for nicotinic.	No.	Topical ocular.	Glaucoma.
			Oral.	Xerostomia.

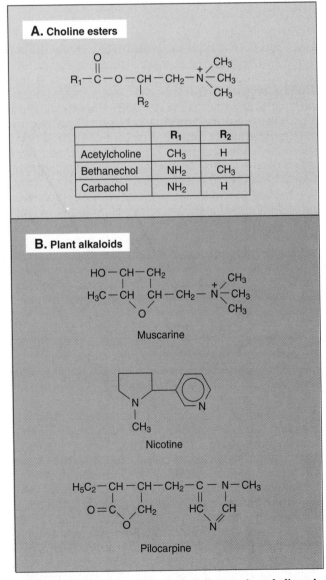

FIGURE 6–1. Structures of selected direct-acting cholinergic receptor agonists. (A) The choline esters include acetylcholine, bethanechol, and carbachol. **(B)** The plant alkaloids include muscarine, nicotine, and pilocarpine.

gastrointestinal motility. While muscarinic receptor agonists stimulate the bladder detrusor muscle, they relax the internal sphincter of the bladder, and these effects promote emptying of the bladder (micturition). High or toxic doses of these agonists can therefore produce excessive salivation and cause diarrhea, intestinal cramps, and urinary incontinence.

Acetylcholine

Chemistry and Pharmacokinetics. Acetylcholine is the choline ester of acetic acid. It is rapidly hydrolyzed by cholinesterase and has an extremely short duration of action.

Effects and Indications. Because of its limited absorption, short duration of action, and lack of specificity for muscarinic or nicotinic receptors, acetylcholine has limited clinical applications.

An ophthalmic solution of acetylcholine is available for intraocular use during **cataract surgery** and produces miosis after extraction of the lens. The solution also can be used in other types of **ophthalmic surgery** that require rapid and complete miosis. Topical ocular administration of acetylcholine is not effective, because acetylcholine is hydrolyzed by corneal cholinesterase before it can penetrate to the iris and ciliary muscle.

In patients undergoing **diagnostic coronary angiography,** acetylcholine can be administered by direct intracoronary injection to produce coronary vasodilation or to provoke coronary artery spasm. The **vasodilative effect** of acetylcholine is mediated by M_3 receptors located in vascular endothelial cells, where muscarinic stimulation causes the calcium-mediated activation of nitric oxide synthetase and the conversion of L-arginine to citrulline and nitric oxide. Nitric oxide is a gas that diffuses into vascular smooth muscle cells and activates guanylyl cyclase so as to increase cyclic GMP formation. Cyclic GMP then inactivates myosin light-chain kinase, leading to vascular smooth muscle relaxation and vasodilation.

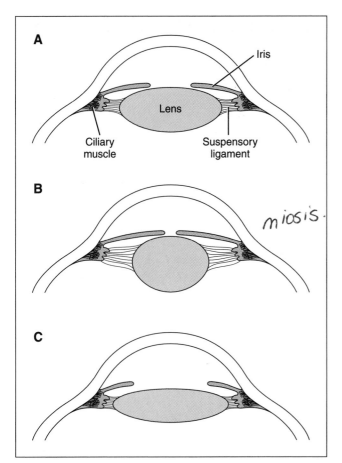

m iosis .

FIGURE 6–2. Effects of pilocarpine and atropine on the eye. (A) The relationship between the iris sphincter and ciliary muscle is shown in the normal eye. **(B)** When pilocarpine, a muscarinic receptor agonist, is administered, contraction of the iris sphincter produces pupillary constriction (miosis). Contraction of the ciliary muscle causes the muscle to be displaced centrally. This relaxes the suspensory ligaments connected to the lens, and the internal elasticity of the lens allows it to increase in thickness. As the lens thickens, its refractive power increases so that it focuses on close objects. **(C)** When atropine, a muscarinic receptor antagonist, is administered, the iris sphincter and ciliary muscles relax. This produces pupillary dilatation (mydriasis) and increases the tension on the suspensory ligaments so that the lens becomes thinner and focuses on distant objects.

The **vasospastic effect** of acetylcholine is apparently due to stimulation of muscarinic receptors that are located on vascular smooth muscle and mediate smooth muscle contraction. In most situations, the vasodilative effect of acetylcholine is more pronounced than the vasoconstrictive effect. However, in patients with vasospastic angina pectoris, intracoronary injection of acetylcholine can provoke a localized vasoconstrictive response, and this helps establish the diagnosis of vasospastic angina.

Bethanechol and Carbachol

Chemistry and Pharmacokinetics. Bethanechol and carbachol are choline esters of carbamic acid. They are resistant to hydrolysis by cholinesterase, and their duration of action is relatively short, lasting for several hours after topical ocular or systemic administration.

Effects and Indications. Because bethanechol activates muscarinic but not nicotinic receptors, it can be used to stimulate bladder or gastrointestinal muscle without significantly affecting the heart rate or blood pressure. Bethanechol is given postoperatively or postpartum to increase bladder muscle tone in patients who suffer from **urinary retention** after receiving anesthetics or other drugs administered during surgery or childbirth. Therapeutic doses of bethanechol given orally or subcutaneously have little effect on blood pressure, but the drug should never be administered intravenously, because this may cause hypotension and bradycardia.

Carbachol is effective in the treatment of **chronic open-angle glaucoma,** but it is usually used in cases in which a patient does not respond adequately to pilocarpine (see below). Carbachol may also be used to produce miosis during **ophthalmic surgery.**

Plant Alkaloids

The plant alkaloids include muscarine, nicotine, and pilocarpine. Their structures are shown in Fig. 6–1B.

Muscarine and Nicotine

Chemistry and Effects. Muscarine is found in mushrooms of the genera *Inocybe* and *Clitocybe,* and the consumption of these poisonous mushrooms may cause diarrhea, sweating, salivation, and lacrimation. Muscarine is also found in trace amounts in *Amanita muscaria,* the original source of muscarine, but the toxicity of this mushroom is largely due to its content of ibotenic acid. Nicotine is derived from *Nicotiana* plants and is contained in cigarettes and other tobacco products. The effects of nicotine dependence are discussed in Chapter 24.

Indications. Muscarine has no current medical use. Nicotine is available in chewing gum, transdermal patches, and other products designed for use in **smoking cessation programs.**

Pilocarpine

Chemistry and Pharmacokinetics. Pilocarpine is a tertiary amine alkaloid that is obtained from *Pilocarpus,* a small shrub. The drug is well absorbed after topical ocular and oral administration.

Effects and Indications. Pilocarpine has greater affinity for muscarinic receptors than for nicotinic receptors and can produce all of the effects of muscarinic receptor stimulation described above.

Pilocarpine is primarily used for the treatment of **chronic open-angle glaucoma,** in which it lowers intraocular pressure by increasing the outflow of aqueous humor (Box 6–1). It is also used in the treatment of **acute angle-closure glaucoma,** a medical emergency in which blindness may result if the intraocular pressure is not lowered immediately. The main side effects of ocular pilocarpine administration are decreased night vision, which is due to miosis, and difficulty in focusing on distant objects, which

---

BOX 6–1. Treatment of Chronic Open-Angle Glaucoma

In the normal eye, aqueous humor is secreted by the ciliary processes and flows through the pupillary aperture of the iris and into the anterior chamber. It then drains through the trabecular meshwork in Schlemm's canal. In patients with open-angle glaucoma, persistently elevated intraocular pressure is associated with narrowing of the anterior chamber angle, a decrease in the rate of aqueous outflow, and the gradual loss of peripheral vision. Various types of drugs can be used to reduce intraocular pressure before irreversible optic nerve damage occurs. The sites of action of these drugs are shown below.

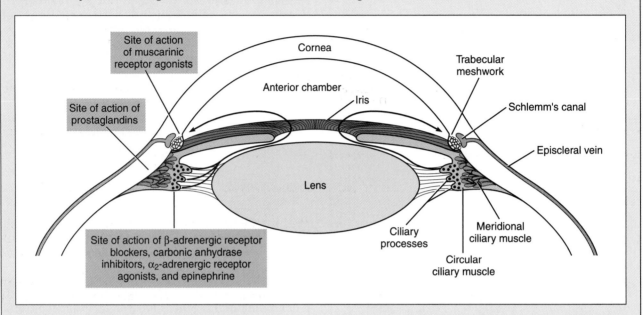

Some types of drugs act by enhancing the drainage of aqueous humor. **Muscarinic receptor agonists,** such as **pilocarpine,** stimulate the contraction of meridional ciliary muscle fibers that insert near the trabecular meshwork. Contraction of these fibers opens the trabecular spaces so that aqueous humor drains more easily. **Prostaglandins,** such as **latanoprost,** increase aqueous drainage through an alternative pathway known as the uveoscleral route. In this pathway, aqueous humor flows through the ciliary muscles into the suprachoroidal space.

Other types of drugs act by reducing the amount of aqueous humor produced by the ciliary processes. The **β-adrenergic receptor blockers,** such as **timolol,** limit the formation of cyclic adenosine monophosphate (cyclic AMP), a substance that stimulates aqueous humor production. **Carbonic anhydrase inhibitors,** such as **dorzolamide,** block the formation of bicarbonate by carbonic anhydrase, an enzyme that is required for aqueous humor secretion. The biochemical mechanisms by which α_2-**adrenergic receptor agonists,** such as **apraclonidine,** reduce aqueous humor production are not known. **Epinephrine** probably acts by reducing blood flow in the ciliary processes.

---

occurs because the lens is accommodated for close vision.

In patients with **xerostomia** (dry mouth), pilocarpine is administered orally to stimulate salivary gland secretion. Low doses can be used to produce this effect without significant side effects in most patients because of the high sensitivity of the salivary glands to muscarinic stimulation.

INDIRECT-ACTING CHOLINERGIC RECEPTOR AGONISTS

One group of indirect-acting agonists functions by inhibiting cholinesterase, while another group exerts its effects by increasing the release of acetylcholine.

Drugs That Inhibit Cholinesterase

The cholinesterase inhibitors prevent the breakdown of acetylcholine at all cholinergic synapses. The shorter-acting types are referred to as **reversible cholinesterase inhibitors,** while the longer-acting types are called **irreversible cholinesterase inhibitors.** The properties and clinical uses of inhibitors from each group are outlined in Table 6–3.

Reversible Cholinesterase Inhibitors
Edrophonium

Chemistry and Pharmacokinetics. Edrophonium (Fig. 6–3A) is a positively charged quaternary alcohol that reversibly binds to a negatively charged (anionic) site on cholinesterase, but it is not a substrate for the enzyme. The reversible binding and rapid renal excretion of the drug are responsible for its short duration of action (about 10 minutes).

Mechanisms and Effects. Edrophonium prevents the hydrolysis of acetylcholine while it is bound to cholinesterase, and it rapidly increases acetylcholine concentrations at cholinergic synapses such as the somatic neuromuscular junction.

TABLE 6–3. Properties and Clinical Uses of Reversible and Irreversible Cholinesterase Inhibitors

Drug	Duration of Action	Route of Administration	Clinical Use
Reversible inhibitors			
Donepezil	24 hours.	Oral.	Alzheimer's disease.
Edrophonium	10 minutes.	Intravenous.	Myasthenia gravis (diagnosis).
Neostigmine	2–4 hours.	Oral, subcutaneous, or intramuscular.	Myasthenia gravis, postoperative urinary retention, and postoperative abdominal distention.
		Intravenous.	Antidote for curariform drug toxicity.
Physostigmine	1–5 hours.	Topical ocular.	Glaucoma.
		Intramuscular or intravenous.	Reversal of central nervous system effects of antimuscarinic drugs such as atropine.
Pyridostigmine	3–6 hours.	Oral, intramuscular, or intravenous.	Myasthenia gravis.
		Intravenous.	Antidote for curariform drug toxicity.
Tacrine	4–6 hours.	Oral.	Alzheimer's disease.
Irreversible inhibitors			
Echothiophate	1 week or more.	Topical ocular.	Glaucoma and accommodative esotropia.
Isoflurophate	1 week or more.	Topical ocular.	Glaucoma and accommodative esotropia.
Malathion	1 week or more.	Topical.	Pediculosis (lice).

Indications. Edrophonium is primarily used in the differential diagnosis of muscle weakness in patients suspected of having **myasthenia gravis.** In this autoimmune disease, antibodies are directed against nicotinic receptors in skeletal muscle. The antibodies can inactivate and destroy nicotinic receptors and thereby impair neuromuscular transmission. This causes severe fatigue and may affect any muscle, although it especially affects the muscles of the face, throat, and neck.

The muscle weakness of myasthenia gravis may result from either a deficiency or an excess of

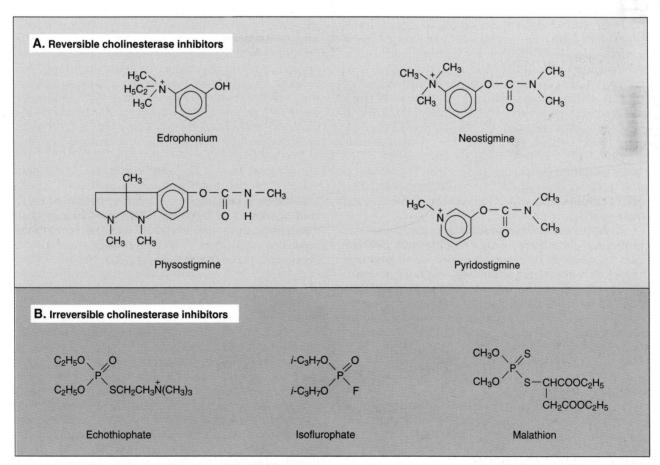

FIGURE 6–3. Structures of selected cholinesterase inhibitors. (A) The reversible cholinesterase inhibitors include edrophonium, neostigmine, physostigmine, and pyridostigmine. **(B)** The irreversible cholinesterase inhibitors are organophosphates and include echothiophate, isoflurophate, and malathion.

acetylcholine. In the untreated state, called a **myasthenic crisis,** muscle weakness is due to an acetylcholine deficiency. Use of edrophonium in this situation can improve neuromuscular transmission, restore eyelid and facial tone, and improve hand grip strength. If patients with myasthenia gravis are treated with excessive doses of a cholinesterase inhibitor, however, muscle weakness may result from an acetylcholine excess that causes prolonged depolarization of skeletal muscle. This is called a **cholinergic crisis** and should be managed by reducing the dosage of the cholinesterase inhibitor.

Neostigmine, Physostigmine, and Pyridostigmine

Chemistry and Pharmacokinetics. Neostigmine, physostigmine, and pyridostigmine (see Fig. 6–3A) are esters of carbamic acid. Physostigmine is a plant alkaloid that contains a tertiary amine, is well absorbed from the gut, and penetrates the blood-brain barrier. Neostigmine and pyridostigmine are synthetic quaternary amine compounds that are less well absorbed from the gut and do not cross the blood-brain barrier.

Mechanisms and Effects. The manner in which ۱stigmine and related carbamates bind to cholin-ˀase is similar to that in which acetylcholine to cholinesterase (Fig. 6–4). The carbamates ۱ly hydrolyzed by the enzyme and prevent the breakdown of acetylcholine for several hours.

Indications. When used in the long-term treatment of **myasthenia gravis,** neostigmine or pyridostigmine improves muscle tone and reduces eyelid and facial ptosis. Although either drug may also reduce diplopia (double vision) and blurred vision, diplopia is relatively resistant to treatment with tolerated doses of the cholinesterase inhibitors. If excessive doses are used, the muscle weakness may increase as a result of depolarizing neuromuscular blockade (see above). Corticosteroids and other immunosuppressant drugs reduce the formation of antibodies to the nicotinic receptor and are often used in combination with cholinesterase inhibitors to treat myasthenia gravis.

Neostigmine or pyridostigmine can be used to counteract **curariform drug toxicity,** and neostigmine is used in the treatment of **postoperative urinary retention and abdominal distention.**

Physostigmine has been used to treat **glaucoma.** In addition, it has been used to counteract seizures and other central nervous system effects caused by an **atropine overdose** or an overdose of another antimuscarinic drug.

Donepezil and Tacrine

Donepezil and tacrine are new, centrally acting, reversible cholinesterase inhibitors that readily cross the blood-brain barrier and act to increase the concentration of acetylcholine at central cholinergic synapses. These drugs are used in the treatment of **Alzheimer's disease** and are discussed in Chapter 21.

Irreversible Cholinesterase Inhibitors

The irreversible cholinesterase inhibitors are all **organophosphates.** A few of them—including **echothiophate, isoflurophate,** and **malathion**—have been employed as therapeutic agents. However, most of them are used as pesticides, and some of them (such as soman) were developed as chemical warfare agents. Because of the widespread use of organophosphates as pesticides, they are responsible for a number of cases of accidental poisoning every year.

Chemistry and Pharmacokinetics. The irreversible cholinesterase inhibitors (see Fig. 6–3B) are esters of phosphoric acid. Most of these organophosphates are highly lipid-soluble and are effectively absorbed from all sites in the body, including the skin, mucous membranes, and gut. Organophosphate toxicity may occur after dermal or ocular exposure or following the oral ingestion of these compounds.

Mechanisms and Effects. The organophosphates form a covalent bond with the catalytic site of cholinesterase. They are hydrolyzed slowly by the enzyme, and this accounts for their long duration of action. The covalent bonding of organophosphates with cholinesterase is further stabilized through a process called "aging," in which one of the organic groups (the "leaving group") is hydrolyzed from the phosphate.

Organophosphate compounds augment cholinergic neurotransmission at both central and peripheral cholinergic synapses. Systemic exposure to these compounds can produce all of the effects of muscarinic receptor activation, including salivation, lacrimation, miosis, accommodative spasm, bronchoconstriction, bradycardia, intestinal cramps, and urinary incontinence. Excessive activation of nicotinic receptors by organophosphate compounds leads to a depolarizing neuromuscular blockade and muscle paralysis. Seizures, respiratory depression, and coma may result from cholinergic receptor activation in the central nervous system.

Clinical Use of Organophosphates. The clinical use of organophosphates is primarily in the treatment of ocular conditions. Echothiophate or isoflurophate has been used to treat **chronic glaucoma** that does not respond adequately to more conservative therapy. The long duration of action of these drugs can provide 24-hour control of intraocular pressure, a condition that may be difficult to achieve with shorter-acting agents. Echothiophate or isoflurophate has also been used to treat a form of strabismus (ocular deviation) called **accommodative esotropia.** In affected patients, the cholinesterase inhibitors reduce strabismus by increasing the accommodation to convergence ratio.

Although malathion is primarily used as a pesticide, it has also been used to treat **pediculosis (lice).** It is administered as a shampoo for head lice and as a lotion for body and pubic lice. It kills the ova as well as the adult lice, and resistance to the drug has not been reported.

Management of Organophosphate Poisoning. Poisoning often results from accidental exposure to

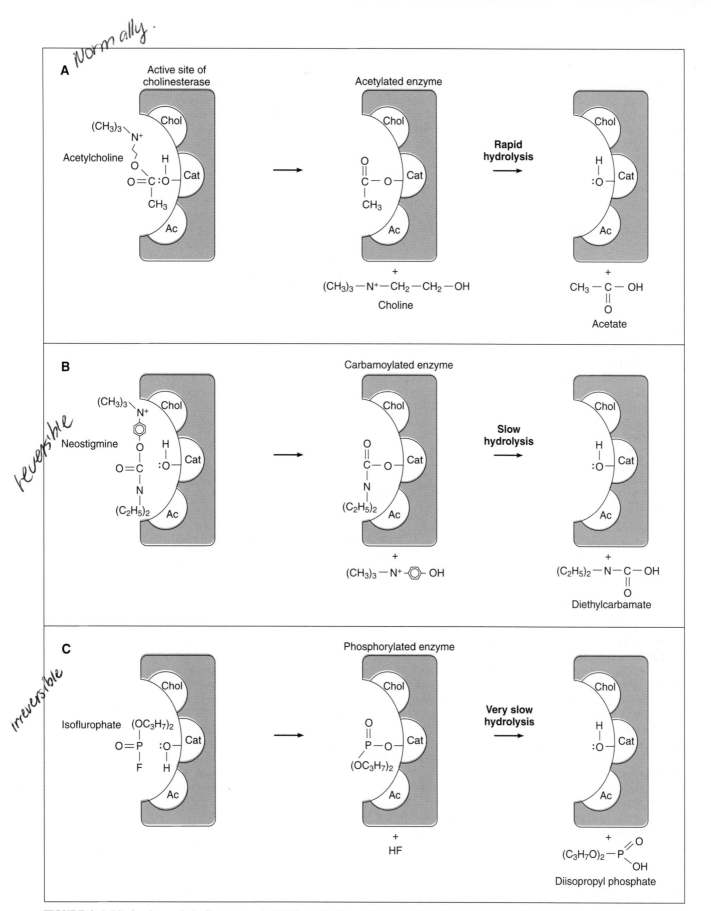

FIGURE 6–4. Mechanisms of cholinesterase inhibition. (A) The active site of cholinesterase includes the choline subsite (Chol), the catalytic subsite (Cat), and the acyl subsite (Ac). Acetylcholine binds to these subsites, and the acetate moiety forms a covalent bond with a serine hydroxyl group at the catalytic subsite as choline is released. The acetylated enzyme is then rapidly hydrolyzed to release acetate. **(B)** Carbamates such as neostigmine also bind to the active site and form a carbamoylated enzyme that is slowly hydrolyzed by cholinesterase. **(C)** Organophosphates such as isoflurophate form a strong covalent bond with the catalytic site of cholinesterase and are very slowly hydrolyzed by the enzyme. HF = hydrofluoric acid.

organophosphate pesticides used in agricultural and gardening applications or from exposure to chemical warfare agents such as soman. Management involves the following: decontamination of the patient; support of cardiovascular and respiratory function; use of a cholinergic receptor antagonist, such as **atropine,** to block excessive acetylcholine; and use of **pralidoxime** (2-PAM) to regenerate cholinesterase. Atropine can effectively counteract the muscarinic effects caused by organophosphates and other cholinesterase inhibitors. However, because of the need to counteract the extremely high levels of acetylcholine at cholinergic synapses, the atropine doses required in the management of organophosphate poisoning are usually much higher than those used in the treatment of other medical conditions. Pralidoxime is used solely for the purpose of regenerating cholinesterase following organophosphate poisoning. Its high affinity for phosphorus enables it to break the phosphorus bond with cholinesterase and thereby regenerate the enzyme. It is important to administer pralidoxime as soon as possible after organophosphate exposure, because "aging" of the organophosphate reduces the ability of pralidoxime to regenerate cholinesterase.

Drugs That Increase Acetylcholine Release

Cisapride and **metoclopramide** increase the release of acetylcholine from myenteric neurons in the enteric nervous system and thereby increase gastrointestinal motility. These effects can be blocked by atropine, a muscarinic receptor antagonist. The uses and adverse effects of cisapride and metoclopramide are discussed in Chapter 28.

OTHER CHOLINERGIC RECEPTOR AGONISTS

Sildenafil is a new drug for treating erectile dysfunction in men. It potentiates the vasodilative effect of acetylcholine and thereby increases penile blood flow and facilitates penile erection during sexual stimulation. Sildenafil acts by inhibiting the breakdown of cyclic GMP by type 5 phosphodiesterase. This action leads to elevated levels of cyclic GMP in the corpus cavernosum of the penis and to increased vasodilation.

Pharmacokinetics. Sildenafil is rapidly absorbed after oral administration and has an oral bioavailability of about 40%. The drug is widely distributed to tissues and is extensively metabolized by cytochrome P450 enzymes. The *N*-desmethyl metabolite has about half the pharmacologic activity of the parent compound. The metabolites of sildenafil are excreted primarily in the feces.

Indications. Sildenafil is used in the treatment of **male erectile dysfunction.** Its effectiveness has been established in a number of double-blind, placebo-controlled crossover studies. The response to the drug is maximal 1–2 hours after its administration, and it is significantly diminished after 4 hours.

Adverse Effects and Interactions. The adverse effects of sildenafil are usually mild and transient.

Headache, blurred vision, and nasal congestion are among the more frequent side effects.

Sildenafil should not be used by men who take organic nitrates, such as nitroglycerin, because these nitrates also increase cyclic GMP formation (see Chapter 11). Concurrent administration of sildenafil and nitroglycerin may lead to profound hypotension, reflex tachycardia, and worsening of angina pectoris. A number of deaths have occurred in men who took both sildenafil and nitroglycerin.

Sildenafil is primarily metabolized by CYP3A4, and inhibitors of this cytochrome P450 isozyme may reduce the drug's clearance and elevate its plasma concentrations. CYP3A4 inhibitors include cimetidine, cisapride, erythromycin, and ketoconazole.

Summary of Important Points

- The direct-acting cholinergic receptor agonists include choline esters (such as bethanechol) and plant alkaloids (such as pilocarpine). Bethanechol is resistant to cholinesterase and is sufficiently selective for gut and bladder muscle to be used in treating urinary retention. Pilocarpine is primarily used to treat open-angle glaucoma.
- The cholinesterase inhibitors indirectly activate cholinergic receptors by increasing the synaptic concentration of acetylcholine. These drugs have both parasympathomimetic and somatic nervous system effects.
- The reversible cholinesterase inhibitors include edrophonium, which is used to diagnose myasthenia gravis, and neostigmine and pyridostigmine, which are used to treat this condition.
- The irreversible cholinesterase inhibitors are organophosphate compounds that are widely used as pesticides and less commonly used in medical therapy. Echothiophate and isoflurophate can be used to treat ocular conditions, and malathion can be used to treat pediculosis.
- Organophosphate toxicity is treated with atropine and a cholinesterase regenerator called pralidoxime.
- Sildenafil inhibits the degradation of cyclic guanosine monophosphate by type 5 phosphodiesterase and thereby potentiates the vasodilative action of acetylcholine. Sildenafil is used to treat male erectile dysfunction.

Selected Readings

Boolell, M., et al. Sildenafil: an orally active type 5 cyclic GMP–specific phosphodiesterase inhibitor for the treatment of penile erectile dysfunction. Int J Impot Res 8:47–52, 1996.

Kanazawa, K., et al. Disparity between serotonin- and acetylcholine-provoked coronary artery spasm. Clin Cardiol 20:146–152, 1997.

Lee, E. J. Pharmacology and toxicology of chemical warfare agents. Ann Acad Med Singapore 26:104–107, 1997.

Lee, S. J., et al. Increased basal tone and hyperresponsiveness to acetylcholine and ergonovine in spasm-related coronary arteries in patients with variant angina. Int J Cardiol 55:117–126, 1996.

Pourmand, R. Myasthenia gravis. Dis Mon 43:65–109, 1997.

CHAPTER SEVEN

CHOLINERGIC RECEPTOR

ANTAGONISTS

CLASSIFICATION OF CHOLINERGIC RECEPTOR ANTAGONISTS

MUSCARINIC RECEPTOR ANTAGONISTS
Belladonna alkaloids
- Atropine
- Hyoscyamine
- Scopolamine

Semisynthetic and synthetic muscarinic receptor antagonists
- Dicyclomine
- Flavoxate
- Ipratropium
- Oxybutynin
- Pirenzepine
- Tolterodine
- Tropicamide

NICOTINIC RECEPTOR ANTAGONISTS
Ganglionic blocking agents
- Trimethaphan

Neuromuscular blocking agents
Nondepolarizing neuromuscular blocking agents
- Atracurium
- Doxacurium
- Mivacurium
- Pancuronium
- Tubocurarine
- Vecuronium

Depolarizing neuromuscular blocking agents
- Succinylcholine

MUSCARINIC RECEPTOR ANTAGONISTS

The muscarinic receptor antagonists compete with acetylcholine for muscarinic receptors at parasympathetic neuroeffector junctions and thereby inhibit the effects of parasympathetic nerve stimulation. Because of these actions, the drugs are frequently called **muscarinic receptor blockers** or **parasympatholytic drugs.**

Some muscarinic receptor antagonists are **belladonna alkaloids** obtained from plants, while others are **semisynthetic or synthetic drugs.** The drugs in these two subgroups have similar effects on target organs, but they differ in their pharmacokinetic properties and clinical uses.

Belladonna Alkaloids

The belladonna alkaloids are extracted from a number of solanaceous plants found in temperate climates around the world, including *Atropa belladonna* (the deadly nightshade), *Datura stramonium* (jimson weed, or Jamestown weed), and *Hyoscyamus niger.* Belladonna is Italian for "fair lady" and originally referred to the pupillary dilatation that was produced by extracts of these plants and was considered cosmetically attractive during the Renaissance.

Atropine, scopolamine, and hyoscyamine are examples of belladonna alkaloids. Because they are esters of tropic acid, they are also known as the **tropane alkaloids.** The belladonna alkaloids can be highly toxic and are sometimes the cause of accidental or intentional poisonings. In fact, atropine was named after Atropos, who was one of the Fates in Greek mythology and was responsible for cutting the thread of life.

Atropine and Scopolamine

Chemistry and Pharmacokinetics. Fig. 7–1A shows the structures of atropine and scopolamine. Each drug is an ester of tropic acid and a tertiary amine. Atropine and scopolamine are well absorbed from the gut and are distributed to the central nervous system. After systemic administration, they are excreted in the urine and have a fairly short half-life of about 2 hours. After topical ocular administration, they have longer-lasting effects because they bind to pigments in the iris, which slowly release the drugs over many days. People with darker irises bind more atropine and experience a more prolonged effect than do people with lighter irises. The ocular effects of atropine gradually subside over time but are still perceptible after several days.

Pharmacologic Effects. The muscarinic receptor antagonists inhibit the effects of parasympathetic nerve stimulation and thereby relax smooth muscle, increase the heart rate and cardiac conduction, and

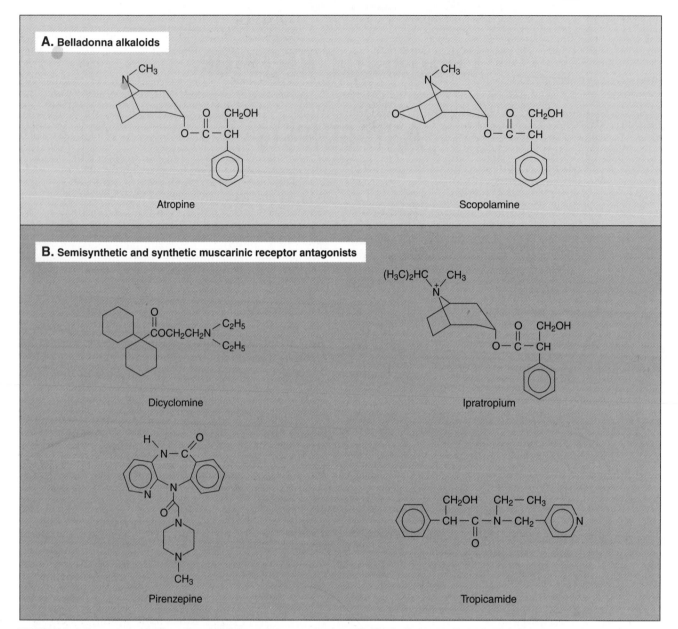

FIGURE 7–1. Structures of selected muscarinic receptor antagonists. (A) The belladonna alkaloids include atropine and scopolamine. **(B)** The semisynthetic and synthetic muscarinic receptor antagonists include dicyclomine, ipratropium, pirenzepine, and tropicamide. Ipratropium is the isopropyl derivative of atropine, and the other three antagonists are synthetic tertiary amines.

inhibit exocrine gland secretion. As shown in Fig. 7–2, as the dose of atropine increases, the severity of effects increases.

(1) Ocular Effects.   Atropine and other muscarinic receptor blockers relax the iris sphincter muscle, and this leads to pupillary dilatation (mydriasis). They also relax the ciliary muscle, thereby increasing the tension on the suspensory ligaments attached to the lens and causing the lens to flatten so that it is focused on distant objects. This inhibits the ability of the eye to focus on near objects, a condition that is called cycloplegia (paralysis of accommodation). Atropine also inhibits lacrimal gland secretion and may cause dry eyes.

(2) Cardiac Effects.   Standard doses of atropine and related drugs increase the heart rate and atrioventricular conduction velocity by blocking the effects of the vagus nerve on the sinoatrial and atrioventricular nodes. When intravenous administration of atropine is begun, however, the low dose of the drug causes a paradoxical slowing of the heart rate. This effect is probably due to stimulation of the vagal motor nucleus in the brain stem. After the full therapeutic dose has been administered, the increase in heart rate is observed.

(3) Respiratory Tract Effects.   In addition to producing bronchial smooth muscle relaxation and bronchodilation, atropine and other muscarinic receptor antagonists act as potent inhibitors of secretions in the upper and lower respiratory tract.

(4) Gastrointestinal and Urinary Tract Effects. Atropine reduces lower esophageal muscle tone and may cause gastroesophageal reflux. Atropine and other muscarinic receptor blockers relax gastrointestinal muscle, except sphincters, and reduce intestinal motility, thereby increasing gastric emptying time and intestinal transit time. They also inhibit gastric acid secretion. Sufficient doses of these drugs may cause constipation. Atropine relaxes the detrusor muscle of the urinary bladder and may cause urinary retention.

(5) Central Nervous System Effects. Atropine, scopolamine, and other tertiary amines are distributed to the central nervous system, where they may block muscarinic receptors and produce either sedation or excitement. Scopolamine is more sedating than is atropine and has been used as an adjunct to anesthesia. Standard doses of atropine typically cause mild stimulation, followed by a slower and longer-lasting sedative effect. With higher doses of atropine, patients may experience an acute confusional state known as delirium. Higher doses of atropine or related drugs may also cause hallucinations.

(6) Other Effects. The muscarinic receptor antagonists inhibit sweating. This may reduce heat loss and lead to hyperthermia, especially in children. The increased body temperature may cause cutaneous vasodilatation, and the skin may become hot, dry, and flushed.

Indications

(1) Ocular Indications. To obtain a relatively localized effect on ocular tissues, atropine and other muscarinic receptor blockers are administered via topical instillation of a solution or ointment. These drugs are typically used to produce mydriasis and facilitate **ophthalmoscopic examination** of the peripheral retina. They can also be used to produce cycloplegia and permit the accurate determination of refractive errors, especially in younger patients with a strong accommodation. Because muscarinic receptor blockers are able to reduce muscle spasm and pain caused by inflammation, they are useful in the treatment of **iritis** and **cyclitis** (inflammation of the iris and ciliary muscles) associated with infection, trauma, or surgery.

(2) Cardiac Indications. Atropine can be used to treat **sinus bradycardia** in cases in which the slow sinus rhythm reduces the cardiac output and blood pressure and produces symptoms of hypotension or ischemia. This type of symptomatic bradycardia sometimes occurs after a myocardial infarction. Atropine is usually administered intravenously for this purpose, but it may be injected endotracheally if a vein is not accessible. In patients with symptomatic **atrioventricular block,** atropine can be used to increase the atrioventricular conduction velocity.

(3) Respiratory Tract Indications. Because of its bronchodilating effects, atropine was once used to treat asthma and other obstructive lung diseases. It is no longer used for this purpose, however, because of its many adverse effects. For example, it impairs

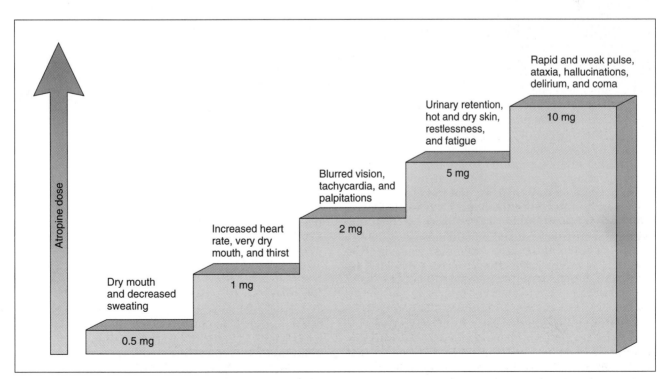

FIGURE 7–2. Dose-dependent effects of atropine. Low doses of atropine inhibit salivation and sweating, and the magnitude of these effects increases as the dosage increases. Higher doses produce tachycardia, urinary retention, and central nervous system effects.

ciliary activity, thereby reducing the clearance of mucus from the lungs and causing accumulation of viscid material in the airways. As discussed below, ipratropium is now used instead of atropine for the treatment of obstructive lung diseases. In the past, atropine and other muscarinic receptor blockers were used to reduce salivary and respiratory secretions and thereby prevent airway obstruction in patients who were receiving general anesthetics. This practice is uncommon today because modern anesthetics are less irritating to lung tissue and usually are not associated with a significant increase in respiratory secretions.

(4) Gastrointestinal and Urinary Tract Indications. Atropine and related drugs are used to relieve **intestinal spasms and pain** associated with several gastrointestinal disorders, and they are also used to relieve **urinary bladder spasms** that may cause dysuria and incontinence. In the past, atropine was frequently used to reduce gastric acid secretion in patients with peptic ulcers. However, large doses were required, and these doses often produced intolerable side effects, such as dry mouth, blurred vision, and urinary retention. For this reason, atropine and other nonselective muscarinic receptor blockers are seldom used to treat peptic ulcers today. As discussed below, a selective muscarinic M_1 receptor blocker, pirenzepine, is now used instead.

(5) Central Nervous System Indications. A transdermal formulation of scopolamine can be used to prevent **motion sickness.** The skin patch slowly releases scopolamine over a period of 3 days and is thought to work by blocking cholinergic neurotransmission from the vestibular apparatus to the vomiting center in the brain stem. As discussed in Chapter 21, muscarinic receptor blockers are also used in the treatment of **Parkinson's disease.**

(6) Other Indications. Atropine is used in two other clinical contexts. First, it is used to prevent muscarinic side effects when cholinesterase inhibitors are given to patients with **myasthenia gravis.** Second, as discussed in Chapter 6, it is used to reverse the muscarinic effects of **cholinesterase inhibitor overdose.** In this setting, supranormal doses of atropine may be required to counteract the large concentrations of acetylcholine that have accumulated at cholinergic synapses, and the atropine dosage must be titrated to the patient's response. Atropine will not counteract the effects of nicotinic receptor activation caused by cholinesterase inhibition. However, the muscle weakness resulting from nicotinic receptor stimulation can be attenuated by adding pralidoxime to the treatment regimen.

Hyoscyamine

Hyoscyamine, the levorotatory isomer of racemic atropine, is the natural form of the alkaloid that occurs in plants and is primarily responsible for the pharmacologic effects of atropine. Hyoscyamine is primarily used to treat **intestinal spasms** and other

gastrointestinal disorders, and it is available in preparations intended for oral or sublingual administration.

Semisynthetic and Synthetic Muscarinic Receptor Antagonists

In the search for a more selective muscarinic receptor antagonist, investigators have developed a large number of semisynthetic and synthetic blocking agents. Fig. 7–1B shows examples of their chemical structures. Although the pharmacologic effects of these agents are similar to those of atropine, their unique pharmacokinetic properties are advantageous in specific situations.

Ipratropium

Ipratropium, a quaternary amine derivative of atropine, is administered by inhalation to patients with **obstructive lung diseases.** Because ipratropium is not well absorbed from the lungs into the systemic circulation, it produces few adverse effects. For example, unlike atropine, it does not impair the ciliary clearance of secretions from the airways. This makes it particularly useful in treating patients with **emphysema** and **chronic bronchitis.** The respiratory effects and uses of this compound are discussed more thoroughly in Chapter 27.

Dicyclomine, Oxybutynin, Flavoxate, and Tolterodine

Dicyclomine and oxybutynin are synthetic tertiary amines that block muscarinic receptors and are useful in the treatment of **intestinal hypermotility and spasms** and **urinary bladder spasms,** such as those occurring secondary to infection or trauma. Flavoxate is a similar compound that is primarily used to relieve bladder spasms. These drugs are well absorbed after oral administration and are primarily eliminated by renal excretion.

Tolterodine is a newer antimuscarinic drug for the treatment of **urinary frequency, urgency, and incontinence.** Like other antimuscarinic drugs, tolterodine inhibits detrusor muscle contractions and reduces the urge to void. It is no more effective than oxybutynin for these indications. However, tolterodine is more selective for the bladder and less likely to produce dry mouth than are other antimuscarinic drugs. Tolterodine is administered orally twice a day. Erythromycin and ketoconazole inhibit the metabolism of tolterodine and may increase its serum levels.

Tropicamide

Tropicamide is a tertiary amine that was developed for topical ocular administration as a mydriatic. It is given just prior to ophthalmoscopy to facilitate **examination of the peripheral retina.** It has a short duration of action (about 1 hour) and is often preferable to atropine and scopolamine for short-term mydriasis.

Pirenzepine

Pirenzepine is a muscarinic receptor antagonist that is selective for M_1 receptors and was developed for the purpose of reducing vagally stimulated gastric acid secretion in patients with **peptic ulcers.** The drug appears to act by blocking M_1 receptors on paracrine cells and thereby inhibiting the release of histamine, a potent gastric acid stimulant. The effects and uses of pirenzepine are discussed in Chapter 28.

NICOTINIC RECEPTOR ANTAGONISTS

The nicotinic receptor antagonists include ganglionic blocking agents and neuromuscular blocking agents.

Ganglionic Blocking Agents

The ganglionic nicotinic receptor blockers, such as **trimethaphan,** selectively block N_N receptors at sympathetic and parasympathetic ganglia. Their effect on a particular tissue depends on whether the sympathetic or parasympathetic system is dominant in that tissue. Blockade of sympathetic ganglia causes hypotension, while blockade of parasympathetic ganglia produces dry mouth, blurred vision, and urinary retention.

Ganglionic blockers were used in the past for treating chronic hypertension, but their side effects have limited their use in patients with this disorder. Trimethaphan is occasionally used in cases of **hypertensive emergency,** when extremely high blood pressures must be lowered rapidly. It is also used to produce **"controlled hypotension" during neurosurgery** and thereby provide a bloodless surgical field.

Neuromuscular Blocking Agents

The neuromuscular blocking agents inhibit neurotransmission at skeletal neuromuscular junctions, causing muscle weakness and paralysis. These agents can be divided into two groups, one consisting of **nondepolarizing blockers** and the other consisting of **depolarizing blockers.**

Nondepolarizing Neuromuscular Blocking Agents
Drug Properties

The nondepolarizing neuromuscular blocking agents are also known as **curariform drugs** and include **atracurium, doxacurium, mivacurium, pancuronium, tubocurarine,** and **vecuronium.** The curariform drugs were originally extracted from plants used by native South Americans as arrow poisons for hunting wild game. **Curare** is another name for the arrow poisons and their chemical derivatives.

Chemistry and Pharmacokinetics. Chemical structures and pharmacologic properties of numerous curariform drugs are shown in Fig. 7–3A and Table 7–1. The curariform drugs are positively charged quaternary amines that are not well absorbed from the gut and do not cross the blood-brain barrier. Hence, they do not cause poisoning when meat containing these substances is ingested. Some of the curariform drugs, such as atracurium and vecuronium, are rapidly metabolized by plasma

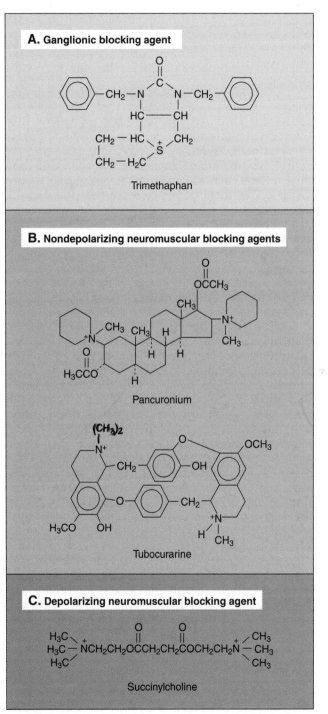

FIGURE 7–3. Structures of selected nicotinic receptor antagonists. **(A)** Ganglionic blocking agents include trimethaphan. **(B)** Nondepolarizing neuromuscular blocking agents include pancuronium, which is an ammonio steroid, and tubocurarine, which is a benzylisoquinoline. **(C)** Succinylcholine, the only depolarizing neuromuscular blocking agent available for clinical use today, is composed of two molecules of acetylcholine.

TABLE 7–1. Properties of Neuromuscular Blocking Agents

Drug	Depolarizing Agent	Histamine Release*	Ganglionic Blockade†	Effects Reversed by Cholinesterase Inhibitors	Duration of Action (Minutes)
Atracurium	No	Medium	Low	Yes	30–40
Doxacurium	No	Low	Low	Yes	90–120
Mivacurium	No	Medium	Low	Yes	10–20
Pancuronium	No	Low	Medium	Yes	120–180
Succinylcholine	Yes	Medium	None‡	No	5–10
Tubocurarine	No	High	High	Yes	60–120
Vecuronium	No	Low	Low	Yes	30–40

*May cause bronchospasm, hypotension, and excessive salivary and bronchial secretions.
†May cause hypotension and tachycardia.
‡May cause bradycardia (by stimulating vagal ganglia) or may cause tachycardia and hypertension (by stimulating sympathetic ganglia).

cholinesterase and therefore have a short duration of action. Other drugs, including tubocurarine and doxacurium, are eliminated by renal and biliary excretion of their parent compounds and hepatic metabolites.

Mechanisms and Effects. Curariform agents act as competitive antagonists of acetylcholine at N_M receptors in skeletal muscle, and this accounts for their muscle-relaxing effects. After a curariform drug is administered, it first paralyzes the small and rapidly moving muscles of the eyes and face and then paralyzes the larger muscles of the limbs and trunk. Finally, it paralyzes the intercostal muscles and diaphragm, causing respiration to cease. This sequence of paralysis is fortunate in that it enables relaxation of abdominal muscles for surgical procedures without producing apnea. However, respiratory function should always be closely monitored in patients receiving a neuromuscular blocking agent.

Curariform drugs stimulate the release of histamine from mast cells, and they block autonomic ganglia and muscarinic receptors (see Table 7–1). These actions may cause bronchospasm, hypotension, and tachycardia. Newer drugs, such as atracurium, doxacurium, mivacurium, and vecuronium, tend to cause less histamine release and fewer autonomic side effects than do tubocurarine and pancuronium.

Interactions. The muscle-relaxing effects of curariform drugs are potentiated by various inhalational anesthetic agents (including halothane and isoflurane) and by the aminoglycoside antibiotics, tetracycline antibiotics, and calcium channel blockers. The effects are also more pronounced in patients who have neuromuscular disorders such as myasthenia gravis than they are in healthy individuals. The muscle-relaxing effects of curariform drugs can be reversed by administering a cholinesterase inhibitor, such as neostigmine, which acts by increasing acetylcholine levels at the neuromuscular junction and counteracting the neuromuscular blockade.

Indications. The neuromuscular blockers are primarily used to induce **muscle relaxation during surgery** and thereby facilitate surgical manipulations. These drugs are sometimes used as an **adjunct to electroconvulsive therapy** so as to prevent injuries that might be caused by involuntary muscle contractions. They have also been used to facilitate intubation of the respiratory tract and thereby facilitate **endoscopic procedures** such as bronchoscopy. During the clinical use of neuromuscular blocking agents, the degree of neuromuscular blockade can be determined by monitoring the contraction of a small limb muscle in response to nerve stimulation.

Specific Drugs

The selection of a nondepolarizing agent for a particular clinical application is usually based on the relative duration of action and safety of the various drugs. Atracurium, mivacurium, and vecuronium are often preferred because of their short duration of action and minimal effects on cardiovascular and respiratory function. Doxacurium might be selected when a longer duration of action is required.

Depolarizing Neuromuscular Blocking Agents

Succinylcholine, the only depolarizing agent available for clinical use today, is composed of two molecules of acetylcholine (see Fig. 7–3B). Succinylcholine binds to nicotinic receptors in skeletal muscle and causes persistent depolarization of the motor end plate. When the drug is first administered, it produces transient muscle contractions called fasciculations. The fasciculations are quickly followed by a sustained muscle paralysis. Succinylcholine is not hydrolyzed as rapidly by cholinesterase as acetylcholine is, and this appears to partly account for the persistent depolarization and muscle paralysis.

Table 7–1 compares the properties of succinylcholine with those of the curariform drugs. Succinylcholine has a relatively short duration of action (5–10 minutes), owing to its hydrolysis by plasma cholinesterase. The sequence of muscle paralysis produced by succinylcholine is similar to that produced by the curariform drugs. However, the effects of succinylcholine are not reversed by cholinesterase inhibitors, and there is no pharmacologic antidote to reverse an overdose of succinylcholine.

Succinylcholine is used to produce **muscle relaxation during surgery.** Before the drug is administered, patients should be screened for atypical cholinesterase. Individuals with this inherited disorder cannot metabolize succinylcholine at normal rates and are susceptible to prolonged neuromuscular paralysis and apnea after receiving the usual dosage of the drug.

Summary of Important Points

- The muscarinic receptor antagonists relax smooth muscle, increase the heart rate and cardiac conduction, and inhibit exocrine gland secretion. They include belladonna alkaloids (such as atropine and scopolamine) and semisynthetic and synthetic drugs (such as ipratropium).
- The muscarinic receptor blockers are used to treat bradycardia, obstructive lung diseases, intestinal spasms, urinary bladder spasms, and peptic ulcers. They are also used to reduce salivary and respiratory secretions and to produce mydriasis and cycloplegia.
- Atropine toxicity may cause dryness of the mouth and skin, blurred vision, tachycardia, palpitations, urinary retention, delirium, and hallucinations.
- The nicotinic receptor antagonists include ganglionic blocking agents (such as trimethaphan) and neuromuscular blocking agents (such as the curariform drugs, which are nondepolarizing, and succinylcholine, which is depolarizing).
- Trimethaphan is used to produce controlled hypotension during surgery and to treat hypertensive emergencies.
- Neuromuscular blockers are primarily used to produce muscle relaxation during surgery.
- Curariform drugs competitively block nicotinic receptors in skeletal muscle. They do not cause muscle fasciculations, and their effects can be reversed by cholinesterase inhibitors.
- Succinylcholine produces muscle fasciculations that are followed by muscle paralysis. The effects cannot be reversed by cholinesterase inhibitors.

Selected Readings

Alabaster, V. A. Discovery and development of selective M_3 antagonists for clinical use. Life Sci 60:1053–1060, 1997.

Gyermek, L. Pharmacology of Antimuscarinic Agents. Boca Raton, Fla., CRC Press, 1997.

Kaiser, H. B., et al. An anticholinergic agent, ipratropium bromide, is useful in the treatment of rhinorrhea associated with perennial allergic rhinitis. Allergy Asthma Proc 19:23–29, 1998.

Nilvebrant, L., et al. Tolterodine: a new bladder-selective antimuscarinic agent. Eur J Pharmacol 327:195–207, 1997.

Reeves, S. T., and N. M. Turcasso. Nondepolarizing neuromuscular blocking drugs in the intensive care unit: a clinical review. South Med J 90:769–794, 1997.

CHAPTER EIGHT

ADRENERGIC RECEPTOR AGONISTS

CLASSIFICATION OF ADRENERGIC RECEPTOR AGONISTS

DIRECT-ACTING ADRENERGIC RECEPTOR AGONISTS
  Catecholamines
  • Dobutamine
  • Dopamine
  • Epinephrine
  • Isoproterenol
  • Norepinephrine
  Noncatecholamines
  • Albuterol
  • Apraclonidine
  • Clonidine
  • Oxymetazoline
  • Phenylephrine
  • Ritodrine
  • Terbutaline

INDIRECT-ACTING ADRENERGIC RECEPTOR AGONISTS
  • Amphetamine
  • Cocaine

MIXED-ACTING ADRENERGIC RECEPTOR AGONISTS
  • Ephedrine
  • Phenylpropanolamine
  • Pseudoephedrine

OVERVIEW OF ADRENERGIC PHARMACOLOGY

The adrenergic receptor agonists are a large group of drugs whose diverse pharmacologic effects make them valuable in the treatment of a wide spectrum of clinical conditions, ranging from cardiovascular emergencies to the common cold. While some of the agonists exert their effects on multiple organ systems, others target a specific organ. The spectrum of effects produced by a particular adrenergic receptor agonist depends on its affinity for different types of adrenergic receptors.

Adrenergic Receptors

Adrenergic receptors (adrenoceptors) have been classified as **α-adrenergic receptors** and **β-adrenergic receptors,** based on their reactions to epinephrine, norepinephrine, and other adrenergic receptor agonists in cardiac and smooth muscle.

Epinephrine and norepinephrine are more potent than isoproterenol at α-adrenergic receptors located in smooth muscle, whereas isoproterenol is more potent than epinephrine and norepinephrine at β-adrenergic receptors located in cardiac muscle.

As shown in Table 8–1 and Fig. 8–1, subtypes of α- and β-adrenergic receptors have also been identified on the basis of several criteria, including differences in signal transduction and physiologic effects and differences in agonist potency and affinity at particular receptor sites. The receptor subtypes have been cloned, and their molecular structures have been determined.

α-Adrenergic Receptors

The subtypes of α-adrenergic receptors can be differentiated on the basis of their location at sympathetic neuroeffector junctions. The α_1-**adrenergic receptors** are primarily located in postjunctional smooth muscle, whereas α_2-**adrenergic receptors** are located on presynaptic neurons as well as in some postsynaptic tissues and blood platelets (see Fig. 8–1).

The α_1 receptors mediate contraction of the vascular smooth muscle, iris dilator muscle, and bladder sphincter muscle. The α_2 receptors located on sympathetic postganglionic neurons serve as **autoreceptors** whose activation leads to feedback inhibition of norepinephrine release from nerve terminals. The α_2 receptors are also found in blood platelets and in ocular, adipose, intestinal, hepatic, renal, and endocrine tissue. In blood platelets, α_2 receptors mediate platelet aggregation. In the pancreas, α_2 receptors mediate the inhibition of insulin secretion that occurs when the sympathetic nervous system is activated.

β-Adrenergic Receptors

Table 8–1 summarizes the effects of three subtypes of β-adrenergic receptors.

Activation of β_1-**adrenergic receptors** produces cardiac stimulation, leading to a positive **chronotropic effect** (increased heart rate), a positive **inotropic effect** (increased contractility), and a positive **dromotropic effect** (increased cardiac impulse conduction velocity). Activation of β_1 receptors also increases renin secretion from renal juxtaglomerular cells.

TABLE 8–1. Properties of Adrenergic, Dopamine, and Imidazoline Receptors

Type of Receptor	Mechanism of Signal Transduction	Effects
Adrenergic		
α_1	Increased inositol triphosphate (IP$_3$) and diacylglycerol (DAG).	Contraction of smooth muscles.
α_2	Decreased cyclic adenosine monophosphate (cAMP).	Inhibition of norepinephrine release, decrease in secretion of aqueous humor, decrease in secretion of insulin, mediation of platelet aggregation, and mediation of central nervous system effects.
β_1	Increased cAMP.	Increase in secretion of renin and increase in heart rate, contractility, and conduction.
β_2	Increased cAMP.	Glycogenolysis, relaxation of smooth muscles, and uptake of potassium in skeletal muscles.
β_3	Increased cAMP.	Lipolysis.
Dopamine		
D$_1$	Increased cAMP.	Relaxation of vascular smooth muscles.
D$_2$	Decreased cAMP, increased potassium currents, and decreased calcium influx.	Modulation of neurotransmission in the sympathetic and central nervous systems.
Imidazoline	Uncertain; possibly increased DAG.	Natriuresis and decrease of sympathetic outflow from the central nervous system.

The **β_2-adrenergic receptors** mediate relaxation of bronchial, uterine, and vascular smooth muscle. In skeletal muscle, β_2 receptors mediate potassium uptake. In the liver, they mediate **glycogenolysis,** which increases the glucose concentration in the blood. Whereas epinephrine and norepinephrine are equally potent at β_1 receptors in cardiac tissue, epinephrine is more potent than norepinephrine at β_2 receptors in smooth muscle.

Activation of **β_3-adrenergic receptors** produces **lipolysis,** a process in which the hydrolysis of triglycerides in adipose tissue leads to the release of fatty acids into the circulation. Investigators are currently searching for selective β_3-adrenergic recep-

tor agonists because they believe that the lipolytic effect of these agonists would be useful in the treatment of obesity.

Dopamine Receptors

Dopamine receptors are activated by dopamine but not by other adrenergic receptor agonists. There are several subtypes, including the **D$_1$ receptors,** which mediate muscle relaxation in vascular smooth muscle, and the **D$_2$ receptors,** which modulate neurotransmitter release. As discussed below, the vasodilative effect of dopamine is useful in the treatment of circulatory shock.

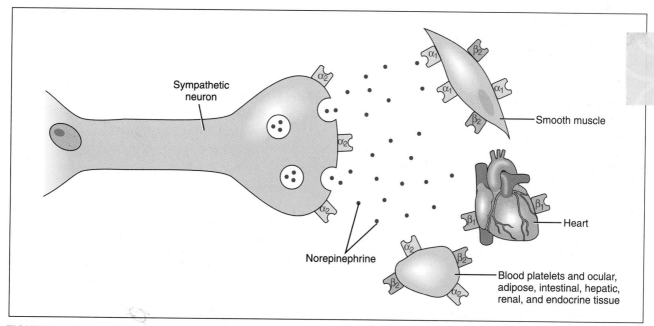

FIGURE 8–1. Primary tissue locations of α-adrenergic and β-adrenergic receptors. While α_1- and β_2-adrenergic receptors are primarily located in smooth muscle, β_1-adrenergic receptors are predominantly found in cardiac tissue. Some α_2-adrenergic receptors are located on sympathetic neurons, where they produce feedback inhibition of neurotransmitter release. Other α_2- and β_2-adrenergic receptors are located in blood platelets and a variety of organ tissues. The α- and β-adrenergic receptors are also found in the central nervous system.

Imidazoline Receptors

Imidazoline receptors are activated by adrenergic receptor agonists and other substances that contain an imidazoline structure. One of the best-studied examples of these substances is clonidine. The imidazoline receptors are found in the central nervous system and a number of peripheral tissues. While the antihypertensive effects of clonidine may be partly attributable to the activation of α_2-adrenergic receptors, investigators have postulated that they are also partly due to the effects of imidazoline receptors, which act in the central nervous system to reduce sympathetic outflow to the heart and vascular smooth muscle. The pharmacologic properties of antihypertensive imidazoline drugs are discussed in greater detail in Chapter 10.

Signal Transduction

The adrenergic, dopamine, and imidazoline receptors are guanine nucleotide protein–binding (G protein–binding) receptors that are located in cell membranes of target tissues.

Activation of α_1-adrenergic receptors is coupled with activation of **phospholipase C,** which catalyzes the release of **inositol triphosphate** (IP_3) and **diacylglycerol** (DAG) from membrane phospholipids. In smooth muscle, IP_3 stimulates the release of calcium from the sarcoplasmic reticulum, and this leads to muscle contraction. This is the mechanism by which a drug can produce vasoconstriction and increased blood pressure in a patient with severe hypotension. Activation of α_2-adrenergic receptors leads to inhibition of adenylyl cyclase and a decrease in the levels of cyclic adenosine monophosphate (cyclic AMP) in sympathetic neurons and other tissues. This is the mechanism responsible for a decrease in aqueous humor secretion and for other effects of α_2-adrenergic receptor agonists. Activation of D_2 receptors also inhibits cyclic AMP formation.

Activation of β-adrenergic receptors and D_1 receptors leads to stimulation of adenylyl cyclase and an increase in the levels of cyclic AMP in cardiac tissue and smooth muscle. Cyclic AMP activates **protein kinases,** which phosphorylate other proteins and enzymes. The cellular response depends on the specific type of proteins that are phosphorylated in each tissue. In cardiac tissue, calcium channels are phosphorylated, thereby augmenting calcium influx and cardiac contractility. In smooth muscle, cyclic AMP–activated kinases produce muscle relaxation.

Classification of Adrenergic Receptor Agonists

The adrenergic receptor agonists mimic the effect of sympathetic nervous system stimulation and are therefore also called **sympathomimetic drugs.** These drugs can be divided into three groups on the basis of their mode of action. The **direct-acting agonists** bind to and activate adrenergic receptors. As shown in Fig. 8–2, the **indirect-acting agonists** increase the stimulation of adrenergic receptors by elevating the concentration of norepinephrine at sympathetic neuroeffector junctions in one of two ways: either by increasing the release of norepinephrine from sympathetic neurons (as occurs, for example, with amphetamine) or by inhibiting the neuronal reuptake of norepinephrine (as occurs with cocaine). The **mixed-acting agonists,** such as ephedrine, have both direct and indirect actions.

DIRECT-ACTING ADRENERGIC RECEPTOR AGONISTS

The direct-acting agonists can be subdivided into catecholamines and noncatecholamines.

Catecholamines

The naturally occurring catecholamines include **norepinephrine,** an endogenous sympathetic neurotransmitter; **epinephrine,** the principal hormone of the adrenal medulla; and **dopamine,** the precursor to norepinephrine and epinephrine. Synthetic catecholamines include **isoproterenol** and **dobutamine.**

Drug Properties

Chemistry and Pharmacokinetics. Each catecholamine consists of the catechol moiety and an ethylamine side chain (Fig. 8–3A). The catecholamines are rapidly inactivated by **monoamine oxidase**

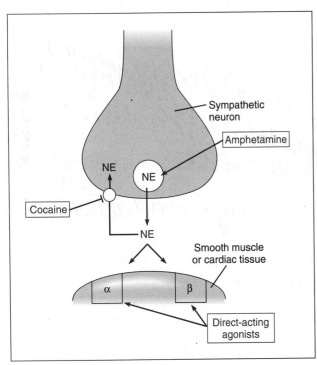

FIGURE 8–2. Mechanisms of indirect-acting and direct-acting adrenergic receptor agonists. Some indirect-acting agonists (such as cocaine) block norepinephrine reuptake, while other indirect-acting agonists (such as amphetamine) increase norepinephrine release from sympathetic neurons. Direct-acting agonists bind to and activate adrenergic receptors. NE = norepinephrine; α = α-adrenergic receptor; and β = β-adrenergic receptor.

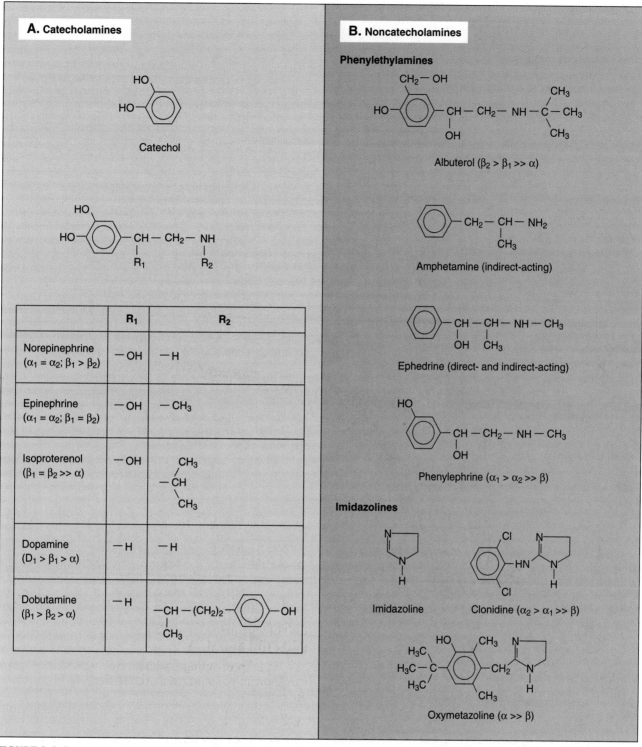

FIGURE 8–3. Structures of selected adrenergic receptor agonists. (A) Catecholamines contain the catechol moiety and an ethylamine side chain. The amine nitrogen substitution determines the relative affinity for α- and β-adrenergic receptors, with larger substitutions (such as in isoproterenol and dobutamine) decreasing the affinity for α-adrenergic receptors and increasing the affinity for β-adrenergic receptors. Note that dopamine has an even higher affinity for dopamine D_1 receptors than for adrenergic receptors. **(B)** One group of noncatecholamines consists of phenylethylamines, which lack one or both of the hydroxyl groups of the catechol moiety. Another group of noncatecholamines consists of imidazolines.

(MAO) and **catechol-*O*-methyltransferase** (COMT), enzymes found in the gut, liver, and other tissues. The drugs have low oral bioavailabilities and short plasma half-lives. For these reasons, they must be administered parenterally when a systemic action is required (for example, in the treatment of patients who are in anaphylactic shock).

Mechanisms and Effects. As shown in Fig. 8–3A and Table 8–2, the various catecholamines differ in their affinities and specificities for receptors. The

TABLE 8–2. Pharmacologic Effects and Clinical Uses of Adrenergic Receptor Agonists

Drug	Pharmacologic Effect (and Receptor)	Clinical Use
Direct-acting catecholamines		
Dobutamine	Cardiac stimulation (β_1) and vasodilation (β_2).	Cardiogenic shock, acute heart failure, and cardiac stimulation during heart surgery.
Dopamine*	Renal vasodilation (D_1), cardiac stimulation (β_1), and increased blood pressure (β_1 and α_1).	Cardiogenic shock, septic shock, heart failure, and adjunct to fluid administration in hypovolemic shock.
Epinephrine	Vasoconstriction and increased blood pressure (α_1), cardiac stimulation (β_1), and bronchodilation (β_2).	Anaphylactic shock, cardiac arrest, ventricular fibrillation, reduction in bleeding during surgery, and prolongation of the action of local anesthetics.
Isoproterenol	Cardiac stimulation (β_1) and bronchodilation (β_2).	Asthma, refractory atrioventricular block, and refractory bradycardia.
Norepinephrine	Vasoconstriction and increased blood pressure (α_1).	Hypotension and shock.
Direct-acting noncatecholamines		
Albuterol	Bronchodilation (β_2).	Asthma.
Apraclonidine	Decreased aqueous humor formation (α_2).	Chronic open-angle glaucoma.
Clonidine	Decreased sympathetic outflow from central nervous system (α_2 and imidazoline).	Chronic hypertension.
Oxymetazoline	Vasoconstriction (α_1).	Nasal and ocular decongestion.
Phenylephrine	Vasoconstriction, increased blood pressure, and mydriasis (α_1).	Nasal decongestion in viral and allergic rhinitis, ocular decongestion in allergic conjunctivitis, mydriasis during ophthalmologic examination, maintenance of blood pressure during surgery, and treatment of drug-induced and neurogenic shock.
Ritodrine	Bronchodilation and uterine relaxation (β_2).	Asthma and premature labor.
Terbutaline	Bronchodilation and uterine relaxation (β_2).	Asthma and premature labor.
Indirect-acting agents		
Amphetamine	Increase in norepinephrine release.	Central nervous system effects.
Cocaine	Inhibition of norepinephrine uptake.	Local anesthesia.
Mixed-acting agents		
Ephedrine	Vasoconstriction (α_1).	Nasal decongestion in viral and allergic rhinitis.
Phenylpropanolamine	Vasoconstriction (α_1).	Nasal decongestion in viral and allergic rhinitis.
Pseudoephedrine	Vasoconstriction (α_1).	Nasal decongestion in viral and allergic rhinitis.

*Dopamine is a catecholamine with mixed action.

size of the alkyl substitution on the amine nitrogen determines the relative affinity for α- and β-adrenergic receptors. Drugs with a large alkyl group (such as isoproterenol) have greater affinity for β-adrenergic receptors than do drugs with a small alkyl group (such as epinephrine). Epinephrine is a potent agonist at all α- and β-adrenergic receptors. Norepinephrine differs from epinephrine only in that it has greater affinity for β_1-adrenergic than for β_2-adrenergic receptors. Because of this difference, norepinephrine constricts all blood vessels, whereas epinephrine constricts some blood vessels but dilates others. Isoproterenol is considered to be a selective β_1- and β_2-adrenergic receptor agonist because it has little affinity for α receptors. Dobutamine primarily stimulates β_1 receptors but has minor stimulatory effects on β_2 and α receptors. Dopamine activates D_1, β_1, and α receptors. Unlike the other catecholamines, dopamine also stimulates the release of norepinephrine from sympathetic neurons. For this reason, dopamine is both a direct-acting and an indirect-acting receptor agonist.

(1) Cardiovascular Effects. Fig. 8–4 compares the cardiovascular effects when norepinephrine, epinephrine, isoproterenol, and dopamine are given by intravenous infusion.

The cardiovascular effects of norepinephrine are primarily due to activation of α_1-adrenergic receptors. Activation produces vasoconstriction and increased peripheral resistance, and this in turn increases the systolic and diastolic blood pressure. Norepinephrine may cause reflex bradycardia if blood pressure increases sufficiently to activate the baroreceptor reflex.

Epinephrine increases the systolic blood pressure but may decrease the diastolic blood pressure. Increased systolic pressure is due to an increased heart rate and cardiac output. The effect on diastolic pressure depends on the relative stimulation of α_1- and β_2-adrenergic receptors, which mediate vasoconstriction and vasodilation, respectively. Lower doses of epinephrine produce greater stimulation of β_2 receptors than α_1 receptors, thereby causing vasodilation and decreasing diastolic blood pressure. Higher doses produce more vasoconstriction and may increase diastolic pressure.

Isoproterenol activates β-adrenergic receptors and produces vasodilation and cardiac stimulation. It usually lowers the diastolic and mean arterial pressure, but it may increase the systolic pressure by increasing the heart rate and contractility. Its potent chronotropic effect may cause tachycardia and cardiac arrhythmias. For this reason, an alternative drug, such as dobutamine or dopamine, is usually administered to increase cardiac output in cases of heart failure and shock.

Dobutamine and dopamine selectively increase myocardial contractility and stroke volume while producing a smaller increase in heart rate. These actions increase cardiac output and are highly beneficial in the treatment of hypotension and shock. Dobutamine also reduces vascular resistance by activating β_2-adrenergic receptors and thereby decreasing cardiac afterload. In patients with heart failure, a reduction in afterload contributes to an increased stroke volume and cardiac output.

When given in low doses, dopamine selectively activates D_1 receptors in renal and other vascular beds, thereby causing vasodilation and an increase in renal blood flow. At slightly higher doses, dopamine activates β_1-adrenergic receptors in the heart, thereby stimulating cardiac contractility and increasing cardiac output and tissue perfusion. At even higher doses, dopamine activates α_1-adrenergic receptors and causes vasoconstriction.

(2) Respiratory Tract Effects. Epinephrine and isoproterenol are potent bronchodilators. Although they have been used in the treatment of asthma, more selective β_2-adrenergic receptor agonists are usually employed for this purpose today.

(3) Adverse Effects. Catecholamines may cause excessive vasoconstriction, leading to tissue ischemia and necrosis. Localized tissue ischemia may result from extravasation of an intravenous drug infusion or from the accidental injection of epinephrine into a finger when a patient is trying to stop an allergic reaction by self-injecting epinephrine into the arm or other site. The administration of excessive doses of catecholamines may reduce blood flow to vital organs, such as the kidneys, or cause excessive cardiac stimulation that leads to myocardial ischemia or cardiac arrhythmias. The β-adrenergic receptor agonists may cause hyperglycemia secondary to glycogenolysis, and this is usually undesirable in diabetic patients.

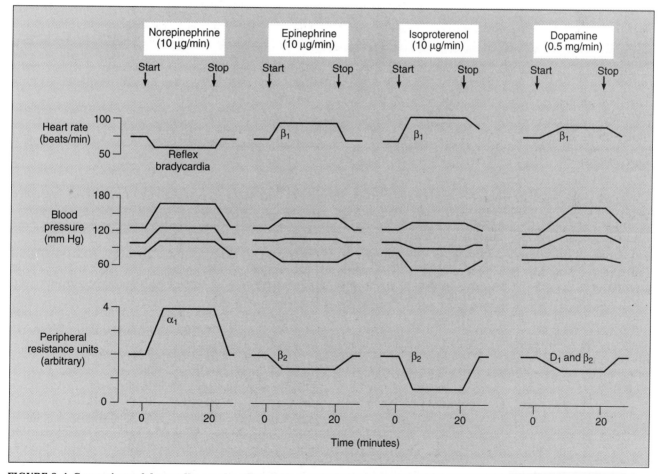

FIGURE 8–4. Comparison of the cardiovascular effects of four catecholamines when a low dose of each drug is given by intravenous infusion. Arrows indicate when the infusion was started and stopped. The blood pressure recordings show systolic, diastolic, and mean arterial pressure. Peripheral resistance is expressed on an arbitrary scale, ranging from 0 to 4 units. The reflex mechanism, adrenergic (α_1, β_1, and β_2) receptors, or dopamine (D_1) receptors responsible for changes in the heart rate and peripheral resistance are illustrated. Norepinephrine increases peripheral resistance and blood pressure, and this leads to reflex bradycardia. Epinephrine increases heart rate while reducing peripheral resistance, and the mean arterial blood pressure increases slightly. Isoproterenol increases the heart rate but significantly lowers peripheral resistance, and the mean arterial pressure declines. Dopamine increases the heart rate (and increases the cardiac output) while lowering vascular resistance, and the mean arterial pressure increases.

Specific Drugs

Catecholamines are used in the treatment of several types of **shock.** Shock is a condition in which the circulation to vital organs is profoundly reduced as a result of inadequate blood volume **(hypovolemic shock),** inadequate cardiac function **(cardiogenic shock),** or inadequate vasomotor tone **(neurogenic shock and septic shock).** Septic shock is associated with massive vasodilation secondary to the production of toxins by pathogenic microorganisms. It is sometimes called "warm shock" to distinguish it from hypovolemic and cardiogenic shock, in which the patient's extremities are usually cold owing to inadequate blood flow. **Anaphylactic shock** is a manifestation of immediate hypersensitivity reactions.

Dopamine is particularly useful in treating **cardiogenic shock** and **septic shock,** and it may be used as an adjunct to fluid administration in the treatment of **hypovolemic shock.** Dopamine is often the preferred catecholamine for treating shock because it stimulates cardiac output while increasing renal blood flow. Dopamine is also used in the treatment of **heart failure.**

In cases of **anaphylactic shock,** epinephrine is the treatment of choice. By producing bronchodilation and increasing blood pressure, it counteracts the effects of histamine that is released during immediate hypersensitivity reactions. Epinephrine is used as a vasoconstrictor to **reduce bleeding** during surgery and to **prolong the action of local anesthetics** by retarding their absorption into the general circulation. Epinephrine is also used as a cardiac stimulant in the treatment of **cardiac arrest** and **ventricular fibrillation.**

Norepinephrine can be used to treat **hypotension** that is caused by decreased peripheral resistance and occurs, for example, in patients undergoing treatment with vasodilators. Although it is sometimes used to treat **shock,** the relatively pure vasoconstrictive effect of norepinephrine is often undesirable in patients with shock, because it may reduce blood flow to vital organs.

Isoproterenol is used to treat refractory **bradycardia** and **atrioventricular block** when other measures have not been successful. Although it has been used to treat **asthma,** selective β_2-adrenergic receptor agonists are usually preferred for this indication because they do not increase the heart rate as much as isoproterenol.

Dobutamine is used as a **cardiac stimulant during heart surgery** and in the short-term management of **acute heart failure** and **cardiogenic shock.**

Noncatecholamines

The structures of representative examples of noncatecholamines are shown in Fig. 8–3B. Because these drugs do not contain a catechol moiety, they are not substrates for COMT. Some of the noncatecholamines are also resistant to degradation by MAO. For this reason, noncatecholamines are effective after oral administration and have a longer duration of action than do the catecholamines.

Phenylephrine

Chemistry and Pharmacokinetics. Phenylephrine is a phenylethylamine (see Fig. 8–3B) and a selective α_1-adrenergic receptor agonist. It is adequately absorbed after oral or topical administration and may also be administered parenterally. The drug is partly metabolized by MAO in the intestine and liver.

Mechanisms and Effects. When phenylephrine activates α_1-adrenergic receptors, the smooth muscles contract. This produces vasoconstriction and increases vascular resistance and blood pressure. Ocular administration of phenylephrine leads to contraction of the iris dilator muscle and dilation of the pupil (mydriasis).

Indications. Phenylephrine is used as a **nasal decongestant** in patients with **viral rhinitis,** an infection that can be caused by more than a hundred serotypes of rhinovirus and is usually referred to as the common cold. It is also used by patients with **allergic rhinitis,** an inflammation of the nasal mucosa that is caused by histamine released from mast cells during allergic reactions. The drug's vasoconstrictive effect on the nasal mucosa reduces vascular congestion and mucus secretion and thereby opens the nasal passages so patients can breathe easier. Both topical and oral preparations are available for this purpose.

In patients with **allergic conjunctivitis,** an inflammation of the eyes associated with hay fever or other allergies, phenylephrine can be used as a topical **ocular decongestant.** The ocular preparation of phenylephrine is also used to induce **mydriasis** and thereby facilitate ophthalmoscopic examination. In contrast to the muscarinic receptor antagonists used for this purpose, such as tropicamide, phenylephrine does not affect the ciliary muscle and cause cycloplegia.

Phenylephrine can be used to treat forms of **hypotension** and **shock** that are caused by decreased peripheral vascular resistance. These include hypotension due to excessive doses of vasodilator drugs, drug-induced shock, and neurogenic shock. Phenylephrine is also used for the **maintenance of blood pressure during surgery.**

Albuterol, Ritodrine, and Terbutaline

Chemistry and Pharmacokinetics. Albuterol (see Fig. 8–3B), ritodrine, and terbutaline are selective β_2-adrenergic receptor agonists that can be administered orally, parenterally, or by inhalation. Their oral bioavailability ranges from 30% to 50% because of their incomplete absorption and hepatic first-pass metabolism. They are partly metabolized to inactive compounds before undergoing renal excretion. About 50% of albuterol, for example, is converted to an inactive sulfate conjugate. To reduce their systemic absorption and adverse effects, albuterol and the related agonists are usually administered by inhalation in the treatment of asthma. The duration of action of these agonists is about 4–6 hours after inhalation or oral administration and is about 2–3 hours after intravenous administration.

Mechanisms, Effects, and Indications. The β₂-adrenergic receptor agonists act by causing smooth muscle relaxation. As discussed in greater detail in Chapter 27, these drugs are helpful in the treatment of **asthma** and other obstructive lung diseases because they produce bronchodilation. They are also helpful in the treatment of **premature labor,** which is defined as labor that begins before the 37th week of gestation and is believed to be due to an imbalance in hormonal regulation caused by physiologic or environmental influences. The administration of one of these agonists to a pregnant woman in premature labor will cause relaxation of the uterus so as to bring the pregnancy as close to term as possible.

The adverse effects of albuterol and other selective β₂-adrenergic receptor agonists include tachycardia, muscle tremor, and nervousness caused by activation of β-adrenergic receptors in the heart, skeletal muscle, and central nervous system.

Imidazolines

Chemistry and Pharmacokinetics. The imidazoline compounds (see Fig. 8–3B) activate α-adrenergic and imidazoline receptors. Some imidazolines are administered by topical ocular or nasal administration, while others are administered by systemic routes. After systemic administration, the imidazolines have a duration of action of several hours and are partly metabolized and excreted in the urine.

Mechanisms, Effects, and Indications. Based on their clinical use, the imidazolines can be divided into three groups. The first group consists of **oxymetazoline** and similar drugs that activate α₁-adrenergic receptors so as to produce vasoconstriction. These drugs are used as topical **nasal and ocular decongestants.** The second group consists of **apraclonidine** and other agents that activate ocular α₂-adrenergic receptors in the ciliary body and thereby reduce the level of aqueous humor secretion. These agents are used to lower intraocular pressure in patients with **chronic open-angle glaucoma,** a condition in which elevated intraocular pressure can damage the optic nerve and eventually cause blindness. The third group consists of **clonidine** and other imidazolines that activate α₂-adrenergic and imidazoline receptors in the central nervous system. The imidazoline receptors are believed to mediate a reduction in sympathetic outflow from the vasomotor center in the medulla. The drugs in this third group are used to treat **chronic hypertension** and are discussed in greater detail in Chapter 10.

The activation of α₂-adrenergic receptors in the central nervous system is believed to be responsible for the sedative and other central nervous system side effects of clonidine and related drugs. Oxymeta-

zoline and similar decongestants may also cause central nervous system and cardiovascular depression if they are absorbed into the systemic circulation and distributed to the brain. For this reason, imidazolines should be used with caution in children under 6 years of age and in the elderly.

INDIRECT-ACTING ADRENERGIC RECEPTOR AGONISTS
Amphetamine and Tyramine

Amphetamine (see Fig. 8–3B) and related compounds increase the Ca²⁺-independent (nonexocytic) release of norepinephrine from sympathetic neurons. After norepinephrine enters the synapse, it activates adrenergic receptors and causes a sympathomimetic effect. By this mechanism, amphetamine produces vasoconstriction, cardiac stimulation, and increased blood pressure. Amphetamine and related drugs also penetrate into the central nervous system and produce central nervous system stimulation. The various **central nervous system effects** are discussed in greater detail in Chapter 24.

Tyramine is a naturally occurring amine found in a number of foods, including bananas. Under normal conditions, tyramine is rapidly degraded by MAO in the gut and liver. In patients receiving MAO inhibitors, however, tyramine may be absorbed from foods in a quantity that is high enough to exert a sympathomimetic effect and increase blood pressure. The interaction between foods containing tyramine and MAO inhibitors is discussed in greater detail in Chapter 22. Tyramine is not used as a drug.

Cocaine

Cocaine, a naturally occurring drug, acts as a local anesthetic and also stimulates the sympathetic nervous system by blocking the neuronal reuptake of norepinephrine at both peripheral and central synapses. The sympathomimetic effects of cocaine are similar to those of amphetamine. Cocaine produces both vasoconstriction and cardiac stimulation and thereby elevates blood pressure. When the drug is used as a local anesthetic, its vasoconstrictive effect serves to retard its absorption into the systemic circulation, and this prolongs its duration of action. However, the vasoconstrictive effect may also cause ischemia and necrosis of the nasal mucosa in people who abuse cocaine. The sympathomimetic effects of cocaine also appear to be responsible for the severe hypertension and cardiac damage that occur in susceptible people who abuse cocaine. The **central nervous system effects** and **local anesthetic effects** of cocaine are discussed further in Chapters 24 and 25, respectively.

MIXED-ACTING ADRENERGIC RECEPTOR AGONISTS

Among the drugs that activate adrenergic receptors via both direct and indirect mechanisms are dopamine (see above), ephedrine, pseudoephedrine, and phenylpropanolamine. These four agents act indirectly by increasing the release of norepinephrine from sympathetic neurons and thereby increasing the concentration of norepinephrine in the synapse.

Ephedrine and Pseudoephedrine

Chemistry and Pharmacokinetics. Ephedrine (see Fig. 8–3B) is a naturally occurring compound obtained from plants of the genus *Ephedra*. It has been used as a natural remedy for centuries and can be purchased in health food stores today. Ephedrine is well absorbed from the gut and has sufficient lipid solubility to enter the central nervous system. It is relatively resistant to metabolism by MAO and COMT and has a duration of action of several hours. Pseudoephedrine is one of the stereoisomers of ephedrine and has been widely used as a decongestant.

Mechanism, Effects, and Indications. Ephedrine and related drugs activate both α- and β-adrenergic receptors by direct and indirect mechanisms. Via the activation of α_1-adrenergic receptors, these drugs produce vasoconstriction. This makes them useful as **nasal decongestants** in the treatment of **viral and allergic rhinitis.** Via the action of β-adrenergic receptors, the drugs produce bronchodilation. Although they have been used as a bronchodilator, a selective β_2-adrenergic receptor agonist such as albuterol is now preferred for this indication.

Side effects of ephedrine and pseudoephedrine include tachycardia, increased blood pressure, and urinary retention. The latter is due to stimulation of the sphincter muscle of the bladder.

Phenylpropanolamine

Phenylpropanolamine is a synthetic drug whose pharmacologic properties are similar to those of ephedrine. It is contained in preparations used for treating **nasal decongestion** in patients with **viral and allergic rhinitis.** Because phenylpropanolamine is a mild central nervous system stimulant, it has also been used as an appetite suppressant.

Summary of Important Points

- Activation of α_1-adrenergic receptors mediates smooth muscle contraction, leading to vasoconstriction, dilation of the pupils, and contraction of the bladder sphincter muscle.
- Activation of α_2-adrenergic receptors inhibits the release of norepinephrine from sympathetic neurons, decreases the secretion of aqueous humor, and decreases the secretion of insulin.
- Activation of β_1-adrenergic receptors produces cardiac stimulation and increases the secretion of renin, whereas activation of β_2-adrenergic receptors mediates smooth muscle relaxation.
- The catecholamines include norepinephrine, epinephrine, isoproterenol, dopamine, and dobutamine. These drugs are rapidly metabolized, must be administered parenterally, and are primarily used to treat cardiac disorders and various types of shock.
- In addition to activating adrenergic receptors, dopamine activates D_1 receptors and thereby increases renal blood flow.
- Noncatecholamines such as phenylephrine and albuterol are resistant to degradation by catechol-*O*-methyltransferase (COMT). They are effective when given orally, have a longer duration of action than do catecholamines, and have a wide range of uses.
- Imidazoline compounds are agents that activate both α-adrenergic and imidazoline receptors. Examples include oxymetazoline, a topical decongestant; clonidine, an antihypertensive agent; and apraclonidine, an agent used in the treatment of glaucoma.
- The indirect-acting adrenergic receptor agonists increase the synaptic concentration of norepinephrine. Amphetamine increases norepinephrine release, whereas cocaine blocks norepinephrine reuptake.
- Mixed-acting agonists have both direct and indirect actions. Ephedrine, pseudoephedrine, and phenylpropanolamine are examples, and they are used as nasal decongestants.

Selected Readings

Bylund, D. B. Pharmacologic characteristics of α_2-adrenergic receptor subtypes. Ann NY Acad Sci 763:1–7, 1995.

Girbes, A. R., and A. J. Smit. Use of dopamine in the ICU: hope, hype, beliefs, and facts. Clin Exp Hypertens 19:191–199, 1997.

Kleerup, E. C. Bronchodilators: new drugs and controversies. Curr Opin Pulm Med 3:17–22, 1997.

Meier-Hellmann, A., and K. Reinhart. Recommendations for the treatment of patients with septic shock. Acta Anaesthesiol Scand Suppl 111:177–180, 1997.

Papatsonis, D. N., et al. Nifedipine and ritodrine in the management of preterm labor: a randomized multicenter trial. Obstet Gynecol 90:230–234, 1997.

CHAPTER NINE

ADRENERGIC RECEPTOR

ANTAGONISTS

CLASSIFICATION OF ADRENERGIC RECEPTOR ANTAGONISTS

α-ADRENERGIC RECEPTOR ANTAGONISTS
Nonselective α-blockers
- Phenoxybenzamine
- Phentolamine

Selective α_1-blockers
- Doxazosin
- Prazosin
- Terazosin

β-ADRENERGIC RECEPTOR ANTAGONISTS
Nonselective β-blockers
- Nadolol
- Pindolol
- Propranolol
- Timolol

Selective β_1-blockers
- Acebutolol
- Atenolol
- Esmolol
- Metoprolol

α- AND β-ADRENERGIC RECEPTOR ANTAGONISTS
- Carvedilol
- Labetalol

OVERVIEW

Excessive sympathetic nervous system activity is a pathogenic factor in a number of diseases, including common cardiovascular disorders such as hypertension, angina pectoris, and cardiac arrhythmias. Drugs that reduce sympathetic stimulation are called **sympatholytics** and are used in the management of cardiovascular diseases and other diseases such as glaucoma, migraine headache, and urinary retention. The most important group of sympatholytics consists of the adrenergic receptor antagonists. Other drugs that have a sympatholytic effect include the ganglionic blocking agents (discussed in Chapter 7) and the sympathetic neuronal blocking agents (discussed in Chapters 5 and 10).

Adrenergic receptor antagonists may block α-adrenergic receptors, β-adrenergic receptors, or both. The **therapeutic effects** of the antagonists are primarily due to blockade of α_1 or β_1 receptors, whereas the **adverse effects** tend to be related to blockade of α_2 or β_2 receptors. Drugs that selectively block either α_1 or β_1 receptors have been developed in an effort to avoid the adverse effects caused by α_2 or β_2 receptor blockade. Blockade of α_1 receptors relaxes vascular and other smooth muscles in tissues innervated by the sympathetic nervous system, whereas blockade of β_1 receptors reduces sympathetic stimulation of the heart.

α-ADRENERGIC RECEPTOR ANTAGONISTS

The α-adrenergic receptor antagonists, or **α-blockers,** can be distinguished on the basis of their selectivity for α receptor subtypes and by their noncompetitive or competitive blockade of α receptors.

Nonselective α-Blockers

Agents that block both α_1 and α_2 receptors are called nonselective α-blockers. Phenoxybenzamine and phentolamine are examples. While phenoxybenzamine is a noncompetitive antagonist, phentolamine is a competitive receptor antagonist.

Phenoxybenzamine

Chemistry and Mechanisms. Phenoxybenzamine is a haloalkylamine (Fig. 9–1A) whose chemical structure and mechanisms of action are similar to those of cyclophosphamide and other nitrogen mustard alkylating agents that are used in cancer chemotherapy. In the body, phenoxybenzamine undergoes spontaneous chemical transformation to an active electrophilic carbonium ion. The carbonium ion forms a stable covalent bond with the α-adrenergic receptor, and this results in the noncompetitive antagonism of epinephrine and other adrenergic agonists (Fig. 9–2).

Pharmacokinetics. When phenoxybenzamine is administered orally, it exhibits a gradual onset of action. This is because time is needed to form

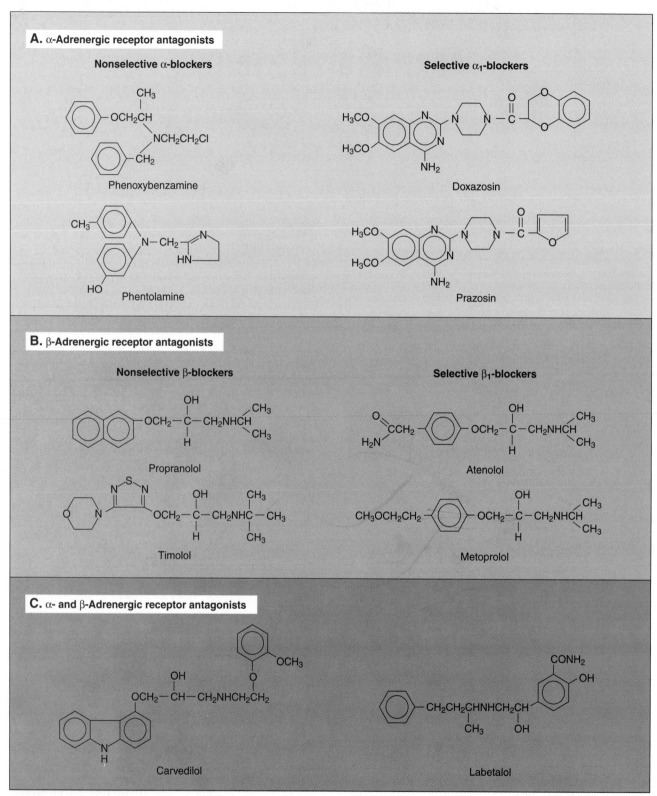

FIGURE 9–1. Structures of selected adrenergic receptor antagonists. (A) The α-adrenergic receptor antagonists include phenoxybenzamine, which is a haloalkylamine; phentolamine, which is an imidazoline; and doxazosin and prazosin, which are quinazolines. While phenoxybenzamine and phentolamine are nonselective α-blockers, doxazosin and prazosin are selective α_1-blockers. **(B)** The β-adrenergic receptor antagonists include propranolol and timolol, which are nonselective β-blockers, and atenolol and metoprolol, which are selective β_1-blockers. Each of these drugs contains an isopropyl or isobutyl group on the amine nitrogen, which confers an affinity for β-adrenergic receptors. **(C)** The α- and β-adrenergic receptor antagonists include carvedilol, which is an indole derivative, and labetalol, which is a benzamide. These agents block α_1-, β_1-, and β_2-adrenergic receptors.

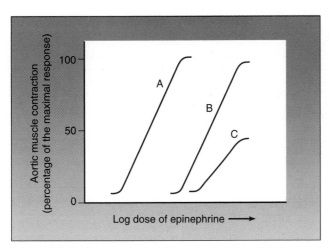

FIGURE 9–2. Competitive and noncompetitive blockade of epinephrine-induced aortic smooth muscle contraction by phentolamine and phenoxybenzamine. Three dose-response curves are compared. A is the curve of epinephrine alone. B is the curve of epinephrine in the presence of phentolamine. Because phentolamine is a competitive α-adrenergic receptor antagonist, epinephrine is able to surmount its effect. C is the curve of epinephrine in the presence of phenoxybenzamine. Because phenoxybenzamine is a noncompetitive antagonist, it reduces the maximal effect of epinephrine.

the active intermediate and bond covalently with α-adrenergic receptors. Phenoxybenzamine is metabolized by dealkylation, is excreted in the urine and bile, and has a half-life of about 24 hours. The drug has a duration of action of 3–4 days because of its stable covalent bonding with α-adrenergic receptors.

Effects and Indications. Because of its noncompetitive and relatively irreversible blockade of α-adrenergic receptors, phenoxybenzamine produces what has been called a **chemical sympathectomy.** It decreases vascular resistance; increases blood flow to the skin, mucosae, and abdominal viscera; and lowers both the supine and the standing blood pressure. It also relaxes smooth muscle in the urinary bladder neck and prostate.

As shown in Table 9–1, phenoxybenzamine is used to treat **hypertensive episodes** in patients with **pheochromocytoma.** Because this tumor of the adrenal medulla secretes huge amounts of catecholamines, patients have extremely high blood pressure and must be treated with an agent such as phenoxybenzamine to control hypertension until surgery can be performed to remove the tumor. Although phenoxybenzamine is sometimes administered to treat **urinary retention** in patients with **benign prostatic hyperplasia** and other disorders of the urinary bladder, the selective α₁-blockers (discussed below) can also be used for this purpose and generally cause fewer adverse effects than phenoxybenzamine.

Phentolamine

Chemistry and Pharmacokinetics. Phentolamine is an imidazoline compound (see Fig. 9–1A) that is structurally related to oxymetazoline and

other agents in the imidazoline class of adrenergic receptor agonists. After intravenous administration of phentolamine, the onset of action is immediate, and the duration of action is 10–15 minutes. After intramuscular or subcutaneous administration, the onset of action is 15–20 minutes, and the duration is 3–4 hours. The drug is chiefly metabolized in the liver before excretion in the urine.

Mechanisms, Effects, and Indications. Phentolamine is a competitive receptor antagonist (see Fig. 9–2) that produces vasodilation, decreases peripheral vascular resistance, and decreases blood pressure. It is used in the diagnosis and treatment of **hypertensive episodes** due to **pheochromocytoma.** In addition, it is used in the treatment of **necrosis and ischemia** due to extravasation or accidental injection of epinephrine or other vasopressor amines. For example, if a patient who carries an epinephrine autoinjector for use in treating acute allergic reactions were to accidentally inject his or her finger and thereby cause ischemia, the patient could be treated by injecting phentolamine into the same site where epinephrine was injected. The phentolamine would competitively block the α-adrenergic receptor stimulation and vasoconstriction produced by the epinephrine.

Phentolamine and other nonselective α-blockers are not useful in treating chronic hypertension, partly because they produce too much reflex tachycardia and are associated with other adverse effects, such as dizziness, headache, and nasal congestion. The adverse effects are mostly caused by excessive vasodilation.

Selective α₁-Blockers

Agents that selectively antagonize α₁-adrenergic receptors are referred to as selective α₁-blockers. Examples include **doxazosin, prazosin,** and **terazosin.** These drugs were developed in the search for α-blockers that could be used to treat chronic hypertension.

Drug Properties

Chemistry and Pharmacokinetics. Doxazosin, prazosin, and terazosin are quinazoline compounds that have similar pharmacologic properties. They are administered orally and undergo varying amounts of first-pass hepatic metabolism. The drugs are highly bound to plasma proteins, including α₁-acid glycoprotein, and they are excreted in the bile, urine, and feces.

Mechanisms, Effects, and Indications. The selective α₁-blockers relax vascular and other smooth muscles, including those of the urinary bladder and prostate. Because they produce vasodilation and decrease blood pressure, they are used to treat **chronic essential (primary) hypertension.** The cardiovascular effects of α- and β-blockers in patients with hypertension are depicted in Fig. 9–3.

**TABLE 9–1. Mechanisms, Pharmacologic Effects, and Clinical Uses
of Adrenergic Receptor Antagonists***

Drug	Mechanism of Action	Pharmacologic Effect	Clinical Use
α-Blockers			
Doxazosin	Competitive α_1-blocker.	Causes vasodilation; decreases vascular resistance and blood pressure; and relaxes bladder neck and prostate.	Hypertension; urinary retention due to benign prostatic hyperplasia.
Phenoxybenzamine	Noncompetitive α_1- and α_2-blocker.	Same as doxazosin.	Hypertensive episodes due to pheochromocytoma; urinary retention due to benign prostatic hyperplasia.
Phentolamine	Competitive α_1- and α_2-blocker.	Causes vasodilation; decreases vascular resistance and blood pressure.	Hypertensive episodes due to pheochromocytoma; necrosis and ischemia after injection of α-adrenergic receptor agonists.
Prazosin	Competitive α_1-blocker.	Same as doxazosin.	Hypertension; urinary retention due to benign prostatic hyperplasia.
Terazosin	Competitive α_1-blocker.	Same as doxazosin.	Hypertension; urinary retention due to benign prostatic hyperplasia.
β-Blockers			
Acebutolol	β_1-Blocker with ISA and MSA.	Decreases cardiac rate, output, AV node conduction, and O_2 demand; decreases blood pressure.	Hypertension; cardiac arrhythmias.
Atenolol	β_1-Blocker.	Same as acebutolol.	Hypertension; angina pectoris; acute myocardial infarction.
Esmolol	β_1-Blocker.	Same as acebutolol.	Acute supraventricular tachycardia.
Metoprolol	β_1-Blocker with MSA.	Same as acebutolol.	Hypertension; angina pectoris; acute myocardial infarction.
Nadolol	β_1- and β_2-Blocker.	Same as acebutolol.	Hypertension; angina pectoris; migraine headache.
Pindolol	β_1- and β_2-Blocker with ISA and MSA.	Same as acebutolol.	Hypertension.
Propranolol	β_1- and β_2-Blocker with MSA.	Same as acebutolol.	Hypertension; angina pectoris; cardiac arrhythmias; hypertrophic subaortic stenosis; essential tremor; migraine headache; acute thyrotoxicosis; acute myocardial infarction; pheochromocytoma.
Timolol	β_1- and β_2-Blocker.	Decreases cardiac rate, output, AV node conduction, and O_2 demand; decreases blood pressure; decreases intraocular pressure.	Hypertension; acute myocardial infarction; migraine headache; glaucoma.
α- and β-Blockers			
Carvedilol	β_1- and β_2-Blocker; α_1-blocker.	Causes vasodilation; decreases heart rate and blood pressure in patients with hypertension; increases cardiac output in patients with heart failure.	Hypertension; heart failure.
Labetalol	β_1- and β_2-Blocker with MSA; α_1-blocker.	Causes vasodilation; decreases heart rate and blood pressure.	Hypertension.

*ISA = intrinsic sympathomimetic activity (partial agonist activity); MSA = membrane-stabilizing activity (local anesthetic activity); and AV = atrioventricular.

The selective α_1-blockers do not cause as much reflex tachycardia as do phentolamine and other agents that nonselectively block both α_1 and α_2 receptors. This is because blockade of α_2 receptors on sympathetic neurons prevents feedback inhibition of norepinephrine release and thereby leads to increased activation of cardiac β_1 receptors and tachycardia (Fig. 9–4). The use of prazosin and other selective α_1-blockers for treating hypertension is discussed in greater detail in Chapter 10.

The ability of selective α_1-blockers to relax the smooth muscle of the bladder neck and prostate has made them useful in treating **urinary retention** due to **benign prostatic hyperplasia** and other conditions. In patients with prostatic hyperplasia, the enlarged prostate gland restricts the outflow of urine from the bladder. By relaxing the smooth muscle, the selective α_1-blockers reduce the obstruction to urine outflow during micturition. This improves the urine flow rate, decreases the amount of urine retained, and reduces the need to urinate at night (Fig. 9–5).

The adverse effects of selective α_1-blockers are mostly due to excessive vasodilation, which may cause hypotension, dizziness, fainting, reflex tachy-

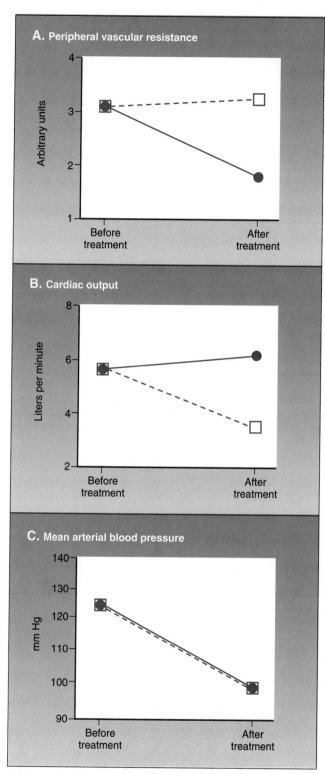

FIGURE 9–3. Cardiovascular effects of α_1-adrenergic receptor antagonists (solid line) and β_1-adrenergic receptor antagonists (dotted line) in patients with hypertension. (A) The α_1-blockers reduce peripheral vascular resistance. The β_1-blockers may cause a slight increase in peripheral vascular resistance, owing to reflex mechanisms. **(B)** The β_1-blockers reduce cardiac output. The α_1-blockers may increase cardiac output by decreasing cardiac afterload and aortic impedance to ventricular ejection of blood. **(C)** Both α_1-blockers and β_1-blockers reduce mean arterial blood pressure.

cardia, palpitations, and edema. The drugs often produce a greater effect on blood pressure when they are initially administered, leading to what has been called **first-dose syncope.** To prevent this phenomenon, patients should be given low doses when they begin treatment. Thereafter, doses may be increased to obtain the desired effect.

Specific Drugs

Prazosin was the first selective α_1-blocker. It undergoes considerable first-pass metabolism and is extensively metabolized before renal and biliary excretion. Its half-life is about 3 hours, and its duration of action is about 6 hours.

Doxazosin is a newer selective α_1-blocker. Its bioavailability and metabolism are similar to those of prazosin, but its half-life is 15 hours, and its duration of action is about 30 hours.

Terazosin has a higher oral bioavailability than other selective α_1-blockers. Its half-life is about 10 hours, and the duration of its pharmacologic effects is about 20 hours.

β-ADRENERGIC RECEPTOR ANTAGONISTS

The β-adrenergic receptor antagonists, or **β-blockers,** can be categorized as nonselective or selective.

Nonselective β-Blockers

The nonselective β-blockers were the first β-blockers to be developed for clinical use. In addition to blocking β_1 receptors in heart tissue, they block β_2 receptors in smooth muscle, liver, and other tissues. Examples include **nadolol, pindolol, propranolol,** and **timolol.**

Drug Properties

Chemistry and Pharmacokinetics. The β-adrenergic receptor antagonists are structural analogues of β-adrenergic receptor agonists. Fig. 9–1B shows the chemical structures and Table 9–2 outlines the pharmacologic properties of various β-blockers. All of the nonselective β-blockers can be administered orally, and propranolol can also be administered parenterally.

Mechanisms and Effects. The nonselective β-blockers competitively block the effects of norepinephrine and other adrenergic agonists at β_1 and β_2 receptors. In addition, some of them exhibit intrinsic sympathomimetic activity (ISA) and membrane-stabilizing activity, as outlined in Table 9–2 and defined below.

Blockade of β_1 receptors reduces sympathetic stimulation of the heart and thereby produces a negative chronotropic, inotropic, and dromotropic effect. Because the β-blockers reduce cardiac output and blood pressure (see Fig. 9–3), they can be used to treat arterial hypertension. In the kidneys, β_1 receptor blockade reduces the secretion of renin from the

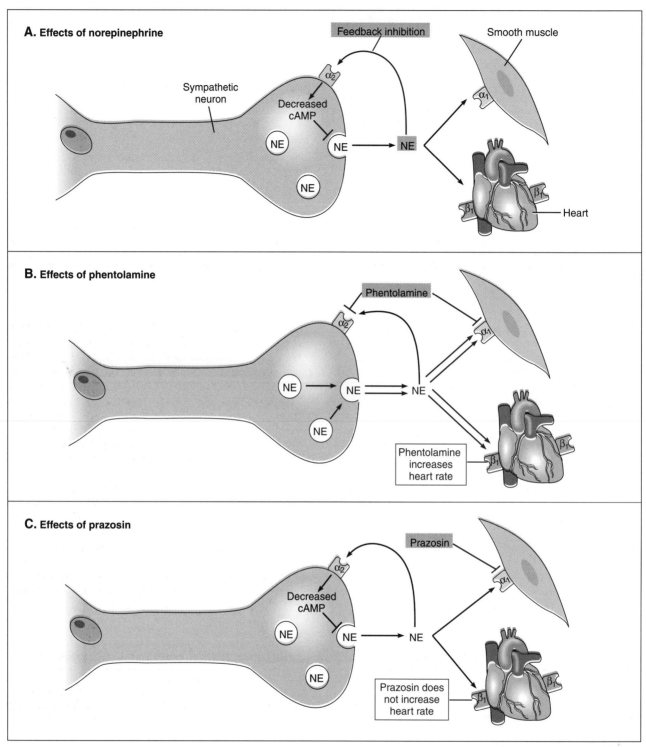

FIGURE 9–4. A comparison of the effects of norepinephrine, phentolamine, and prazosin on heart rate. (A) Norepinephrine (NE) activates presynaptic α_2-adrenergic receptors (α_2), and this inhibits the formation of cyclic adenosine monophosphate (cAMP) and decreases the release of NE. **(B)** Phentolamine blocks α_2 receptor–mediated inhibition of NE release. This increases the stimulation of cardiac β_1-adrenergic receptors (β_1) and results in tachycardia. **(C)** Prazosin, a selective α_1-blocker, does not block α_2 receptor–mediated inhibition of NE release. Therefore, prazosin causes less tachycardia than does phentolamine. α_1 = α_1-adrenergic receptors.

juxtaglomerular cells. In the eye, receptor blockade reduces aqueous humor secretion and intraocular pressure.

Blockade of β_2 receptors produces several effects that may lead to adverse reactions in some patients receiving β-blockers, such as patients with asthma or diabetes. In the lungs, antagonism of β_2 receptors may cause bronchoconstriction in patients with asthma. These patients depend on the bronchodilating effect of endogenous epinephrine to prevent bronchospasm, so agents that block β_2 receptors should be avoided or used with great caution. If a

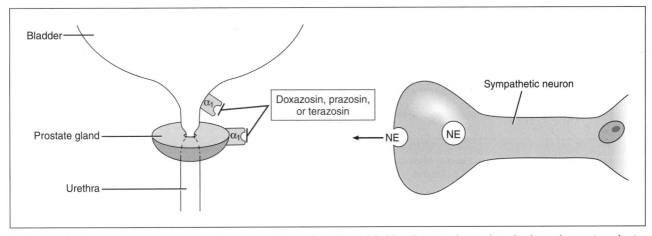

FIGURE 9–5. Effects of α_1-adrenergic receptor antagonists on the urinary bladder. Prostatic hyperplasia leads to obstruction of urine outflow from the bladder through the urethra. An α_1-blocker, such as doxazosin, prazosin, or terazosin, will relax smooth muscle in the prostate and bladder neck and thereby facilitate micturition in patients with prostatic hyperplasia. $\alpha_1 = \alpha_1$-adrenergic receptors; and NE = norepinephrine.

β-blocker is required to treat an asthmatic patient, a selective β_1-blocker should be used. In the liver, β_2 receptor blockade inhibits epinephrine-stimulated glycogenolysis and may thereby slow the recovery of blood glucose after a hypoglycemic episode in a patient with diabetes. The β-blockers may also mask some of the early signs of hypoglycemia, such as tachycardia and sweating, which would otherwise alert the diabetic patient to this problem. For these reasons, β-blockers should be used cautiously in patients with diabetes and particularly in those who have insulin-dependent diabetes and are susceptible to hypoglycemic episodes associated with excessive insulin administration.

Specific Drugs

Tables 9–1 and 9–2 compare the effects, uses, and properties of four nonselective β-blockers: nadolol, pindolol, propranolol, and timolol.

Of these four drugs, only pindolol has **intrinsic sympathomimetic activity (ISA),** or **partial agonist activity,** which enables it to exert a weak agonist effect on β receptors. This effect is observed when the patient is resting and sympathetic tone is low, and it may result in a smaller reduction in heart rate than that caused by β-blockers without ISA. When sympathetic tone is high, pindolol acts as a competitive receptor antagonist to inhibit sympathetic stimulation of the heart in the same manner as other β-blockers.

Although pindolol and propranolol exhibit **membrane-stabilizing activity,** or **local anesthetic activity,** nadolol and timolol do not. Drugs with local anesthetic activity are able to block sodium channels in nerves and heart tissue and thereby slow conduction velocity.

Pindolol is used only for the treatment of **hypertension.** In contrast, propranolol has many clinical applications. Propranolol is used, for exam-

TABLE 9–2. Pharmacokinetic Properties of Drugs That Cause β-Adrenergic Receptor Blockade

Drug	Lipid Solubility	Oral Bioavailability	Elimination Half-Life	Intrinsic Sympathomimetic Activity	Membrane-Stabilizing Activity
Nonselective β-blockers					
Nadolol	Low	35%	15–20 hours	None	None
Pindolol	Medium	75%	3–4 hours	Medium	Low
Propranolol	High	25%	4–6 hours	None	High
Timolol	Medium	50%	4–6 hours	None	None
Selective β_1-blockers					
Acebutolol	Medium	40%	10–12 hours*	Low	Medium
Atenolol	Low	50%	6–7 hours	None	None
Esmolol	Unknown	—	10 minutes	None	None
Metoprolol	Medium	40%	3–4 hours	None	Low
α- and β-Blockers					
Carvedilol	Unknown	30%	6–8 hours	None	None
Labetalol	Unknown	20%	6–8 hours	None	Low

*Includes half-life of active metabolite.

ple, to treat patients with **hypertension, angina pectoris,** or **cardiac arrhythmias** (conditions discussed in detail in the chapters of Section III); patients with **hypertrophic subaortic stenosis** (a form of hypertrophic cardiomyopathy, a condition that impedes the ejection of blood from the ventricles and reduces cardiac output); and patients with **essential tremor** (a benign condition characterized by involuntary trembling of the hands). Propranolol is also used in the prevention of **migraine headache** and as adjunct therapy in the treatment of **acute thyrotoxicosis, acute myocardial infarction,** and **pheochromocytoma.** Patients with thyrotoxicosis often experience tachycardia and palpitations because thyroid hormones increase the effects of sympathetic stimulation on the heart. Propranolol is used to reduce these symptoms until the underlying thyroid disorder can be treated. Propranolol and other β-blockers are frequently administered to patients with acute myocardial infarction because clinical trials have shown that β-blockers reduce the incidence of sudden death and mortality in these patients. In patients with pheochromocytoma, propranolol is used to reduce cardiac stimulation caused by circulating catecholamines released from this adrenal medullary tumor.

Propranolol was the first β-blocker approved for clinical use, and it is distinguished by its high lipid solubility and central nervous system penetration, which may cause a higher incidence of central nervous system side effects in some patients. Propranolol has a greater local anesthetic effect than other β-blockers, but the clinical significance of this activity is uncertain.

Nadolol is a long-acting drug that is largely excreted unchanged in the urine. It is primarily used for the treatment of **hypertension** and **angina pectoris** and for the prevention of **migraine headache.**

Timolol is administered orally to treat **hypertension,** to reduce the risk of death in patients with **acute myocardial infarction,** and to prevent **migraine headache.** Timolol was the first β-blocker to be used for the treatment of **glaucoma** and is available as an ophthalmic solution for topical ocular administration. The drug is absorbed through the cornea and penetrates to the ciliary body. In glaucoma, which is discussed in greater detail in Chapter 6, β-blockers reduce aqueous humor secretion and intraocular pressure. Timolol was selected for ophthalmic use partly because it does not have membrane-stabilizing activity and therefore does not anesthetize the cornea when instilled into the eye.

Selective β₁-Blockers
Drug Properties

Examples of selective β₁-blockers include **acebutolol, atenolol, esmolol,** and **metoprolol.** These drugs have a greater affinity for β₁ receptors than for β₂ receptors. Because β₁ receptors are primarily located in cardiac tissue, the β₁-blockers are also known as **cardioselective β-blockers.**

In comparison with the nonselective β-blockers, the selective β₁-blockers produce less bronchoconstriction and other β₂ receptor–mediated effects. However, their selectivity for β₁ receptors is not absolute, and β₂ receptor blockade increases as the dosage increases. For this reason, selective β₁-blockers should be used with caution in patients who have asthma.

Specific Drugs

Tables 9–1 and 9–2 compare the effects, uses, and properties of four selective β₁-blockers.

Acebutolol is a cardioselective β-blocker with a low degree of ISA. It is converted to an active metabolite, *N*-acetyl acebutolol, which has a longer half-life than the parent compound and accounts for the drug's relatively long duration of action. Acebutolol is administered orally to treat **hypertension** and **cardiac arrhythmias** such as ventricular premature beats.

Atenolol shows less variability in its oral absorption than other β-blockers and is excreted largely unchanged in the urine. It also has a lower lipid solubility and has been associated with a lower incidence of central nervous system side effects, such as vivid dreams, tiredness, and depression. Atenolol is administered orally or parenterally and is primarily used in the treatment of **hypertension, angina pectoris,** and **acute myocardial infarction.**

Esmolol is administered intravenously to treat **acute supraventricular tachycardia** in cases, for example, when this cardiac arrhythmia occurs during surgery. Esmolol is rapidly metabolized to inactive compounds by plasma esterase enzymes and has a much shorter half-life than other β-blockers.

Metoprolol is used in the treatment of **hypertension, angina pectoris,** and **acute myocardial infarction.** It may be administered orally or parenterally, and it is extensively metabolized by cytochrome P450 enzymes before undergoing renal excretion.

α- AND β-ADRENERGIC RECEPTOR ANTAGONISTS

Carvedilol and **labetalol** are agents that block both α- and β-adrenergic receptors. Their chemical structures, effects, uses, and properties are shown in Fig. 9–1C and Tables 9–1 and 9–2.

In addition to causing β₁ and β₂ receptor blockade, carvedilol has a vasodilative effect that is partly due to α₁ receptor blockade. Carvedilol decreases blood pressure and has been used in the treatment of **hypertension.** As discussed further in Chapter 12, it also decreases cardiac afterload and increases cardiac output in patients with **heart failure.**

Labetalol is a nonselective β-blocker and a selective α₁-blocker that is primarily used in the treatment of **hypertension.** It is 5–10 times more potent as a β-blocker than as an α-blocker, but both actions are believed to contribute to its antihypertensive effect. Labetalol decreases the heart rate and cardiac output as a result of β_1 receptor blockade, and it decreases peripheral vascular resistance as a result of α_1 receptor blockade.

Summary of Important Points

- The α-adrenergic receptor antagonists (α-blockers) relax smooth muscle and decrease vascular resistance, whereas the β-adrenergic receptor antagonists (β-blockers) reduce the heart rate and cardiac output. Both α-blockers and β-blockers reduce blood pressure.
- The nonselective α-blockers include phenoxybenzamine (a noncompetitive blocker) and phentolamine (a competitive blocker). These drugs block both α_1 and α_2 receptors and are primarily used to treat hypertensive episodes due to pheochromocytoma.
- The selective α_1-blockers include doxazosin, prazosin, and terazosin. These drugs are used in the treatment of chronic essential (primary) hypertension and in the treatment of urinary retention due to benign prostatic hyperplasia and other conditions.
- The nonselective β-blockers antagonize both β_1 and β_2 receptors and include nadolol, pindolol, propranolol, and timolol. In comparison with other β-blockers, pindolol has a higher degree of intrinsic sympathomimetic activity (partial agonist activity), and propranolol has a higher degree of membrane-stabilizing activity (local anesthetic activity).
- The selective β_1-blockers include acebutolol, atenolol, esmolol, and metoprolol. These drugs cause less bronchoconstriction than do nonselective β-blockers.
- The β-blockers have a variety of clinical applications, including the prevention of migraine headache and the treatment of hypertension, angina pectoris, cardiac arrhythmias, and glaucoma.

Selected Readings

Bousquet, P., L. Monassier, and J. Feldman. Autonomic nervous system as a target for cardiovascular drugs. Clin Exp Pharmacol Physiol 25:446–448, 1998.

Dunn, C. J., et al. Carvedilol: a reappraisal of its pharmacological properties and therapeutic use in cardiovascular disorders. Drugs 54:161–185, 1997.

Hieble, J. P., and R. R. Ruffolo. The use of α-adrenoceptor antagonists in the pharmacological management of benign prostatic hypertrophy: an overview. Pharmacol Res 33:145–160, 1996.

Lepor, H., et al. Doxazosin for benign prostatic hyperplasia: long-term efficacy and safety in hypertensive and normotensive patients. J Urol 157:525–530, 1997.

Sand, J., et al. Preoperative treatment and survival of patients with pheochromocytomas. Ann Chir Gynaecol 86:230–232, 1997.

Schobel, H. P., et al. Treatment and posttreatment effects of α- versus β-receptor blockers on left ventricular structure and function in essential hypertension. Am Heart J 132:1004–1009, 1996.

Silberstein, S. D. Preventive treatment of migraine: an overview. Cephalalgia 17:67–72, 1997.

SECTION III

CARDIOVASCULAR, RENAL,

AND HEMATOLOGIC

PHARMACOLOGY

CHAPTER TEN

ANTIHYPERTENSIVE DRUGS

CLASSIFICATION OF ANTIHYPERTENSIVE DRUGS

DIURETICS
Thiazide and related diuretics
- Hydrochlorothiazide, indapamide, and metolazone

Loop diuretics
- Bumetanide and furosemide

Potassium-sparing diuretics
- Amiloride, spironolactone, and triamterene

SYMPATHOLYTICS
Adrenergic receptor antagonists
- Atenolol, doxazosin, labetalol, metoprolol, nadolol, phenoxybenzamine, pindolol, prazosin, propranolol, and terazosin

Centrally acting drugs
- Clonidine, guanabenz, guanfacine, and methyldopa

Neuronal blocking agents
- Guanethidine and reserpine

Ganglionic blocking agents
- Trimethaphan

ANGIOTENSIN INHIBITORS
Angiotensin-converting enzyme inhibitors
- Benazepril, captopril, enalapril, enalaprilat, fosinopril, lisinopril, quinapril, and ramipril

Angiotensin receptor antagonists
- Losartan and valsartan

VASODILATORS
Calcium channel blockers
- Amlodipine, diltiazem, felodipine, isradipine, nicardipine, nifedipine, and verapamil

Other vasodilators
- Hydralazine, minoxidil, and nitroprusside

OVERVIEW
Hypertension

An estimated 50 million people in the USA have hypertension, commonly defined as a sustained systolic blood pressure of 140 mm Hg or higher or a sustained diastolic blood pressure of 90 mm Hg or higher. About 95% of the cases of hypertension are considered to be **primary (essential) hypertension,** while the remainder are classified as **secondary hypertension.** Although the cause of primary hypertension in any specific patient is usually unknown, numerous genetic and environmental factors have been associated with it. These include obesity, sedentary life-style, excessive dietary sodium intake by individuals with salt sensitivity, excessive intake of alcohol, and stress. Secondary hypertension is most often due to renal disease or endocrine abnormalities (such as increased estrogen, aldosterone, or catecholamine levels), and these causes can often be corrected by medication or surgery.

As shown in Table 10–1, there are **four stages of hypertension,** ranging from mild (stage 1) to very severe (stage 4). Over a long period of time, an increased arterial pressure damages blood vessels, accelerates **atherosclerosis,** and produces **left ventricular hypertrophy.** The rate at which these changes occur is proportional to the severity of hypertension. Eventually, the abnormalities contribute to the development of **ischemic heart disease, stroke, heart failure,** and **renal failure,** which are the most common causes of death in hypertensive patients.

Over the past 20 years, health professionals and public officials have increased their efforts to educate the public about the hazards of untreated hypertension, and this has led to a 55% increase in the number of hypertensive individuals who are aware of their condition and treat it effectively via life-style modifications, pharmacologic agents, and other means. The effective treatment of hypertension appears to be one of the factors that has contributed to a 57% reduction in the incidence of stroke and a 50% reduction in the number of deaths due to coronary artery disease during the past 2 decades.

Regulation of Blood Pressure

Blood pressure is regulated primarily by the **sympathetic nervous system** and the **kidneys** through their influence on cardiac output and peripheral vascular resistance.

Cardiac output, which is the product of stroke volume and heart rate, is increased by sympathetic stimulation via activation of β-adrenergic receptors in the heart. Cardiac output is also influenced by the kidneys via their regulation of blood volume, which is

TABLE 10–1. Blood Pressure Classification and Follow-Up Recommendations*

Category	Systolic Blood Pressure (mm Hg)	Diastolic Blood Pressure (mm Hg)	Follow-Up Recommendations
Normal blood pressure	<130	<85	Check again in 2 years.
High normal blood pressure	130–139	85–89	Check again in 1 year.
Hypertension			
Stage 1 (mild)	140–159	90–99	Confirm within 2 months.
Stage 2 (moderate)	160–179	100–109	Evaluate within 1 month.
Stage 3 (severe)	180–209	110–119	Evaluate in <1 week.
Stage 4 (very severe)	≥210	≥120	Evaluate immediately.

*Data pertain to persons who are 18 years or older, are not acutely ill, and are not taking antihypertensive drugs. When systolic and diastolic pressures fall into different categories, the higher category should be used to classify the patient's stage of hypertension. In addition to classifying hypertension on the basis of average blood pressure levels, the clinician should indicate the presence or absence of target organ damage (such as left ventricular hypertrophy) and other cardiovascular risk factors (such as diabetes or hypercholesterolemia).

one of the factors determining the cardiac filling pressure and stroke volume.

Peripheral vascular resistance (PVR) is chiefly determined by the resistance to blood flow through the arterioles, whose cross-sectional area depends on arteriolar smooth muscle tone in the various vascular beds. Via activation of α-adrenergic receptors, the sympathetic nervous system stimulates arteriolar smooth muscle contraction, and this leads to vasoconstriction. Several blood-borne substances, including vasopressin and angiotensin II, produce vasoconstriction. In addition, adenosine, serotonin, endothelin, prostaglandins, and a number of other substances that are produced locally in various tissues have an effect on arteriolar smooth muscle tone. These substances serve to regulate blood flow through the tissues, and they may also affect systemic arterial pressure.

The sympathetic nervous system provides **short-term regulation** of blood pressure through the **baroreceptor reflex.** This reflex modulates sympathetic stimulation of cardiac output and PVR and adjusts blood pressure in response to postural changes and altered physical activity. The kidneys are primarily responsible for the **long-term control** of blood pressure, via regulation of plasma volume and the renin-angiotensin-aldosterone axis. By these mechanisms, the sympathetic system and kidneys maintain arterial blood pressure within a fairly narrow range when a person is at rest, and they adjust blood pressure appropriately in response to postural changes and physical activity.

In normotensive individuals, an increase in blood pressure leads to a proportional increase in sodium and water excretion by the kidneys, so that blood volume is reduced and blood pressure returns to its normal "set point." In hypertensive patients, the set point at which blood pressure is controlled is higher than normal; the regulation of blood pressure is defective; and an increase in blood pressure is not followed by a proportional increase in sodium and water excretion by the kidneys. Although studies have shown that PVR is elevated in most hypertensive patients, it is not clear whether this is the cause or the result of hypertension.

Sites and Effects of Antihypertensive Drug Action

The four major categories of antihypertensive drugs are the diuretics, sympatholytics, angiotensin inhibitors, and vasodilators. Subcategories and examples are listed at the beginning of the chapter. The various antihypertensive drugs lower blood pressure through actions exerted on one or more of the following sites: kidneys, sympathetic nervous system, renin-angiotensin-aldosterone axis, or vascular smooth muscle (Fig. 10–1).

Antihypertensive drugs can be characterized in terms of their cardiovascular effects (Table 10–2) and their pharmacologic effects on serum potassium and cholesterol measurements, which are important **cardiovascular risk factors** (Table 10–3). They can also be characterized in terms of the **compensatory mechanisms** invoked by their hypotensive effect. The compensatory mechanisms tend to return blood pressure to the pretreatment level and include reflex tachycardia, fluid retention by the kidneys, and activation of the renin-angiotensin-aldosterone axis. Drugs that cause vasodilation tend to invoke compensatory mechanisms to a greater extent than do drugs that suppress cardiac output, cause diuresis, or inhibit angiotensin. For this reason, vasodilators are often combined with other types of drugs that prevent compensatory responses.

While most antihypertensive drugs are taken orally on a long-term basis, some are administered parenterally for the management of **hypertensive emergencies,** which are defined as situations in which the patient's diastolic blood pressure is greater than 120 mm Hg and there is evidence of target organ damage. In these situations, it is important to gradually reduce the diastolic blood pressure to a safe level, usually between 100 and 120 mm Hg, in order to prevent damage to vital organs such as the brain and heart. Nitroprusside, a vasodilator, is frequently used to treat hypertensive emergencies. Other drugs that are used in these emergencies include clonidine, hydralazine, labetalol, methyldopa, nicardipine, nitroglycerin, and trimethaphan.

DIURETICS

Chapter 13 provides detailed information about the various classes of diuretics and their uses, mechanisms of action, and pharmacologic proper-

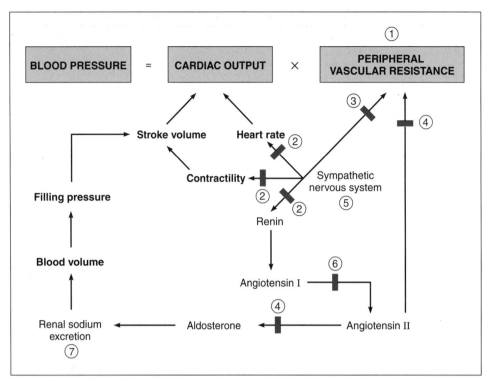

FIGURE 10–1. Physiologic control of blood pressure and sites of drug action. Blood pressure is the product of cardiac output and peripheral vascular resistance. These parameters are regulated on a systemic level by the sympathetic nervous system and the kidneys. Antihypertensive drugs act to suppress excessive sympathetic activity and modify renal function so as to counteract the mechanisms responsible for hypertension. Sites of action of the following drugs are shown: (1) vasodilators; (2) β-adrenergic receptor antagonists (β-blockers); (3) α-adrenergic receptor antagonists (α-blockers); (4) angiotensin receptor antagonists; (5) centrally acting sympatholytics; (6) angiotensin-converting enzyme (ACE) inhibitors; and (7) diuretics. The vasodilators, sympatholytics, and angiotensin inhibitors reduce peripheral vascular resistance; β-adrenergic receptor blockers reduce cardiac output; and diuretics promote sodium excretion and reduce blood volume.

ties. The discussion here focuses on the use of three classes of diuretics to treat hypertension: the thiazide and related diuretics, the loop diuretics, and the potassium-sparing diuretics.

All diuretics cause an increase in renal sodium excretion. This so-called **natriuretic effect,** or **natriuresis,** appears to be responsible for much of their antihypertensive activity. The thiazide diuretics have a moderate natriuretic effect and are the diuretics used most frequently in the treatment of hypertension. The loop diuretics have the greatest natriuretic effect of all classes of diuretics and may be used to treat hypertension when a thiazide diuretic is not effective or is contraindicated. The potassium-sparing diuretics have a relatively low natriuretic effect and are primarily employed in combination with a thiazide or loop diuretic to reduce potassium excretion and prevent hypokalemia.

Thiazide and Related Diuretics

The thiazide and related diuretics reduce blood pressure by two mechanisms, both stemming from their ability to increase sodium and water excretion. When they are first administered to a patient, the drugs decrease blood volume and thereby decrease cardiac output (Fig. 10–2 and Table 10–2). With continued administration over weeks and months, they also decrease PVR, and this appears to account for much of their long-term antihypertensive effect. The decreased PVR may be due to a reduction in the sodium content of arteriolar smooth muscle cells, which decreases muscle contraction in response to vasopressor agents such as norepinephrine and angiotensin. This relationship is supported by the finding that the effect of a thiazide on PVR is reduced if patients ingest enough dietary sodium to counteract the natriuretic effect of the drug.

Use of a thiazide typically reduces the blood pressure by 10–15 mm Hg. **Hydrochlorothiazide** is the thiazide diuretic that is most often used for treating hypertension. **Indapamide, metolazone,** and other thiazide-related diuretics have equivalent efficacy in the treatment of hypertension and differ primarily in their pharmacokinetic properties. Indapamide may also cause vasodilation via calcium channel blockade.

For many patients with mild hypertension, single-drug therapy with a thiazide provides economical and effective treatment. For patients with moderate to severe hypertension, a thiazide diuretic may be used in combination with another type of antihypertensive agent (such as a sympatholytic, an angiotensin inhibitor, or a vasodilator). The two drugs

TABLE 10–2. Cardiovascular Effects of Antihypertensive Drugs

Drug Classification	Peripheral Vascular Resistance	Cardiac Output	Blood Volume	Plasma Renin Activity	Left Ventricular Hypertrophy
Diuretics					
Thiazide and loop diuretics	Decrease	Decrease	Decrease	Increase	No change or decrease
Potassium-sparing diuretics	Decrease	Decrease	Decrease	Increase	No change or decrease
Sympatholytics					
α-Adrenergic receptor antagonists	Decrease	No change or increase	No change or increase	No change or decrease	Decrease
β-Adrenergic receptor antagonists	No change or decrease	Decrease	No change or decrease	Decrease	Decrease
Centrally acting drugs	Decrease	No change or decrease	Increase*	Decrease	Decrease
Neuronal blocking agents	Decrease	No change or decrease	Increase	No change or decrease	Unknown
Ganglionic blocking agents	Decrease	No change or decrease	No change or increase	No change or decrease	Unknown
Angiotensin inhibitors					
Angiotensin-converting enzyme inhibitors	Decrease	No change or increase	No change	Increase	Decrease
Angiotensin receptor antagonists	Decrease	No change or increase	No change or increase	Increase	Decrease
Vasodilators					
Calcium channel blockers	Decrease	No change or increase†	No change	No change or increase	Decrease
Other vasodilators					
Hydralazine	Decrease	Increase	Increase	Increase	Increase
Minoxidil	Decrease	Increase	Increase	Increase	Increase
Nitroprusside	Decrease	Increase	Increase	Increase	No change or increase

*Two exceptions are guanabenz and guanfacine, which either cause no change in blood volume or decrease it slightly.
†An exception is verapamil, which may increase or decrease cardiac output.

TABLE 10–3. Pharmacologic Effects of Antihypertensive Drugs on Serum Potassium and Cholesterol Measurements

Drug Classification	Serum Potassium	Total Cholesterol	Low-Density Lipoproteins	High-Density Lipoproteins	Triglycerides
Diuretics					
Thiazide and loop diuretics	Decrease	Increase	Increase	No change or decrease	Increase
Potassium-sparing diuretics	Increase	Unknown	Unknown	Unknown	Unknown
Sympatholytics					
α-Adrenergic receptor antagonists	No change	Decrease	Decrease	Increase	Decrease
β-Adrenergic receptor antagonists	Slight increase	No change or increase	No change or increase	Variable	No change or increase
Centrally acting drugs	No change	No change	No change	No change	No change
Neuronal blocking agents	No change	No change	No change	No change	No change
Ganglionic blocking agents	No change	Unknown	Unknown	Unknown	Unknown
Angiotensin inhibitors					
Angiotensin-converting enzyme inhibitors	Increase	No change	No change	No change	No change
Angiotensin receptor antagonists	Increase	No change	No change	No change	No change
Vasodilators					
Calcium channel blockers	No change	No change	No change	No change	No change
Other vasodilators					
Hydralazine	No change	No change	No change	No change	No change
Minoxidil	No change	No change	No change	No change	No change
Nitroprusside	No change	Not applicable*	Not applicable*	Not applicable*	Not applicable*

*Nitroprusside is used only for short-term management of hypertension.

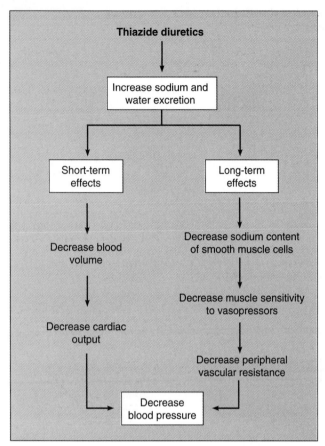

FIGURE 10–2. Antihypertensive actions of thiazide diuretics. Initially, thiazide diuretics decrease blood volume and thereby decrease cardiac output. Over time, the drugs decrease peripheral vascular resistance, an action that may be secondary to a reduction in the sodium content of smooth muscle cells.

usually have an additive effect, and the thiazide prevents the compensatory fluid retention that may otherwise be evoked by the other agent.

The common adverse effects, contraindications, and interactions of thiazide diuretics and other antihypertensive agents are summarized in Table 10–4. The primary disadvantage of thiazide diuretics is their tendency to cause hypokalemia, which may predispose patients with heart disease to cardiac arrhythmias. Using a low dosage of a thiazide diuretic (such as 25–50 mg of hydrochlorothiazide per day) usually produces a maximal antihypertensive effect with minimal hypokalemia. Using a higher dosage causes more hypokalemia but does not have a greater effect on blood pressure. Thiazides elevate plasma levels of glucose, uric acid, and lipids in some patients. Less commonly, they cause hematologic toxicity and aggravate hepatic disease. They may also evoke a compensatory increase in renin secretion, and this reduces their effectiveness in some patients.

An advantage of taking thiazide diuretics is that they appear to offer protection against **osteoporosis,** a condition in which bone demineralization and loss of bone mass make patients more susceptible to fractures. Thiazides are probably beneficial in this condition because they decrease the urinary excretion of calcium.

Loop Diuretics

Despite the greater natriuretic effect of loop diuretics, they are usually less effective than thiazide diuretics in the treatment of hypertensive patients with normal renal function. In patients with poor renal function, however, the thiazide diuretics lose their effectiveness if renal function declines significantly, whereas the loop diuretics continue to work. For these reasons, loop diuretics are usually reserved for use in hypertensive patients who have poor renal function and a serum creatinine level greater than 2.3 mg/dL.

Examples of loop diuretics are **bumetanide** and **furosemide.** Unlike the thiazide diuretics, these agents are not beneficial in patients with osteoporosis. This is because loop diuretics increase calcium excretion.

Potassium-Sparing Diuretics

Examples of potassium-sparing diuretics are **amiloride, spironolactone,** and **triamterene.** These agents exert a mild natriuretic and antihypertensive effect. They also reduce renal potassium excretion and thereby prevent hypokalemia, a common problem caused by other diuretics.

Several drug products that contain both a thiazide diuretic and a potassium-sparing diuretic are available. Potassium chloride tablets may also be used to prevent and treat hypokalemia.

SYMPATHOLYTICS

The sympatholytics used in the treatment of hypertension include adrenergic receptor antagonists, centrally acting drugs, neuronal blocking agents, and ganglionic blocking agents. The pharmacologic effects of these drugs are summarized in Tables 10–2 and 10–3; their common adverse effects, contraindications, and drug interactions are listed in Table 10–4; and the structures of two representative sympatholytics are shown in Fig. 10–3A.

Adrenergic Receptor Antagonists

The sympatholytics used most often to treat hypertension are the α-adrenergic receptor antagonists (α-blockers) and β-adrenergic receptor antagonists (β-blockers). The β-blockers are the preferred first-line therapy for many hypertensive patients, whereas the α-blockers are usually employed as second-line therapy when other agents are ineffective or contraindicated.

α-Adrenergic Receptor Antagonists

The α-blockers act to inhibit sympathetic stimulation of arteriolar contraction. Like other vasodilators, they may cause reflex tachycardia and fluid retention. Selective α1-blockers, such as **doxazosin, prazosin,** and **terazosin,** are preferred for the treatment of chronic essential hypertension because they produce less tachycardia than do nonselective α-

TABLE 10–4. Adverse Effects, Contraindications, and Drug Interactions of Antihypertensive Agents*

Drug Classification	Common Adverse Effects	Contraindications	Common Drug Interactions
Diuretics			
Thiazide and loop diuretics	Blood cell deficiencies, hyperlipidemia, hyperuricemia, hypokalemia, and other electrolyte changes. Aggravation of diabetes.	Hypersensitivity and severe hepatic dysfunction.	Increase serum levels of lithium. Hypotensive effect decreased by NSAIDs and augmented by ACE inhibitors.
Potassium-sparing diuretics	Hyperkalemia.	Hypersensitivity and severe renal disease.	Hyperkalemic effect increased by ACE inhibitors and potassium supplements.
Sympatholytics			
α-Adrenergic receptor antagonists	Dizziness, first-dose syncope, fluid retention, and orthostatic hypotension.	Hypersensitivity.	Hypotensive effect increased by β-adrenergic receptor antagonists and diuretics.
β-Adrenergic receptor antagonists	Bradycardia, bronchoconstriction, depression, fatigue, impaired glycogenolysis, and vivid dreams.	Asthma, atrioventricular block, bradycardia, hypersensitivity, and severe chronic obstructive pulmonary disease.	Cardiac depression increased by diltiazem and verapamil. Hypotensive effect decreased by NSAIDs.
Centrally acting drugs			
Clonidine	Dry mouth, fatigue, rebound hypertension, and sedation.	Hypersensitivity. Use cautiously in patients with ischemic heart disease or stroke.	Hypotensive effect decreased by tricyclic antidepressants. Sedative effect increased by CNS depressants.
Guanabenz	Same as clonidine.	Same as clonidine.	Same as clonidine.
Guanfacine	Same as clonidine but milder.	Same as clonidine.	Same as clonidine.
Methyldopa	Autoimmune hemolytic anemia, hepatitis, and lupuslike syndrome. Other adverse effects same as those of clonidine.	Hypersensitivity.	Hypotensive effect increased by levodopa. Other interactions same as those of clonidine.
Neuronal blocking agents			
Guanethidine	Diarrhea, retrograde ejaculation, and orthostatic hypotension.	Heart failure, hypersensitivity, pheochromocytoma, and recent use of a monoamine oxidase inhibitor.	Hypotensive effect decreased by sympathomimetics and tricyclic antidepressants.
Reserpine	Bradycardia, CNS depression, diarrhea, nasal stuffiness, and nightmares.	CNS depression, hypersensitivity, peptic ulcer, and ulcerative colitis.	Has additive effect with CNS depressants. Hypotensive effect decreased by tricyclic antidepressants.
Ganglionic blocking agents	Orthostatic hypotension and urinary retention.	Hypersensitivity.	None.
Angiotensin inhibitors			
Angiotensin-converting enzyme (ACE) inhibitors	Acute renal failure, angioedema, cough, hyperkalemia, loss of taste, neutropenia, and rash.	Bilateral renal artery stenosis, hypersensitivity, and pregnancy.	Increase serum levels of lithium. Hyperkalemic effect increased by potassium-sparing diuretics and potassium supplements. Hypotensive effect decreased by NSAIDs.
Angiotensin receptor antagonists	Hyperkalemia.	Same as ACE inhibitors.	Serum levels of drug increased by cimetidine and decreased by phenobarbital.
Vasodilators			
Calcium channel blockers			
Dihydropyridines†	Dizziness, edema, gingival hyperplasia, headache, and tachycardia.	Hypersensitivity.	Serum levels of drug increased by azole antifungal agents, cimetidine, and grapefruit juice.
Diltiazem	Atrioventricular block, bradycardia, constipation, dizziness, edema, gingival hyperplasia, headache, and heart failure.	Hypersensitivity, severe atrioventricular block or heart failure, sick sinus syndrome, ventricular tachycardia, and Wolff-Parkinson-White syndrome.	Increases serum levels of carbamazepine, digoxin, and theophylline. Decreases serum levels of lithium.
Verapamil	Same as diltiazem.	Same as diltiazem.	Same as diltiazem.

Continued

**TABLE 10–4. Adverse Effects, Contraindications, and Drug Interactions
of Antihypertensive Agents*** *(Continued)*

Drug Classification	Common Adverse Effects	Contraindications	Common Drug Interactions
Other vasodilators			
Hydralazine	Angina, dizziness, fluid retention, headache, lupuslike syndrome, and tachycardia.	Coronary artery disease, hypersensitivity, and mitral valve disease.	Hypotensive effect decreased by NSAIDs.
Minoxidil	Angina, dizziness, fluid retention, headache, hypertrichosis, pericardial effusion, and tachycardia.	Acute myocardial infarction, aortic aneurysm, hypersensitivity, and pheochromocytoma.	Hypotensive effect decreased by NSAIDs.
Nitroprusside	Dizziness, headache, increased intracranial pressure, methemoglobinemia, and thiocyanate-cyanide toxicity.	Arteriovenous shunt, coarctation of the aorta, decreased cerebral perfusion, and hypersensitivity.	None.

*ACE = angiotensin-converting enzyme; CNS = central nervous system; and NSAIDs = nonsteroidal anti-inflammatory drugs.
†The dihydropyridines include amlodipine, felodipine, isradipine, nicardipine, and nifedipine.

blockers, which inhibit both α_1- and α_2-adrenergic receptors. **Phenoxybenzamine** and other nonselective α-blockers are used to manage patients with hypertensive episodes due to pheochromocytoma.

The α-blockers tend to cause some activation of the sympathetic nervous system and may increase the heart rate, contractile force, circulating norepinephrine level, and myocardial oxygen demand. The drugs do not protect the heart against ventricular arrhythmias and are less useful in patients with ischemic heart disease. Because they also activate the renin-angiotensin-aldosterone system and may cause some fluid retention, they are frequently given in combination with a diuretic. The use of a selective α_1-blocker and a diuretic causes first-dose syncope in some patients, but this can be prevented by beginning treatment with a low dose of the blocker at bedtime and withholding the diuretic for 1 day. The pharmacokinetic properties and other pharmacologic effects and uses of α-blockers are covered in Chapter 9.

β-Adrenergic Receptor Antagonists

The β-blockers are widely employed in the treatment of hypertension because they are relatively safe and effective in most patients and are particularly useful in patients who suffer from angina or have a history of myocardial infarction. The drugs are cardioprotective and only rarely cause orthostatic hypotension or produce hepatic, renal, or hematopoietic toxicity. For these reasons, β-blockers provide effective single-drug therapy for many patients with mild hypertension and can be combined with other drugs to treat more severe forms of hypertension.

The β-blockers produce their therapeutic effects in patients with hypertension and other cardiovascular diseases by blocking β_1-adrenergic receptors in the heart and other tissues. This reduces cardiac output by decreasing the heart rate and contractility. The β-blockers inhibit renin secretion from renal juxtaglomerular cells, and this in turn reduces the

formation of angiotensin II and the subsequent release of aldosterone. The drugs also appear to reduce sympathetic outflow from the central nervous system (CNS). Hence, β-blockers have multiple actions affecting blood pressure.

Chapter 9 compares the properties of **atenolol, metoprolol,** and other cardioselective (β_1-selective) β-blockers with those of **nadolol, pindolol, propranolol,** and other nonselective β-blockers. Although these agents appear to be equally effective in lowering blood pressure, the selective β_1-blockers may be preferred for hypertensive patients with diabetes or obstructive lung disease. Atenolol is less lipophilic than propranolol and usually causes fewer CNS side effects. **Labetalol,** a combined α- and β-adrenergic receptor antagonist, is used to treat both chronic hypertension and hypertensive emergencies. Because of its α-adrenergic receptor–blocking activity, it may cause orthostatic hypotension.

Centrally Acting Drugs

Examples of centrally acting sympatholytics that are used in the treatment of hypertension are **clonidine, guanabenz, guanfacine,** and **methyldopa.** These agents are α_2-adrenergic receptor agonists that reduce sympathetic outflow from the brain stem to the heart, blood vessels, and other tissues. They lower the blood pressure primarily by causing a reduction in PVR while the heart rate and cardiac output are either reduced or remain unchanged. Since tricyclic antidepressant drugs can block the effects of centrally acting sympatholytic drugs, the two classes of drugs should not be used concurrently.

Sedation, dry mouth, and other CNS side effects of centrally acting sympatholytics may be problematic in hypertensive patients whose work requires mental alertness, as well as in those who are elderly or have neurologic diseases. In many cases, the sedative effects subside after a few weeks of treatment, so discontinuation of the drug is not necessary. Because severe rebound hypertension may occur if the drug is discontinued abruptly, the dosage should be tapered gradually over 1–2 weeks if treatment is to be stopped.

In addition to activating α_2-adrenergic receptors, clonidine also activates a recently discovered class of nonadrenergic receptors known as **imidazoline receptors,** and investigators have postulated that stimulation of these receptors is partly responsible for the drug's antihypertensive action. With continued research concerning imidazoline receptors, investigators hope that it will be possible to design drugs that selectively activate imidazoline receptors and thereby avoid sedation, dry mouth, and related side effects associated with the activation of central α_2-adrenergic receptors.

Methyldopa is similar to clonidine in its actions and effects. Unlike clonidine and other centrally

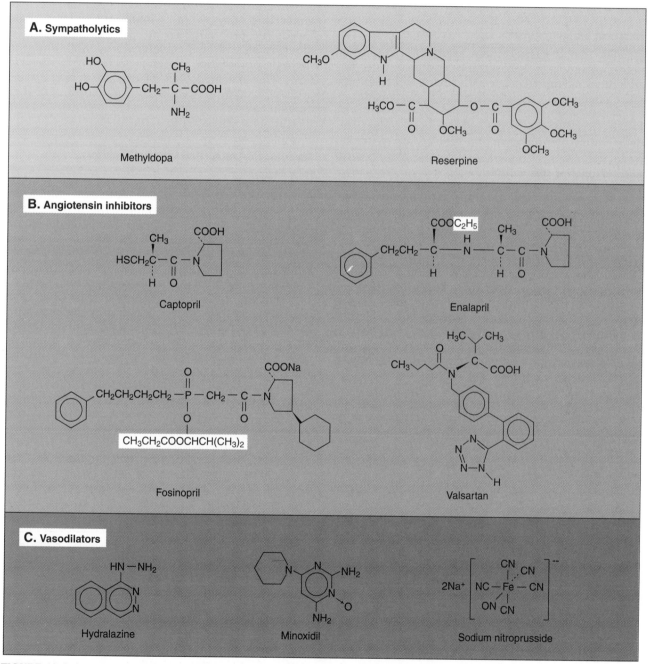

FIGURE 10–3. Structures of selected antihypertensive drugs. (A) The sympatholytics include methyldopa, which is converted in the brain to an active metabolite called methylnorepinephrine; clonidine, whose structure is shown in Fig. 8–3; reserpine, an alkaloid obtained from the snakeroot plant, *Rauwolfia serpentina;* and the adrenergic receptor antagonists, representative structures of which are shown in Fig. 9–1. **(B)** One group of angiotensin inhibitors consists of angiotensin-converting enzyme (ACE) inhibitors and includes captopril, enalapril, and fosinopril. The unshaded portions of enalapril and fosinopril are removed by esterases to form the active metabolites, enalaprilat and fosinoprilat. Another group consists of angiotensin receptor antagonists and includes valsartan. **(C)** The vasodilators include hydralazine; minoxidil; sodium nitroprusside; and the calcium channel blockers, representative structures of which are shown in Fig. 11–3.

acting drugs, however, methyldopa is accumulated by central noradrenergic neurons and is converted to an active metabolite, methylnorepinephrine. Methyldopa is well known for its ability to cause immunologic effects, including a Coombs-positive hemolytic anemia (reported in up to 2% of patients), autoimmune hepatitis, and other organ dysfunction. Methyldopa is often preferred for the treatment of hypertension in pregnant women, since long experience has shown that it does not harm the fetus.

Neuronal Blocking Agents

The use of **guanethidine, reserpine,** and other neuronal blockers has steadily declined with the advent of agents that are safer, more specific, and more effective for the treatment of hypertension.

Guanethidine has been used to treat moderate to severe hypertension but is seldom used today. The drug inhibits neurotransmitter release and reuptake, and its side effects include orthostatic hypotension and retrograde ejaculation.

Reserpine is still used to treat mild hypertension in some patients because it is low in cost, is taken once a day, and does not require titration of the dosage. Often, it is given in combination with a diuretic. Reserpine reduces blood pressure by blocking the storage of norepinephrine in the vesicles of sympathetic neurons, gradually leading to neurotransmitter depletion. Because the drug also depletes norepinephrine in the CNS and may depress the mood, it should be avoided in patients with a history of depression. Reserpine must be used cautiously in patients receiving digitalis and in those with peptic ulcer disease, which can be aggravated by this drug.

Ganglionic Blocking Agents

The use of ganglionic blockers for the treatment of chronic hypertension is essentially obsolete, but **trimethaphan** is still used in hypertensive emergencies. The drug is administered intravenously and lowers the blood pressure by blocking neurotransmission at sympathetic ganglia. Trimethaphan may cause blurred vision, dry mouth, and paresis of the bladder and bowel as a result of blocking parasympathetic ganglia. For this reason, drugs such as clonidine, nitroprusside, and labetalol are used more frequently for treating hypertensive emergencies.

ANGIOTENSIN INHIBITORS

Angiotensin inhibitors include the angiotensin-converting enzyme (ACE) inhibitors and the angiotensin receptor antagonists. β-Adrenergic receptor blockers also reduce angiotensin by inhibiting sympathetic stimulation of renin secretion by the kidneys. The pharmacologic properties of these drugs are summarized in Tables 10–2 and 10–3, and their common adverse effects, contraindications, and drug interactions are listed in Table 10–4.

Angiotensin-Converting Enzyme Inhibitors
Drug Properties

Chemistry and Pharmacokinetics. Molecular techniques were used to model the active site of angiotensin-converting enzyme (ACE) and design the ACE inhibitors. Structures of the original ACE inhibitor, **captopril,** and other drugs in this class are shown in Fig. 10–3B. The various ACE inhibitors have essentially identical mechanisms of action and pharmacologic effects, but they differ in their pharmacokinetic properties (Table 10–5). They undergo varying degrees of first-pass hepatic inactivation after oral administration, and several of the ACE inhibitors have active metabolites. Except for captopril, most of the ACE inhibitors have a duration of action of about 24 hours and may be administered once or twice daily in the treatment of hypertension and other disorders.

Mechanisms and Pharmacologic Effects. The actions of ACE inhibitors and other drugs affecting the renin-angiotensin-aldosterone axis are shown in Fig. 10–4. There are three primary stimuli to renin

TABLE 10–5. Pharmacokinetic Properties of Angiotensin Inhibitors

Drug	Oral Bioavailability	Absorption Reduced by Food	Active Metabolite	Duration of Action (Hours)
Angiotensin-converting enzyme inhibitors				
Benazepril	37%	No	Benazeprilat	24
Captopril	75%	30–40%	None	6–12
Enalapril	60%	No	Enalaprilat*	24
Fosinopril	36%	No	Fosinoprilat	24
Lisinopril	25%	No	None	24
Quinapril	60%	25–30%	Quinaprilat	24
Ramipril	55%	No	Ramiprilat	24
Angiotensin receptor antagonists				
Losartan	33%	10%	E-3174 carboxylic acid	24
Valsartan	25%	40%	None	24

*Enalaprilat is available as a separate drug for intravenous administration.

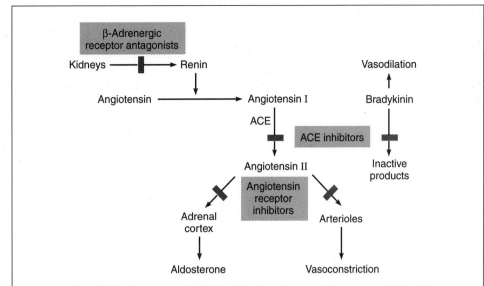

FIGURE 10–4. Actions of antihypertensive drugs on the renin-angiotensin-aldosterone axis. β-Adrenergic receptor antagonists inhibit sympathetic stimulation of renin secretion. Angiotensin-converting enzyme (ACE) inhibitors block the formation of angiotensin II and inhibit the breakdown of bradykinin, a vasodilator. Angiotensin receptor antagonists, such as losartan, block AT_1 receptors in smooth muscle and adrenal cortex.

secretion: (1) sympathetic nervous system activation of β_1-adrenergic receptors on renal juxtaglomerular cells, (2) a reduction in blood pressure and wall tension in renal afferent arterioles, and (3) a reduction in sodium chloride reabsorption by the renal macula densa.

When blood pressure falls and renin is released, this initiates a cascade of events that normally return blood pressure to the preexisting level. In the circulation, renin acts as a protease that converts circulating angiotensinogen to angiotensin I. ACE, a protease primarily located in the pulmonary vasculature, then converts the physiologically inactive angiotensin I to the active angiotensin II. Angiotensin II activates two types of **angiotensin receptors,** called AT_1 and AT_2. The AT_1 receptors are coupled with enzymes that increase the formation of inositol triphosphate (IP_3) and various arachidonic acid metabolites and decrease the formation of cyclic adenosine monophosphate (cAMP). Activation of AT_1 receptors in the adrenal cortex causes the synthesis and release of aldosterone, and activation of AT_1 receptors in vascular smooth muscle causes vasoconstriction. In addition to causing these two effects via IP_3-mediated release of intracellular calcium, AT_1 receptors mediate cardiac, renal, and CNS effects. The functional significance of AT_2 receptors has not been elucidated.

In the normal chain of events, ACE not only converts angiotensin I to angiotensin II but also catalyzes the inactivation of bradykinin, an endogenous vasodilator peptide. Drugs that inhibit ACE therefore exert hypotensive effects by blocking the formation of a vasoconstrictor (angiotensin II) and by blocking the degradation of a vasodilator (bradykinin). Increased renal prostaglandin synthesis may also contribute to the hypotensive effects of these drugs. Some studies have found that angiotensin II levels may return toward pretreatment levels during

long-term ACE inhibitor therapy, even though the blood pressure remains under control. This suggests that the effects on bradykinin and prostaglandins are an important component of the antihypertensive action of these drugs.

The antihypertensive action of ACE inhibitors is primarily due to a reduction in PVR, with little or no change in cardiac output or blood volume (see Table 10–2). ACE inhibitors decrease both arterial pressure and venous pressure, and this in turn reduces cardiac afterload and cardiac preload, respectively. By reducing angiotensin-stimulated aldosterone secretion, ACE inhibitors prevent the compensatory increase in sodium retention and plasma volume that may occur with some other antihypertensive drugs. In patients treated with ACE inhibitors, renal sodium retention is decreased, renal potassium retention is increased, and serum potassium levels typically increase by about 0.5 mEq/L.

Adverse Effects. ACE inhibitors may cause fetal and neonatal morbidity and mortality when administered to pregnant women, especially during the second and third trimesters. Therefore, use of these drugs should be discontinued when pregnancy is detected. ACE inhibitors may also cause renal failure in patients who have bilateral renal artery stenosis, because these patients depend on angiotensin II to maintain renal blood flow and glomerular filtration, as illustrated in Fig. 10–5.

In most other patients, ACE inhibitors are well tolerated, and epidemiologic studies have shown that they do not adversely affect the life-style of patients as much as some other types of antihypertensive drugs do. The most common side effect is a dry, irritating, and nonproductive cough, which occurs in up to 20% of patients and may be due to increased bradykinin levels. A pruritic rash occurs in up to 10% of patients. Infrequently, ACE inhibitors cause an abnormal taste sensation, which appears to be

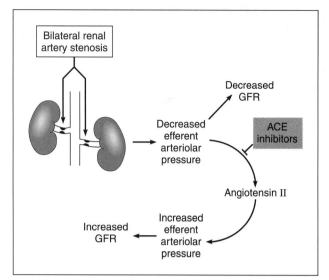

FIGURE 10–5. Effects of angiotensin-converting enzyme (ACE) inhibitors in patients with bilateral renal artery stenosis. Renal blood flow is reduced in the presence of bilateral renal artery stenosis. In affected patients, glomerular filtration is maintained by elevating efferent arteriolar pressure via vasoconstriction produced by angiotensin II. By blocking the formation of angiotensin II, ACE inhibitors may severely impair glomerular filtration and lead to renal failure. GFR = glomerular filtration rate.

related to the binding of zinc by the drugs. Other less common but more severe adverse effects of ACE inhibitors include angioedema and neutropenia.

Interactions. The antihypertensive action of ACE inhibitors is augmented by thiazide and loop diuretics. Both types of diuretics should be used cautiously with ACE inhibitors because of the potential of the drug combination to cause hypotension and renal insufficiency. ACE inhibitors may interact with potassium-sparing diuretics and potassium supplements to increase serum potassium levels significantly and cause hyperkalemia. They may also increase serum lithium levels and provoke lithium toxicity in patients receiving lithium compounds for the treatment of bipolar disorder. Nonsteroidal antiinflammatory drugs (NSAIDs), such as ibuprofen, may impede the effects of ACE inhibitors and other antihypertensive agents.

Indications. Because they have excellent antihypertensive action and few bothersome side effects, ACE inhibitors are used in the management of mild to severe hypertension in patients with a wide variety of traits and concomitant diseases, as outlined in Table 10–6. The drugs are of particular value in treating hypertensive patients with coexisting heart failure, myocardial infarction, or diabetes mellitus.

Studies have shown that ACE inhibitors decrease cardiac afterload, increase cardiac output, and reduce the risk of death in patients with heart failure (see Chapter 12). These agents also increase the survival rate and reduce the incidence of overt heart failure in patients who have myocardial infarction and significant left ventricular dysfunction, as evidenced by a cardiac ejection fraction of less than 40%. (The ejection fraction is the percentage of blood that is ejected from the left ventricle during each systole.)

In diabetic patients who exhibit early signs of renal impairment, such as albuminuria and increased serum creatinine levels, ACE inhibitors exert a renoprotective effect. Studies indicate that the ACE inhibitor **enalapril** reduces the progression of these harbingers of renal failure and the subsequent need for renal dialysis in these patients. Moreover, if enalapril is withdrawn from treatment, the progression of nephropathy resumes quickly. Based on these findings, experts now recommend that ACE inhibitor therapy be considered for diabetic patients with albuminuria or increased serum creatinine levels, regardless of whether they have hypertension.

Specific Drugs

Three classes of ACE inhibitors have been developed. In each class, a different chemical group binds the zinc ion in ACE. The sulfhydryl (mercapto) compounds include **captopril;** the phosphoryl agents include **fosinopril;** and the carboxyl derivatives include **benazepril, enalapril, lisinopril, quinapril,** and **ramipril.** All of these drugs except captopril and lisinopril are enzymatically transformed to active metabolites. **Enalaprilat,** the active metabolite of enalapril, is available for intravenous administration; the other ACE inhibitors are administered orally.

The orally administered ACE inhibitors undergo considerable first-pass inactivation, and their oral bioavailability ranges from 25% to 75% (see Table 10–5). In comparison with other ACE inhibitors, which are administered 1 or 2 times a day, captopril has a shorter half-life and must be administered 2 or 3 times a day. Some studies indicate that captopril causes a higher incidence of rash, and this may be related to its sulfhydryl structure.

Angiotensin Receptor Antagonists

A new approach to angiotensin inhibition has been the development of angiotensin receptor antagonists. These drugs block AT_1 receptors in vascular smooth muscle and in the adrenal cortex, thereby causing vasodilation and decreasing aldosterone secretion.

The first angiotensin receptor antagonists were intravenously administered peptides (such as saralasin, which is no longer used). Orally effective nonpeptide drugs, including **losartan** and **valsartan,** are now available for clinical use. In the treatment of hypertension, these drugs appear to be as effective as the ACE inhibitors but only rarely cause the chronic cough that is a frequent problem with ACE inhibitors. The angiotensin receptor inhibitors are relatively free of other adverse effects, and the vast majority of patients tolerate them well. The drugs do not increase serum glucose, uric acid, or cholesterol levels. Occasional abnormalities in the test results of patients taking these drugs have included hyperkale-

**TABLE 10–6. Selection of Antihypertensive Drugs for Patients
With Specific Traits or Concomitant Diseases**

Characteristics of Patients	Most Preferred Drugs*	Least Preferred Drugs
Demographic traits		
Age under 50 years	α-Adrenergic receptor antagonist (α-blocker); verapamil; diltiazem; angiotensin-converting enzyme (ACE) inhibitor.	—
Age over 65 years	Thiazide diuretic; ACE inhibitor; dihyropyridine calcium channel blocker.	Centrally acting α-adrenergic receptor agonist.
African heritage	Calcium channel blocker; thiazide diuretic.	β-Adrenergic receptor antagonist (β-blocker).
Pregnancy	Methyldopa; hydralazine.	ACE inhibitor; angiotensin receptor antagonist.
Life-style traits		
Physically active	ACE inhibitor; calcium channel blocker; α-blocker.	β-Blocker; thiazide diuretic.
Noncompliant	Drug that can be given once daily.	Centrally acting α-adrenergic receptor agonist.
Concomitant diseases		
Angina pectoris	β-Blocker; diltiazem; verapamil.	Hydralazine; minoxidil.
Asthma	Calcium channel blocker; ACE inhibitor.	β-Blocker.
Benign prostatic hyperplasia	α-Blocker.	—
Collagen disease	ACE inhibitor (not captopril); calcium channel blocker.	Hydralazine; methyldopa.
Congestive heart failure	ACE inhibitor; α-blocker; hydralazine.	Calcium channel blocker.
Depression	—	Centrally acting α-adrenergic receptor agonist; β-blocker; reserpine.
Diabetes mellitus	ACE inhibitor; α-blocker; calcium channel blocker.	β-Blocker; diuretic.
Gout	—	Diuretic.
Hypercholesterolemia	α-Blocker; ACE inhibitor; calcium channel blocker; indapamide.	β-Blocker without intrinsic sympathomimetic activity; other thiazide diuretic.
Migraine headache	β-Blocker; calcium channel blocker.	—
Myocardial infarction	β-Blocker; ACE inhibitor.	—
Osteoporosis	Thiazide diuretic.	—
Peripheral vascular disease	ACE inhibitor; calcium channel blocker; α-blocker.	β-Blocker.

*Drugs are listed in order of preference.

mia, neutropenia, and elevated serum levels of hepatic aminotransferase enzymes. Like the ACE inhibitors, the angiotensin receptor blockers may cause fetal injury and death and should not be used during pregnancy.

VASODILATORS

The vasodilators include the calcium channel blockers and other agents such as hydralazine, minoxidil, and nitroprusside. The pharmacologic effects, adverse effects, contraindications, and drug interactions of these agents are summarized in Tables 10–2, 10–3, and 10–4.

Calcium Channel Blockers

Calcium channel blockers are used in the treatment of hypertension, angina pectoris, and cardiac arrhythmias. While Chapter 11 discusses the pharmacologic properties of these drugs in detail, this chapter focuses on their antihypertensive actions.

By blocking calcium ion channels in the plasma membranes of smooth muscle, the calcium channel blockers relax vascular smooth muscle and thereby cause vasodilation. Calcium channel blockers have a greater effect on arteriolar smooth muscle than on venous smooth muscle, and their effect on blood pressure is primarily due to a reduction in PVR, with relatively little impact on venous capacitance, cardiac filling pressure, and cardiac output. Some studies indicate that calcium channel blockers have a natriuretic effect that may contribute to their ability to lower blood pressure.

While all of the calcium channel blockers relax vascular smooth muscle, **diltiazem** and **verapamil** also have a significant effect on cardiac tissue and reduce the heart rate in some patients. Most of the other calcium channel blockers, including **amlodipine, felodipine, isradipine, nicardipine,** and **nifedipine,** belong to the dihydropyridine class. The dihydropyridines have relatively little effect on cardiac tissue at usual therapeutic levels; however, they may evoke reflex tachycardia, and some of them have been reported to suppress cardiac contractility in patients with heart failure.

The calcium channel blockers are effective in the management of all forms of hypertension and are among the most widely used antihypertensive agents. They do not alter levels of serum glucose, lipids, uric acid, or electrolytes. They are relatively free of adverse effects, and they are particularly useful in treating hypertensive patients who have asthma or are of African heritage (see Table 10–6).

Other Vasodilators
Hydralazine and Minoxidil

Hydralazine and minoxidil (see Fig. 10–3C) are orally effective vasodilators that are primarily used in combination with other antihypertensive drugs for the treatment of moderate to very severe hypertension. When used alone, they often evoke reflex tachycardia and cause fluid retention, and they may precipitate angina in susceptible patients. To prevent these problems, hydralazine or minoxidil is usually given in combination with two other drugs: a diuretic plus either a β-adrenergic receptor antagonist or another sympatholytic agent. Hydralazine has been associated with a lupuslike syndrome, whereas minoxidil may cause hypertrichosis (excessive hair growth), particularly in women. In fact, minoxidil has been marketed as a topical formulation for the treatment of several forms of baldness in men and women.

Nitroprusside

Sodium nitroprusside (see Fig. 10–3C) is commonly used in the management of hypertensive emergencies because it effectively reduces the patient's blood pressure to a safe level. The drug is administered by intravenous infusion and has a short half-life. Nitroprusside is rapidly metabolized to cyanide in erythrocytes and other tissues. Cyanide is then converted to thiocyanate in the presence of a sulfur donor. Both thiocyanate and cyanide gradually accumulate during nitroprusside infusion. For this reason, the duration of therapy with this drug is usually limited to a few days. During drug administration, the patient's blood pressure should be monitored frequently, and thiocyanate levels should be checked every 72 hours to detect potential toxicity.

THE MANAGEMENT OF HYPERTENSION

The stepped care approach to the management of hypertension begins with nonpharmacologic measures before proceeding to single-drug or multiple-drug therapy.

Recommending Life-Style Modifications

Patients with hypertension should be encouraged to pursue life-style changes that will improve their general health and may substantially lower their blood pressure. Effective strategies include exercise and weight loss, stress management, reduction of alcohol intake, and institution of a diet that is low in sodium and provides an adequate intake of potassium, calcium, and magnesium. Unless hypertension is severe, patients should be encouraged to try nondrug therapy for several months before instituting drug therapy.

Choosing and Implementing Drug Therapy

Essential hypertension often requires long-term drug therapy to control blood pressure and prevent damage to target organs. A large number of effective antihypertensive medications are available, and their selection is primarily based on their adverse effect profile, contraindications, cost, and convenience to the patient. Because hypertension is usually asymptomatic, even minor side effects may decrease the patient's compliance and blood pressure control. For this reason, it is important to select a drug that is both effective and well tolerated.

Single- and Multiple-Drug Therapy

The Joint National Committee on Prevention, Detection, Evaluation, and Treatment of High Blood Pressure recommends that physicians begin with single-drug therapy (monotherapy) for patients who require drug treatment, since monotherapy reduces costs, adverse effects, and noncompliance by patients.

The committee recommends that a β-adrenergic receptor antagonist or a diuretic be used initially for most hypertensive patients (see exceptions below and in Table 10–6), although an ACE inhibitor, a calcium channel blocker, or an α_1-adrenergic receptor antagonist can be used as an alternative when β-blockers or diuretics are unsuitable. If the first drug does not provide adequate control, a second drug is added or substituted for the first drug. In some cases, three drugs may be required to effectively control blood pressure.

Unless intolerable side effects occur or hypertension is severe, drugs should be given a trial of several weeks before evaluating their effectiveness and changing medications.

Special Considerations

Treatment of Patients Over 65 Years Old. In hypertensive patients over 65 years old, the use of a thiazide diuretic, an ACE inhibitor, or a dihydropyridine calcium channel blocker is often preferred for initial therapy. Particularly in patients over 70 years old, β-blockers may reduce cardiac output too much. In elderly black patients, β-blockers are often less effective than diuretics, so a diuretic or calcium channel blocker should be used.

Treatment of Patients With Concomitant Diseases. Whenever possible, patients with hypertension and a coexisting disorder should be treated with drugs that are potentially beneficial to both conditions, and agents that may exacerbate the coexisting disorder should be avoided.

Most patients with **ischemic heart disease,** including those with **angina pectoris** or **myocardial infarction,** should be treated with a β-blocker unless it is contraindicated. The β-blockers protect against sudden death in these patients and are among the drugs that reduce ventricular hypertrophy. Diuretics may cause hypokalemia, which predisposes to ventricular arrhythmia, and they are less useful in patients with ischemic heart disease or ventricular hypertrophy.

In patients with **hypercholesterolemia,** treatment with an α-adrenergic receptor antagonist, ACE inhibitor, calcium channel blocker, or indapamide may be preferred, because these agents do not adversely affect serum lipoprotein levels. Diuretics increase levels of low-density lipoprotein (LDL) and decrease levels of high-density lipoprotein (HDL) in some patients; therefore, these levels should be closely monitored in patients who have hypercholesterolemia and require a diuretic. Since β-blockers have little effect on LDL levels, they may still be preferred for patients with hypertension and ischemic heart disease.

In patients with **diabetes mellitus,** treatment with an ACE inhibitor, α-blocker, or calcium channel blocker is often preferred because these agents do not prolong hypoglycemia, as do the β-blockers. Diuretics are not preferred in diabetic patients, because they increase blood glucose levels in many cases.

In patients with **asthma,** treatment with β-blockers should be avoided, because these agents may cause bronchoconstriction. Use of a calcium channel blocker or ACE inhibitor is usually preferred. Calcium channel blockers may relax bronchial smooth muscle and thereby reduce bronchoconstriction in patients with asthma.

Summary of Important Points

- The four major classes of antihypertensive drugs are the diuretics, sympatholytics, angiotensin inhibitors, and vasodilators.
- Thiazide and related diuretics, loop diuretics, and potassium-sparing diuretics are used to treat hypertensive patients. The thiazides initially reduce blood volume and cardiac output, but their long-term effect on blood pressure is primarily due to decreased peripheral vascular resistance (PVR).
- Sympatholytics used in the treatment of hypertension include α-adrenergic receptor antagonists, β-adrenergic receptor antagonists, centrally acting drugs, neuronal blocking agents, and ganglionic blocking agents. Except for the β-blockers, which reduce cardiac output, the sympatholytics reduce blood pressure primarily by decreasing PVR.
- The two types of angiotensin inhibitors are the angiotensin-converting enzyme (ACE) inhibitors, such as captopril, and the angiotensin receptor antagonists, such as losartan. These drugs reduce PVR and aldosterone levels, with little effect on blood volume or cardiac output in patients who do not have heart failure.
- Among the vasodilators used to treat hypertension are the calcium channel blockers, hydralazine, minoxidil, and nitroprusside. These drugs reduce PVR, and some of them provoke reflex tachycardia and fluid retention.
- The stepped care approach to the management of hypertension begins with nonpharmacologic measures and then proceeds to the use of a β-blocker, diuretic, ACE inhibitor, calcium channel blocker, or α-blocker. If a single drug does not control blood pressure, other drugs may be added or substituted.

Selected Readings

Appel, L. J., et al. A clinical trial of the effects of dietary patterns on blood pressure. N Engl J Med 336:1117–1124, 1997.

Criscione, L., et al. Pharmacological profile of valsartan: a potent, orally active, nonpeptide antagonist of the angiotensin AT-1 receptor subtype. Br J Pharmacol 110:761–771, 1993.

Ernsberger, P., et al. The I_1-imidazoline receptor: from binding site to therapeutic target in cardiovascular disease. J Hypertens Suppl 15:S9–S23, 1997.

Joint National Committee. The sixth report of the Joint National Committee on Prevention, Detection, Evaluation, and Treatment of High Blood Pressure. Arch Intern Med 157:2413–2446, 1997.

Kaplan, N. M. Treatment of hypertension: insights from the JNC-VI report. Am Fam Physician 58:1323–1330, 1998.

Koopman, H., et al. Diet or diuretic? Treatment of newly diagnosed mild to moderate hypertension in the elderly. J Hum Hypertens 11:807–812, 1997.

CHAPTER ELEVEN

ANTIANGINAL DRUGS

CLASSIFICATION OF ANTIANGINAL DRUGS

VASODILATORS

Organic nitrites and nitrates
- Amyl nitrite
- Isosorbide dinitrate
- Isosorbide mononitrate
- Nitroglycerin

Calcium channel blockers
- Amlodipine
- Bepridil
- Diltiazem
- Nicardipine
- Nifedipine
- Verapamil

β-ADRENERGIC RECEPTOR ANTAGONISTS
- Atenolol
- Metoprolol
- Nadolol
- Propranolol

OVERVIEW
Ischemic Heart Disease

Ischemic heart disease has two primary forms, angina pectoris and myocardial infarction (Fig. 11–1). **Angina pectoris** is usually a chronic condition and is characterized by episodic chest discomfort that occurs during transient coronary ischemia. In contrast, **myocardial infarction** is the result of an acute and complete occlusion of a coronary artery, which is most frequently caused by coronary thrombosis.

The symptoms of angina pectoris, often described as resembling a heavy weight or pressure on the chest, occur when the oxygen supply to the myocardium is not sufficient to provide the energy required by the tissue. The imbalance between oxygen supply and oxygen demand may result from the following: an acute disruption of coronary blood flow due to coronary vasospasm or platelet aggregation; an increased demand for oxygen evoked by physical exertion in the face of a limited oxygen supply; or a combination of pathophysiologic mechanisms, such as vasospasm and platelet aggregation occurring in association with coronary atherosclerosis.

Typical angina occurs when the myocardial oxygen demand increases in association with exercise or stress but the coronary blood flow and oxygen supply are limited by the presence of coronary atherosclerosis that partially occludes a major coro-

nary vessel. The condition is characterized as **stable angina** if angina attacks have similar characteristics and occur under the same circumstances each time. It is characterized as **unstable angina** if the frequency and severity of attacks increase (crescendo). Unstable angina, which is usually due to the occlusion of coronary vessels by small thrombi and ruptured atheromatous plaque, is often the forerunner of myocardial infarction. **Variant angina (Prinzmetal's angina)** is due to acute coronary vasospasm and often occurs at rest or during sleep. Variant angina is sometimes considered a form of unstable angina.

Table 11–1 lists five classes of drugs and compares their efficacy in treating different forms of ischemic heart disease. This chapter focuses on the first three classes—namely, organic nitrites and nitrates, calcium channel blockers (CCBs), and β-adrenergic receptor antagonists (β-blockers)—which are the primary agents for treating angina. Chapter 16 discusses antiplatelet drugs (such as aspirin) and fibrinolytic drugs that are useful in treating unstable angina and myocardial infarction.

Mechanisms and Effects of Antianginal Drugs

The pharmacologic treatment of angina pectoris seeks to restore the balance between myocardial oxygen supply and demand, either by increasing oxygen supply or decreasing oxygen demand. The factors that determine supply and demand are illustrated in Fig. 11–2.

Myocardial oxygen supply is primarily determined by **coronary blood flow** and **regional flow distribution** but is also influenced by **oxygen extraction.** In patients with coronary artery disease, the subendocardial tissue is more likely to suffer from ischemia because it is not as well perfused as the subepicardial tissue. The use of nitrates or CCBs (vasodilator drugs) may reduce ischemia by increasing the total coronary flow and by increasing the distribution of coronary flow to ischemic subendocardial tissue. The drugs increase the distribution of blood flow to subendocardial tissue by dilating collateral vessels and by decreasing intraventricular pressure and the resistance to perfusion of this tissue. The use of β-blockers may improve the distribution of coronary flow by reducing intraventricular pressure. Cardiac tissue extracts a higher percentage of oxygen from blood than does any other tissue, and this factor is not affected by existing drugs.

Myocardial oxygen demand is largely determined by the amount of energy required to support

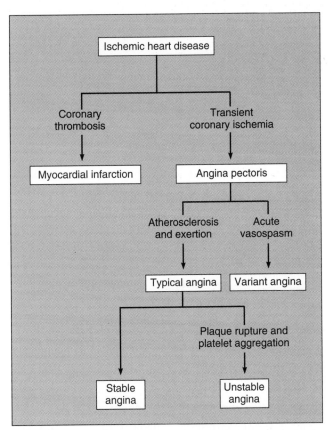

FIGURE 11–1. Classification and pathophysiology of ischemic heart disease. Variant angina, also called Prinzmetal's angina, is considered a form of unstable angina if the angina attacks occur with increasing severity or frequency.

the work of the heart. The factors that influence cardiac work include the **heart rate, cardiac contractility,** and **myocardial wall tension.** Contractility is directly related to the amount of cytosolic calcium that is available to stimulate the shortening of myocardial fibers. As contractility increases, the velocity of fiber shortening and the peak systolic muscle tension also increase. Myocardial wall tension is equal to the product of ventricular volume (radius) and pressure, divided by wall thickness. Ventricular wall tension is primarily determined by arterial and venous blood pressure.

Antianginal drugs act by several mechanisms to reduce myocardial oxygen demand. The β-blockers and some of the CCBs decrease heart rate and con-

tractility, whereas the vasodilators reduce wall tension via their effects on ventricular volume and pressure. Dilation of veins decreases venous pressure, cardiac filling pressure, and ventricular diastolic pressure (preload). Dilation of arteries decreases arterial and aortic pressure and thereby reduces ventricular systolic pressure (afterload). The organic nitrates act primarily on venous tissue and predominantly affect preload, whereas the CCBs act mostly on arteriolar muscle so as to reduce afterload.

In **typical angina,** which is caused by increased oxygen demand in the face of a limited oxygen supply, vasodilators and β-blockers act primarily by decreasing oxygen demand through the mechanisms described above. They may also increase the perfusion of ischemic subendocardial tissue. In **variant angina,** chest pain usually occurs at rest (when oxygen demand is relatively low), and ischemia results in a reduction in oxygen supply secondary to coronary artery spasm. Under these conditions, vasodilators increase oxygen supply by relaxing coronary smooth muscle and restoring normal coronary flow. The β-blockers are not effective in the treatment of variant angina, because they are not able to counteract vasospasm and increase coronary blood flow. The β-blockers may actually reduce coronary blood flow by blocking the vasodilative effect of epinephrine, an effect that is mediated by β_2-adrenergic receptors in coronary smooth muscle.

VASODILATORS

Two classes of vasodilators are used in the management of angina pectoris. The first consists of organic nitrites and nitrates, while the second consists of calcium channel blockers.

Organic Nitrites and Nitrates

The organic nitrites and nitrates are polyol esters of nitrous acid and nitric acid, respectively (Fig. 11–3A). Amyl nitrite is the only nitrite compound used to treat angina and is administered by inhalation. Nitroglycerin (glyceryl trinitrate), isosorbide dinitrate, and isosorbide mononitrate are nitrate compounds with sufficient solubility in water and lipids to enable rapid dissolution and absorption following sublingual, oral, or transdermal administration. The onset and duration of action of these drugs

TABLE 11–1. Efficacy of Drugs Used in the Treatment of Ischemic Heart Disease*

| | Typical Angina Pectoris | | Variant Angina Pectoris | Myocardial Infarction |
Drug or Drug Class	Stable Angina	Unstable Angina		
Organic nitrites and nitrates	++	++	++	+
Calcium channel blockers	++	0 to ++	+++	0
β-Adrenergic receptor antagonists	++	++	0	+++
Aspirin	+	+++	0	++
Fibrinolytic drugs	0	0	0	+++

*Ratings range from 0 (not efficacious) to +++ (highly efficacious).

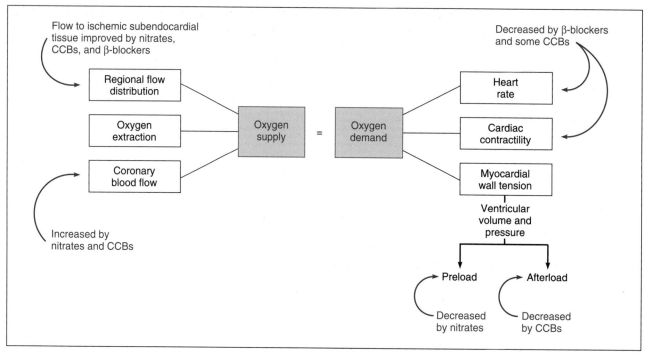

FIGURE 11–2. Effects of organic nitrites and nitrates (nitrates), calcium channel blockers (CCBs), and β-adrenergic receptor antagonists (β-blockers) on myocardial oxygen supply and demand.

varies with their physical properties, route of administration, and rate of biotransformation. Amyl nitrite has the most rapid onset and the shortest duration of action, whereas isosorbide compounds have the slowest onset and the longest duration. Nitroglycerin has an intermediate onset and duration. All of these compounds are extensively metabolized in the liver.

Amyl Nitrite

Amyl nitrite is a volatile liquid that can be inhaled and absorbed through the lungs. Its action is rapid in onset (within 30 seconds) and brief in duration (3–5 minutes). Amyl nitrite is effective in the **treatment of acute angina attacks,** as well as in the **initial management of cyanide poisoning.** In patients with cyanide poisoning, amyl nitrite is used until intravenous sodium nitrite and sodium thiosulfate can be administered. The nitrites oxidize hemoglobin to methemoglobin. In comparison with hemoglobin, methemoglobin has a greater affinity for cyanide, and this allows it to trap the compound in the form of cyanmethemoglobin. Thiosulfate is then administered to convert cyanide to inactive thiocyanate.

Nitroglycerin, Isosorbide Dinitrate, and Isosorbide Mononitrate

Chemistry and Pharmacokinetics. Nitroglycerin and the isosorbide preparations are nitrate compounds used in the **prevention and treatment of angina attacks.**

Nitroglycerin is available in formulations for sublingual, transdermal, topical, oral, and intravenous administration. The drug's solubility in water and lipids permits its rapid dissolution and absorption after sublingual or buccal administration for the treatment of acute angina attacks. Its high lipid solubility and low dosage have enabled the formulation of skin patches for transdermal administration. The patches slowly release the drug for absorption through the skin into the circulation and are used in the prevention of angina attacks. In ointment form, nitroglycerin is absorbed through the skin over a period of several hours. The ointment is primarily used in hospitalized patients with **angina** or **myocardial infarction.** Nitroglycerin is administered orally in the form of sustained-release capsules that are used to prevent angina attacks. The drug is well absorbed from the gut but undergoes considerable first-pass inactivation, thereby necessitating the use of larger doses when administered orally. Nitroglycerin is also available as an intravenous solution that is used chiefly to reduce preload but also to reduce afterload in patients who have **acute heart failure** associated with myocardial infarction and other conditions.

Isosorbide dinitrate may be administered sublingually or orally and is used for both the prevention and the treatment of angina attacks. Isosorbide dinitrate produces the same pharmacologic effects as nitroglycerin, but it has a slightly slower onset of action and a greater duration of action (Fig. 11–4). It is converted to an active compound, isosorbide mononitrate, which is now available as a separate drug preparation for the prevention of angina attacks.

Mechanisms and Pharmacologic Effects. The organic nitrates are believed to act by releasing nitric oxide in vascular endothelial cells (Fig. 11–5). This reaction requires tissue sulfhydryl groups, which may become depleted during continuous exposure to organic nitrates, thereby causing nitrate tolerance. Nitric oxide is a gas that diffuses into vascular smooth muscle cells, where it activates guanylyl cyclase, forming cyclic guanosine monophosphate (cyclic GMP). Cyclic GMP is believed to relax vascular smooth muscle by inactivating myosin light-chain kinase or by stimulating dephosphorylation of myosin phosphate.

The organic nitrates preferentially relax venous smooth muscle and have a relatively smaller effect on arteriolar smooth muscle. This leads to venous pooling of blood, a decrease in venous blood return to the heart, and a decrease in ventricular volume, pressure, and wall tension. By these mechanisms, the nitrates reduce cardiac work and oxygen demand and thereby relieve or prevent angina pectoris. By reducing cardiac preload, the nitrates also reduce cardiac output and thereby contribute to a reduction in blood pressure. If blood pressure falls sufficiently, reflex tachycardia may be invoked. The nitrates do not have any direct effects on myocardial tissue.

Tolerance. Whenever nitroglycerin or an isosorbide compound is administered continuously, nitrate tolerance can occur. This effect is due to depletion of sulfhydryl compounds at the receptor site and is a form of pharmacodynamic tolerance. It has been demonstrated to occur with intravenous, transdermal, and oral administration of the nitrates, including sustained-release preparations of them. To prevent nitrate tolerance and loss of therapeutic effect, skin patches should be removed for at least 10 hours a day, and long-acting oral medications should be administered only once or twice a day.

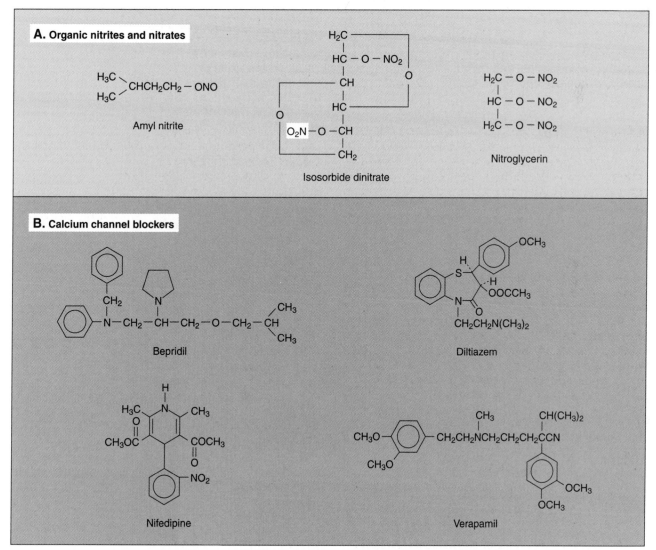

FIGURE 11–3. Structures of selected antianginal drugs. There are three groups of antianginal drugs. Representative structures of one group, the β-adrenergic receptor antagonists, are depicted in Fig. 9–1. Examples of the other two groups are shown here. **(A)** The organic nitrites and nitrates include amyl nitrite, isosorbide compounds, and nitroglycerin. The unshaded portion of isosorbide dinitrate is enzymatically removed in the formation of isosorbide mononitrate. **(B)** The calcium channel blockers belong to several chemical classes. Bepridil is a diarylamine ether; diltiazem is a benzothiazepine compound; nifedipine is a 1,4-dihydropyridine compound; and verapamil is a phenylalkylamine derivative.

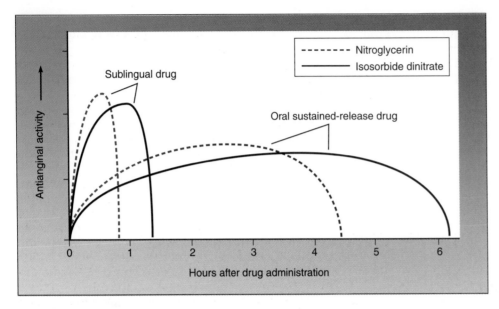

FIGURE 11–4. **Pharmacokinetics of nitroglycerin and isosorbide dinitrate.** Nitroglycerin is more rapidly absorbed and has a shorter duration of action, partly because it is quickly converted to two metabolites that are less active (glyceryl mononitrate and dinitrate). Isosorbide dinitrate is converted to a metabolite that is active and has a longer half-life (isosorbide mononitrate).

Adverse Effects and Interactions. The most common adverse effects of organic nitrates are due to excessive vasodilation and include headache, hypotension, dizziness, and reflex tachycardia. Tachycardia increases oxygen demand and may counteract the beneficial effects of nitrates, so patients should be cautioned to avoid excessive doses of these drugs. To prevent reflex tachycardia, a β-blocker may be used together with an organic nitrate or other type of vasodilator. In combination, the drugs have a synergistic therapeutic effect.

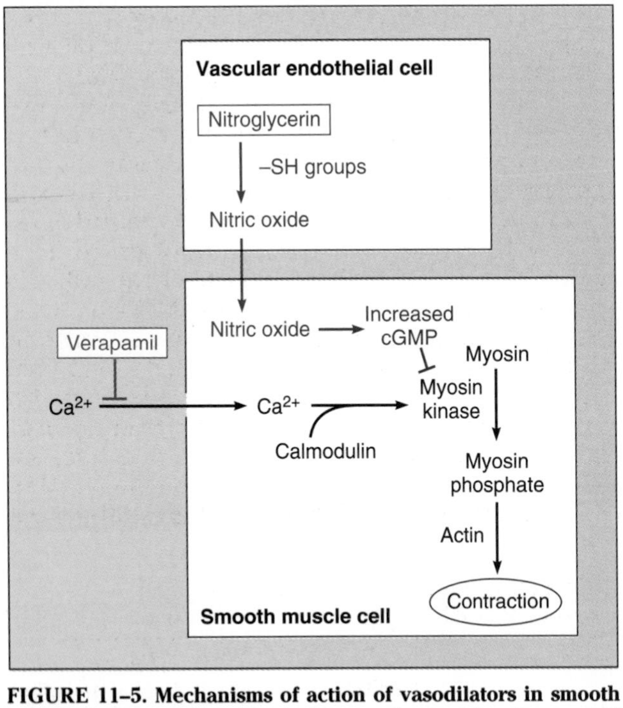

Calcium Channel Blockers

Calcium channel blockers (CCBs) belong to numerous chemical classes. **Amlodipine, felodipine, isradipine, nicardipine, nifedipine,** and **nimodipine** belong to the dihydropyridine class and have similar pharmacologic properties. **Bepridil, diltiazem,** and **verapamil** each belong to a different chemical class and are the only member of their class that is currently available for clinical use.

All of the CCBs except bepridil and nimodipine are indicated for the treatment of **hypertension** (see Chapter 10). Diltiazem and verapamil are also used to treat certain types of **cardiac arrhythmias** (see Chapter 14). Nimodipine is indicated for the treatment of **subarachnoid hemorrhage,** which is one of the causes of stroke. In this setting, the drug is believed to dilate small cerebral vessels and thereby increase collateral circulation. Nimodipine may also reduce neuronal damage caused by an excessive release of calcium invoked by cerebral ischemia.

The discussion below focuses on the CCBs that are used in the management of **angina pectoris.** These antianginal CCBs include three dihydropyridines (amlodipine, nicardipine, and nifedipine), bepridil, diltiazem, and verapamil.

Drug Properties

Chemistry and Pharmacokinetics. Structures of selected CCBs are shown in Fig. 11–3B, and the pharmacokinetic properties of the six antianginal CCBs are summarized in Table 11–2. These CCBs are

FIGURE 11–5. **Mechanisms of action of vasodilators in smooth muscle.** Actions of nitroglycerin (an organic nitrate) and verapamil (a calcium channel blocker) are shown. Organic nitrates form nitric oxide in the presence of tissue sulfhydryl (SH) groups. Nitric oxide diffuses into smooth muscle cells, where it activates guanylyl cyclase and thereby stimulates the formation of cyclic guanosine monophosphate (cGMP). Investigators believe that cGMP causes smooth muscle relaxation either by inactivating myosin kinase or by dephosphorylating myosin phosphate. When calcium (Ca^{2+}) enters the smooth muscle via calcium channels, it binds to calmodulin and thereby activates myosin kinase. Myosin kinase phosphorylates the light chains of myosin, enabling it to interact with actin to cause muscle contraction. Verapamil works by blocking calcium channels.

TABLE 11–2. Pharmacokinetic Properties of Calcium Channel Blockers Used in the Treatment of Angina Pectoris*

Drug	Oral Bioavail-ability	Excreted Unchanged in Urine	Elimination Half-Life (Hours)
Dihydropyridines			
Amlodipine	75%	10%	40
Nicardipine	35%	1%	3
Nifedipine	60%	1%	3
Other calcium channel blockers			
Bepridil	60%	5%	25
Diltiazem	55%	3%	5
Verapamil	25%	3%	5

*Values shown are the mean of values reported in the literature.

well absorbed after oral administration, but most of them undergo significant first-pass metabolism. Diltiazem, nicardipine, nifedipine, and verapamil have relatively short half-lives and are available in immediate-release preparations (which require multiple daily doses) and in sustained-release preparations (which require one or two doses a day). Amlodipine and bepridil have longer half-lives and are administered once or twice a day.

Mechanisms and Pharmacologic Effects. The **calcium ion channels** are located in the plasma membrane of smooth muscle and cardiac tissues. The influx of calcium through these channels leads to membrane depolarization and initiates or strengthens muscle contraction. CCBs bind to these channels and alter their conformation in a way that prevents the entry of calcium into cells (see Fig. 11–5). By this mechanism, CCBs produce smooth muscle relaxation and suppress cardiac activity.

Calcium channels are classified on the basis of their electrophysiologic properties. The two main types of voltage-activated calcium channels are the L (long) type and the T (transient) type. **L-type calcium channels** are high-voltage channels that are slowly inactivated, and their calcium influx has a relatively long duration. **T-type calcium channels** are low-voltage channels that are rapidly inactivated, and

their calcium influx is more transient. Both L-type and T-type channels are found in vascular smooth muscle and in the sinoatrial (SA) and atrioventricular (AV) nodes. However, only L-type channels are found in the muscle cells of the heart. The CCBs that are currently available act to selectively block L-type channels. **Mibefradil,** a drug that selectively blocked T-type channels, was approved for treating angina and hypertension in 1997, but it was withdrawn from the market in 1998 because of potentially dangerous interactions with other drugs.

While all CCBs cause vascular smooth muscle to relax, they differ markedly in their effects on cardiac tissue (Table 11–3). The dihydropyridines are potent vasodilators and may reduce blood pressure sufficiently to evoke reflex tachycardia. At therapeutic doses, the dihydropyridines do not suppress cardiac function as much as the other CCBs do. Diltiazem and verapamil decrease SA node automaticity, cardiac contractility, and AV node conduction velocity to a greater degree than the other CCBs do and may significantly reduce cardiac output in patients with heart failure.

Adverse Effects. The most common side effects of CCBs in general are fatigue, headache, dizziness, flushing, edema, and other manifestations of vasodilation and hypotension. Several epidemiologic studies have suggested that CCBs are also associated with an increased risk of adverse cardiovascular events, gastrointestinal bleeding, and cancer.

In retrospective case-control studies, investigators found a higher incidence of myocardial infarction, congestive heart failure, and deaths due to coronary heart disease in the group of patients who took immediate-release forms of nifedipine and other short-acting CCBs than in the control group. In a prospective clinical trial called the Multicenter Isradipine Diuretic Atherosclerosis Study (MIDAS), investigators found a statistically significant increase in angina attacks, transient ischemic attacks, and nonfatal arrhythmias in the group of patients treated with isradipine. They also found a higher rate of myocardial infarction, stroke, congestive heart failure, angina, and sudden death in the isradipine-treated group than in the control group, but these differences

TABLE 11–3. Cardiovascular Effects of Calcium Channel Blockers Used in the Treatment of Angina Pectoris

Drug	Coronary Blood Flow	Sinoatrial Node Automaticity*	Cardiac Contractility*	Atrioventricular Node Conduction Velocity*
Dihydropyridines				
Amlodipine	Increases	None	None	None
Nicardipine	Increases	None	None	None
Nifedipine	Increases	None	Decreases slightly	None
Other calcium channel blockers				
Bepridil	Increases	Decreases slightly	Decreases slightly	Dereases slightly
Diltiazem	Increases	Decreases	Decreases slightly	Decreases
Verapamil	Increases	Decreases	Decreases	Decreases

*Direct effects may be counteracted by reflex activity.

were not statistically significant. The association of CCBs and adverse cardiovascular events is currently being evaluated in other prospective clinical trials.

The CCBs are reported to have antiplatelet effects. In a retrospective case-control study of various drugs, the risk of gastrointestinal bleeding in patients treated with diltiazem or verapamil was found to be higher than that in patients treated with β-blockers or angiotensin-converting enzyme (ACE) inhibitors. Although this study does not prove that CCBs cause gastrointestinal bleeding, CCBs are not recommended for patients who have other risk factors for bleeding, such as peptic ulcers.

Various studies have explored the possible link between CCB use and cancer. One retrospective case-control study found that patients taking nifedipine or verapamil have a higher risk of cancer than those taking β-blockers or ACE inhibitors. This is a complex subject, since some in vitro studies suggest that CCBs have anticancer effects and others indicate that CCBs inhibit apoptosis (programmed cell death), which is a defense mechanism against cancer.

Additional adverse effects of specific CCBs are described below.

Amlodipine, Nicardipine, and Nifedipine

Amlodipine, nicardipine, and nifedipine are the dihydropyridine CCBs approved for the treatment of angina. Amlodipine has a long elimination half-life and is administered once a day. It has little or no direct effect on the heart rate, AV node conduction, and cardiac contractility. Nicardipine and nifedipine have relatively short half-lives, and the immediate-release preparations must be administered several times a day in the treatment of angina. Nifedipine is more likely than other dihydropyridines to depress cardiac contractility.

The dihydropyridines are potent vasodilators and may evoke reflex tachycardia and cause cardiac arrhythmias in some patients. Unlike diltiazem and verapamil, the dihydropyridines do not affect digoxin serum levels significantly.

Bepridil

Unlike the other CCBs, which block only calcium channels, bepridil also blocks sodium channels in cardiac tissue. Bepridil slows the heart rate slightly and reduces AV node conduction while increasing the AV node refractory period. Bepridil also causes prolongation of the QT interval, which may evoke cardiac arrhythmias such as torsade de pointes (polymorphic ventricular tachycardia). For this reason, the drug is usually reserved for use in patients who have not responded to other antianginal drugs.

Diltiazem and Verapamil

Diltiazem or verapamil may be used in the treatment of typical or variant angina. However, because these drugs are able to suppress cardiac contractility, caution should be exercised when administering either of them to patients with heart failure. In patients who have typical angina without heart failure, the drugs have the advantage of reducing the heart rate and contractility in addition to their effects on myocardial wall tension.

Verapamil may cause constipation, probably due to relaxation of gastrointestinal smooth muscle and reduced peristalsis. Both verapamil and diltiazem reduce the clearance of digoxin and may thereby increase serum digoxin levels and precipitate digoxin toxicity. Digoxin doses should be reduced in patients receiving these drugs.

β-ADRENERGIC RECEPTOR ANTAGONISTS

The pharmacologic properties of β-adrenergic receptor antagonists, or β-blockers, are discussed in Chapter 9, and their use in the treatment of hypertension and arrhythmias is discussed in Chapters 10 and 14, respectively.

Among the β-blockers used in the management of angina are **atenolol, metoprolol, nadolol,** and **propranolol.** These β-blockers have a significant role in the management of **typical angina pectoris** and **acute myocardial infarction,** but they are not used in the management of variant angina or acute anginal attacks. In typical angina, they are used as prophylactic agents because of their ability to prevent exercise-induced tachycardia and increased myocardial oxygen demand. They can also prevent reflex tachycardia induced by organic nitrates or dihydropyridine CCBs.

Atenolol, metoprolol, and propranolol are often used in myocardial infarction to reduce the risk of sudden death due to acute ventricular arrhythmias.

The β-blockers have a negative inotropic effect that may be hazardous to patients with heart failure. Because the combination of verapamil and a β-blocker is particularly likely to reduce cardiac contractility and cardiac output, it should be used with great caution. The combination of a β-blocker and diltiazem is less hazardous.

THE MANAGEMENT OF ANGINA PECTORIS

In patients with a history of angina pectoris, the primary objectives of drug therapy are to relieve acute symptoms, to prevent ischemic attacks, and to reduce the risks of myocardial infarction and other potential cardiovascular problems, as illustrated in Box 11–1.

If a patient has only an occasional angina episode, sublingual nitroglycerin may be used as needed to relieve acute symptoms. If episodes occur predictably with exertion, sublingual nitroglycerin or isosorbide dinitrate may be taken as a prophylactic measure just prior to exertion. If the severity of angina requires regular use of sublingual nitroglycerin, however, long-term prophylactic therapy should be considered. In some cases, angiography should

BOX 11–1.   Typical Angina Pectoris

Case Presentation

A 57-year-old construction worker who is a heavy smoker complains of a pressure-like discomfort in the retrosternal area. He says the problem began about a month ago and occurs two or three times a week. When questioned about the discomfort, he says that it only occurs when he is working, disappears when he rests, does not radiate to his left arm or jaw, and has never lasted for more than 15 minutes. Except for a blood pressure of 150/100 mm Hg, his results on physical examination and electrocardiogram are normal.

Case Management

After ruling out other causes of the patient's chest discomfort, the physician makes a provisional diagnosis of typical angina pectoris and prescribes sublingual nitroglycerin, 0.3 mg, as needed for acute chest discomfort. Because the patient has hypertension and angina but does not have diabetes, asthma, or heart failure, the physician also prescribes a β-adrenergic receptor antagonist, atenolol, for the treatment of hypertension and the prevention of angina. The patient is encouraged to monitor his blood pressure regularly and is scheduled to see his physician again in 3 weeks.

Case Comments

β-Adrenergic receptor antagonists are the preferred therapy for patients with hypertension and angina, because these drugs are effective in the management of both conditions and provide protection against ischemia-induced arrhythmias. Patients with chronic stable angina should be evaluated for hypercholesterolemia and treated appropriately with dietary restrictions and drug therapy to retard the progression of atherosclerosis. Control of blood pressure will also reduce atherogenesis. Patients with angina should be considered for angiographic evaluation of their coronary arteries to determine whether angioplasty or coronary artery bypass grafting is appropriate.

also be performed to determine if angioplasty or coronary artery bypass grafting is appropriate.

For patients who have stable angina and require long-term treatment, either a β-blocker, a long-acting nitrate, or a CCB may be chosen for initial therapy, with other drugs added or substituted depending on the response. The β-blockers are the only antianginal drugs that have been proved to reduce the incidence of ventricular arrhythmias that cause sudden death in patients who have had a myocardial infarction.

Because of this cardioprotective effect, some authorities consider β-blockers the drug of choice in treating most patients who have angina pectoris (see exceptions below and in Table 11–4) and especially those who have unstable angina. Patients with unstable angina have a high risk of myocardial infarction and should also receive aspirin or other antithrombotic drugs to prevent platelet aggregation and thrombus formation. CCBs are less suitable than β-blockers for patients with unstable angina or a recent myocardial infarction, because the dihydropyridine CCBs have the potential to cause reflex tachycardia and because verapamil and diltiazem have the potential to suppress cardiac contractility.

The β-blockers are ineffective in treating variant angina, which is caused by coronary vasospasm. This condition can be treated with amlodipine, nifedipine, diltiazem, or verapamil. Bepridil and nicardipine are not approved for the treatment of vasospastic angina.

In patients who have angina and concomitant asthma, diabetes, or heart failure, the β-blockers should be avoided or used with great caution. In patients with asthma, a CCB is usually preferred because of its potential ability to relax bronchial smooth muscle. In patients with diabetes, a CCB is often used; however, if a β-blocker is chosen, it should be a cardioselective (β_1-selective) blocker such as atenolol, which has less potential to interfere with β_2-mediated glycogenolysis and slow the recovery from insulin-induced hypoglycemia. Other guidelines for patients with angina and concomitant diseases are presented in Table 11–4.

Summary of Important Points

- In patients with typical angina, the antianginal drugs act by decreasing myocardial oxygen demand. The organic nitrites and nitrates and the calcium channel blockers (CCBs) decrease myocardial wall tension, whereas the β-adrenergic receptor antagonists (β-blockers) and some CCBs decrease the heart rate and contractility.
- Nitrates and dihydropyridine CCBs have the potential to cause reflex tachycardia, but this effect can be prevented by concurrent administration of a β-blocker.

TABLE 11–4.   Selection of Antianginal Drugs for Patients With Angina Pectoris and Concomitant Diseases

Concomitant Disease	Most Preferred Drugs	Least Preferred Drugs
Asthma	Calcium channel blocker; organic nitrite or nitrate.	β-Adrenergic receptor antagonist.
Diabetes mellitus	Calcium channel blocker; organic nitrite or nitrate.	β-Adrenergic receptor antagonist.
Heart failure	Organic nitrite or nitrate.	β-Adrenergic receptor antagonist; diltiazem; verapamil.
Hypertension	β-Adrenergic receptor antagonist; calcium channel blocker.	Organic nitrite or nitrate.
Peptic ulcer	β-Adrenergic receptor antagonist; organic nitrite or nitrate.	Calcium channel blocker.

- Continuous exposure to nitrates leads to tolerance. Nitrate tolerance is due to depletion of sulfhydryl groups at the receptor site where nitric oxide is released.
- All CCBs have similar vasodilative activity. Verapamil and diltiazem also produce significant cardiac depression, and verapamil has a greater effect than diltiazem on cardiac contractility. Verapamil and diltiazem may increase serum digoxin levels and cause digitalis toxicity.
- In patients with a history of myocardial infarction, the β-blockers have been found to reduce the incidence of ventricular arrhythmias that cause sudden death. This cardioprotective effect adds to their value in the treatment of angina.
- Some vasodilators are effective in the treatment of variant angina, but β-blockers are not.

Selected Readings

Borhani, N. O., et al. Final outcome results of the Multicenter Isradipine Diuretic Atherosclerosis Study (MIDAS). JAMA 276:785–791, 1996.

Ertel, S. I., and E. A. Ertel. Low-voltage–activated T-type Ca^{2+} channels. Trends Pharmacol Sci 18:37–42, 1997.

Pahor, M., et al. Calcium channel blockade and incidence of cancer in aged populations. Lancet 348:493–497, 1996.

Pahor, M., et al. Risk of gastrointestinal haemorrhage with calcium antagonists in hypertensive patients over 67 years old. Lancet 347:1061–1065, 1996.

Parker, J. D., and J. O. Parker. Nitrate therapy for stable angina pectoris. N Engl J Med 338:520–531, 1998.

Savonitto, S., and D. Ardissino. Selection of drug therapy in stable angina pectoris. Cardiovasc Drug Ther 12:197–210, 1998.

Spaulding, C., et al. Pharmacologic and therapeutic basis for combined administration of beta blockers and calcium channel blockers in the treatment of stable chronic angina. Br J Clin Pract 88(supplement):17–22, 1997.

CHAPTER TWELVE

DRUGS FOR HEART FAILURE

CLASSIFICATION OF DRUGS FOR HEART FAILURE

POSITIVELY INOTROPIC DRUGS
Digitalis glycosides
- Digitoxin
- Digoxin

Adrenergic receptor agonists
- Dobutamine
- Dopamine

Phosphodiesterase inhibitors
- Amrinone
- Milrinone

VASODILATORS
Angiotensin-converting enzyme inhibitors
- Captopril
- Enalapril
- Lisinopril

Calcium channel blockers
- Amlodipine

Other vasodilators
- Hydralazine
- Isosorbide dinitrate
- Nitroprusside

DIURETICS
- Bumetanide
- Furosemide
- Hydrochlorothiazide
- Torsemide

OTHER DRUGS FOR HEART FAILURE
- Amiodarone
- Carvedilol

OVERVIEW

In the USA, **congestive heart failure** affects from 2 million to 3 million individuals, is the primary cause of 38,000 deaths per year, and is a contributing factor in another 225,000 deaths. The overall mortality rate in patients with congestive heart failure is about eight times as high as that in the normal population, and the 2-year mortality rate for patients with severe heart failure approaches 70%.

Pathophysiology of Heart Failure

Heart failure is usually a consequence of underlying cardiovascular disorders. At the present time, **myocardial infarction** is the most common cause of heart failure. Frequent cardiovascular causes include acute and chronic coronary artery disease, chronic hypertension, valvular disorders, arrhythmias, viral cardiomyopathy, and other conditions that reduce ventricular ejection during systole (such as hypertrophic subaortic stenosis and constrictive pericarditis). Noncardiac causes of heart failure include severe anemia, thiamine deficiency, and use of certain anticancer drugs, such as doxorubicin (see Chapter 45).

The hallmark of heart failure is a **reduction in stroke volume and cardiac output** at any given diastolic muscle fiber length, as determined by measuring the ventricular end-diastolic pressure (preload). The reduced stroke volume may be caused by **diastolic dysfunction** or **systolic dysfunction** and is manifested as an inability of the ventricles either to properly fill or to properly empty, respectively. Systolic dysfunction may be due to decreased cardiac contractility secondary to a dilated or ischemic myocardium. Diastolic dysfunction may be due to decreased compliance (increased stiffness) of ventricular tissue secondary to left ventricular hypertrophy or fibrosis.

In cases of **left ventricular failure (left-sided heart failure),** the left ventricle does not adequately pump blood forward, so the pressure in the pulmonary circulation increases. When the increased pressure forces fluid into the lung interstitium, this causes **congestion** and **edema** (Fig. 12–1). **Pulmonary edema** reduces the diffusion of oxygen and carbon dioxide between alveoli and the pulmonary capillaries. This causes **hypoxemia** (deficient oxygenation of the blood) and can lead to **dyspnea** (difficulty in breathing), including **exertional dyspnea** (dyspnea provoked by exercise), **orthopnea** (intensified dyspnea when lying flat), and **paroxysmal nocturnal dyspnea** (edema-induced bronchoconstriction when sleeping).

The combination of edema-related hypoxemia and the failure of the heart to pump sufficient blood to adequately perfuse the tissues may lead to generalized tissue hypoxia and organ dysfunction. For this reason, patients with heart failure often experience symptoms of weakness and fatigue and have reduced exercise capacity.

In cases of **right ventricular failure (right-sided heart failure),** congestion in the peripheral veins leads to **ankle edema** in the ambulatory patient and to **sacral edema** in the bedridden patient. It also leads

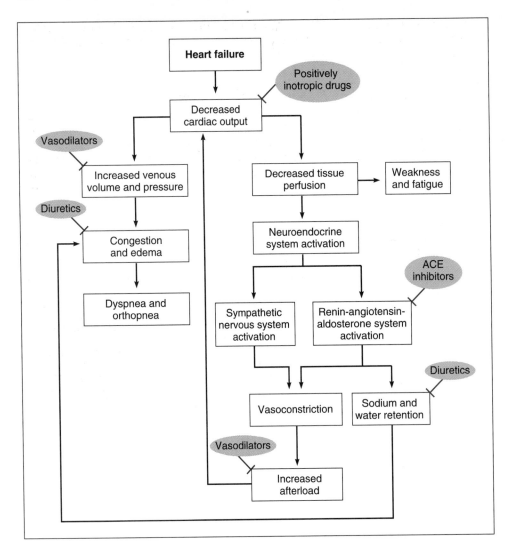

FIGURE 12–1. Pathophysiology and treatment of congestive heart failure. ACE = angiotensin-converting enzyme.

to **hepatojugular reflux,** characterized by an increase in jugular vein distention when pressure is applied over the liver. Ultimately, right-sided failure may lead to left-sided failure as the left ventricle is forced to work harder in an attempt to maintain cardiac output.

The reduction in cardiac output that occurs in heart failure triggers a cascade of **compensatory neurohumoral responses.** Although these responses attempt to restore cardiac output via the Frank-Starling mechanism (see Fig. 12–1), they are often maladaptive and counterproductive. The reduction in tissue perfusion activates the sympathetic nervous system and renin-angiotensin-aldosterone system, both of which in turn stimulate vasoconstriction. Arterial vasoconstriction increases aortic impedance to left ventricular ejection and thereby decreases cardiac output, especially in patients with a weak, dilated heart. When angiotensin II stimulates the secretion of aldosterone and antidiuretic hormone, this increases the amount of sodium and water retention, the plasma volume, and the venous pressure. In addition, angiotensin II may activate cardiac remodeling and wall thinning, which often reduce systolic and diastolic function. Hence, the net result

of the neurohumoral responses is often a further reduction in cardiac output and an increase in circulatory congestion.

Mechanisms and Effects of Drugs for Heart Failure

Among the pharmacologic agents currently used to treat heart failure are several positively inotropic drugs, numerous vasodilators and diuretics, and a few other types of drugs whose ultimate role is still being determined. The positively inotropic drugs and arterial vasodilators all increase stroke volume, but they do so by different mechanisms. In addition, some vasodilators may reduce venous pressure, congestion, and edema. Diuretics are used to mobilize edematous fluid and reduce plasma volume, thereby decreasing venous congestion.

Table 12–1 compares the cardiovascular effects of drugs discussed in this chapter. Each of these drugs partly counteracts the loss of myocardial function and the maladaptive responses that occur during heart failure; however, none of the current therapies, either alone or in combination, has been completely satisfactory. Because congestive heart failure has such a high incidence and poor prognosis, a great deal of effort has been expended in the search for better means to treat it. The most significant development in the last 2 decades has been the introduction and gradual acceptance of the use of vasodilators for this purpose. In fact, several vasodilators have been shown to reduce the mortality rate in patients with heart failure. Other drugs that are currently under investigation for use in these patients include β-adrenergic receptor antagonists. Ultimately, however, the successful treatment of pa-

tients with heart failure may require the development of novel drugs that activate genes capable of repairing or replacing myocardial tissue.

POSITIVELY INOTROPIC DRUGS

Derived from the Greek words for fiber (*inos*) and changing (*tropikos*), the term *inotropic* refers to a change in muscle contractility. Drugs that increase cardiac contractility are said to have a **positive inotropic effect,** while drugs that decrease contractility have a **negative inotropic effect.** Drugs with a

TABLE 12–1.   Cardiovascular Effects of Drugs Used in the Treatment of Heart Failure*

Drug	Cardiac Contractility	Heart Rate	Preload Reduction	Afterload Reduction	Risk of Arrhythmia	Other Effects
Positively inotropic drugs						
Digitalis glycosides						
Digoxin	+	–	++	0 to +	++	Increases parasympathetic tone and decreases sympathetic tone
Digitoxin	+	–	++	0 to +	++	Increases parasympathetic tone and decreases sympathetic tone.
Adrenergic receptor agonists						
Dobutamine	++	+ to ++	0 to +	+ to ++	+ to ++	
Dopamine	++	+ to ++	0 to +	+ to ++	+ to ++	
Phosphodiesterase inhibitors						
Amrinone	+	0 to ++	++	++	++	
Milrinone	+	0 to ++	++	++	++	
Vasodilators						
Angiotensin-converting enzyme inhibitors						
Captopril	0	0	++	++	0	
Enalapril	0	0	++	++	0	
Lisinopril	0	0	++	++	0	
Calcium channel blockers						
Amlodipine	0	0	0 to +	++	0	Blocks L-type calcium channels.
Other vasodilators						
Hydralazine	0	+ (R)	0	++	+	Reduces blood pressure.
Isosorbide dinitrate	0	+ (R)	++	+	0	Reduces pulmonary congestion.
Nitroprusside	0	+ (R)	++	+	0	Reduces pulmonary congestion.
Diuretics						
Bumetanide	0	0	+	0	0	Reduces edema and congestion.
Furosemide	0	0	+	0	0	Reduces edema and congestion.
Hydrochlorothiazide	0	0	+	+	0	Reduces edema and congestion.
Torsemide	0	0	+	0	0	Reduces edema and congestion.
Other drugs						
Amiodarone	0	–	0 to +	+	–	Reduces blood pressure.
Carvedilol	0	0 to –	0	+	0	Blocks α- and β-adrenergic receptors.

*Effects are indicated as follows: decrease (–); no change or variable (0); increase ranging from small (+) to large (++); and reflex (R).

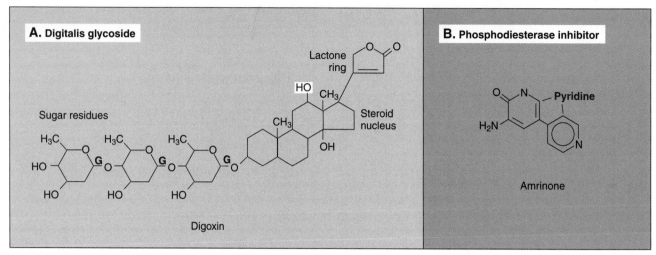

FIGURE 12–2. Structures of two examples of positively inotropic drugs for heart failure. (A) One group of positively inotropic drugs, the digitalis glycosides, includes digoxin and digitoxin. The portion of digoxin that is unshaded in this figure is absent in digitoxin. G denotes a glycosidic bond. **(B)** Two other groups of positively inotropic drugs consist of phosphodiesterase inhibitors (such as amrinone, a bipyridine, shown here) and adrenergic receptor agonists (such as dobutamine and dopamine, shown in Fig. 8–3).

positive effect include members of three groups: digitalis glycosides, adrenergic receptor agonists, and phosphodiesterase inhibitors.

Digitalis Glycosides

Despite the fact that the digitalis glycosides have been used to treat heart failure for over 200 years, their effectiveness and place in therapy remain controversial. A number of recent clinical trials indicate that digitalis provides a definite, yet limited, benefit to patients with congestive heart failure.

Drug Properties

A large number of digitalis glycosides have been isolated from plant and animal sources, including the leaves of *Digitalis* (foxglove) plants and the skin secretions of certain toads. Digoxin is the only digitalis glycoside that is extensively used today, having largely replaced digitoxin and crude digitalis leaf

preparations in the treatment of heart failure and other cardiac disorders.

Chemistry and Pharmacokinetics. The digitalis glycosides are composed of a steroid nucleus, a lactone ring, and three sugar residues linked by glycosidic bonds (Fig. 12–2A). The stereochemical configuration of the steroid nucleus of digitalis glycosides is different than that of human steroids, and the digitalis glycosides lack most of the effects produced by gonadal or adrenal steroids.

As shown in Table 12–2, digitalis glycosides are adequately absorbed from the gut and have half-lives that are relatively long. Digoxin has a half-life of 35 hours and is primarily eliminated by renal excretion of the parent compound, whereas digitoxin has a half-life of more than a week and is extensively metabolized before excretion. Because the digitalis glycosides have a low therapeutic index, serum concentrations are useful in assessing the adequacy of the dosage and evaluating potential digitalis toxicity. Serum concentrations of digoxin should be

TABLE 12–2. Pharmacokinetic Properties of Positively Inotropic Drugs*

Drug	Oral Bioavailability	Onset of Action	Duration of Action	Elimination Half-Life	Excreted Unchanged in Urine	Therapeutic Serum Level
Digitalis glycosides						
Digoxin	75%	1 hour	24 hours	35 hours	60%	0.5–2 ng/mL
Digitoxin	90%	2 hours	36 hours	180 hours	30%	15–30 ng/mL
Adrenergic receptor agonists						
Dobutamine	NA	1 minute	<10 minutes	2 minutes	0%	NA
Dopamine	NA	1 minute	<10 minutes	6 minutes	Negligible amount	NA
Phosphodiesterase inhibitors						
Amrinone	NA	3 minutes	Variable	4 hours	60%	NA
Milrinone	NA	3 minutes	Variable	4 hours	60%	NA

*Values shown are the mean of values reported in the literature. NA = not applicable (not administered orally).

in the range of 0.5–2 ng/mL, and those of digitoxin should be in the range of 15–30 ng/mL.

Mechanisms and Pharmacologic Effects. The direct and indirect actions of digitalis glycosides produce a unique constellation of effects on the cardiovascular system. They have a **positive inotropic effect** (an increase in the force of contraction), a **negative chronotropic effect** (a decrease in the heart rate), and a **negative dromotropic effect** (a decrease in conduction velocity). Among the various types of positively inotropic drugs, only the digitalis glycosides have the ability to strengthen cardiac contraction while decreasing heart rate. Moreover, the digitalis glycosides indirectly increase parasympathetic tone while reducing sympathetic tone. This contributes to their effects on heart rate and conduction velocity and may account in part for their important role in the treatment of heart failure and other cardiac disorders.

(1) Positive Inotropic Effect. Digitalis produces a modest positive inotropic effect that is due to an increase in intracellular calcium and is secondary to inhibition of the sodium pump (Na$^+$,K$^+$-ATPase) in the plasma membrane (sarcolemma). When the sodium pump is inhibited, the concentration of intracellular sodium is increased, thereby increasing the activity of the sodium-calcium exchanger and causing more calcium to enter the cardiac myocyte (Fig. 12–3). The increase in cytoplasmic calcium stimulates the release of additional calcium from the sarcoplasmic reticulum and leads to greater myofibril shortening (contraction).

The positive inotropic effect of digitalis increases the velocity of cardiac muscle contraction and the peak systolic muscle tension. These actions increase stroke volume and cardiac output at any given diastolic fiber length (preload), as shown in Fig. 12–4. The stroke volume is the amount of blood pumped by the ventricle during each systole, and the cardiac output is the amount of blood ejected from either ventricle of the heart per minute.

(2) Electrophysiologic and Electrocardiographic Effects. Digitalis has several indirect effects on cardiac electrophysiology. It causes an increase in parasympathetic (vagal) tone, and this decreases the heart rate and atrioventricular (AV) node conduction velocity while increasing the AV node refractory period (Fig. 12–5). At the same time, it causes a decrease in sympathetic tone. In patients with heart failure, the reduction in sympathetic tone is partly due to the withdrawal of reflex sympathetic stimulation secondary to the improved cardiac output produced by digitalis. The drug also appears to directly inhibit sympathetic nerve activity. The reduction in sympathetic tone augments the effect of vagal activation on the sinoatrial and AV nodes, and it also decreases sympathetic vasoconstriction and thereby counteracts the direct vasoconstrictive effect of digitalis. The effects of digitalis on the AV node account for its ability to slow the ventricular rate in patients with atrial fibrillation (see below).

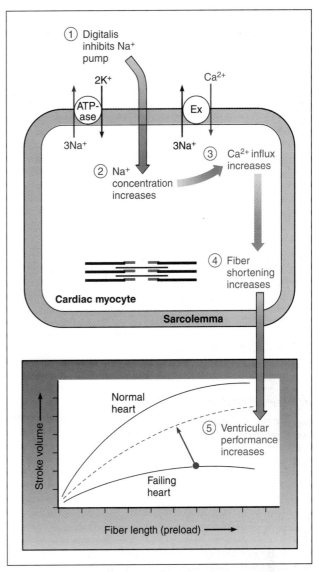

FIGURE 12–3. Mechanisms by which digitalis exerts its positive inotropic effect on the heart. Digitalis inhibits the sodium pump (ATPase) in the sarcolemma and increases the concentration of intracellular sodium. The high sodium concentration increases the activity of the sodium-calcium exchanger (Ex), thereby causing more calcium to enter the cardiac myocyte. Calcium activates muscle fiber shortening and increases cardiac contractility, and this in turn increases stroke volume at any given fiber length (preload).

Digitalis also has direct effects on cardiac electrophysiology. Of particular importance is the drug's ability to increase abnormal impulse formation by evoking spontaneous **afterdepolarizations** (see Fig. 12–5). These abnormal depolarizations occur during or immediately after normal cardiac repolarization and lead to **extrasystoles** (premature or coupled beats) and **tachycardia** (rapid beating of the heart). The afterdepolarizations appear to be caused by excessive calcium influx into cardiac cells, and they are more likely to occur after higher doses of digitalis are given.

Digitalis has several effects on the electrocardiogram (see Fig. 12–5). It shortens the ventricular

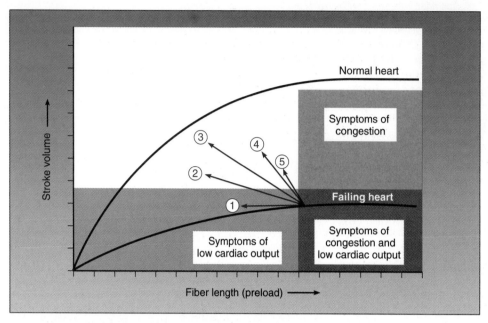

FIGURE 12–4. Effect of drug treatment on ventricular performance. Effects of the following drugs or drug combinations are shown: (1) a diuretic or a nitrate; (2) nitroprusside or an angiotensin-converting enzyme (ACE) inhibitor; (3) a positively inotropic drug plus a vasodilator; (4) dobutamine; and (5) a digitalis glycoside. The positively inotropic drugs increase stroke volume at any given fiber length and thereby decrease venous pressure and preload. Some vasodilators, such as the angiotensin-converting enzyme (ACE) inhibitors, decrease afterload and thereby increase stroke volume. Vasodilators may also decrease preload.

FIGURE 12–5. Electrophysiologic and electrocardiographic effects of digitalis. Digitalis causes an increase in parasympathetic (vagal) tone and a decrease in sympathetic tone. These actions slow the heart rate by decreasing sinoatrial (SA) node automaticity. The increased vagal tone and decreased sympathetic tone also slow the atrioventricular (AV) node conduction velocity while increasing the AV node refractory period. The reduced AV conduction velocity increases the PR interval on the electrocardiogram (ECG). In ventricular tissue, digitalis shortens the action potential duration, and this decreases the QT interval. Toxic concentrations of digitalis may evoke afterdepolarizations throughout the heart and thereby cause extrasystoles and tachycardia. Digitalis also causes ST segment depression, which gives rise to the so-called hockey stick configuration on the ECG.

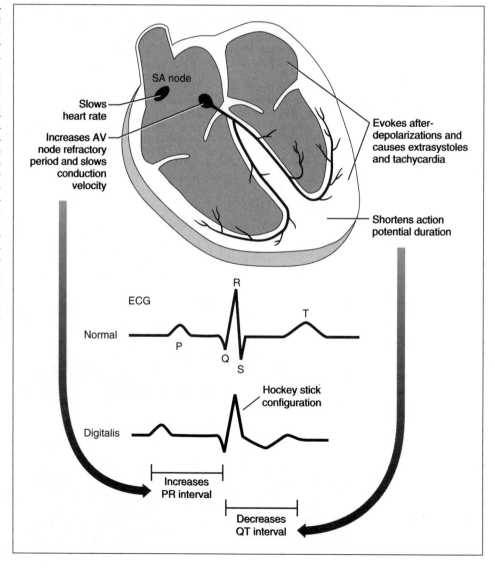

action potential duration by accelerating repolarization, and this decreases the QT interval. It reduces the AV node conduction velocity and thereby increases the PR interval. Finally, it causes ST segment depression, which gives rise to the so-called hockey stick configuration of the ST segment.

Adverse Effects. The most common adverse effects of the digitalis glycosides are gastrointestinal, cardiac, and neurologic reactions. Frequently, the earliest signs of digitalis toxicity are anorexia, nausea, and vomiting. These reactions are often associated with elevated serum concentrations of digitalis glycosides and may forewarn of more serious toxicity.

Arrhythmias are usually the most serious manifestation of digitalis toxicity and may include AV block and various tachyarrhythmias. Atrial tachycardia with 2:1 or 3:1 AV block is one of the most common types of digitalis-induced arrhythmia, but digitalis can also cause ventricular arrhythmias. Hypokalemia can precipitate arrhythmias in patients receiving digitalis, and the serum potassium level should be determined immediately if arrhythmias occur in these patients.

The neurologic effects of digitalis include blurred vision and yellow, green, or blue chromatopsia (a condition in which objects appear unnaturally colored). Severe digitalis toxicity can precipitate seizures.

Because digitalis has some estrogenic activity, it occasionally causes gynecomastia (excessive growth of male mammary glands).

Interactions. Several drugs may interact with digoxin and thereby affect its efficacy and toxicity (Table 12–3). Because antacids and cholestyramine may reduce the absorption of digoxin and decrease its therapeutic effects, their administration should be separated from the administration of digoxin by at least 2 hours. Diltiazem, quinidine, and verapamil reduce digoxin clearance and increase serum digoxin levels, and this may cause digitalis toxicity. When digoxin is used concurrently with these drugs, only 50% of the usual dose of digoxin should be given, and serum digoxin levels should be monitored. Diuretics should be used cautiously with digoxin. Diuretic-induced hypokalemia may precipitate digitalis toxicity because the reduced serum potassium concentration increases digitalis binding to the sodium pump. Hypokalemia may also contribute directly to arrhythmias.

Indications. Digitalis glycosides have been used to treat **congestive heart failure** for centuries, but their benefits have been uncertain while their toxicity has been substantial. The improvement produced by digitalis glycosides in patients with heart failure is probably due to a combination of a modest positive inotropic effect and attenuation of the neurohumoral consequences of heart failure. As discussed above, digitalis augments parasympathetic tone while reducing sympathetic tone, and these actions reduce heart rate, sympathetic vasoconstriction, and cardiac afterload.

In patients with heart failure, clinical trials have shown that although digitalis treatment does not prolong survival, it reduces symptoms and the need for hospitalization. Moreover, patients who have been withdrawn from digitalis exhibit worsening of

TABLE 12–3. Adverse Effects, Contraindications, and Drug Interactions of Positively Inotropic Drugs

Drug	Common Adverse Effects	Contraindications	Common Drug Interactions
Digitalis glycosides			
Digoxin	Anorexia, nausea, and vomiting; arrhythmias; blurred vision; chromatopsia; gynecomastia; and seizures.	Hypersensitivity to digitalis; obstructive and restrictive cardiomyopathy; and ventricular arrhythmia.	Digitalis absorption inhibited by antacids and cholestyramine. Digitalis clearance reduced by diltiazem, quinidine, and verapamil. Diuretic-induced hypokalemia precipitates digitalis toxicity.
Digitoxin	Same as digoxin.	Same as digoxin.	Same as digoxin.
Adrenergic receptor agonists			
Dobutamine	Excessive vasoconstriction and tachyarrhythmias.	Atrial fibrillation; cardiomyopathy; and hypersensitivity to dobutamine.	Activity affected by other agonists and antagonists.
Dopamine	Same as dobutamine.	Arrhythmia; hypersensitivity to dopamine; and pheochromocytoma.	Same as dobutamine.
Phosphodiesterase inhibitors			
Amrinone	Arrhythmias; hypotension; and thrombocytopenia.	Acute myocardial infarction; hypersensitivity to amrinone or bisulfites; and severe valvular disease.	Incompatible with furosemide in intravenous solutions.
Milrinone	Arrhythmias; hepatotoxicity; hypotension; and thrombocytopenia.	Acute myocardial infarction; hypersensitivity to milrinone; and severe valvular disease.	Unknown.

heart failure. Hence, digitalis will probably continue to have a role in treating heart failure in combination with vasodilators, diuretics, and other drugs.

The most certain indication for digitalis, however, appears to be the treatment of patients with **both heart failure and atrial fibrillation.** In these patients, the ventricular rate is often rapid and irregular, thereby causing palpitations and reducing cardiac output. By slowing the AV node conduction velocity and increasing the AV node refractory period, digitalis reduces the number of ectopic impulses that are transmitted from the atria to the ventricles and thereby slows the ventricular rate.

Digoxin

Over the past several decades, digoxin has become the most widely used cardiac glycoside. One of the reasons that it is used more frequently than digitoxin is that its half-life is shorter. This enables steady-state concentrations to be achieved more rapidly without the administration of loading doses. The more rapid elimination of digoxin is also an advantage if toxicity occurs. An antidote for serious digoxin toxicity is available in the form of **digoxin immune Fab.** This antibody preparation is administered intravenously and can rapidly reverse severe digoxin toxicity.

Digitoxin

Digitoxin is less polar than digoxin because it lacks one of the hydroxyl groups on the steroid nucleus of digoxin (see Fig. 12–2A). For this reason, digitoxin is better absorbed from the gut and crosses the blood-brain barrier more easily. Digitoxin is eliminated primarily by hepatic metabolism, and it has a much longer half-life than digoxin.

Adrenergic Receptor Agonists

Dobutamine and **dopamine** are the adrenergic receptor agonists most frequently used in patients with heart failure. Each of these agents must be administered by continuous intravenous infusion, and this usually restricts their use to the short-term management of **acute heart failure** and **cardiogenic shock.**

Dobutamine and dopamine are β-adrenergic receptor agonists that selectively stimulate cardiac contractility and usually cause less tachycardia than do other β-adrenergic receptor agonists, such as isoproterenol. Dobutamine activates β_2 receptors more than it activates α receptors in vascular smooth muscle. For this reason, it produces a mild vasodilative effect. Dopamine dilates renal and splanchnic vessels by activating dopamine receptors in these vascular beds.

The properties and effects of dobutamine and dopamine are summarized in Tables 12–1, 12–2, and 12–3 and are described in greater detail in Chapter 8.

Phosphodiesterase Inhibitors

The phosphodiesterase inhibitors currently used in the treatment of heart failure are **amrinone** (see Fig. 12–2B) and **milrinone.** These bipyridine drugs inhibit **type III phosphodiesterase,** an enzyme that normally catalyzes the conversion of cyclic adenosine monophosphate (cyclic AMP, or cAMP) to the inactive 5'-AMP. By inhibiting phosphodiesterase, the drugs increase the concentration of cAMP in cardiac tissue and smooth muscle and thereby increase cardiac contractility and relax vascular smooth muscle.

Amrinone and milrinone are used only for the short-term management of **acute heart failure** or **acute exacerbations of chronic heart failure** in patients who are not responsive to other drugs. Amrinone and milrinone are administered intravenously for this purpose. Clinical studies have shown that the long-term use of these drugs may cause serious adverse effects, including thrombocytopenia and ventricular arrhythmias, and is associated with an increased mortality rate in patients with severe heart failure (Table 12–4).

VASODILATORS

Vasodilators are useful in the treatment of congestive heart failure because of their ability to reduce venous and arterial pressure. The reduction in venous pressure decreases edema, while the dilation of arteries increases cardiac output. The vasodilators that inhibit angiotensin also counteract some of the adverse neurohumoral changes that occur in heart failure.

Angiotensin-Converting Enzyme Inhibitors

Angiotensin-converting enzyme (ACE) inhibitors reduce the formation of angiotensin II and are used in the treatment of **diabetic nephropathy, hypertension,** and **heart failure.** The general pharmacologic properties of these drugs are described in Chapter 10.

Angiotensin II has several actions that contribute to the pathogenesis of heart failure, including vasoconstriction and increased secretion of aldosterone and antidiuretic hormone. **Captopril, enalapril, lisinopril,** and other ACE inhibitors act by producing venous and arterial dilation and decreasing the secretion of these two hormones. These actions in turn reduce the plasma volume, venous pressure, and level of edema, and they may increase cardiac output by reducing arterial pressure and cardiac afterload. In addition, ACE inhibitors may counteract the adverse effects of angiotensin that contribute to ventricular remodeling and diastolic dysfunction in patients with chronic heart failure.

As described in Table 12–4, enalapril and other vasodilators have been shown to decrease the mortality rate in patients with heart failure. The CONSENSUS trial found that enalapril reduced the mortality rate by 40% in patients with **severe heart failure.** The V-HeFT-II trial showed that treatment with enalapril reduced the mortality rate more than did treatment

TABLE 12–4. Findings in Clinical Studies of Drugs Used in the Treatment of Heart Failure

Drug	Study	Findings
Positively inotropic drugs		
Amrinone	Packer et al.[1]	Amrinone increased mortality rate in patients with severe heart failure.
Digoxin versus milrinone	DiBianco et al.[2]	Digoxin was superior to milrinone; milrinone caused arrhythmia in more patients.
Digoxin versus placebo	DIG[3]	Digoxin did not decrease mortality rate but decreased rate of hospitalization admissions for heart failure and other causes.
Digoxin withdrawal	PROVED[4]	Clinical worsening of heart failure occurred with digoxin withdrawal.
	RADIANCE[5]	Clinical worsening of heart failure occurred with digoxin withdrawal.
Milrinone	PROMISE[6]	Milrinone increased mortality rate in patients with severe heart failure.
Vasodilators		
Captopril	SAVE[7]	Captopril decreased risk of congestive heart failure by 37% in post–myocardial infarction patients with left ventricular dysfunction.
Enalapril	CONSENSUS[8]	Enalapril decreased mortality rate by 40% at 6 months in patients with severe heart failure.
Enalapril	SOLVD[9]	Enalapril decreased mortality rate by 18% in patients with mild to moderate heart failure; also decreased risk of congestive heart failure by 37% in patients with asymptomatic left ventricular dysfunction.
Enalapril versus combination of nitrate plus hydralazine versus placebo	V-HeFT-II[10]	Enalapril decreased risk of sudden death by 36% in patients with chronic heart failure; nitrate plus hydralazine decreased mortality rate more than placebo did but less than enalapril did.
Other drugs		
Amiodarone	CHF-STAT[11]	Amiodarone did not decrease overall mortality rate in patients with congestive heart failure but did improve ejection fractions, especially in patients with nonischemic disease.
Amiodarone	GESICA[12]	Amiodarone decreased mortality rate and rate of hospital admissions for worsening congestive heart failure; also improved ejection fractions and reduced heart rates.
Carvedilol	AUZ-NZ[13]	Carvedilol decreased mortality rate and improved ejection fractions but did not change exercise tolerance or global assessment in patients with congestive heart failure.
Carvedilol	PRECISE[14]	Carvedilol increased exercise tolerance and improved ejection fractions in patients with congestive heart failure.
Carvedilol	US mild CHF[15]	Carvedilol decreased mortality rate, decreased rate of hospital admissions, increased exercise tolerance, and improved global assessment in patients with mild congestive heart failure.
Carvedilol versus metoprolol	COMET	Study is under way.

[1]Packer, M., et al. Circulation 70:1038–1047, 1984.
[2]DiBianco, R., et al. N Engl J Med 320:677–683, 1989.
[3]Digitalis Investigational Group. N Engl J Med 336:525–533, 1997.
[4]Uretsky, B. F., et al. J Am Coll Cardiol 22:955–962, 1993.
[5]Packer, M., et al. N Engl J Med 329:1–7, 1993.
[6]Packer, M., et al. N Engl J Med 325:1468–1475, 1991.
[7]Pfeffer, M. A., et al. N Engl J Med 327:669–677, 1992.
[8]CONSENSUS Trial Study Group. N Engl J Med 316:1429–1435, 1987.
[9]SOLVD Investigators. N Engl J Med 325:293–302, 1991.
[10]Cohn, J. N., et al. N Engl J Med 325:303–310, 1991.
[11]Massie, B. M., et al. Circulation 93:2128–2134, 1995.
[12]Doval, H. C., et al. Lancet 344:493–498, 1994.
[13]Australia–New Zealand Heart Failure Research Collaborative Group. Lancet 349:375–380, 1997.
[14]Packer, M., et al. Circulation 94:2793–2799, 1996.
[15]Packer, M., et al. N Engl J Med 334:1349–1355, 1996.

with the combination of a nitrate and hydralazine in patients with **chronic heart failure.** The SAVE and SOLVD studies showed that treatment with captopril or enalapril can prevent the transition from asymptomatic to overt heart failure, thereby supporting the early use of an ACE inhibitor in patients with **asymptomatic heart failure.**

In patients with **acute myocardial infarction,** treatment with an ACE inhibitor has been found to improve the survival rate when it is administered within 24 hours of the onset of symptoms. Investigators believe that this benefit is partly due to the inhibition of angiotensin-induced ventricular remodeling, which would otherwise lead to ventricular thinning and expansion of the infarct zone in these patients.

Calcium Channel Blockers

Calcium channel blockers (CCBs) are drugs that prevent the entry of calcium into smooth muscle and cardiac cells. All of them produce vasodilation, and some of them reduce the heart rate and cardiac contractility. These cardiovascular effects are discussed in greater detail in Chapter 11, as are the differences between calcium channels of the L (long) type and the T (transient) type.

Traditional CCBs selectively block L-type calcium channels, and their use in the treatment of heart failure appears to be limited or contraindicated. **Verapamil** and **diltiazem,** for example, have significant negative inotropic effects and may reduce cardiac output significantly in patients with heart failure. **Nifedipine** and **amlodipine,** two dihydropyridine CCBs, cause less suppression of cardiac function at therapeutic doses and have been evaluated in patients with heart failure. Because nifedipine was found to worsen the clinical outcome, it is not currently recommended for use in these patients. Its deleterious effect in patients with heart failure may be partly due to reflex activation of the sympathetic nervous system. In contrast, amlodipine was found to reduce the mortality rate in a group of patients who had **nonischemic heart failure** and were receiving standard therapy.

Other Vasodilators

The **organic nitrates,** such as **isosorbide dinitrate,** relax venous smooth muscle more than arterial smooth muscle, and **hydralazine** is an arterial vasodilator. Isosorbide dinitrate is sometimes used alone to reduce **pulmonary congestion,** and the combination of a nitrate plus hydralazine may be used in patients who have **chronic heart failure** and cannot tolerate an ACE inhibitor. The combination increases cardiac output and reduces venous pressure and edema.

Nitroprusside is used for the short-term treatment of **acute heart failure** and **cardiogenic shock** because of its rapid onset of action. However, the drug must be administered by continuous intravenous infusion, and it requires frequent monitoring of blood pressure.

The pharmacologic properties of nitroprusside and organic nitrates are discussed in Chapter 10 and Chapter 11, respectively.

DIURETICS

In patients with heart failure, diuretics are used to reduce plasma volume and edema and thereby relieve the symptoms of circulatory congestion.

Loop diuretics, such as **bumetanide, furosemide,** and **torsemide,** have more natriuretic activity than other types of diuretics and are used in **most cases of heart failure.** Loop diuretics must be used carefully in order to avoid excessive diuresis, dehydration, and electrolyte imbalances. Hypokalemia predisposes patients to digitalis toxicity, and there is some evidence that torsemide may cause less kaliuresis than do the other loop diuretics.

Thiazide diuretics, such as **hydrochlorothiazide,** may be used in cases of **mild heart failure,** when a less powerful natriuretic agent will suffice.

The pharmacologic properties of diuretics are described in Chapter 13.

OTHER DRUGS FOR HEART FAILURE
β-Adrenergic Receptor Antagonists

Once contraindicated in heart failure because of their negative inotropic effect, the β-adrenergic receptor antagonists (β-blockers) have emerged as one of the new treatments for this cardiac condition. The shift in attitude is largely due to advances in the understanding of heart failure and to an increased emphasis on counteracting the adverse neurohumoral consequences of it.

The potential benefits of therapy with β-blockers are due to the ability of these drugs to reduce excessive sympathetic stimulation of the heart and circulation in patients with heart failure. Sympathetic stimulation causes acute adverse effects, such as tachycardia and increased myocardial oxygen demand, as well as chronic adverse effects, including cardiac hypertrophy, impaired myocyte function, and myocyte death. In addition, sympathetic stimulation increases renin release and angiotensin formation, and angiotensin II may have adverse effects on the heart.

While early trials with β-blockers that have intrinsic sympathomimetic activity were disappointing, more recent studies with a new β-blocker called **carvedilol** have been quite promising. Carvedilol is an unusual β-blocker in that it has considerable vasodilative activity, some of which is due to α-adrenergic receptor blockade. It also has antioxidant properties and has been called a **multiple-action neurohormonal antagonist** (MANA). Other pharmacologic properties of this drug are discussed in Chapter 9.

In several clinical studies, carvedilol has been found to increase exercise tolerance, increase the ventricular ejection fraction, reduce the severity of heart failure, and improve the global assessment of patients with this condition. Moreover, the mortality rate in patients with heart failure has been found to be significantly reduced when carvedilol is added to a standard treatment regimen that includes an ACE inhibitor and a diuretic. Based on these studies, carvedilol is currently recommended for patients who have **mild to moderate heart failure,** do not have significant hypotension or pulmonary congestion, and are already receiving an ACE inhibitor, a diuretic, and digoxin. Patients should be monitored for the adverse effects of carvedilol, which include bradycardia, worsening heart failure, and dizziness or light-headedness due to vasodilation and decreased blood pressure.

Two meta-analyses of β-blocker studies have been completed. One found that other β-blockers are as effective as carvedilol in reducing the mortality rate associated with heart failure, while the other found that carvedilol is superior. Clinical trials are currently under way to further examine the effects of various β-blockers on heart failure.

Amiodarone

Amiodarone is a class III antiarrhythmic agent whose pharmacologic properties include β-adrenergic receptor blockade and vasodilation. Its effectiveness in heart failure has been studied in several clinical trials (see Table 12–4), most of which have shown that amiodarone improves ventricular performance and reduces the mortality rate. In the GESICA trial, amiodarone reduced the heart rate, improved ejection fractions, decreased the risk of death by 28%, and decreased the rate of hospital admissions associated with worsening congestive heart failure by 31%. In the CHF-STAT trial, amiodarone did not show any effect on overall survival and sudden death rates; however, this trial had a much larger percentage of patients with ischemic congestive heart failure than did several other trials.

Although amiodarone appears to be useful in the treatment of patients who have **heart failure with ventricular arrhythmias,** its overall role in the treatment of heart failure remains uncertain.

THE MANAGEMENT OF HEART FAILURE

In patients with heart failure, the goals are to relieve the symptoms of disease and to prolong survival. Acute heart failure usually requires hospitalization and the administration of intravenous medications and oxygen. Chronic heart failure of lesser severity may be treated with oral medications, dietary restrictions, and exercise guidelines. While bed rest may relieve symptoms of heart failure during the early course of therapy, many patients benefit from an incremental exercise program after they are stabilized on medications.

The selection of medications for heart failure depends on the severity of the condition and the particular signs and symptoms exhibited by the patient. The initial treatment of heart failure often includes a diuretic to mobilize edematous fluid and reduce venous pressure and symptoms of circulatory congestion. Symptoms of low cardiac output, such as weakness and fatigue, may be relieved by the administration of digoxin, an ACE inhibitor, or other arterial vasodilator. The long-term therapy of heart failure may also include the judicious use of carvedilol or other β-blocker, as this type of drug appears to reduce the adverse effects of excessive sympathetic stimulation seen in patients with heart failure. Other drugs, such as amiodarone, may also benefit selected patients, and ongoing clinical trials will help guide their usage. The treatment of heart failure will continue to evolve as new drugs with unique mechanisms of action are developed.

Summary of Important Points

- Heart failure is a common manifestation of ischemic heart disease, chronic hypertension, valvular disorders, and other cardiovascular conditions.
- In patients with heart failure, digitalis glycosides increase cardiac contractility and cardiac output while decreasing heart rate, venous pressure, and congestion.
- Digitalis glycosides augment parasympathetic tone and thereby slow the atrioventricular (AV) node conduction velocity and increase the AV node refractory period. These actions slow the ventricular rate in patients with atrial fibrillation.
- Digoxin is primarily eliminated by renal excretion and has a relatively short half-life, whereas digitoxin is eliminated by hepatic metabolism and has a much longer half-life.
- The adverse gastrointestinal, cardiac, and neurologic effects of digitalis glycosides include anorexia, nausea, vomiting, arrhythmias, blurred vision, chromatopsia, and seizures.
- Digoxin immune Fab can be used to treat life-threatening digoxin toxicity.
- Angiotensin-converting enzyme (ACE) inhibitors and other vasodilators have been shown to improve cardiac output and reduce the mortality rate in patients with heart failure.
- Diuretics are used to mobilize edematous fluid in patients with heart failure.

Selected Readings

Cohn, J. N. The management of chronic heart failure. N Engl J Med 335:490–498, 1996.

Cohn, J. N. Overview of the treatment of heart failure. Am J Cardiol 80:2–6, 1997.

Hobbs, R. E. Digoxin's effect on mortality and hospitalization in heart failure: implications of the DIG study. Cleve Clin J Med 64:234–237, 1997.

Linn, W. D. Angiotensin-converting enzyme inhibitors in left ventricular dysfunction. Pharmacotherapy 16:50S–58S, 1996.

McAlister, F. A., and K. K. Teo. The management of congestive heart failure. Postgrad Med J 73:194–200, 1997.

McKelvie, R. S. Community management of heart failure. Can Fam Physician 44:2689–2692, 1998.

Naccarelli, G. V., et al. A decade of clinical trial developments in postmyocardial infarction, congestive heart failure, and sustained ventricular tachyarrhythmia patients: from CAST to AVID and beyond. J Cardiovasc Electrophysiol 9:864–891, 1998.

Packer, M., et al. The effect of carvedilol on morbidity and mortality in patients with chronic heart failure. N Engl J Med 334:1349–1355, 1996.

Singh, S. N., et al. Amiodarone in patients with congestive heart failure and symptomatic ventricular arrhythmias. N Engl J Med 333:77–82, 1995.

Young, J. B. Carvedilol for heart failure: renewed interest in beta blockers. Cleve Clin J Med 64:414–422, 1997.

CHAPTER THIRTEEN

DIURETICS

CLASSIFICATION OF DIURETICS

Thiazide and related diuretics
- Hydrochlorothiazide
- Indapamide
- Metolazone
- Polythiazide

Loop diuretics
- Bumetanide
- Ethacrynic acid
- Furosemide
- Torsemide

Potassium-sparing diuretics
- Amiloride
- Spironolactone
- Triamterene

Osmotic diuretics
- Glycerol
- Mannitol

Carbonic anhydrase inhibitors
- Acetazolamide
- Dorzolamide

OVERVIEW

Diuretics are used in the management of edema associated with cardiovascular, renal, and endocrine abnormalities, as well as in the treatment of hypertension, glaucoma, and several other clinical disorders (Table 13–1). The drugs act at various sites in the nephron to cause **diuresis** (an increase in urine production). Most diuretics inhibit the reabsorption of sodium from the nephron into the circulation and thereby cause an increase in **natriuresis** (the excretion of sodium in the urine). Several types of diuretics also cause an increase in **kaliuresis** (the excretion of potassium in the urine). Members of a new group of experimental drugs, the **aquaretics,** act to increase free water excretion by blocking receptors for antidiuretic hormone (arginine vasopressin receptors of the V_2 type). These receptors are discussed briefly in Chapter 31.

NEPHRON FUNCTION AND SITES OF DRUG ACTION

Sodium and other electrolytes are reabsorbed into the circulation at various sites throughout the nephron by active and passive processes that involve **ion channels, transport proteins,** and the **sodium pump** (Na^+,K^+-ATPase). Ion channels are unique membrane proteins through which a specific ion moves across the cell membrane in the direction that is determined by the electrochemical gradient for the ion. The transport proteins include **symporters,** which transport two or more ions in the same direction, and **antiporters,** which transport ions in opposite directions across cell membranes. Most diuretics act by blocking a specific ion channel or transporter in the tubular epithelial cells. The effects of diuretics on ion reabsorption and secretion in the nephron are illustrated in Box 13–1.

Glomerular Filtration

Urine formation begins with glomerular filtration, a process in which an ultrafiltrate of blood is forced out of the glomerular capillaries and into the nephron lumen by the hydrostatic pressure in these capillaries. In healthy individuals, this filtrate is essentially free of blood cells and plasma proteins. **Digitalis glycosides** and other cardiac stimulants may indirectly cause diuresis by increasing cardiac output, renal blood flow, and the glomerular filtration rate. The renal actions of these drugs are described in greater detail in Chapter 12. The diuretic drugs described in this chapter do not increase the glomerular filtration rate, and some of them may indirectly reduce it by decreasing plasma volume and renal blood flow.

Proximal Tubule

The proximal tubule is an important site of tubular reabsorption and secretion. Essentially all of the filtered glucose, amino acids, and other organic solutes are reabsorbed in the early portion of the proximal tubule. About 85% of filtered sodium bicarbonate is reabsorbed in the proximal tubule, and this reabsorption is inhibited by a class of diuretics known as **carbonic anhydrase inhibitors.** For reasons described later in this chapter, these drugs are relatively weak diuretics and are seldom employed for this purpose, though their actions are useful in the treatment of glaucoma and other conditions.

About 40% of filtered sodium chloride is reabsorbed in the proximal tubule. However, this is a relatively unimportant site of diuretic action because inhibition of sodium chloride reabsorption in the proximal tubule almost invariably leads to increased

TABLE 13–1. Usefulness of Diuretics in the Management of Various Clinical Disorders*

Disorder	Thiazide and Related Diuretics	Loop Diuretics	Potassium-Sparing Diuretics	Osmotic Diuretics	Carbonic Anhydrase Inhibitors
Cerebral edema	0	0	0	+	0
Cirrhosis	+	++	+	0	0
Congestive heart failure	+	++	+	0	0
Diabetes insipidus	++	0	0	0	0
Epilepsy	0	0	0	0	+
Glaucoma	0	0	0	+	++
High-altitude sickness	0	0	0	0	++
Hyperaldosteronism	0	0	+	0	0
Hypercalcemia	0	++	0	0	0
Hypertension	++	+	+	0	0
Hypokalemia	0	0	++	0	0
Nephrolithiasis	++	0	0	0	0
Nephrotic syndrome	+	++	+	0	0
Pulmonary edema	+	++	+	0	0
Renal impairment	+	++	0	+	0

*Ratings range from 0 (not useful) to ++ (highly useful).

sodium chloride reabsorption in more distal segments of the nephron.

The proximal tubule is the major site of the active tubular secretion of organic acids and bases into the nephron lumen, including natural compounds such as uric acid and drugs such as penicillins. The **loop diuretics** and **thiazide diuretics** are also secreted by proximal tubular cells, and then these drugs are carried in the tubular fluid to their site of action in the loop of Henle and the distal tubule, respectively.

Loop of Henle

The loop of Henle is responsible for the reabsorption of about 35% of the filtered sodium chloride. This segment also participates in the formation of a concentrated urine by transporting sodium chloride into the surrounding interstitium, where a hypertonic interstitial fluid is formed. This fluid attracts water from the collecting duct under the influence of antidiuretic hormone. The reabsorption of sodium from the thick ascending limb is inhibited by **loop diuretics,** which produce a greater diuretic effect than any other class of diuretics.

Distal Tubule

The early distal tubule is responsible for the reabsorption of 5–10% of the filtered sodium chloride, and this reabsorption is inhibited by **thiazide and related diuretics.** Because a relatively small percentage of sodium reabsorption can be inhibited by these drugs, they have a more modest diuretic action than the loop diuretics.

Collecting Duct

The collecting duct serves to adjust the final composition and volume of urine in order to regulate extracellular fluid composition and pH and thereby maintain physiologic homeostasis. The collecting duct is the site of action of **aldosterone** and **antidiuretic hormone.** Aldosterone is a mineralocorticoid that increases sodium reabsorption, thereby promoting sodium retention by the body. Antidiuretic hormone increases the reabsorption of water from the collecting duct, which conserves body water and concentrates the urine. The actions of these hormones are partly responsible for maintaining plasma volume and osmolality in the normal range.

The collecting duct is responsible for the reabsorption of about 3% of the filtered sodium chloride. This reabsorption is coupled with potassium and hydrogen excretion. The **potassium-sparing diuretics** inhibit these processes and are used to reduce potassium excretion and prevent hypokalemia.

DIURETIC AGENTS
Thiazide and Related Diuretics

The thiazides and related diuretics are the most commonly used diuretics. They are orally efficacious, have a moderate natriuretic effect, and have few adverse effects in most patients.

Drug Properties

Chemistry and Pharmacokinetics. Thiazides are sulfonamide compounds that contain a benzothiadiazide (thiazide) moiety (Fig. 13–1A). They exhibit good oral bioavailability and were the first orally administered diuretics to be widely used for the treatment of hypertension and edema. Thiazides are actively secreted into the nephron by proximal tubular cells, and they travel through the nephron lumen to reach their site of action in the distal tubule. Some of the thiazides are partially metabolized before excretion in the urine (Table 13–2).

Mechanisms and Pharmacologic Effects. Thiazide diuretics act primarily on the early portion of the distal tubule to inhibit the Na^+,Cl^- symporter that participates in the reabsorption of sodium and chloride from this segment of the nephron (see Box

BOX 13–1. Sites and Mechanisms of Action of Diuretics*

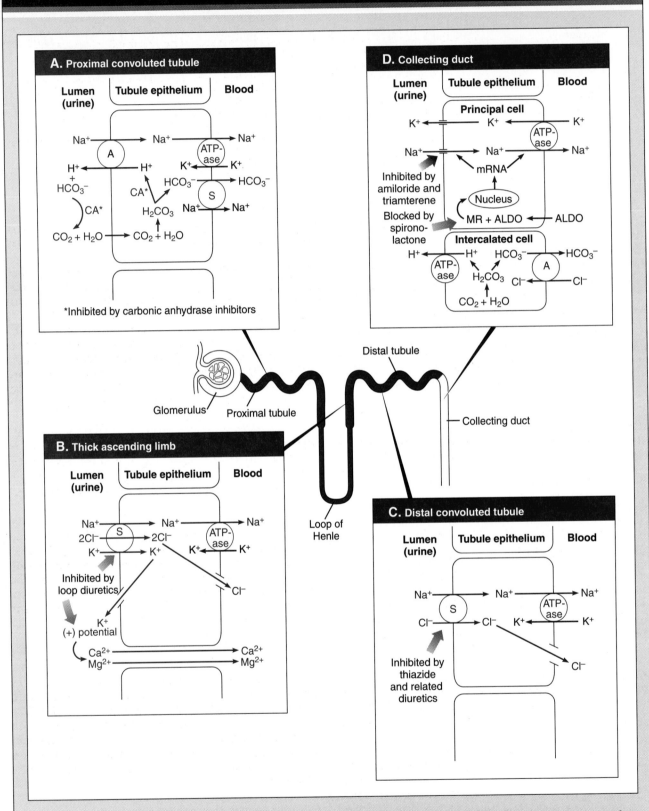

In the proximal tubule **(A)**, carbonic anhydrase catalyzes the reversible conversion of hydrogen ion and bicarbonate to carbon dioxide and water, thereby enabling the reabsorption of sodium bicarbonate. This process is inhibited by **carbonic anhydrase inhibitors,** such as **acetazolamide.**

In the thick ascending limb of the loop of Henle **(B),** the Na$^+$,K$^+$,2Cl$^-$ symporter transports sodium, potassium, and chloride ions into the tubular cells, and then sodium is transferred to the interstitial fluid by the sodium pump. Potassium back-diffuses into the

Continued

lumen and contributes to the positive transepithelial potential that drives paracellular calcium and magnesium reabsorption. By inhibiting the symporter, the **loop diuretics** reduce the back-diffusion of potassium and increase the excretion of calcium and magnesium.

In the distal tubule **(C)**, sodium is transported into tubular epithelial cells by the Na^+,Cl^- symporter and then is transferred to interstitial fluid by the sodium pump. The Na^+,Cl^- symporter is inhibited by **thiazide and related diuretics.**

In the collecting duct **(D)**, sodium enters the principal cells through sodium channels. Sodium is then transferred into the interstitial fluid by the sodium pump, while potassium is pumped in the opposite direction and then moves through potassium channels into the tubular fluid. Aldosterone stimulates these processes by increasing the synthesis of messenger RNA that encodes for sodium channel and sodium pump proteins. The **potassium-sparing diuretics** exert their effects via two mechanisms: **amiloride** and **triamterene** inhibit the entrance of sodium into the principal cells, whereas **spironolactone** blocks the mineralocorticoid receptor and thereby inhibits sodium reabsorption and potassium secretion.

*A = antiporter; ALDO = aldosterone; CA = carbonic anhydrase; MR = mineralocorticoid receptor; mRNA = messenger RNA; and S = symporter.

13–1). This action leads to the delivery of a greater volume of sodium chloride–enriched tubular fluid to the late distal tubule and collecting duct, and this in turn stimulates the exchange of sodium and potassium at these sites. In the process, a small amount of sodium is reabsorbed as potassium is secreted into urine in the tubules. By this mechanism, thiazides have a kaliuretic effect that leads to hypokalemia in some patients.

As shown in Table 13–3, thiazides increase magnesium excretion, but (unlike many diuretics) they decrease calcium excretion in the urine. The exact mechanism of these effects is uncertain. The ability of thiazides to reduce calcium excretion is the basis for their use in the treatment of kidney stones caused by excessive calcium in the urine.

Adverse Effects and Interactions.   Table 13–4 lists the common adverse effects and interactions of thiazides and other diuretics.

Thiazide diuretics sometimes cause hypokalemia, particularly in patients whose dietary potassium intake is inadequate. Hypokalemia may eventually lead to hypokalemic metabolic alkalosis (Fig. 13–2). In this disorder, hydrogen ions enter body cells as potassium leaves these cells in an attempt to correct the plasma potassium deficiency. As the plasma potassium level falls, more hydrogen ions are secreted into urine in the tubules in exchange for sodium, and this further contributes to the development of metabolic alkalosis. In cases of hypokalemic metabolic alkalosis, potassium chloride is administered intravenously and orally. Correction of the serum potassium level then leads to correction of the acid-base disturbance as potassium displaces hydrogen ions from body cells and fewer hydrogen ions are secreted by the collecting duct.

In addition to causing electrolyte and acid-base disturbances, the thiazides may cause several metabolic abnormalities, including elevated blood glucose, uric acid, and lipid levels. An increase in blood glucose levels may be caused in part by diuretic-induced potassium deficiency, because hypokalemia reduces the secretion of insulin by pancreatic beta cells and thereby increases plasma glucose concentrations. Hyperuricemia is caused by inhibition of uric acid secretion from the proximal tubule and may

lead to the development of gout. The effects of thiazide diuretics on serum lipid levels are discussed in greater detail in Chapter 10.

Indications.   Thiazide diuretics are widely used in the management of cardiovascular and renal diseases (see Table 13–1). They are often prescribed for **hypertension** and may be used for the treatment of **edema** associated with **congestive heart failure, cirrhosis, corticosteroid and estrogen therapy,** and **renal disorders** such as **nephrotic syndrome.** Because thiazides reduce calcium excretion and decrease urinary calcium levels, they are helpful in treating patients with **nephrolithiasis** (kidney stones) associated with **hypercalciuria.**

Thiazides are also used to treat nephrogenic **diabetes insipidus.** In this disorder, the kidneys are not responsive to circulating antidiuretic hormone, and patients may excrete from 10 to 20 L of urine per day. Thiazides exert a paradoxical antidiuretic effect in these patients and reduce the excessive urine volume dramatically. In cases of diabetes insipidus, the effectiveness of thiazides is believed to stem from a reduction in plasma volume caused by these drugs. The reduced plasma volume serves to increase sodium and water reabsorption from the proximal tubule, so that less water is delivered to the diluting segments of the nephron. As a result, the urine output falls.

Hydrochlorothiazide and Polythiazide

The numerous thiazide compounds that are available have almost identical actions but differ in their potency and pharmacokinetic properties. Hydrochlorothiazide is the most frequently prescribed thiazide. Polythiazide has a much longer half-life and duration of action than hydrochlorothiazide, and this is advantageous in the management of some disorders.

Thiazide-Like Diuretics

There are several thiazide-like diuretics whose structures are slightly different from those of the thiazide compounds but whose actions and uses are generally similar. One of them is **indapamide,** an

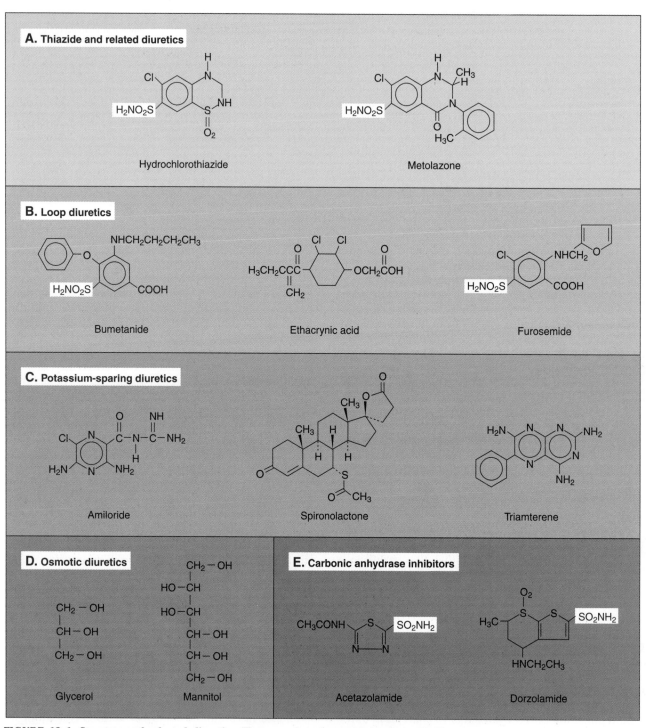

FIGURE 13–1. Structures of selected diuretics. There are five classes of diuretics. **(A)** The thiazide and related diuretics include hydrochlorothiazide and metolazone. These diuretics are sulfonamide derivatives, as are the carbonic anhydrase inhibitors and all of the loop diuretics except ethacrynic acid. The sulfonamide moiety is unshaded. **(B)** Loop diuretics include bumetanide, ethacrynic acid, and furosemide. **(C)** Potassium-sparing diuretics include amiloride, spironolactone, and triamterene. **(D)** Osmotic diuretics include glycerol and mannitol. **(E)** Carbonic anhydrase inhibitors include acetazolamide and dorzolamide.

agent primarily used in the treatment of **hypertension** and **congestive heart failure.** Another is **metolazone,** a diuretic that may be more effective than thiazide compounds in the treatment of patients with **impaired renal function.** Metolazone is sometimes combined with a loop diuretic to treat patients with **diuretic resistance.** Patients with diuretic resistance do not adequately respond to any single diuretic agent, but they may respond to the combination of a thiazide-like diuretic and a loop diuretic. The combined use of these diuretics produces **sequential nephron blockade,** in which the drugs inhibit the reabsorption of sodium in the ascending limb and the early distal tubule.

TABLE 13–2. Pharmacokinetic Properties of Diuretics*

Drug	Oral Bioavailability	Elimination Half-Life (Hours)	Route of Elimination	Duration of Action (Hours)
Thiazide and related diuretics				
Hydrochlorothiazide	70%	5	60% R and 40% M	12 for oral
Indapamide	90%	16	70% R and 30% M	30 for oral
Metolazone	65%	8	80% R and 20% M	18 for oral
Polythiazide	U	26	25% R and 75% U	36 for oral
Loop diuretics				
Bumetanide	85%	1.25	65% R and 35% M	5 for oral 1 for IV
Ethacrynic acid	100%	1	65% R and 35% M	7 for oral 2 for IV
Furosemide	60%	2	60% R and 40% M	7 for oral 2 for IV
Torsemide	80%	3.5	30% R and 70% M	7 for oral 7 for IV
Potassium-sparing diuretics				
Amiloride	20%	8	R	24 for oral
Spironolactone	65%	1.5	M	60 for oral
Triamterene	50%	4	M	14 for oral
Osmotic diuretics				
Glycerol	95%	0.7	M	1 for oral
Mannitol	NA	1	R	7 for IV
Carbonic anhydrase inhibitors				
Acetazolamide	70%	7.5	R	10 for oral
Dorzolamide	NA	Biphasic†	R and M	8 for topical

*Values shown are the mean of values reported in the literature. IV = intravenous; M = metabolism; NA = not applicable (not administered orally); R = renal; and U = unknown.
†Dorzolamide is eliminated in a biphasic manner, with a rapid decline in serum levels followed by a much slower release from erythrocytes, and has a half-life of 4 months.

Loop Diuretics
Drug Properties

Chemistry and Pharmacokinetics. The structures of several loop diuretics are shown in Fig. 13–1B, and their pharmacokinetic properties are summarized in Table 13–2.

Mechanisms and Pharmacologic Effects. Loop diuretics inhibit the $Na^+,K^+,2Cl^-$ symporter in the ascending limb of the loop of Henle and thereby exert a powerful natriuretic effect. In comparison with other diuretics, loop diuretics are able to inhibit the reabsorption of a greater percentage of filtered sodium. Loop diuretics are sometimes called **high-ceiling diuretics** because they produce a dose-dependent diuresis throughout their potential dos-

age range. This property can be contrasted with the rather flat dose-response curve and limited diuretic efficacy of thiazides and other diuretic drugs (Fig. 13–3).

In addition to their natriuretic effect, the loop diuretics produce kaliuresis by increasing the exchange of sodium and potassium in the late distal tubule and collecting duct via the same mechanisms as those described for the thiazide diuretics. Loop diuretics also increase magnesium and calcium excretion by reducing the reabsorption of these ions in the ascending limb (see Box 13–1). This action results from inhibition of the $Na^+,K^+,2Cl^-$ symporter, which reduces the back-diffusion of potassium into the nephron lumen. The reduction of potassium back-diffusion decreases the transepithelial electrical po-

TABLE 13–3. Effects of Diuretics on Plasma pH and Urinary Excretion of Electrolytes*

Drug	Plasma pH	Electrolytes Excreted				
		Ca^{2+}	HCO_3^-	K^+	Mg^{2+}	Na^+
Thiazide and related diuretics	0 or +	−	0 or +	++	++	++
Loop diuretics	0 or +	++	0	++	++	+++
Potassium-sparing diuretics	0 or −	−	0	−	−	+
Osmotic diuretics	0	+	+	+	++	+++
Carbonic anhydrase inhibitors	−	0 or +	+++	+	−	+

*Acute effects are shown and are indicated as follows: decrease (−); no change or variable (0); and increase ranging from small (+) to large (+++).

TABLE 13–4. Adverse Effects, Contraindications, and Drug Interactions of Diuretics*

Drug	Common Adverse Effects	Contraindications	Common Drug Interactions
Thiazide and related diuretics			
Hydrochlorothiazide	Blood cell deficiencies; electrolyte imbalances; and increased blood cholesterol, glucose, or uric acid levels.	Hypersensitivity to hydrochlorothiazide or sulfonamides.	Potentiates the diuretic effect of loop diuretics.
Indapamide	Electrolyte imbalances and increased blood cholesterol, glucose, or uric acid levels.	Hypersensitivity to indapamide or sulfonamides.	Same as hydrochlorothiazide.
Metolazone	Blood cell deficiencies; electrolyte imbalances; and increased blood cholesterol or glucose levels.	Hypersensitivity to metolazone or sulfonamides.	Same as hydrochlorothiazide.
Polythiazide	Same as hydrochlorothiazide.	Hypersensitivity to polythiazide or sulfonamides.	Same as hydrochlorothiazide.
Loop diuretics			
Bumetanide	Blood cell deficiencies; electrolyte imbalances; hearing impairment; and hypersensitivity reactions.	Anuria and hypersensitivity to bumetanide or sulfonamides.	Diuretic effect decreased by NSAIDs. Administration with ACE inhibitors may cause excessive hypotension.
Ethacrynic acid	Blood cell deficiencies; electrolyte imbalances; hearing impairment; and rash.	Anuria and hypersensitivity to ethacrynic acid.	Diuretic effect decreased by NSAIDs.
Furosemide	Blood cell deficiencies; electrolyte imbalances; hearing impairment; hypersensitivity reactions; increased blood cholesterol, glucose, or uric acid levels; and photosensitivity.	Anuria and hypersensitivity to furosemide or sulfonamides.	Same as bumetanide.
Torsemide	Electrolyte imbalances and increased blood cholesterol, glucose, or uric acid levels.	Anuria and hypersensitivity to torsemide or sulfonamides.	Same as bumetanide.
Potassium-sparing diuretics			
Amiloride	Blood cell deficiencies; gastrointestinal distress; and hyperkalemia.	Anuria and hypersensitivity to amiloride.	Administration with ACE inhibitors or potassium supplements may cause hyperkalemia. Administration with NSAIDs may cause renal failure.
Spironolactone	Gynecomastia; hyperkalemia; and impotence.	Anuria; hyperkalemia; hypersensitivity to spironolactone; and severe renal disease.	Administration with ACE inhibitors or potassium supplements may cause hyperkalemia.
Triamterene	Same as amiloride.	Anuria; history of renal stones; and hypersensitivity to triamterene.	Same as amiloride.
Osmotic diuretics			
Glycerol	Heart failure; nausea and vomiting; and pulmonary congestion and edema.	Anuria; hypersensitivity to glycerol; intestinal pain or obstruction; pulmonary congestion; and severe dehydration.	Potentiates effects of other diuretics.
Mannitol	Same as glycerol.	Anuria; hypersensitivity to mannitol; intracranial bleeding; pulmonary congestion; and severe dehydration.	Same as glycerol.
Carbonic anhydrase inhibitors			
Acetazolamide	Blood cell deficiencies; drowsiness; hepatic insufficiency; hyperglycemia; hypokalemia; metabolic acidosis; paresthesia; and uremia.	Electrolyte abnormalities; hypersensitivity to acetazolamide or sulfonamides; and severe hepatic or renal disease.	Serum levels of weak bases, such as amphetamine, ephedrine, and quinidine, are increased by CA inhibitors. Serum levels of CA inhibitors are increased by salicylates.
Dorzolamide	Bitter taste; blurred vision; and ocular discomfort and allergic reactions.	Hypersensitivity to dorzolamide or sulfonamides; and severe renal impairment.	Unknown.

*ACE = angiotensin-converting enzyme; CA = carbonic anhydrase; and NSAIDs = nonsteroidal anti-inflammatory drugs.

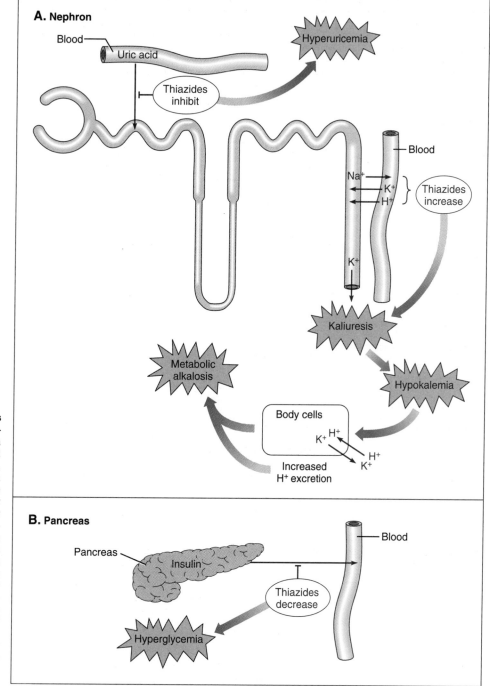

FIGURE 13–2. Adverse effects of thiazide diuretics. (A) Inhibition of uric acid secretion in the proximal tubule may lead to hyperuricemia and gout. Increased potassium secretion in the collecting duct may cause hypokalemia. Hypokalemia may lead to metabolic alkalosis by promoting the exchange of intracellular potassium for hydrogen ions and by increasing the excretion of hydrogen ions. The increased excretion is due to lack of availability of potassium for exchange with sodium in the collecting duct. **(B)** In the presence of hypokalemia, the amount of insulin secreted by the pancreas may be reduced, thereby leading to hyperglycemia. Other mechanisms may also be involved in the development of hyperglycemia.

tential that normally drives the paracellular reabsorption of magnesium and calcium. Inhibition of this process thereby increases magnesium and calcium excretion.

Adverse Effects and Interactions. Loop diuretics can produce a variety of electrolyte abnormalities, including hypokalemia, hypocalcemia, hypomagnesemia, and metabolic alkalosis. These diuretics may also increase blood glucose and uric acid levels in the same manner as the thiazide diuretics. In some patients, use of loop diuretics causes ototoxicity with manifestations such as tinnitus, ear pain, vertigo, and hearing deficits. In most cases, the hearing loss is

reversible. Other adverse effects, contraindications, and drug interactions are listed in Table 13–4.

Indications. Loop diuretics are used when intensive diuresis is required and cannot be achieved with other diuretics. Loop diuretics are highly effective in the treatment of **pulmonary edema,** partly because of the vasodilation that occurs when they are administered intravenously. They are preferred in the treatment of **renal impairment,** because (unlike thiazide and other diuretics) they are effective in patients whose creatinine clearance drops below 30 mL/min. Loop diuretics are often the drugs of choice for patients with edema due to **congestive**

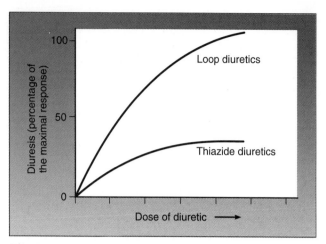

FIGURE 13–3. Dose-response curves of loop and thiazide diuretics. Loop diuretics produce dose-dependent diuresis throughout their therapeutic dosage range, whereas thiazide diuretics have a relatively flat dose-response curve and a limited maximal response.

heart failure, cirrhosis, and other disorders. Although they are prescribed for patients with **hypertension,** the thiazide diuretics are usually preferred for this condition. Loop diuretics can be used to treat **hypercalcemia,** whereas the thiazide diuretics may increase serum calcium levels slightly.

Bumetanide, Furosemide, and Torsemide

Bumetanide, furosemide, and torsemide are sulfonamide derivatives with similar pharmacologic actions and effects. These drugs may be administered orally or intravenously. In comparison with other loop diuretics, torsemide has a somewhat longer half-life and a significantly longer duration of action after intravenous administration (see Table 13–2). All three of the drugs are partly metabolized before they are excreted in the urine.

Ethacrynic Acid

Ethacrynic acid is the only loop diuretic that is not a sulfonamide derivative. It is available for use when patients are hypersensitive to other drugs in this class. Otherwise, it is seldom used because it produces more ototoxicity than do the other loop diuretics.

Potassium-Sparing Diuretics

There are two types of potassium-sparing diuretics: the epithelial sodium channel blockers and the aldosterone receptor antagonists.

Amiloride and Triamterene

Amiloride and triamterene (see Fig. 13–1C) are epithelial sodium channel antagonists. By blocking the entry of sodium into the principal tubular cells of the late distal tubule and collecting duct (see Box 13–1), these drugs prevent sodium reabsorption at this site and indirectly reduce the secretion of potassium into the tubular filtrate and urine. Through these actions, the potassium-sparing diuretics produce a modest amount of natriuresis while decreasing kaliuresis, and they are primarily used for the prevention and treatment of **hypokalemia** induced by thiazide and loop diuretics. The properties, effects, and uses of amiloride, triamterene, and other potassium-sparing diuretics are outlined in Tables 13–1 to 13–4.

The most characteristic adverse effect of the potassium-sparing diuretics is hyperkalemia, but this is unlikely to occur unless the patient also ingests potassium supplements or other drugs that increase serum potassium levels or unless the patient has a renal disorder that predisposes to hyperkalemia.

Spironolactone

Spironolactone, a steroid congener of aldosterone, competitively blocks the binding of aldosterone to the mineralocorticoid receptor in tubular epithelial cells of the late distal convoluted tubule and collecting duct. Normally, the mineralocorticoid receptor is activated by aldosterone and then interacts with nuclear DNA to promote the transcription of genes that encode proteins of the epithelial sodium channels, sodium pump, and related compounds involved in the reabsorption of sodium and secretion of potassium in these tubular segments. By blocking these actions, spironolactone reduces sodium reabsorption and the coupled secretion of potassium.

Spironolactone is adequately absorbed from the gut and has a long duration of action, despite its short elimination half-life, indicating that its cellular actions persist longer than its circulating drug levels (see Table 13–2). Spironolactone is used to prevent **hypokalemia** in the same manner as amiloride and triamterene, and it has a special role in the treatment of **primary hyperaldosteronism.** Because of its antiandrogenic effect, it is also used in the treatment of **polycystic ovary disease** and **hirsutism** in women.

The adverse effects of spironolactone include gynecomastia and impotence in men (caused by the drug's antiandrogenic effects) and hyperkalemia.

Osmotic Diuretics

Glycerol and **mannitol** (see Fig. 13–1D) are examples of osmotic diuretics. These diuretics increase the osmotic pressure of the plasma and thereby attract water from interstitial and transcellular fluids. Because of this action, mannitol is used to treat **cerebral edema** and reduce intracranial pressure. Glycerol and mannitol are both used in the treatment of **acute glaucoma.** By attracting water from ocular fluids into the circulation, the drugs reduce intraocular volume and pressure. Glycerol is administered orally for this purpose, whereas mannitol is administered intravenously.

Mannitol is also used as a diuretic. Following intravenous administration, it is filtered at the glomerulus but is not reabsorbed from the renal tubules. It osmotically attracts and retains water as it moves through the nephron and into the urine. This action reduces the tubular sodium concentration and the concentration gradient between the tubular fluid and cells and thereby retards the reabsorption of sodium. Hence, mannitol has both direct and indirect actions that promote diuresis. The diuretic effect of mannitol has been used to improve renal function in the oliguric phase of **acute renal failure** and to promote the excretion of toxic substances. It has been administered along with intravenous fluids to maintain renal function and reduce the renal toxicity of antineoplastic platinum compounds, such as cisplatin.

The primary adverse effect of mannitol is excessive plasma volume expansion, which is most likely to occur if the drug is administered too rapidly or with too large a volume of intravenous fluid. Excessive plasma volume may lead to heart failure and pulmonary congestion and edema in susceptible patients.

Carbonic Anhydrase Inhibitors
Drug Properties

The carbonic anhydrase (CA) inhibitors were the first sulfonamide derivatives to be used as diuretics, and their discovery eventually led to the development of the thiazide and loop diuretics. **Acetazolamide, dorzolamide,** and other CA inhibitors are relatively weak diuretics and are seldom used to promote diuresis today. Instead, their ability to inhibit CA has led to their use in the treatment of disorders such as high-altitude sickness and glaucoma.

Specific Drugs

Chemistry and Pharmacokinetics. Acetazolamide is one of several orally administered CA inhibitors, whereas dorzolamide is used as an ophthalmic solution for treating glaucoma. Dorzolamide is partly absorbed from the eye into the circulation and undergoes some metabolic transformation before it is excreted in the urine. The drug is eliminated in a biphasic manner, with a rapid decline in serum levels followed by a much slower release from erythrocytes, and it has a half-life of 4 months. The structures and pharmacokinetic properties of acetazolamide and dorzolamide are outlined in Fig. 13–1E and Table 13–2.

Mechanisms, Pharmacologic Effects, and Indications. Acetazolamide and other drugs in this class inhibit CA throughout the body. This enzyme catalyzes the conversion of carbon dioxide and water to carbonic acid, which spontaneously decomposes to bicarbonate and hydrogen ions:

$$CO_2 + H_2O \rightleftharpoons H_2CO_3 \longrightarrow HCO_3^- + H^+$$

When the ciliary process forms aqueous humor, CA participates by catalyzing the formation of bicarbonate, which is secreted into the posterior chamber of the eye, along with water and other substances that make up the aqueous humor. In patients with **glaucoma,** inhibition of CA reduces aqueous humor secretion and intraocular pressure. The CA inhibitors are used in the treatment of both the acute and the chronic form of glaucoma, although they must be combined with other drugs to treat the acute form. Traditionally, the CA inhibitors have been administered orally to patients with glaucoma. Now one of these drugs, dorzolamide, is available for topical ocular administration. It is administered every 8 hours in the treatment of **chronic ocular hypertension** and **open-angle glaucoma.**

CA is also required for the reabsorption of sodium bicarbonate from the proximal tubule and for the secretion of hydrogen ion in the collecting duct. In the reabsorption of sodium bicarbonate, bicarbonate must be converted to carbon dioxide and water by CA, because the apical cell membrane of the tubular epithelial cells is impermeable to bicarbonate. The carbon dioxide and water are able to diffuse into the tubular cells, where CA converts them back to bicarbonate, which is then transported into the interstitial fluid for diffusion into the circulation (see Box 13–1). Inhibition of this process by acetazolamide and other CA inhibitors causes a marked reduction in the reabsorption of sodium bicarbonate and a corresponding increase in its renal excretion. This leads to alkalinization of the urine and produces a mild form of hyperchloremic metabolic acidosis. The hyperchloremia results from the increased reabsorption of chloride as a compensation for reduced bicarbonate reabsorption.

CA inhibitors are seldom used as **diuretics,** although they are employed occasionally to **alkalinize the urine.** They are effective in the prevention and treatment of a form of **high-altitude sickness** called **mountain sickness,** because the metabolic acidosis produced by the drugs counteracts the respiratory alkalosis that may result from hyperventilation in this condition. By counteracting respiratory alkalosis, the drugs enhance ventilation acclimatization and maintain oxygenation during sleep at a high altitude. The drugs also counteract fluid retention and cause a decrease in cerebral spinal fluid (CSF) pressure, which may be elevated with acute high-altitude sickness. At the same time, CA inhibitors prevent the fall in CSF pH that occurs in this disorder.

Inhibition of CA in the central nervous system elevates the seizure threshold. For this reason, CA inhibitors have been used occasionally for the treatment of **epilepsy.**

Adverse Effects and Interactions. Acetazolamide and other orally administered CA inhibitors may cause drowsiness, paresthesia, and other central nervous system effects. They may also cause hypokalemia and hyperglycemia. Less commonly, they are associated with various hypersensitivity reactions and blood cell deficiencies. By increasing the pH of the renal tubular fluid and alkalinizing the urine, the CA inhibitors decrease the excretion of weak bases, such as amphetamine, ephedrine, and quinidine, and thereby increase their serum levels and cause drug toxicity.

THE MANAGEMENT OF EDEMA

Edema is a condition in which fluid accumulates in the interstitial space and body cavities, either because of increased hydrostatic pressure in the capillary beds or because of inadequate colloid osmotic pressure in the plasma. The plasma osmotic pressure is primarily influenced by the osmotic attraction of water by sodium and plasma proteins. Conditions that cause edema as a result of increased hydrostatic pressure include congestive heart failure and certain renal diseases, all of which cause sodium and water retention. Conditions that cause edema as a result of inadequate colloid osmotic pressure include severe dietary protein deficiency and hepatic diseases, such as cirrhosis. In conditions such as cirrhosis, the liver is unable to synthesize adequate albumin and other plasma proteins to maintain plasma osmotic pressure.

Nephrotic syndrome is a renal disease that leads to excessive protein excretion in the urine (protein-uria) and may cause edema by this mechanism. Infection, neoplasms, and thromboembolism may also cause edema by various mechanisms that include inflammation, increased capillary fluid permeability, and increased hydrostatic pressure due to obstruction of blood vessels.

The primary treatment of edema is to **correct the underlying disorder** and restore plasma osmotic pressure and hydrostatic pressure to normal values. In acute life-threatening situations, such as cerebral edema and pulmonary edema, **diuretics** and other drugs must be administered immediately to prevent tissue hypoxia, injury, and death. In milder forms of edema, diuretics may be used as short-term adjunct treatments that serve to mobilize edematous fluid while an attempt is made to correct the underlying cause. However, most cases of mild peripheral edema can be managed without pharmacologic therapy by correcting the underlying disorder or discontinuing a causative drug.

Summary of Important Points

- Diuretics are drugs that increase urine production. Most diuretics inhibit the reabsorption of sodium from various sites in the nephron.
- Thiazide diuretics inhibit sodium chloride reabsorption from the distal tubule. They cause natriuresis and kaliuresis, but they decrease calcium excretion. They are primarily used to treat hypertension, edema, hypercalciuria, and nephrogenic diabetes insipidus.
- Loop diuretics inhibit the $Na^+, K^+, 2Cl^-$ symporter in the ascending limb and thereby increase sodium, potassium, calcium, and magnesium excretion. They are chiefly used to treat congestive heart failure, renal failure, pulmonary edema, and hypercalcemia.
- Thiazide and loop diuretics may cause hypokalemia and other electrolyte disturbances, as well as hyperglycemia and hyperuricemia.
- Potassium-sparing diuretics inhibit potassium secretion in the collecting duct and are primarily used to prevent hypokalemia, which may be caused by thiazide and loop diuretics.
- Osmotic diuretics increase the osmotic pressure of plasma and retain water in the nephron. They are used to treat cerebral edema, glaucoma, and the oliguria of acute renal failure.
- Carbonic anhydrase inhibitors are weak diuretics that inhibit sodium bicarbonate reabsorption from the proximal tubule and may cause a mild form of metabolic acidosis. They reduce aqueous humor secretion and are primarily used to treat glaucoma.

Selected Readings

Brater, D. C. Diuretic therapy. N Engl J Med 339:387–395, 1998.

Gines, P., and W. Jimenez. Aquaretic agents: a new potential treatment of dilutional hyponatremia in cirrhosis. J Hepatol 24:506–512, 1996.

Ikeda, K., et al. Molecular and clinical implications of loop diuretic ototoxicity. Hear Res 107:1–8, 1997.

Kellum, J. A. Use of diuretics in the acute care setting. Kidney Int Suppl 66:S67–S70, 1998.

Morrison, R. T. Edema and principles of diuretic use. Med Clin North Am 81:689–704, 1997.

Moser, M. Diuretics in the prevention and treatment of congestive heart failure. Cardiovasc Drugs Ther 11(supplement 1):273–277, 1997.

Sica, D. A., and T. W. Gehr. Diuretic combinations in refractory oedema states: pharmacokinetic-pharmacodynamic relationships. Clin Pharmacokinet 30:229–249, 1996.

Suki, W. N. Use of diuretics in chronic renal failure. Kidney Int Suppl 59:S33–S35, 1997.

CHAPTER FOURTEEN

ANTIARRHYTHMIC DRUGS

CLASSIFICATION OF ANTIARRHYTHMIC DRUGS

SODIUM CHANNEL BLOCKERS
Class IA drugs
- Disopyramide
- Procainamide
- Quinidine

Class IB drugs
- Lidocaine
- Mexiletine
- Tocainide

Class IC drugs
- Flecainide
- Propafenone

Other class I drugs
- Moricizine

OTHER ANTIARRHYTHMIC DRUGS
Class II drugs
- Esmolol
- Metoprolol
- Propranolol

Class III drugs
- Amiodarone
- Bretylium
- Ibutilide
- Sotalol

Class IV drugs
- Diltiazem
- Verapamil

Miscellaneous drugs
- Adenosine
- Digoxin
- Magnesium sulfate

OVERVIEW

In a healthy adult with a normal heart, each heartbeat originates in the sinoatrial (SA) node, the rhythm of heartbeats is regular, and the heart rate is about 70 beats per minute at rest. If the origin, rhythm, or rate of heartbeats is abnormal, the condition is called an **arrhythmia (dysrhythmia).** Arrhythmias occur primarily because of disturbances in cardiac impulse formation or conduction, and they may originate in any part of the heart. Those arising in the atria or atrioventricular (AV) node are called **supraventricular arrhythmias,** whereas those arising in the ventricles are called **ventricular arrhythmias.** Those in which the heart rate is too rapid are called **tachyarrhythmias,** and those in which the heart rate is too slow are called **bradyarrhythmias.**

Some arrhythmias are benign and do not necessarily require treatment. Others require treatment because they reduce cardiac output and blood pressure significantly or because they may precipitate more serious and even lethal rhythm disturbances. Both pharmacologic and electrophysiologic methods are used to terminate and prevent arrhythmias. This chapter describes the pathophysiology of arrhythmias and the mechanisms by which antiarrhythmic drugs work.

Cardiac Action Potentials and Electrocardiographic Findings

Fig. 14–1 depicts the relationships between ion currents, cardiac action potentials in phases 0 through 4, and findings on the surface electrocardiogram (ECG).

The SA node, located in the right atrium, is the site of origin of the normal heartbeat. The SA node spontaneously depolarizes to form an impulse that is conducted through the atrium to the AV node and then through the bundle of His, bundle branches, and Purkinje fibers to the ventricular muscle.

The spontaneous depolarization of the SA node is due to the influx of sodium and calcium as the efflux of potassium subsides. When the threshold potential (TP) is reached at about –40 mV, the SA node is more rapidly depolarized by sodium and calcium influx so as to generate an impulse that can be conducted to the rest of the heart. As the impulse is conducted to atrial and ventricular muscle cells, these cells are rapidly depolarized by the influx of sodium through the fast sodium channel. As the cells depolarize to about –40 mV, the slow calcium channels open. The influx of calcium through these channels during phase 2 serves to activate muscle contraction. Cardiac tissues become repolarized during phase 3 as a result of the efflux of potassium through several types of rectifier potassium channels (I_K), an efflux that occurs when the influx of calcium declines.

As shown in Fig. 14–1, the surface ECG is a summation of action potentials generated by the heart during the cardiac cycle. The **P wave** represents atrial depolarization, while the **PR interval** corresponds to the time required to conduct the action potential through both the atria and the AV node. The **QRS complex** and the **T wave** represent ventricular depolarization and ventricular repolari-

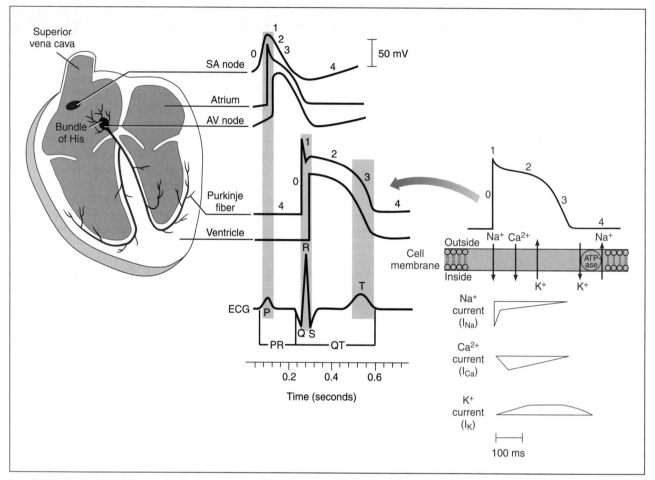

FIGURE 14–1. Relationships between ion currents, cardiac action potentials, and the findings on surface electrocardiogram (ECG). The normal heartbeat originates in the sinoatrial (SA) node. The impulse is conducted through internodal fibers to the atrioventricular (AV) node and then through the bundle of His, bundle branches, and Purkinje fibers to the ventricular muscle. On the ECG, the P wave represents atrial depolarization, the QRS complex represents ventricular depolarization, and the T wave represents ventricular repolarization. The PR interval is primarily related to the conduction time through the AV node, and the QT interval represents the time between ventricular depolarization and repolarization. In phase 0, ventricular depolarization is due to sodium influx through the fast sodium channel. In phase 1, the membrane is transiently repolarized as a result of potassium efflux. In phase 2, the membrane potential is relatively stable because of the concurrent influx of calcium and efflux of potassium. In phase 3, repolarization is due to continued potassium efflux as calcium influx declines. In phase 4, the ion balance is returned to normal by the action of the sodium pump (Na$^+$,K$^+$-ATPase). Calcium is removed from the cell by the sodium-calcium exchanger and the calcium ATPase (not shown).

zation, respectively. Hence, the **QT interval** represents the duration of the ventricular action potential.

Pathophysiology of Arrhythmias

Arrhythmias may be caused by the following: coronary ischemia and tissue hypoxia; electrolyte disturbances; overstimulation of the sympathetic nervous system; general anesthetics; and other conditions or drugs that perturb cardiac transmembrane potentials and lead to abnormal impulse formation or abnormal impulse conduction.

Abnormal Impulse Formation

Abnormal impulse formation may generate extrasystoles and result in tachycardia. The two mechanisms that are primarily responsible for abnormal impulse formation are increased automaticity and the occurrence of afterdepolarizations. These are depicted in Box 14–1.

Increased Automaticity. Spontaneous phase 4 depolarization generates an action potential that can be propagated to other parts of the heart. The SA node is the usual site of spontaneous impulse initiation (automaticity), but other cardiac tissues, including the AV node and the His-Purkinje system tissues, are also capable of spontaneous depolarization. Pathologic conditions or drugs may cause these tissues to depolarize more rapidly and thereby generate abnormal impulses. For example, overstimulation of the sympathetic nervous system or use of sympathomimetic drugs increases automaticity and may cause tachyarrhythmia.

The rate at which action potentials are generated in the SA node and elsewhere in the heart depends on the time required to depolarize the tissue from the maximum diastolic potential (MDP) to the TP. Automaticity is increased if the MDP becomes more positive or if the TP becomes more negative. Serum electrolyte abnormalities, hypoxia, and other patho-

BOX 14–1.   The Electrophysiologic Basis of Arrhythmias

Abnormal Impulse Formation

The two mechanisms that are primarily responsible for abnormal impulse formation are increased automaticity and afterdepolarizations.

Increased automaticity can be caused by any change that decreases the time required for depolarization from the maximum diastolic potential (MDP) to the threshold potential (TP). Increased automaticity occurs if the rate of diastolic depolarization (the slope of phase 4) in the sinoatrial node or in latent pacemakers is increased. It also occurs if there is a shift of the TP to a more negative value or if there is a shift of the MDP to a more positive value.

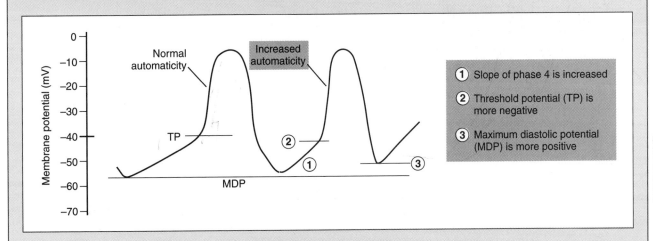

Afterdepolarizations are believed to result from abnormal calcium influx into cardiac cells during or immediately after phase 3 of the ventricular action potential. Afterdepolarizations may lead to extrasystoles and tachycardia.

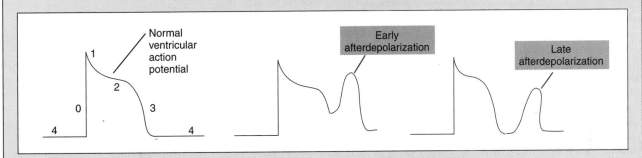

Abnormal Impulse Conduction

Reentry is characterized by the retrograde conduction of an impulse into previously depolarized tissue. It is usually due to the presence of a unidirectional conduction block in a bifurcating conduction pathway. For reentry to occur, the conduction time through the retrograde pathway must exceed the refractory period of the reentered tissue.

In **ventricular tissue**, the unidirectional block is often due to decremental conduction of the impulse in the anterograde direction, with normal conduction of the impulse in the retrograde direction.

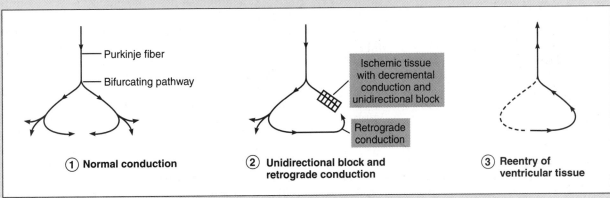

Continued

Abnormal Impulse Conduction (*Continued*)

Reentry in the **atrioventricular (AV) node** is the most common electrophysiologic mechanism responsible for paroxysmal supraventricular tachycardia (PSVT). Reentry occurs when a premature atrial depolarization arrives at the AV node and finds that one pathway (β) is still refractory from the previous depolarization. However, the other pathway (α) is able to conduct the impulse to the ventricle. Retrograde conduction of the impulse through pathway β leads to reentry of the atrium and results in tachycardia. In the AV node, the unidirectional block results from the β pathway's longer refractory period, which blocks anterograde conduction but permits retrograde conduction after it has recovered its excitability.

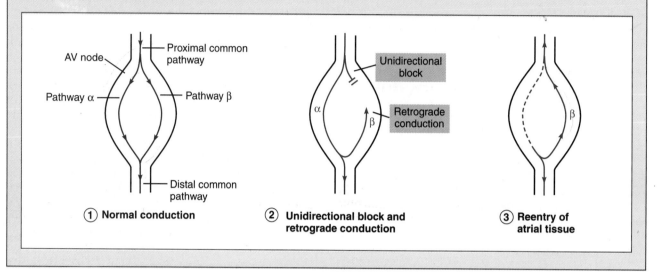

① **Normal conduction** ② **Unidirectional block and retrograde conduction** ③ **Reentry of atrial tissue**

logic changes may affect the MDP or TP in this manner and lead to arrhythmias.

Afterdepolarizations. Afterdepolarizations are abnormal impulses resulting from the spontaneous generation of action potentials during or immediately after phase 3 repolarization. Depending on their time of occurrence, the abnormal impulses are designated as **early afterdepolarizations** or **late afterdepolarizations.** Afterdepolarizations are believed to be triggered by abnormal calcium influx and may be provoked by digitalis glycosides and by other drugs or pathologic events that prolong cardiac repolarization and the QT interval.

Abnormal Impulse Conduction

Abnormal impulse conduction is the basis for the formation of arrhythmias by the process of **reentry,** a process that involves reexcitation of a particular zone of cardiac tissue by the same impulse. Reentry is believed to be the most common mechanism responsible for the genesis of arrhythmias. It is usually due to the presence of a **unidirectional conduction block** in a bifurcating conduction pathway (see Box 14–1).

Reentry in Ventricular Tissue. In ventricular tissue, ischemia and tissue hypoxia may cause a reduction in the resting membrane potential and a decrease in membrane responsiveness. Under these conditions, the cells do not depolarize as rapidly or completely during phase 0, and this reduces the rate at which the impulse is conducted to surrounding ventricular tissue. When a cardiac impulse is con-

ducted through ischemic or infarcted tissue, the conduction velocity gradually slows until conduction ceases. This phenomenon is called **decremental conduction** and is the most common cause of a unidirectional block in ventricular tissue. If the unidirectional block occurs in one arm of a bifurcating pathway, the impulse may continue through the other arm in the normal (anterograde) direction and then reenter the ventricular tissue by retrograde conduction.

The reason that the impulse is blocked in the anterograde direction but is conducted in the retrograde direction is related to the characteristics of decremental conduction. In this type of conduction, the impulse encounters increasing resistance as it moves in the anterograde direction, and its velocity slows until the impulse is finally extinguished. The retrograde impulse has full velocity as it encounters the area of greatest resistance, and this enables it to jump across the ischemic area without being extinguished.

Reentry in the Atrioventricular Node. Reentry in the AV node is the most common electrophysiologic mechanism responsible for **paroxysmal supraventricular tachycardia** (PSVT). There are several forms of PSVT. The form that occurs in patients with Wolff-Parkinson-White syndrome involves an accessory AV node conduction pathway through the bundle of Kent. However, in patients with the most common form of PSVT, the reentrant circuit is located entirely within the AV node. In the common form of PSVT, a premature atrial impulse is blocked in one pathway, is conducted through the AV node via the other pathway, and reenters the atrium by retrograde conduction. In AV node reentry, the unidirectional block is not due to decremental conduction but is instead due to the difference in the refractory periods of the two pathways.

Drug-Induced Arrhythmias

Drugs can induce arrhythmias by several mechanisms.

Sympathomimetic drugs can increase the automaticity of the SA node, AV node, or His-Purkinje fibers and thereby produce tachyarrhythmias.

Digitalis glycosides sometimes evoke afterdepolarizations by increasing calcium influx into cardiac cells, and they may also impair AV node conduction and cause AV block.

Other drugs cause arrhythmias via their effects on ventricular conduction and repolarization. Drugs that slow ventricular repolarization and cause QT prolongation may evoke a form of polymorphic ventricular tachycardia called **torsade de pointes** (based on a French term meaning "fringe of pointed tips" and often called torsades de pointes). In this disorder, each QRS complex has a configuration that differs from the preceding one, and QT prolongation probably predisposes the ventricular tissue to afterdepolarizations that produce extrasystoles and tachycardia. Types of drugs that have been reported to induce torsade de pointes include **antiarrhythmic drugs** (such as quinidine and sotalol), **psychotropic drugs** (such as phenothiazines), and other agents (such as cisapride).

Mechanisms and Classification of Antiarrhythmic Drugs

Antiarrhythmic drugs act primarily by suppressing or preventing abnormal impulse formation or conduction. Drugs that block sodium or calcium channels can reduce abnormal automaticity and slow conduction of the cardiac impulse. Drugs that block potassium channels can prolong repolarization and the action potential duration and thereby increase the refractory period of cardiac tissue. Drugs that block β-adrenergic receptors reduce the sympathetic stimulation of cardiac automaticity and conduction velocity and thereby prevent the overstimulation that contributes to some arrhythmias.

On the basis of these mechanisms, Vaughan-Williams has divided the antiarrhythmic drugs into four main classes, with **class I** consisting of sodium channel blockers, **class II** consisting of β-adrenergic receptor antagonists (β-blockers), **class III** consisting of potassium channel blockers and other drugs that prolong the action potential duration, and **class IV** consisting of calcium channel blockers. Although this classification system is helpful, a few drugs (such as adenosine) do not fit into any of these categories, and some drugs (such as amiodarone) could be included in more than one category.

SODIUM CHANNEL BLOCKERS

Class I, the largest group of antiarrhythmic drugs, consists of sodium channel blockers. These drugs bind to sodium channels when the channels are in the open and inactivated states, and they dissociate from the channels during the resting state (Box 14–2). The sodium channel blockers have the most pronounced effect on cardiac tissue that is firing rapidly, because sodium channels in this tissue spend a greater amount of time in the open and inactivated states than in the resting state. This is called **use-dependent blockade**. Because of use-dependent blockade, sodium channel blockers suppress cardiac conduction more in a patient with tachycardia than in a person with a normal heart rate.

The drugs in class I have been subdivided into three groups (IA, IB, and IC), based on whether they have greater affinity for the open state or the inactivated state and based on their rate of dissociation from sodium channels (rate of recovery). As shown in Box 14–2, **class IA drugs** have greater affinity for the open state and have a slow recovery; **class IB drugs** have greater affinity for the inactivated state and have a rapid recovery; and **class IC drugs** have greater affinity for the open state and a very slow recovery.

Class IB drugs have a more pronounced effect on ischemic tissue than on nonischemic tissue. In ischemic tissue, cells are partly depolarized because they lack the amount of adenosine triphosphate (ATP) needed to operate the sodium pump. As a result, these cells spend more time in the inactivated state than do cells in nonischemic tissue.

Class IC drugs have a greater effect on ventricular conduction than do class IA or IB drugs. This is because class IC drugs show an affinity for the open state and because they have the slowest recovery from blockade.

Class IA Drugs

Disopyramide, procainamide, and quinidine are class IA drugs. These drugs have similar electrophysiologic effects and clinical indications, but they differ in their pharmacokinetic properties and adverse effects.

Drug Properties

The class IA drugs block the fast sodium channel and also block potassium channels. Therefore, they slow phase 0 depolarization and phase 3 repolarization in ventricular tissue (Fig. 14–2). These actions decrease the ventricular conduction velocity and prolong the ventricular action potential duration and refractory period (Table 14–1). On the ECG, this increases the QRS duration and prolongs the QT interval. Class IA drugs suppress abnormal (ectopic) automaticity, but they usually do not significantly affect SA node automaticity and the heart rate.

BOX 14–2.   Electrophysiologic Properties of Sodium Channel Blockers

During phase 0 of the ventricular action potential, the sodium channels open to depolarize the cell. The channels are then inactivated and no longer permit sodium entry during phases 1, 2, and 3. The channels must return to the resting state (phase 4) before they can open again during the next action potential.

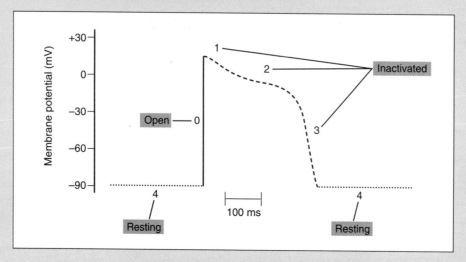

Drugs dissociate from the sodium channels at different rates (recovery). Drugs with a slow recovery have a greater effect on cardiac conduction velocity.

Drug Class	Example	Sodium Channel Affinity	Rate of Dissociation
Class IA	Quinidine	Open > inactivated	Slow
Class IB	Lidocaine	Inactivated > open	Rapid
Class IC	Flecainide	Open > inactivated	Very slow

All of the class IA drugs have some degree of antimuscarinic (atropine-like) activity and may inhibit parasympathetic (vagal) effects on the SA and AV nodes. Disopyramide has the greatest antimuscarinic effect, procainamide has the least, and quinidine has an intermediate effect.

Quinidine

Chemistry and Pharmacokinetics. Quinidine is a quinoline derivative whose structure is shown in Fig. 14–3A. The drug is the dextrorotatory isomer of quinine, an alkaloid that is obtained from the bark of the cinchona tree and has been used to treat fever and malaria for centuries. The pharmacokinetic properties of quinidine and other antiarrhythmic drugs are summarized in Table 14–2. Quinidine is usually administered orally and is adequately absorbed from the gut. It undergoes considerable hepatic biotransformation and is excreted in the urine as the parent compound and metabolites. It has a moderately short half-life and is often administered as a sustained-release preparation.

Adverse Effects. The most common adverse effect of quinidine is diarrhea, which occurs in up to 30% of patients taking the drug and is often responsi-

ble for their discontinuation of its use. A less common adverse effect is torsade de pointes, which may cause syncope secondary to a reduction in cardiac output and blood pressure. Thrombocytopenia has also been reported with quinidine use. Higher doses of quinidine may cause cinchonism, characterized by a constellation of neurologic symptoms that include tinnitus, dizziness, and blurred vision.

Indications. Quinidine is most often used orally on a long-term basis for the suppression of **supraventricular and ventricular arrhythmias.** It is seldom used parenterally, because intravenous administration may cause considerable hypotension owing to the drug's antagonism of α-adrenergic receptors. Because quinidine may increase the AV node conduction velocity and ventricular rate in patients with atrial fibrillation, these patients should be given a drug that decreases AV node conduction, such as digoxin, before they are given quinidine.

Procainamide

Procainamide produces the same electrophysiologic effects as quinidine and has many of the same clinical indications.

Chemistry and Pharmacokinetics. Procainamide is the amide derivative of the local anesthetic procaine (see Fig. 14–3A). Both compounds have antiarrhythmic activity, but procaine has less effect on the heart and produces more central nervous system side effects than does procainamide. Therefore, procaine is not used as an antiarrhythmic drug. Procainamide is well absorbed from the gut and is converted to an active metabolite, N-acetylprocainamide (NAPA), in the liver. NAPA exerts class III antiarrhythmic activity and is being investigated as an antiarrhythmic drug.

Adverse Effects. Long-term use of procainamide may cause a syndrome that resembles lupus erythematosus, presents with arthralgia and a butterfly rash on the face, and is reversible. This syndrome can be distinguished from idiopathic lupus on the basis of serologic tests for anti-DNA antibodies.

Indications. Procainamide produces less hypotension after intravenous administration than does quinidine and is sometimes administered by this route for the treatment of **acute ventricular arrhythmias.** Like quinidine, procainamide is given orally on

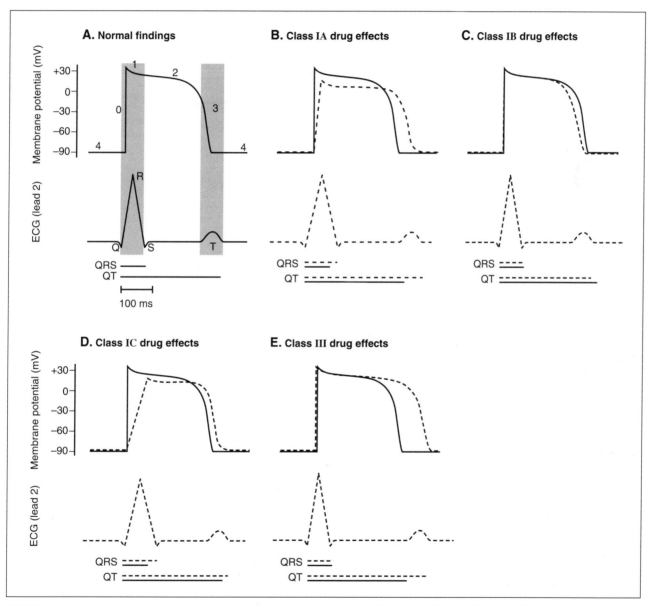

FIGURE 14–2. **Effects of class I and class III antiarrhythmic drugs on the ventricular action potential duration and on the electrocardiogram (ECG).** In each panel, the membrane potential scale is in millivolts (mV), and the time scale is in milliseconds (ms). Solid black tracings and lines for the time scale depict normal findings, while dotted tracings and lines depict the effects of drug administration. **(A)** Lightly shaded vertical bars show the relationship between the ventricular action potential duration and the findings on ECG in the normally functioning heart. **(B)** Class IA drugs slow phase 0 depolarization and phase 3 repolarization, thereby increasing the QRS duration and the QT interval. **(C)** Class IB drugs have little effect on normal cardiac tissue, but they may accelerate phase 3 repolarization and decrease the QT interval slightly. **(D)** Class IC drugs have the greatest effect on phase 0 depolarization and increase the QRS duration markedly, but they have little effect on phase 3 and the QT interval. **(E)** Class III drugs have little effect on phase 0, but they markedly prolong phase 3 and increase the QT interval.

TABLE 14–1. Electrophysiologic Properties of Antiarrhythmic Drugs*

Drug	Ectopic Auto-maticity	Atrioventricular (AV) Node		His-Purkinje System and Ventricle		Electrocardiogram			
		Con-duction Velocity	Refractory Period	Con-duction Velocity	Refractory Period	Heart Rate	PR Interval	QRS Duration	QT Interval
Class I drugs									
IA drugs	D	±	0/I	D	I	±	±	I	I
IB drugs	D	0	0	0/D†	±	0	0	0	0/D
IC drugs	D	D	0/I	D	I	0	I	I	0/I
Moricizine	D	D	0	D	0/I	0/I	I	I	0/D
Class II drugs	D	D	I	0	0	D	I	0	0/D
Class III drugs									
Amiodarone	D	D	I	D	I	D	I	I	I
Bretylium	I	0	0/±	0/I	I	0	0	0	0
Ibutilide	U	0/D	I	0	I	0/D	0/I	0	I
Sotalol	D	D	I	0	I	D	I	0	I
Class IV drugs	D	D	I	0	0	D	I	0	0
Other drugs									
Adenosine	D	D	I	0	0	I	I	0	0
Digoxin	I	D	I	0	D	D	I	0	D
Magnesium sulfate	D	0	0	0	0	0	0	0	0

*Effects are indicated as follows: decrease (D); increase (I); variable increase or decrease (±); no change (0); and unknown (U).
†Slow conduction in ischemic tissue.

a long-term basis for the suppression of **supraventricular and ventricular arrhythmias.**

Disopyramide

Disopyramide is administered orally for the prevention of **ventricular arrhythmias** and is sometimes effective in patients who have not responded to other drugs. Disopyramide has electrophysiologic effects similar to those of quinidine. Because it has greater negative inotropic and antimuscarinic effects than do other class IA drugs, it should be used with caution in patients with heart failure and in elderly patients, who are often more susceptible to blurred vision, urinary retention, and other antimuscarinic side effects.

Class IB Drugs

Lidocaine, mexiletine, and tocainide are class IB drugs. Their electrophysiologic properties make them particularly suitable for the treatment of ventricular arrhythmias.

Drug Properties

Chemistry and Pharmacokinetics. Lidocaine is a local anesthetic that also has antiarrhythmic activity. It undergoes extensive first-pass hepatic inactivation after oral administration and is not suitable for administration by this route. The other class IB drugs, mexiletine and tocainide, are lidocaine congeners that are not susceptible to first-pass inactivation and are intended for oral administration. Lidocaine is rapidly inactivated by hepatic enzymes,

whereas mexiletine and tocainide are more slowly metabolized and have much longer half-lives (see Table 14–2). The fraction of tocainide that is excreted unchanged in the urine is much greater than the fraction of lidocaine and mexiletine.

Mechanisms and Effects. Lidocaine has a strong affinity for sodium channels in depolarized ischemic tissue but a relative lack of effect on sodium channels in normal cardiac tissue. Therefore, in nonischemic tissue, it has little effect on electrophysiologic and electrocardiographic findings when given at therapeutic levels. Lidocaine is not very effective in the treatment of supraventricular arrhythmias, because these arrhythmias usually arise in nonischemic tissue. The lidocaine congeners, mexiletine and tocainide, have electrophysiologic properties similar to those of lidocaine, but they are less selective for inactivated sodium channels in ischemic tissue and may produce greater effects on normal cardiac tissue than does lidocaine.

Lidocaine

Lidocaine is usually administered intravenously as a loading dose (bolus) followed by a continuous intravenous infusion in the treatment of **ventricular tachycardia and other acute ventricular arrhythmias.** It has a rapid onset of action, and its effects subside quickly when the infusion is stopped.

A high serum concentration of lidocaine may cause central nervous system side effects such as nervousness, tremor, and paresthesia. It may also slow the conduction velocity in normal cardiac tissue. Because lidocaine is extensively metabolized, concurrent use of a drug that inhibits cytochrome P450 enzymes, such as cimetidine, may increase the serum concentration of lidocaine and precipitate lidocaine toxicity.

Mexiletine and Tocainide

Mexiletine and tocainide are administered orally on a long-term basis for the suppression of **ventricular arrhythmias.**

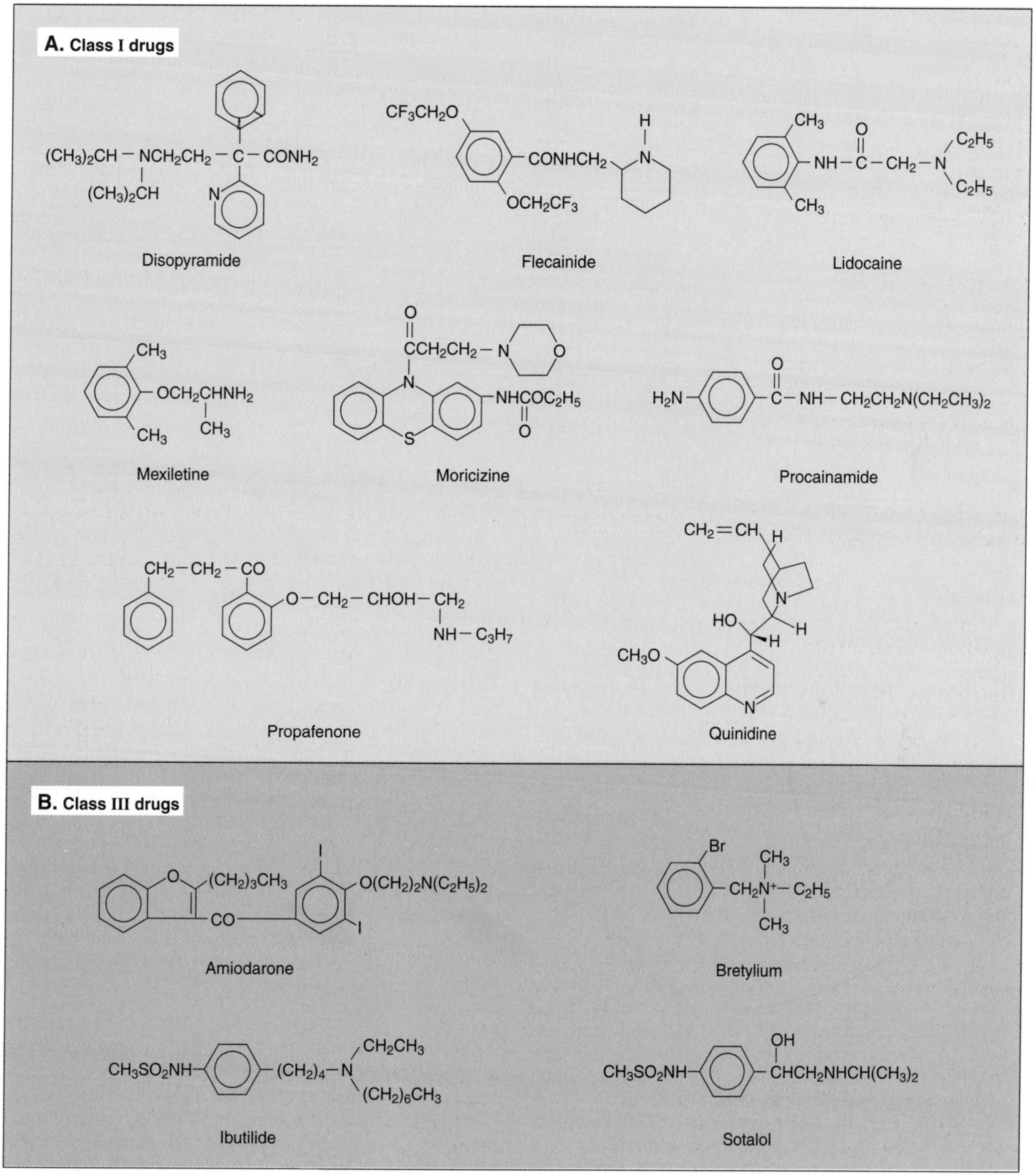

FIGURE 14–3. Structures of selected class I and class III antiarrhythmic drugs. There are four classes of antiarrhythmics. **(A)** Class I consists of sodium channel blockers and is divided into three main groups. Disopyramide, procainamide, and quinidine are in class IA; lidocaine and mexiletine are in class IB; flecainide and propafenone are in class IC; and moricizine is a class I drug that does not fall into any of these three groups. **(B)** Class III consists of potassium channel blockers and other drugs that prolong the action potential duration. It includes amiodarone, bretylium, ibutilide, and sotalol. Both ibutilide and sotalol are methane sulfonamide derivatives. Class II consists of β-adrenergic receptor antagonists (see Fig. 9–1). Class IV consists of calcium channel blockers (see Fig. 11–3).

TABLE 14–2. Pharmacokinetic Properties of Antiarrhythmic Drugs*

Drug	Oral Bioavail-ability	Onset of Action	Duration of Action	Elimination Half-Life	Excreted Unchanged in Urine	Therapeutic Serum Concentration
Class IA drugs						
Disopyramide	90%	1 hour	6 hours	7 hours	50%	2–7 µg/mL
Procainamide	85%	1 hour	5 hours	3.5 hours	55%	4–8 µg/mL
Quinidine	75%	1 hour	7 hours	6 hours	30%	2–5 µg/mL
Class IB drugs						
Lidocaine	NA	See text	See text	1.5 hours	1%	1.5–6 µg/mL
Mexiletine	90%	1 hour	10 hours	11 hours	10%	0.5–2 µg/mL
Tocainide	92%	1 hour	12 hours	12 hours	40%	4–10 µg/mL
Class IC drugs						
Flecainide	75%	3 hours	21 hours	14 hours	30%	0.2–1 µg/mL
Propafenone	10%	3 hours	10 hours	6 hours	<1%	0.06–0.1 µg/mL
Other class I drugs						
Moricizine	35%	2 hours	16 hours	2.5 hours	<1%	0.2–3.6 µg/mL
Class II drugs						
Esmolol	NA	<5 minutes	20–30 minutes	0.15 hour	<2%	0.5–1 µg/mL
Metoprolol	35%	1 hour	15 hours	3.5 hours	7%	15–25 ng/mL
Propranolol	35%	0.5 hour	4 hours	4 hours	<0.5%	0.2–1 µg/mL
Class III drugs						
Amiodarone	45%	2 weeks	4 weeks	40 days	0%	0.5–2.5 µg/mL
Bretylium	NA	5 minutes	8 hours	8 hours	80%	0.5–2 µg/mL
Ibutilide	NA	5 minutes	Unknown	6 hours	<10%	NA
Sotalol	90%	2 hours	15 hours	12 hours	90%	1–4 µg/mL
Class IV drugs						
Diltiazem	55%	2 hours	8 hours	5 hours	3%	0.1–0.2 µg/mL
Verapamil	25%	2 hours	9 hours	5 hours	3%	0.1–0.3 µg/mL
Miscellaneous drugs						
Adenosine	NA	30 seconds	1.5 minutes	<10 seconds	0%	NA
Digoxin	75%	1 hour	24 hours	35 hours	60%	0.5–2 ng/mL
Magnesium sulfate	NA	<5 minutes	NA	NA	100%	NA

*Values shown are the mean of values reported in the literature. NA = not applicable (not administered orally).

Because use of tocainide can lead to agranulocytosis and other blood cell deficiencies, patients receiving this drug should have blood counts performed periodically. Mexiletine is less frequently associated with these adverse effects.

Class IC Drugs

Flecainide and propafenone are class IC drugs and are administered orally. Their properties and chemical structures are outlined in Table 14–1, Table 14–2, and Fig. 14–3A.

Class IC drugs block fast sodium channels and block the rate of rise of the action potential during phase 0 to a greater extent than do other class I drugs. By this mechanism, the class IC drugs slow conduction throughout the heart and especially in the His-Purkinje system. Flecainide and propafenone usually have less effect on the potassium rectifier current (I_K) and do not prolong the QT interval as much as do class IA drugs, such as quinidine.

Flecainide

Flecainide is indicated for the treatment of **supraventricular arrhythmias** and **documented life-threatening ventricular arrhythmias.** In the past, it was also routinely used to suppress ventricular arrhythmias in patients with cardiac disorders. However, this practice has changed since a clinical study called the Cardiac Arrhythmia Suppression Trial (CAST) showed that flecainide actually increased the mortality rate in patients who were recovering from myocardial infarction.

Although flecainide does not cause afterdepolarizations and torsade de pointes, it is capable of increasing the ventricular rate and causing reentrant ventricular tachycardia. Other adverse effects of flecainide include bronchospasm, leukopenia, thrombocytopenia, and seizures.

Propafenone

The effect of propafenone on fast sodium channels and cardiac conduction is similar to that of flecainide. Like flecainide, propafenone prolongs the PR interval and QRS duration, but it has little effect on the QT interval. Propafenone also has weak β-adrenergic receptor–blocking activity.

Propafenone is administered orally on a long-term basis to suppress **supraventricular tachycardia.** The drug is also used to treat life-threatening forms of ventricular arrhythmia, such as **sustained ventricular tachycardia.**

Propafenone has the potential to cause ventricular arrhythmias and several hematologic abnormalities, including agranulocytosis, anemia, and thrombocytopenia.

Other Class I Drugs

Moricizine is a class I drug whose unusual properties do not permit its assignment to one of the three main subgroups, although it is probably most similar to the class IC drugs. Moricizine is a phenothiazine analogue that blocks sodium channels in a manner similar to flecainide. It slows both the AV node conduction velocity and the ventricular conduction velocity, thereby increasing the QRS duration. However, it may shorten the ventricular action potential duration and QT interval in a manner similar to lidocaine.

In the CAST II study, long-term use of moricizine to suppress arrhythmias was found to increase the mortality rate in patients with a history of myocardial infarction. For this reason, the drug is approved only for the treatment of **documented life-threatening ventricular arrhythmias.**

OTHER ANTIARRHYTHMIC DRUGS

Tables 14–1 and 14–2 compare the electrophysiologic and pharmacokinetic properties of the various groups and subgroups of antiarrhythmic drugs.

Class II Drugs
Drug Properties

The class II antiarrhythmics include esmolol, metoprolol, and propranolol. These drugs are β-adrenergic receptor antagonists (β-blockers) used for the prevention and treatment of supraventricular arrhythmias and for their ability to reduce ventricular ectopic depolarizations and sudden death in patients with myocardial infarction.

The β-blockers have antiarrhythmic effects because of their ability to inhibit sympathetic activation of cardiac automaticity and conduction. The β-blockers slow the heart rate, decrease the AV node conduction velocity, and increase the AV node refractory period (Fig. 14–4). They have little effect on ventricular conduction and repolarization. The general pharmacologic properties of β-blockers are discussed in Chapter 9.

Esmolol

Esmolol is a β-blocker that is given intravenously, is rapidly metabolized by plasma esterase, and has a very short half-life. Its pharmacologic properties make it ideally suited for the treatment of patients who suffer from **acute supraventricular tachycardia** during or immediately after surgery.

Metoprolol and Propranolol

Metoprolol and propranolol can be administered orally or intravenously for the treatment and sup-

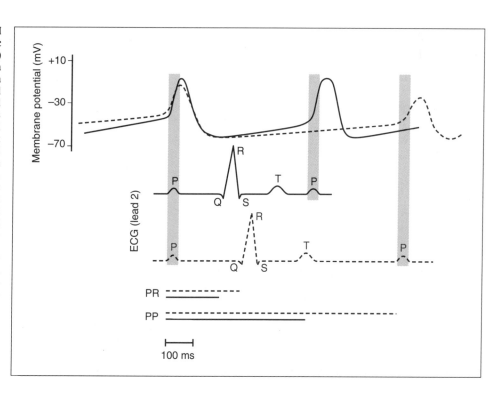

FIGURE 14–4. Effects of class II and class IV antiarrhythmic drugs on the sinoatrial (SA) node action potential duration and on the electrocardiogram (ECG). The membrane potential scale is in millivolts (mV), and the time scale is in milliseconds (ms). Solid black tracings and lines for the time scale depict normal findings, while dotted tracings and lines depict the effects of drug administration. Lightly shaded vertical bars show the relationship between the action potential duration and the findings on ECG. Class II drugs (β-adrenergic receptor antagonists) and class IV drugs (calcium channel blockers) slow phase 4 depolarization in the SA node and increase the PP interval. They also slow the atrioventricular node conduction velocity and increase the PR interval.

pression of **supraventricular and ventricular arrhythmias.** In patients with **myocardial infarction,** metoprolol is often administered intravenously during the early phase of treatment, followed by oral maintenance therapy that may continue for several months. The β-blockers have been demonstrated to protect the heart against the damage caused by ischemia and free radicals that may be formed during reperfusion of the coronary arteries when fibrinolytic drugs are used.

Class III Drugs

Amiodarone, bretylium, ibutilide, and sotalol are class III antiarrhythmics. The most common attribute of this heterogeneous group of drugs is the prolongation of the ventricular action potential duration and refractory period. Some class III drugs act by blocking the potassium rectifier current (I_K) that repolarizes the heart during phase 3 of the action potential, but other class III drugs have different mechanisms. Most of these drugs do not slow the ventricular conduction velocity or increase the QRS duration significantly.

Amiodarone

Chemistry and Pharmacokinetics. Amiodarone is an organic iodine compound that is structurally related to thyroid hormones (see Fig. 14–3B), can be administered orally or intravenously, and has unusual pharmacokinetic properties. After oral administration, amiodarone is slowly and variably absorbed and is primarily eliminated by biliary excretion. As shown in Table 14–2, the drug's action does not begin for about 2 weeks, and its half-life is about 40 days (with a range of 26–107 days).

Mechanisms and Pharmacologic Effects. Although amiodarone has class III antiarrhythmic activity, it also blocks sodium channels, calcium channels, and β-adrenergic receptors. Hence, it is difficult to assign its antiarrhythmic activity to a specific mechanism. As shown in Table 14–1, amiodarone decreases SA node automaticity, decreases AV node conduction velocity, and prolongs AV node and ventricular refractory periods. It causes a greater prolongation of the QT interval than other antiarrhythmic drugs, and it causes a slight prolongation of the QRS duration.

Adverse Effects and Interactions. Amiodarone can cause a number of adverse cardiovascular effects, including hypotension, AV block, and various arrhythmias. However, it is reported to cause drug-induced arrhythmias in only 2% of patients, and it is infrequently associated with torsade de pointes, despite its ability to cause QT prolongation. Although amiodarone has a mild negative inotropic effect, it has been successfully used to treat arrhythmias in patients with heart failure (see Chapter 12).

Amiodarone produces a constellation of other adverse effects, including blue-gray skin discoloration, thyroid abnormalities, and potentially fatal pulmonary fibrosis and pneumonitis. The thyroid abnormalities are due to the iodine content of the drug and include both hypothyroidism and hyperthyroidism. Amiodarone can also cause corneal deposits, blurred vision, photosensitivity, and gastrointestinal disturbances. Fortunately, low doses of the drug are effective in many patients and are associated with fewer adverse effects.

Amiodarone inhibits the metabolism of a number of pharmacologic agents and significantly elevates the plasma concentrations of drugs such as digoxin, flecainide, phenytoin, procainamide, and warfarin. The dosage of these drugs should be decreased in patients receiving concurrent amiodarone therapy. Amiodarone also interacts with inhalational anesthetics and other central nervous system depressants to cause an increased incidence of adverse cardiovascular effects such as bradycardia.

Indications. Amiodarone is used orally on a long-term basis for the suppression of both **supraventricular and ventricular arrhythmias,** including **atrial fibrillation, atrial flutter, supraventricular tachycardia,** and **life-threatening ventricular tachycardia.** Because of its profile of adverse effects, the drug is usually used when other treatments have not been successful. However, its role as a first-line drug appears to be increasing. Amiodarone is used intravenously to treat **acute life-threatening ventricular fibrillation** or **symptomatic, sustained ventricular tachycardia.** In this setting, the drug may be given as a loading infusion followed by a maintenance infusion.

Ibutilide

Unlike most other class III drugs, ibutilide does not block outward potassium channels. Instead, it prolongs the action potential duration by promoting the influx of sodium through slow inward sodium channels. The sodium influx counteracts the outward potassium current and thereby prolongs repolarization.

Ibutilide is administered by intravenous infusion. It is rapidly biotransformed in the liver, and its metabolites are eliminated in the urine and feces, with an average half-life of 6 hours. The drug is indicated for the rapid conversion of **atrial fibrillation or flutter** to normal sinus rhythm. It does not significantly affect the heart rate, blood pressure, QRS duration, or PR interval. However, it can induce torsade de pointes and should be avoided in patients with a history of this condition.

Sotalol

Sotalol is a nonselective β-adrenergic receptor antagonist that prolongs the cardiac action potential duration and QT interval by blocking the delayed potassium rectifier current (I_K) during phase 3 of the ventricular action potential (see Fig. 14–2). The drug also decreases automaticity, slows the AV node conduction velocity, and increases the AV node refractory period without affecting the ventricular conduction and QRS duration.

Sotalol is approved for the treatment of **ventricular arrhythmias** and is also effective in the management of **atrial arrhythmias,** including **atrial fibrillation.** It produces a dose-dependent incidence of torsade de pointes, which most likely is due to QT prolongation. Some of its adverse effects, such as bronchospasm, are due to β-adrenergic receptor blockade.

Bretylium

Bretylium prolongs the ventricular action potential duration in normal cardiac tissue to a greater extent than it does in ischemic tissue. This reduces the heterogeneity of action potential durations that occurs during focal cardiac ischemia, and the synchronization of action potentials is believed to suppress reentry.

Bretylium is administered intravenously to suppress **ventricular fibrillation** and prevent its recurrence. The drug exerts several effects on sympathetic nerve terminals, and these actions may produce transient hypertension followed by prolonged hypotension.

Class IV Drugs

Diltiazem and **verapamil** are calcium channel blockers that have significant effects on cardiac tissue. They primarily act to decrease the AV node conduction velocity and increase the AV node refractory period, and they have a smaller effect on the SA node and heart rate. As shown in Table 14–1, they have little effect on the ventricular conduction velocity and refractory period.

Diltiazem and verapamil can be administered intravenously for the termination of **acute supraventricular tachycardia.** They are also used to reduce the ventricular rate in patients who have **atrial fibrillation** with a rapid ventricular response. These drugs can exacerbate ventricular tachycardia, so it is important that arrhythmias be correctly diagnosed before treatment with diltiazem or verapamil is begun. Other calcium channel blockers (including dihydropyridines such as amlodipine) have less effect on cardiac tissue and no role in the treatment of arrhythmias.

Miscellaneous Drugs
Adenosine

Adenosine is a naturally occurring nucleoside composed of adenine and ribose. When administered as a rapid intravenous bolus, it has an extremely short half-life of 10 seconds or less. In the body, adenosine is derived from ATP and activates specific G protein–coupled adenosine receptors. Stimulation of these receptors leads to activation of acetylcholine-sensitive potassium channels and blockade of calcium influx in the SA node, atrium, and AV node. It thereby causes cell hyperpolarization, slows the AV node conduction velocity, and increases the AV node refractory period. In fact, AV node conduction may be completely blocked for a few seconds, resulting in a brief period of asystole. These actions serve to terminate supraventricular tachycardia by preventing the retrograde conduction of reentrant impulses through the AV node. Because of its brief duration of action, adenosine has been termed a pharmacologic counterpart to electrical cardioversion.

Adenosine is primarily used to terminate **acute paroxysmal supraventricular tachycardia,** including the type associated with Wolff-Parkinson-White syndrome. It is not indicated for the treatment of atrial fibrillation or flutter.

Digoxin

Like all digitalis glycosides, digoxin acts indirectly to increase vagal tone and thereby slow the AV node conduction velocity and increase the AV node refractory period. Thus, the effects of digoxin on cardiac tissue are similar to the effects of β-blockers and calcium channel blockers, and the clinical indications are also similar. Digoxin is often used to slow the ventricular rate in patients with **atrial fibrillation.** It may be preferable to β-blockers for this indication because it does not cause as much bradycardia, and it may be preferable to calcium channel blockers because it does not have a negative inotropic effect. In fact, digoxin and other digitalis glycosides have a positive inotropic effect and are also used in the treatment of **heart failure** (see Chapter 12).

Magnesium Sulfate

The magnesium ion is the second most common intracellular cation and has a number of roles in normal cardiac function. Magnesium deficiency may be caused by use of drugs such as loop diuretics or by pathologic states, and this deficiency may contribute to the development of arrhythmias and congestive heart failure, as well as to gastrointestinal and renal disorders.

Magnesium sulfate is administered intravenously to suppress **drug-induced torsade de pointes,** to treat **digitalis-induced ventricular arrhythmias,** and to treat **supraventricular arrhythmias associated with magnesium deficiency.** Magnesium has been studied as a treatment for other arrhythmias, but its efficacy is not yet established.

THE MANAGEMENT OF SUPRAVENTRICULAR ARRHYTHMIAS
Atrial Fibrillation and Flutter

Atrial fibrillation is thought to be caused by a disorganized form of reentry in atrial tissue, a form in which atrial cells are continuously reexcited as soon as they have repolarized. Under these conditions, the

AV node is continuously bombarded with atrial impulses, some of which are conducted to the ventricles, so that the ventricular rate is often rapid and irregular.

The first objective of treatment is to control the rapid ventricular rate. This is accomplished by administering drugs that slow the conduction velocity and increase the refractory period of the AV node, so that fewer atrial impulses are transmitted to the ventricles. Drugs used for this purpose include digoxin, calcium channel blockers, and β-blockers. Digoxin may be preferred for this purpose because it does not reduce cardiac contractility or slow the sinus rate as much as the calcium channel blockers or β-blockers do. While digoxin and these other drugs usually slow the ventricular rate, they usually do not affect the underlying atrial fibrillation.

After the ventricular rate is controlled, the atrial fibrillation can be converted to normal sinus rhythm by the use of direct current (DC) cardioversion or by the intravenous administration of ibutilide. Unfortunately, many patients who are successfully converted will undergo relapse. Long-term suppression of atrial fibrillation with class I or class III drugs may be effective in some patients after conversion to normal sinus rhythm. However, these drugs are not always efficacious and have numerous adverse effects. For this reason, many patients with chronic atrial fibrillation are treated with a drug to control the ventricular rate and with an anticoagulant to prevent thromboembolism, which is often associated with atrial fibrillation (see Chapter 16). Patients who have Wolff-Parkinson-White syndrome and develop atrial fibrillation should not be treated with digoxin or verapamil, because these drugs may decrease accessory pathway refractoriness and lead to ventricular tachycardia.

Atrial flutter is usually treated in the same manner as atrial fibrillation. Surgical ablation of the arrhythmogenic tissue may be effective in some patients with atrial flutter.

Supraventricular Tachycardia

Paroxysmal supraventricular tachycardia, or PSVT, is most frequently due to a reentrant circuit in the AV node. Acute PSVT is often treated with intravenous adenosine, which causes AV block and interrupts the reentrant pathway. Alternatively, AV block may be produced by a calcium channel blocker such as verapamil or by a β-blocker such as esmolol. Esmolol is a short-acting drug whose use is often preferred in perioperative patients. Long-term suppression is usually accomplished by use of a calcium channel blocker, β-blocker, or digitalis glycoside. Surgical ablation of the arrhythmogenic tissue may also be effective.

Patients with Wolff-Parkinson-White syndrome exhibit an atypical form of PSVT that is due to reentry through an accessory bypass conduction pathway between the atria and ventricles. This form of PSVT can also be terminated with drugs that cause AV

block. Long-term treatment may consist of surgical ablation of arrhythmogenic tissue or use of a sodium or potassium channel blocker to suppress the arrhythmia.

THE MANAGEMENT OF VENTRICULAR ARRHYTHMIAS
Ventricular Tachycardia

Ventricular tachycardia is an arrhythmia with a monomorphic, regular, wide QRS complex. It is often associated with myocardial infarction and is thought to be caused by decremental conduction and reentry in ventricular tissue, phenomena that are described earlier in this chapter. If the patient with ventricular tachycardia does not have a pulse or is hemodynamically unstable, DC cardioversion is often employed to terminate the arrhythmia. If the patient has a pulse and is stable, intravenous lidocaine is usually administered. Recently, intravenous amiodarone has been used to suppress ventricular tachycardia.

For long-term therapy, a sodium or potassium channel blocker may be used to prevent recurrences. Amiodarone and sotalol are among the current choices for this purpose, and amiodarone is distinguished by its relative lack of arrhythmogenic activity.

Patients who have taken an overdose of a tricyclic antidepressant drug, such as imipramine, may develop tachycardia that has a wide QRS complex and is believed to result from the blockade of cardiac sodium channels by the antidepressant. The treatment for this particular form of ventricular tachycardia is the intravenous administration of sodium bicarbonate, which increases the ratio of the nonionized form to the ionized form of imipramine and thereby causes dissociation of the drug from sodium channels.

Torsade de Pointes

Torsade de pointes is a polymorphic ventricular tachycardia that is induced by drugs or pathologic states that prolong the QT interval and predispose cardiac cells to afterdepolarizations. Patients with this arrhythmia may be treated by intravenous administration of magnesium sulfate, cardiac pacing, or intravenous administration of isoproterenol (a β-adrenergic receptor agonist). These treatments act in part by shortening the QT interval.

Ventricular Fibrillation

Ventricular fibrillation is thought to be caused by a disorganized reentry circuit in the ventricles. DC cardioversion is the treatment of choice for patients with this disorder. Lidocaine, procainamide, or bretylium has been used as an adjunct treatment and is usually administered before and between attempts at electrical defibrillation. Recently, amiodarone has also been used for this purpose. Long-term preventive therapy may include an implantable cardioverter-defibrillator and the administration of a sodium or potassium channel blocker. One clinical study found that patients treated with amiodarone had an improved survival rate, experienced fewer episodes of syncope, and required fewer shocks from an implanted cardioverter-defibrillator.

Summary of Important Points

- Antiarrhythmic drugs suppress the abnormal impulse formation or conduction that causes arrhythmias.
- Antiarrhythmic drugs are divided into four main classes, with class I consisting of sodium channel blockers, class II consisting of β-adrenergic receptor antagonists (β-blockers), class III consisting of potassium channel blockers and other drugs that prolong the action potential duration, and class IV consisting of calcium channel blockers.
- Class IA drugs, such as quinidine, slow conduction and prolong refractory periods, thereby increasing the QRS duration and the QT interval. They are primarily used for the long-term suppression of arrhythmias.
- Class IB drugs have little effect on normal cardiac tissue and electrocardiographic findings, but they may decrease the QT interval slightly. Lidocaine is administered intravenously for the treatment of acute ventricular arrhythmias. Mexiletine and tocainide are oral congeners of lidocaine and are used for long-term therapy.
- Class IC drugs have a greater effect than other sodium channel blockers on cardiac conduction but have little effect on the action potential duration. Flecainide and propafenone are used to treat supraventricular arrhythmias and life-threatening ventricular arrhythmias.
- Class II drugs (β-blockers) slow the AV node conduction velocity and prolong the AV node refractory period and are used to treat supraventricular arrhythmias. They also reduce the incidence of fatal ventricular arrhythmias in patients with myocardial infarction.
- Class III drugs, such as amiodarone, ibutilide, and sotalol, prolong the action potential duration,

refractory periods, and QT interval. They are used in treating supraventricular and ventricular arrhythmias.
- Class IV drugs (calcium channel blockers) slow the AV node conduction velocity, prolong the AV node refractory period, and thereby terminate the AV node reentry that is responsible for supraventricular tachycardia.
- Adenosine is administered as a rapid intravenous bolus to terminate acute supraventricular tachycardia.

Selected Readings

Bauman, J. L. Class III antiarrhythmic agents: the next wave. Pharmacotherapy 17:76S–83S, 1997.
Cairns, J. A. Antiarrhythmic therapy in the postinfarction setting: update from major amiodarone studies. Int J Clin Pract 52:422–424, 1998.
Desai, A. D., et al. The role of intravenous amiodarone in the management of cardiac arrhythmias. Ann Intern Med 127:294–303, 1997.
Foster, R. H., et al. Ibutilide: a review of its pharmacologic properties and clinical potential in the acute management of atrial flutter and fibrillation. Drugs 54:312–330, 1997.
Gallik, D. M., et al. Efficacy and safety of sotalol in patients with refractory atrial fibrillation or flutter. Am Heart J 134:155–160, 1997.
Guerra, P. G., et al. Is there a future for antiarrhythmic drug therapy? Drugs 56:767–781, 1998.
Kowey, P. R. Safety and risk-benefit analysis of ibutilide for acute conversion of atrial fibrillation-flutter. Am J Cardiol 78:46–52, 1996.
Nair, L. A., and A. O. Grant. Emerging class III antiarrhythmic agents: mechanism of action and proarrhythmic potential. Cardiovasc Drugs Ther 11:149–167, 1997.
Nolan, P. E. Pharmacokinetics and pharmacodynamics of intravenous agents for ventricular arrhythmias. Pharmacotherapy 17:65S–75S, 1997.
Pinto, J. V., et al. Amiodarone therapy in chronic heart failure and myocardial infarction: a review of the mortality trials with special attention to STAT-CHF and the GESICA trials. Prog Cardiovasc Dis 40:85–93, 1997.
Reasor, M. J., and S. Kacew. An evaluation of possible mechanisms underlying amiodarone-induced pulmonary toxicity. Proc Soc Exp Biol Med 212:297–304, 1996.
Reiffel, J. A., et al. Sotalol for ventricular tachyarrhythmias: beta-blocking and class III contributions and relative efficacy versus class I drugs after prior drug failure. Am J Cardiol 79:1048–1053, 1997.
Singh, B. N. Amiodarone: the expanding antiarrhythmic role and how to follow a patient on chronic therapy. Clin Cardiol 20:608–618, 1997.

CHAPTER FIFTEEN

DRUGS FOR HYPERLIPIDEMIA

CLASSIFICATION OF DRUGS FOR HYPERLIPIDEMIA

DRUGS FOR HYPERCHOLESTEROLEMIA
HMG-CoA reductase inhibitors
- Atorvastatin
- Fluvastatin
- Lovastatin
- Pravastatin
- Simvastatin

Bile acid–binding resins
- Cholestyramine
- Colestipol

DRUGS FOR HYPERCHOLESTEROLEMIA, HYPERTRIGLYCERIDEMIA, OR SPECIAL INDICATIONS
Fibric acid derivatives
- Bezafibrate
- Fenofibrate
- Gemfibrozil

Miscellaneous drugs and natural compounds
- Estrogens
- Niacin
- Vitamin E and other antioxidants

OVERVIEW

Lipids are essential molecules for human life. **Cholesterol** is an essential component of cell membranes and is the precursor to the sterol and steroid compounds that are synthesized in the body. **Triglycerides** are the main storage form of fuel to support the generation of high-energy compounds in the body. Despite the vital functions of these lipids, elevated concentrations of them play an important role in the development of heart disease and other disorders.

While **hyperlipidemia** and **hyperlipoproteinemia** are general terms for elevated concentrations of lipids and lipoproteins in the blood, **hypercholesterolemia** and **hypertriglyceridemia** refer specifically to elevated concentrations of cholesterol and triglycerides, respectively. Hypercholesterolemia contributes to the pathogenesis of **atherosclerosis** and has been causally associated with **coronary artery disease** and other atherosclerotic vascular diseases (Fig. 15–1). Hypertriglyceridemia is associated with **pancreatitis** and is also believed to have a role in the development of atherosclerosis and heart disease in

some patients, although its role in cardiovascular disorders appears to be less significant than that of hypercholesterolemia.

Because **coronary heart disease** is the main cause of premature death in industrialized countries, it is important to detect and eliminate modifiable risk factors associated with it. In addition to hyperlipidemia, these risk factors for coronary heart disease include hypertension, cigarette smoking, and diabetes mellitus. Unmodifiable risk factors include male gender and advanced age. Women have a lower risk of heart disease until after menopause, and this lower risk is primarily due to the favorable effect of estrogens on serum lipoprotein levels. Estrogens may also have beneficial effects on the microcirculation and energy metabolism. For these reasons, there has been an increased emphasis on giving estrogen replacement therapy to postmenopausal women as a means of protecting them against heart disease.

After discussing lipoproteins, lipid transport, and the causes and types of hyperlipoproteinemia, this chapter describes how dietary restrictions, alone or in combination with drug treatment, can reduce serum lipoprotein levels and thereby reduce the risk of coronary heart disease.

Lipoproteins and Lipid Transport

Because lipids are insoluble in plasma, they must be transported in the circulation in the form of lipoproteins. There are numerous **types of lipoproteins,** including chylomicrons, very low density lipoproteins (VLDL), low-density lipoproteins (LDL), intermediate-density lipoproteins (IDL), high-density lipoproteins (HDL), and lipoprotein(a). The various types are distinguished in terms of their buoyant density, lipid and protein composition, and role in lipid transport. Moreover, each type is associated with a unique group of **apoproteins.** Some of the apoproteins are exchanged between different types of lipoproteins as they transport lipids to various tissues. The composition and metabolism of lipoproteins is depicted in Box 15–1.

Chylomicrons

Chylomicrons are primarily involved in the transport of dietary lipids from the gut to the adipose tissue and liver. When cholesterol and triglycerides are ingested, they are emulsified in the intestines by

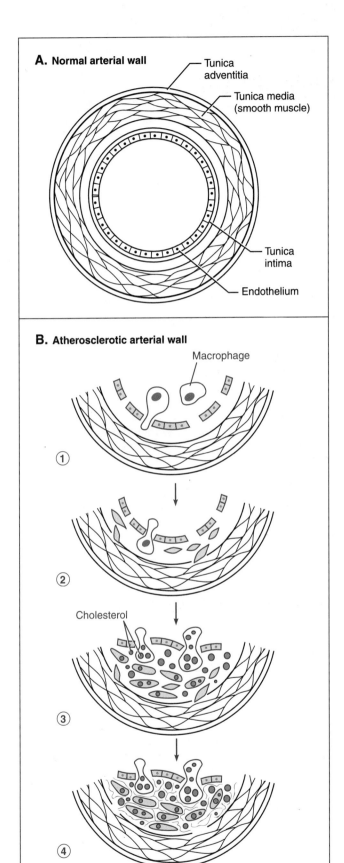

A. Normal arterial wall

- Tunica adventitia
- Tunica media (smooth muscle)
- Tunica intima
- Endothelium

B. Atherosclerotic arterial wall

Macrophage

① ② Cholesterol ③ ④

FIGURE 15–1. Comparison of normal (A) and atherosclerotic (B) arterial walls. Steps in the pathogenesis of atherosclerosis are as follows: (1) Damage to the endothelium is followed by invasion of macrophages. (2) Endothelial and macrophage growth factors stimulate smooth muscle cells to migrate into the tunica intima and to proliferate. (3) Oxidized cholesterol accumulates in and around macrophages (foam cells) and muscle cells. (4) Collagen and elastic fibers form a connective tissue matrix that results in a fibrous plaque.

the bile acids and other bile secretions, and the emulsified lipids are combined with proteins to form chylomicrons in the gut wall. After chylomicrons are secreted into the circulation, they deliver triglycerides to adipose tissue via the action of a lipoprotein lipase located in the vascular endothelial cells. By this process, chylomicrons are converted to a cholesterol-rich chylomicron remnant, which transports cholesterol to the liver.

Very Low Density and Low-Density Lipoproteins

Golgi bodies in the liver form VLDL from triglycerides, cholesterol, and protein and then secrete the VLDL into the circulation. The VLDL deliver triglycerides to adipose tissue in the same manner as do the chylomicrons. During the process, the VLDL are transformed into IDL and LDL that contain a high percentage of cholesterol.

The LDL transport cholesterol to peripheral tissues for incorporation into cell membranes and steroids. In this process, the LDL bind to specific LDL receptors that are located in the plasma membrane of cells and recognize apoprotein B-100 on the surface of LDL molecules. After binding to their receptors, the LDL undergo endocytosis and are incorporated into lysosomes for further processing of cholesterol and protein.

LDL may also deliver cholesterol to nascent atheromas and thereby contribute to the development of atherosclerosis (see Fig. 15–1). In atheromas, cholesterol is phagocytosed by macrophages, which are transformed into foam cells as they become filled with oxidized cholesterol.

High-Density Lipoproteins

HDL are small lipoproteins that are secreted the gut and liver. The nascent HDL contain prote and a small quantity of phospholipid, with relative little cholesterol or triglycerides. Their high density is due to the large ratio of protein to lipid in HDL molecules. As the HDL circulate in the blood, they exchange apoproteins C and E with VLDL, and they acquire cholesterol from peripheral tissues and atheromas. The exchange of apoproteins is related to the delivery of VLDL and triglycerides to adipose tissue via lipoprotein lipase.

HDL also serve to transport cholesterol from atheromas and peripheral tissues to the liver. During this process of **reverse cholesterol transport,** the HDL acquire cholesterol from peripheral tissues and esterify the cholesterol with fatty acids via an enzyme called lecithin–cholesterol acyltransferase (LCAT). The cholesteryl esters either are transported by HDL

BOX 15–1.   Lipoprotein Metabolism and Atherosclerosis

The liver is the central processing site for lipoprotein metabolism. Cholesterol is derived from three sources: (1) biosynthesis from acetyl-CoA, (2) delivery of dietary cholesterol by chylomicron remnants, and (3) endocytosis of low-density lipoprotein (LDL) cholesterol by LDL receptors.

Triglycerides are formed in the liver from fatty acids, which are derived from lipolysis of triglycerides in adipose tissue. Triglycerides, cholesterol, and protein are packaged by Golgi bodies in the liver to form very low density lipoproteins (VLDL), which are secreted into the circulation. The VLDL accept apoproteins C and E from high-density lipoproteins (HDL) and then return these apoproteins to HDL as they deliver triglycerides (as fatty acids) to adipose and other tissues via the action of lipoprotein lipase (LL) located in the capillary endothelium.

Composition of Lipoproteins

Lipoprotein	Core Lipids*	Apoproteins*
Chylomicron	Dietary triglycerides and cholesteryl esters	B-48, C, E, and A
VLDL	Endogenous triglycerides and cholesteryl esters	C, B-100, and E
LDL	Cholesteryl esters	B-100
HDL	Cholesteryl esters and phospholipids	A-I, A-II, C, E, and D

*Listed in order of quantitative importance.

With the removal of apoproteins and triglycerides, VLDL are transformed into LDL and intermediate-density lipoproteins (IDL). The LDL deliver cholesterol to various sites in the body, including peripheral tissues and the liver via endocytosis by LDL receptors. LDL cholesterol is also incorporated into atherosclerotic plaques.

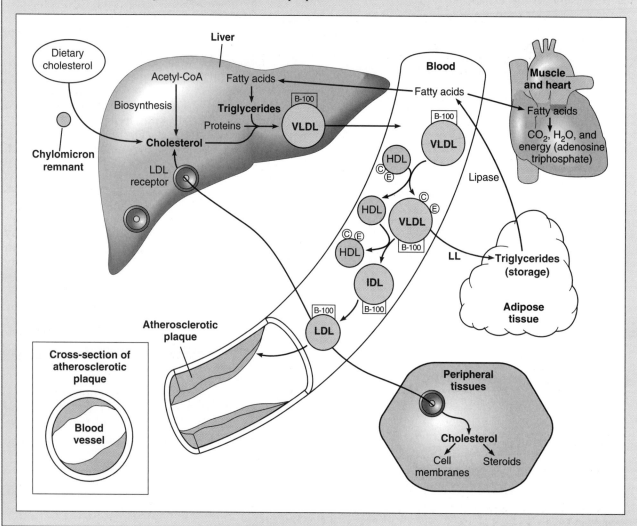

to the liver or are transferred to LDL for transport to the liver. The contribution of reverse cholesterol transport to coronary artery disease has been supported by epidemiologic studies that show an inverse correlation between HDL cholesterol levels and the risk of this disease. Moreover, the protective effect of estrogen against coronary artery disease is believed to be due primarily to the ability of estrogen to increase levels of HDL cholesterol.

Lipoprotein(a)

Lipoprotein(a) is a unique lipoprotein whose physiologic function is unknown and whose occurrence is genetically determined. It is found in atherosclerotic plaques of some individuals, and plasma levels of lipoprotein(a) are highly correlated with angiographically demonstrable coronary artery disease.

Causes and Types of Hyperlipoproteinemia

Hyperlipoproteinemia occurs as a result of genetic or environmental factors that increase the formation of lipoproteins or reduce the clearance of lipoproteins from the circulation. These factors include biochemical defects in lipoprotein metabolism, excessive dietary intake of lipids, endocrine abnormalities, and use of drugs that perturb lipoprotein formation or catabolism. Table 15–1 provides information about the characteristics and types of hyperlipoproteinemia.

Primary hyperlipoproteinemias are relatively rare disorders, each of which is caused by a **monogenic defect** (a specific defect at a single gene). In some disorders, LDL cholesterol levels are severely elevated because of a deficiency of LDL receptors or a defect in the structure of apoprotein B. In the latter case, LDL receptors do not recognized LDL, so LDL removal from the circulation is markedly impaired. In another disorder, VLDL and triglyceride levels are severely elevated because of a lipoprotein lipase deficiency that prevents delivery of triglycerides to adipose tissue.

Most cases of hyperlipoproteinemia are not due to a single gene defect but instead result from the influence of several genes that predispose the patient to milder forms of hyperlipoproteinemia, particularly in the presence of excessive dietary intake of lipids. These milder forms, called **polygenic-environmental hyperlipoproteinemias,** are much more common than primary hyperlipoproteinemias and are responsible for most cases of accelerated atherosclerosis.

Secondary hyperlipoproteinemias are commonly caused by the presence of alcoholism, diabetes mellitus, or uremia or by the use of drugs such as β-adrenergic receptor antagonists, isotretinoin, oral contraceptives, or thiazide diuretics. They are less commonly caused by hypothyroidism, nephrotic syndrome, or obstructive liver disease.

General Approach to the Management of Hyperlipidemia

Secondary causes of hyperlipoproteinemia should be excluded before treatment is considered, because abnormal levels of cholesterol or triglycerides can often be corrected by proper management of the underlying condition or by replacing the offending drug with an alternative.

The treatment of hyperlipidemia may consist of instituting dietary restrictions and changes, with or without drug therapy. As shown in Table 15–2, the approach is based on an assessment of the patient's lipid levels and risk factors for heart disease.

TABLE 15–1. Types and Characteristics of Hyperlipoproteinemia

Types	Incidence	Total Cholesterol Concentration (mg/dL)	Triglyceride Concentration (mg/dL)
Primary (monogenic) types			
Hypercholesterolemia	Rare	>300	<250
Hypertriglyceridemia	Rare	<250	>300
Mixed hyperlipidemia	Rare	>250	>300
Polygenic-environmental types			
Hypercholesterolemia	Common	200–270	<250
Mixed hyperlipidemia	Less common	>200	>300
Secondary types			
Hyperlipoproteinemia due to alcoholism, diabetes mellitus, uremia, or use of β-adrenergic receptor antagonists,† isotretinoin, oral contraceptives, or thiazide diuretics	Common	Usually normal*	Increased
Hyperlipoproteinemia due to hypothyroidism, nephrotic syndrome, or obstructive liver disease	Less common	Increased	Normal or slightly increased

*Use of thiazide diuretics may increase the total cholesterol concentration.
†Use of β-adrenergic receptor antagonists may decrease the high-density lipoprotein (HDL) cholesterol concentration.

TABLE 15–2.   Classification of Cholesterol Measurements and Guidelines for the Management of Hypercholesterolemia

Category	Total Cholesterol Concentration (mg/dL)	Low-Density Lipoprotein (LDL) Cholesterol Concentration (mg/dL)	Presence of Other Risk Factors*	Management
Desirable cholesterol concentrations	<200	<130	No	Repeat lipid measurements in 5 years.
	<200	<100	Yes	Recommend dietary modifications; review other methods to reduce risk factors; and repeat lipid measurements in 1–5 years.
Borderline to high cholesterol concentrations	200–239	130–159	No	Recommend dietary modifications and repeat lipid measurements annually.
	200–239	130–159	Yes	Recommend dietary modifications; review other methods to reduce risk factors; consider drug therapy; and repeat lipid measurements as needed.
High cholesterol concentrations	≥240	≥160	No	Recommend dietary modifications; institute drug therapy if the LDL cholesterol concentration exceeds 190 mg/dL; and repeat lipid measurements as needed.
	≥240	≥160	Yes	Recommend dietary modifications; review other methods to reduce risk factors; institute drug therapy; and repeat lipid measurements as needed.

*Elevated total cholesterol and LDL cholesterol concentrations increase the risk of atherosclerosis and are causally associated with coronary artery disease and other atherosclerotic vascular diseases. Other risk factors include male gender, advanced age (>45 years in men or >55 years in women), hypertension, cigarette smoking, diabetes mellitus, decreased high-density lipoprotein (HDL) cholesterol concentration (<35 mg/dL), and family history of coronary artery disease at a young age.

Guidelines for Dietary Modifications

Dietary modifications are the cornerstone of treatment for hyperlipidemia and may be effective by themselves in patients with mildly elevated cholesterol or triglyceride levels.

The diet of patients with hypercholesterolemia should be low in cholesterol, saturated fat, and calories. **Saturated fat** and **cholesterol** are restricted because each independently increases LDL cholesterol levels, and **calories** are restricted to help the patient achieve or maintain an ideal body weight. Cholesterol intake should be under 200 mg a day, and calories from fat should be limited to 20–25% of total calories, with saturated fat limited to less than 8% of total calories. Even more severe restrictions may be considered in patients with multiple risk factors or angiographic evidence of coronary artery disease. Studies have shown that restricted diets are effective in reversing the angiographic evidence and reducing the mortality rate in patients with coronary artery disease.

In some patients with hypertriglyceridemia, supplementing the diet with fish oils that contain **omega-3 fatty acids** may be useful in lowering the triglyceride levels. These high-molecular-weight fatty acids contain a double bond between the third and fourth carbon from the end of the molecule.

Guidelines for Drug Therapy

In patients who do not respond adequately to dietary modifications, drugs are usually indicated. The drugs for hyperlipidemia can be divided into two broad groups, based on their therapeutic use. The HMG-CoA reductase inhibitors and the bile acid–binding resins are primarily used to treat hypercholesterolemia, whereas the fibric acid derivatives and niacin are used to treat both hypercholesterolemia and hypertriglyceridemia. Another drug, probucol, has limited use for specialized purposes that are described below.

DRUGS FOR HYPERCHOLESTEROLEMIA

Tables 15–3, 15–4, and 15–5 outline the effects and pharmacokinetic properties of the drugs used to treat hypercholesterolemia and compare them with the effects and properties of other drugs discussed in this chapter.

HMG-CoA Reductase Inhibitors

Among the HMG-CoA reductase inhibitors are **atorvastatin, fluvastatin, lovastatin, pravastatin,** and **simvastatin.** These drugs have demonstrated a high degree of effectiveness in the treatment of

TABLE 15–3. Effects of Diet and Drug Therapy on Serum Lipid Concentrations

Therapy	Low-Density Lipoprotein (LDL) Cholesterol Concentration	High-Density Lipoprotein (HDL) Cholesterol Concentration	Total Triglyceride Concentration	Other Effects
Dietary modifications alone	↓10–15%	0%	↓20%	Reduction of weight and decrease in blood pressure.
Drug therapy HMG-CoA reductase inhibitors	↓20–40%	↑10%	↓10–20%	Increase in hepatic LDL receptors.
Bile acid–binding resins	↓10–20%	↑0–2%	↑0–5%	Increase in hepatic LDL receptors.
Fibric acid derivatives	↓10%*	↑10–25%	↓40–50%	Activation of lipoprotein lipase.
Other drugs Niacin	↓10–15%	↑10%	↓20–80%	Decrease in lipolysis and lipoprotein(a) levels.
Probucol	↓10–15%	↓10–15%	↓2%	Prevention of cholesterol oxidation.

*Bezafibrate and fenofibrate have a greater effect than gemfibrozil on the LDL cholesterol concentration.

hypercholesterolemia and have a good safety record. Their once-daily dosage regimen is highly convenient and fosters patient compliance.

Drug Properties

Chemistry and Pharmacokinetics. The reductase inhibitors are structurally related to 3-hydroxy-3-methylglutaryl–coenzyme A (HMG-CoA), which is the substrate for HMG-CoA reductase (Fig. 15–2A). The drugs have a relatively low bioavailability, largely owing to extensive first-pass metabolism. Lovastatin and simvastatin are prodrugs that must be converted to an active metabolite in the liver, whereas the other reductase inhibitors are active compounds. All of the drugs except atorvastatin have a relatively short

TABLE 15–4. Pharmacokinetic Properties of Drugs for Hyperlipidemia*

Drug	Oral Bioavailability	Elimination Half-Life (Hours)	Major Routes of Elimination	Other Properties
HMG-CoA reductase inhibitors				
Atorvastatin	12%	14	M and F	Does not cross the blood-brain barrier.
Fluvastatin	25%	<1	M and F	Does not cross the blood-brain barrier.
Lovastatin	5%	3.5	M and F	Is a prodrug; crosses the blood-brain barrier.
Pravastatin	17%	1.8	M and F	Does not cross the blood-brain barrier.
Simvastatin	<5%	3	M and F	Is a prodrug; crosses the blood-brain barrier.
Bile acid–binding resins				
Cholestyramine	0%	NA	F	Is a high-molecular-weight polymer.
Colestipol	0%	NA	F	Is a high-molecular-weight polymer.
Fibric acid derivatives				
Bezafibrate	90%	2	R	—
Fenofibrate	≈100%	23	M	Is a prodrug.
Gemfibrozil	≈100%	2	M (98%)	Undergoes enterohepatic cycling.
Other drugs				
Niacin	≈100%	0.5	M and R	—
Probucol	<10%	Variable†	F	Accumulates in adipose tissue.

*F = fecal; M = metabolism; NA = not applicable; and R = renal.
†The half-life of probucol is long (hours to days) and highly variable.

TABLE 15–5. Adverse Effects, Contraindications, and Interactions of Drugs for Hyperlipidemia

Drug	Common Adverse Effects	Contraindications	Common Drug Interactions
HMG-CoA reductase inhibitors	Elevated serum levels of hepatic enzymes; hepatitis; and myalgia, rhabdomyolysis, and other myopathies.	Hepatic disease and hypersensitivity.	Cause slight increase in serum levels of warfarin. Increase risk of myopathies when taken with erythromycin, gemfibrozil, or niacin.*
Bile acid–binding resins	Constipation; fecal impaction; and rash.	Hypersensitivity.	Decrease absorption of digoxin, thyroxin, warfarin, and other drugs.
Fibric acid derivatives	Allergic reactions; blood cell deficiencies; and myalgia, rhabdomyolysis, and other myopathies.	Biliary and gallbladder disease; hypersensitivity; severe hepatic disease; and severe renal disease.	Increase risk of myopathy when taken with HMG-CoA reductase inhibitors or niacin.
Other drugs			
Niacin	Gastric irritation; glucose intolerance; myalgia, rhabdomyolysis, and other myopathies; and vasodilation, flushing, and pruritus.	Diabetes mellitus; hepatic disease; hypersensitivity; and peptic ulcers.	Increases risk of myopathy when taken with gemfibrozil or HMG-CoA reductase inhibitors.*
Probucol	Decreased serum levels of high-density lipoprotein (HDL) cholesterol; prolongation of QT interval; and torsade de pointes.	Arrhythmias; hypersensitivity; and myocardial damage.	None important.

*If niacin must be used in combination with an HMG-CoA reductase inhibitor, the safest combination is niacin plus fluvastatin and the combination that poses the greatest risk is niacin plus lovastatin.

half-life (see Table 15–4). The reductase inhibitors are metabolized by two cytochrome P450 isozymes (CYP3A and CYP2C), and they may interact with other drugs metabolized by these isozymes (see below).

Mechanisms and Pharmacologic Effects. HMG-CoA reductase normally converts HMG-CoA to mevalonic acid and is the rate-limiting enzyme in cholesterol biosynthesis (Figs. 15–3 and 15–4). By competitively inhibiting HMG-CoA reductase, pravastatin and other drugs in this class reduce hepatic cholesterol biosynthesis. This increases the number of hepatic LDL receptors and enables more LDL to be delivered to the liver. As a result, there is a reduction in the level of LDL cholesterol in the serum and a reduction in the amount of cholesterol available for the formation of VLDL. In patients with hypercholesterolemia, these actions usually cause a decrease of 20–40% in serum LDL cholesterol levels and an increase of 10% in serum HDL cholesterol levels (see Table 15–3). The reductase inhibitors also reduce serum triglyceride levels.

Adverse Effects and Interactions. The HMG-CoA reductase inhibitors are relatively free of adverse effects, but they may elevate serum levels of hepatic enzymes and cause hepatitis (see Table 15–5). Less frequently, they cause myalgia and rhabdomyolysis. In rhabdomyolysis, muscle cells are destroyed, thereby releasing myoglobin into the circulation.

Myoglobin may accumulate in the kidneys and cause acute renal failure. For this reason, patients taking a reductase inhibitor should be asked to report any sign of unusual, diffuse, or persistent muscle tenderness, pain, or weakness, especially if it is accompanied by malaise or fever. Use of the reductase inhibitor must be discontinued if myopathy is diagnosed or if levels of creatine phosphokinase are found to be elevated.

Because fibric acid derivatives may also cause myopathies, the combination of these drugs and HMG-CoA reductase inhibitors should be avoided or used with great caution. Other drugs, such as erythromycin, can inhibit the metabolism of HMG-CoA reductase inhibitors and thereby increase the incidence of adverse effects such as myositis.

The reductase inhibitors may interact with other drugs that are metabolized by cytochrome P450. For example, they increase warfarin levels slightly by inhibiting warfarin metabolism.

Indications. The reductase inhibitors are used to treat **hypercholesterolemia** when diet therapy is inadequate. They are capable of reducing serum cholesterol levels to a greater extent than any other drug that is currently available for this purpose. Of the reductase inhibitors, atorvastatin has the greatest effect on triglyceride levels and may be particularly useful in treating patients with **mixed hyperlipidemia.**

Clinical trials of reductase inhibitors have demonstrated that these drugs slow the progression of atherosclerosis, reduce the risk of coronary heart disease and other atherosclerotic vascular diseases, and reduce the cardiac mortality rate. A large prospective study of over 4000 patients in Scandinavia showed that simvastatin reduced the cardiac disease–related mortality rate by 42% and the total

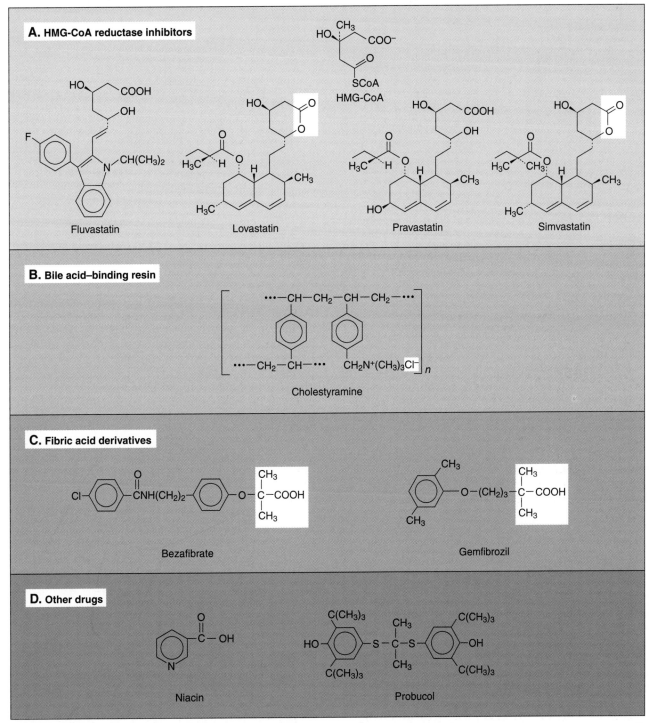

FIGURE 15–2. Structures of selected drugs for hyperlipidemia. (A) Fluvastatin, lovastatin, pravastatin, and simvastatin are structurally related to 3-hydroxy-3-methylglutaryl–coenzyme A (HMG-CoA), which is the substrate for HMG-CoA reductase. The portion of the lovastatin and simvastatin molecules that is opened up during enzymatic activation of the drugs is unshaded. (B) Cholestyramine is a bile acid–binding resin. The chloride that is exchanged for bile acids is unshaded. (C) The fibric acid derivatives include bezafibrate (available in Europe) and gemfibrozil (available in the USA and elsewhere). The fibric acid moiety is unshaded. (D) Other drugs used in the treatment of hyperlipidemia include niacin (nicotinic acid) and probucol (an antioxidant compound).

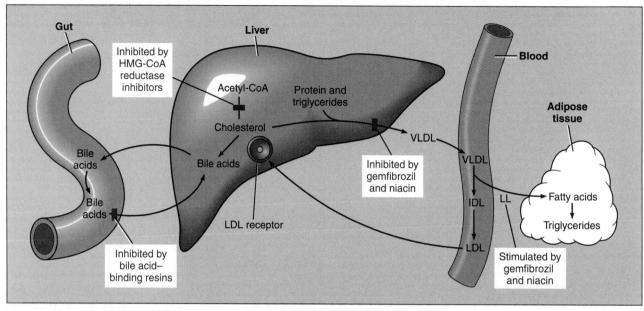

FIGURE 15–3. Sites and mechanisms of drugs for hyperlipidemia. The HMG-CoA reductase inhibitors block the rate-limiting step in cholesterol biosynthesis. The bile acid–binding resins inhibit the reabsorption of bile acids from the gut. Gemfibrozil and niacin inhibit the secretion of very low density lipoproteins (VLDL) from the liver, and they stimulate lipoprotein lipase (LL) so as to increase the delivery of fatty acids to adipose and other tissues. IDL = intermediate-density lipoprotein.

mortality rate by 30% in men with a history of myocardial infarction.

Specific Drugs

Most of the reductase inhibitors are taken in the evening or at bedtime in order to inhibit nocturnal cholesterol biosynthesis. Lovastatin should be taken with the evening meal to facilitate its absorption, whereas the other drugs may be taken without regard to food. Atorvastatin has a longer half-life than the other drugs and may be taken at any time of day. Lovastatin and simvastatin cross the blood-brain barrier and may cause sleep disturbances in some patients, whereas the other drugs do not. Fluvastatin appears to be less likely to cause myopathy than other reductase inhibitors, especially when combined with niacin.

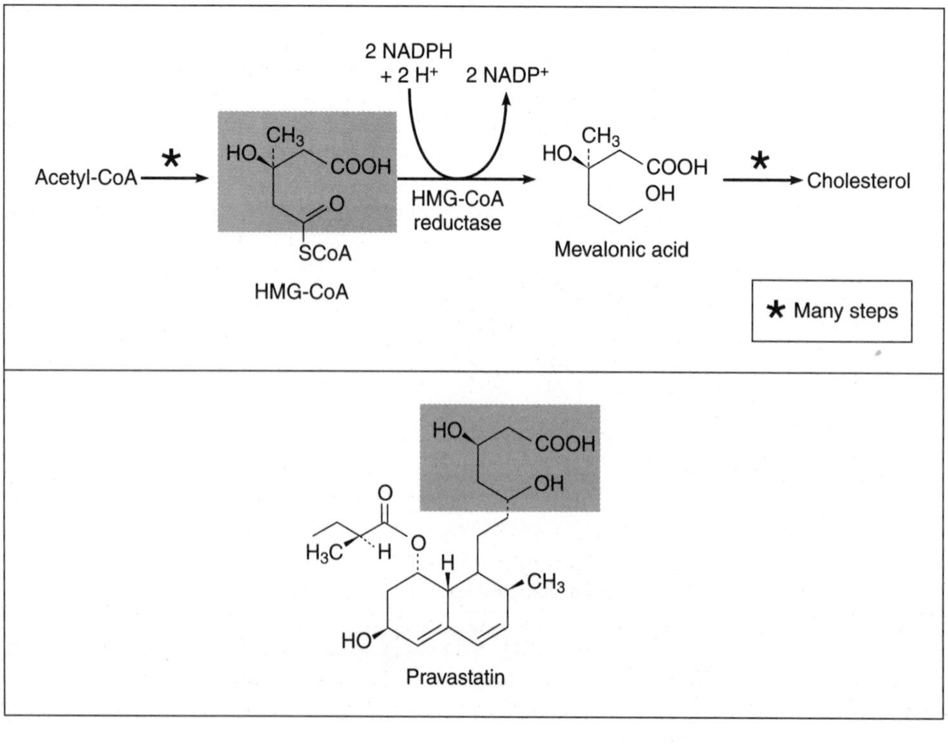

FIGURE 15–4. The inhibition of cholesterol biosynthesis by HMG-CoA reductase inhibitors. HMG-CoA reductase catalyzes the conversion of 3-hydroxy-3-methylglutaryl–coenzyme A (HMG-CoA) to mevalonic acid, the rate-limiting enzyme in cholesterol biosynthesis. The reductase inhibitors contain a structure that is similar to the structure of HMG-CoA (the shaded portions of pravastatin and HMG-CoA), and they compete with the substrate for the catalytic site of the enzyme.

Bile Acid–Binding Resins
Drug Properties

Bile acid–binding resins are moderately effective drugs for hypercholesterolemia and have an excellent safety record. They are especially valuable for patients who cannot tolerate other drugs and for patients who are young and therefore may need to take drug therapy for a long time.

Chemistry and Pharmacokinetics. The bile acid–binding resins are large-molecular-weight polymers containing a chloride ion that can be exchanged for bile acids in the gut (see Fig. 15–2B). The resins are not absorbed from the gut and are excreted in the feces.

Mechanisms and Pharmacologic Effects. After the resins bind to bile acids, the bile acid–resin complex is excreted. This action prevents the enterohepatic cycling of bile acids and obligates the liver to synthesize replacement bile acids from cholesterol. To obtain more cholesterol for this purpose, the liver increases the number of LDL receptors. Then the levels of LDL cholesterol in the serum are reduced as more cholesterol is delivered to the liver. As shown in Table 15–3, the resins have relatively little effect on levels of HDL cholesterol and triglycerides, which are usually increased slightly.

Adverse Effects and Interactions. The bile acid–binding resins have few adverse effects. They may cause constipation, fecal impaction, and other gastrointestinal side effects, some of which can be prevented by taking the drugs with a full glass of water. Occasionally, they cause irritation of the perianal area and a skin rash. In the gut, the resins can bind to digoxin, thyroxin, warfarin, and other drugs. For this reason, it is best to take resins 2 hours before or after taking other medications.

Indications. The resins are indicated for the treatment of **hypercholesterolemia** and are particularly useful in patients who cannot tolerate other drugs. Although the resins are less effective and convenient to use than the HMG-CoA reductase inhibitors, they do not cause hepatitis or myopathy, and they can be given in combination with other drugs to produce an additive effect on serum cholesterol levels. The resins have also been used to treat **diarrhea** caused by excessive bile acid secretion.

Cholestyramine and Colestipol

Cholestyramine and colestipol are bile acid–binding resins that are available in powder (granular) form for mixing with water or juice just prior to administration. To obtain the maximal effect on serum cholesterol levels, these drugs must be taken before each meal and at bedtime.

DRUGS FOR HYPERCHOLESTEROLEMIA, HYPERTRIGLYCERIDEMIA, OR SPECIAL INDICATIONS

Fibric acid derivatives, niacin, probucol, and several other drugs and natural compounds are used in the treatment of various forms of hyperlipidemia. The structures, effects, and properties of these drugs are shown in Fig. 15–2 and in Tables 15–3, 15–4, and 15–5.

Fibric Acid Derivatives
Drug Properties

Fibric acid derivatives are primarily used for the treatment of hypertriglyceridemia or marked HDL deficiency. Some of the newer ones have unique properties that may add to their utility in patients with heart disease.

Chemistry and Pharmacokinetics. The drugs are derivatives of a branched-chain carboxylic acid known as fibric acid or **fibrate** (see Fig. 15–2C). The first drug in this class, clofibrate, is largely obsolete because of its high incidence of adverse effects. Gemfibrozil is the only other member of the class that is currently available in the USA, but other drugs, such as bezafibrate and fenofibrate, are under development and review by regulatory agencies.

Mechanisms and Pharmacologic Effects. Gemfibrozil and other fibrates have two actions that reduce serum VLDL and triglyceride levels (see Table 15–3). They activate lipoprotein lipase and thereby promote the delivery of triglycerides to adipose tissue, and they interfere with the formation of VLDL in the liver in a manner similar to niacin (see Fig. 15–3). The reduction in triglyceride levels produced by these drugs is accompanied by an impressive increase in HDL cholesterol levels. However, the effect of fibrates on LDL cholesterol is more variable and drug-specific. Gemfibrozil reduces LDL cholesterol levels modestly in most patients but may increase it in some, probably because it promotes the conversion of VLDL to LDL. The newer fibrates appear to have a greater effect on serum cholesterol levels than does gemfibrozil.

Adverse Effects and Interactions. The fibrates may cause blood cell deficiencies and other hypersensitivity reactions. Like the HMG-CoA reductase inhibitors, the fibrates can also cause rhabdomyolysis and other myopathies (see Table 15–5). For this reason, the combination of reductase inhibitors and fibrates should be avoided or used with great caution. Fibrates may be given with bile acid–binding resins, but the doses must be separated by more than 2 hours, because the resins reduce fibrate absorption.

Gemfibrozil

Gemfibrozil is primarily indicated for the treatment of **hypertriglyceridemia.** It is also useful in patients with **mixed hyperlipidemia** and can be administered to increase HDL cholesterol in patients with an isolated **HDL deficiency.**

The Helsinki Heart Study, which involved 2000 men with hypercholesterolemia, found that gemfibrozil increased HDL cholesterol levels and decreased LDL cholesterol and triglyceride levels. It also reduced the coronary artery disease–related mortality rate, but the overall mortality rate was not affected because of an increase in deaths due to other diseases, accidents, and violence.

Bezafibrate and Fenofibrate

Both bezafibrate and fenofibrate are available in Europe, and bezafibrate is being reviewed by the Food and Drug Administration in the USA. These drugs reduce LDL cholesterol levels to a greater extent than do other fibrates, and bezafibrate also lowers blood glucose levels and affects fibrinogen and platelet levels. For this reason, bezafibrate may benefit patients who have **hyperlipidemia in the presence of a thrombotic disorder.**

Miscellaneous Drugs and Natural Compounds
Niacin

Pharmacologic doses of niacin have profound effects on serum lipid levels. Although the drug is capable of causing a number of adverse effects, it nevertheless has a valuable role in the treatment of many patients with hyperlipidemia.

Chemistry and Pharmacokinetics. Niacin, or **nicotinic acid,** is a vitamin whose structure is shown in Fig. 15–2D. The small amount of niacin that is ingested in food is converted in the body to enzyme cofactors required for oxidative reactions in intermediary metabolism. These cofactors are nicotinamide adenine dinucleotide (NAD) and its phosphate derivative (NADP). Niacin is well absorbed from the gut and is extensively metabolized before undergoing renal excretion.

Mechanisms and Pharmacologic Effects. The quantity of niacin ingested in food does not have any measurable effect on serum lipid levels. The action of niacin on lipids is a pharmacologic effect that requires the administration of several grams of the compound each day. These large doses of niacin produce effects that are similar to those of gemfibrozil. Niacin reduces hepatic VLDL secretion, and it enhances VLDL clearance by activating lipoprotein lipase (see Fig. 15–3). The effect on VLDL secretion is partly due to inhibition of lipolysis in adipose tissue. This action reduces the supply of circulating free fatty acids that the liver uses to synthesize triglycerides for incorporation into VLDL. Although niacin may significantly decrease serum LDL cholesterol and triglyceride levels, it usually increases HDL cholesterol levels (see Table 15–3).

Adverse Effects and Interactions. The large doses of niacin that are required to lower serum lipid levels sometimes produce marked vasodilation and flushing of the skin, accompanied by pruritus and a feeling of warmth and tingling. This effect can be significantly reduced by pretreatment with aspirin, and some tolerance to this effect develops with continued drug administration. Although niacin is effective and well tolerated by many patients, it has a

number of more serious adverse effects that preclude its use by others. Niacin can elevate serum transaminase levels and cause hepatitis. It also produces gastric distress and may activate a peptic ulcer. Finally, niacin causes glucose intolerance in some patients and may aggravate diabetes mellitus. For these reasons, niacin use should usually be avoided in patients with hepatic disorders, peptic ulcers, or diabetes mellitus.

Indications. Niacin is probably the most effective single drug that is currently available for the treatment of **mixed hyperlipidemia.** It favorably influences the serum levels of VLDL, LDL, and HDL, and it may be used in combination with bile acid–binding resins and other drugs to treat more severe cases of hyperlipidemia. Niacin can also be used to treat patients who have either **hypertriglyceridemia** or **hypercholesterolemia,** and it has been found to be effective in the treatment of patients who have lipoprotein(a) levels that put them at increased risk for heart disease.

Estrogens

Estrogens have been demonstrated to protect women against atherosclerosis, largely by increasing HDL cholesterol levels. Moreover, **estrogen replacement therapy** in menopausal women has demonstrated value in preventing coronary artery disease in this population. This subject is discussed in more detail in Chapter 34.

Vitamin E and Other Antioxidants

Vitamin E and other naturally occurring antioxidants may have a protective effect against atherosclerosis and coronary artery disease by preventing the oxidation of LDL cholesterol. Two large clinical trials have supported the protective role of vitamin E, and other studies have suggested a protective role for **beta-carotene,** especially in cigarette smokers. Moderate dietary supplementation with these agents has not been associated with adverse effects.

Dietary **flavonoids,** such as those contained in tea, may also exert an antioxidant effect and protect against atherosclerosis.

The role of **vitamin C** in atherosclerosis remains uncertain.

DRUG COMBINATIONS

Drugs may be used in combination to treat hyperlipidemia in patients who do not respond to a single drug. The safest combinations are those consisting of a bile acid–binding resin and either an HMG-CoA reductase inhibitor, niacin, or gemfibrozil. The effective treatment of primary hyperlipoproteinemias may require the use of niacin and either gemfibrozil or an HMG-CoA reductase inhibitor, and the most severe cases of hyperlipidemia may require the use of a three-drug regimen.

Some drug combinations should be avoided or only used with great caution. The combination of gemfibrozil plus an HMG-CoA reductase inhibitor has a greater tendency to cause myopathy than does the use of either drug alone. For the same reason, lovastatin should not be used in combination with niacin, but other HMG-CoA reductase inhibitors appear to be safer with niacin.

Summary of Important Points

- Cholesterol and triglycerides are secreted by the liver in the form of very low density lipoproteins (VLDL). After delivering triglycerides to adipose tissue, VLDL become low-density lipoproteins (LDL). The LDL deliver cholesterol to peripheral tissues, the liver, and atheromas. High-density lipoproteins (HDL) transport cholesterol from tissues and atheromas to the liver.
- Hypercholesterolemia is a risk factor for atherosclerosis and coronary artery disease. Hypertriglyceridemia is associated with pancreatitis and is also believed to have a role in the development of heart disease in some patients.
- All patients with hypercholesterolemia and hypertriglyceridemia should be given dietary counseling, and some may also require drug therapy.
- Lovastatin and other HMG-CoA reductase inhibitors block the rate-limiting enzyme in cholesterol biosynthesis and lead to a secondary increase in hepatic LDL receptors.
- Cholestyramine and colestipol are bile acid–binding resins that prevent the enterohepatic cycling of bile acids and increase hepatic cholesterol conversion to replacement bile acids.
- Niacin (nicotinic acid) and gemfibrozil (a fibric acid derivative) reduce hepatic VLDL secretion and increase VLDL clearance by activating lipoprotein lipase. These drugs reduce serum triglyceride levels more than they reduce cholesterol levels.

Selected Readings

Bertolini, S., et al. Efficacy and safety of atorvastatin compared to pravastatin in patients with hypercholesterolemia. Atherosclerosis 130:191–197, 1997.

Davignon, J., and J. S. Cohn. Triglycerides: a risk factor for coronary heart disease. Atherosclerosis 124(supplement):S57–S64, 1996.

de-Faire, U., et al. Retardation of coronary atherosclerosis: the Bezafibrate Coronary Atherosclerosis Intervention Trial (BECAIT) and other angiographic trials. Cardiovasc Drugs Ther 11(supplement 1):257–263, 1997.

Furberg, C. D., et al. Effect of lovastatin on early carotid atherosclerosis and cardiovascular events. Circulation 90:1679–1687, 1994.

Furberg, C. D., et al. Pravastatin, lipids, and major coronary events. Am J Cardiol 73:1133–1134, 1994.

Guyton, J. R., and D. M. Capuzzi. Treatment of hyperlipidemia with combined niacin-statin regimens. Am J Cardiol 82:82U–84U, 1998.

Hertog, M. G., et al. Dietary antioxidant flavonoids and risk of coronary heart disease. Lancet 342:1007–1011, 1993.

Illingworth, D. R., and J. A. Tobert. A review of clinical trials comparing HMG-CoA reductase inhibitors. Clin Ther 16:366–385, 1994.

Jones, P. H., et al. Effect of gemfibrozil on levels of lipoprotein(a) in type II hyperlipoproteinemic subjects. J Lipid Res 37:1298–1308, 1996.

Morgan, J. M., et al. A new extended-release niacin (Niaspan): efficacy, tolerability, and safety in hypercholesterolemic patients. Am J Cardiol 82:29U–34U, 1998.

Rimm, E. B., et al. Vitamin E consumption and the risk of coronary heart disease in men. N Engl J Med 328:1450–1456, 1993.

Scandinavian Simvastatin Survival Study Group. Randomized trial of cholesterol lowering in 4444 patients with coronary heart disease: the Scandinavian Simvastatin Survival Study (4S). Lancet 344:1383–1389, 1994.

Sinzinger, H., et al. Atherogenic risk reduction in patients with dyslipidaemia: comparison between bezafibrate and lovastatin. Eur Heart J 16:1491–1501, 1995.

Waters, D., et al. Effects of monotherapy with an HMG-CoA reductase inhibitor on the progression of coronary atherosclerosis as assessed by serial quantitative arteriography. Circulation 89:959–968, 1994.

CHAPTER SIXTEEN

ANTICOAGULANT, ANTIPLATELET,

AND FIBRINOLYTIC DRUGS

CLASSIFICATION OF ANTICOAGULANT, ANTIPLATELET, AND FIBRINOLYTIC DRUGS

ANTICOAGULANT DRUGS
  Oral anticoagulants
- Anisindione
- Dicumarol
- Warfarin

  Parenteral anticoagulants
- Dalteparin
- Enoxaparin
- Heparin
- Hirudin and related drugs

ANTIPLATELET DRUGS
- Abciximab
- Aspirin
- Dipyridamole
- Ticlopidine

FIBRINOLYTIC DRUGS
- Alteplase
- Anistreplase
- Reteplase
- Streptokinase
- Urokinase

BLOOD COAGULATION
Normal Hemostasis

When a small blood vessel is injured, hemorrhage is prevented by the occurrence of **vasospasm,** the formation of a **platelet plug,** and the formation of a **fibrin clot** (Fig. 16–1). After the vessel is repaired, the clot is removed via the process of **fibrinolysis.**

Vasospasm reduces bleeding and blood flow and thereby facilitates platelet adhesion and coagulation. Exposure of the blood to extravascular collagen causes adherence of platelets to the injured vessel wall and initiates the sequential activation of numerous **coagulation factors,** or **blood clotting factors.** These factors and their synonyms are listed in Table 16–1, and the **coagulation pathways** are illustrated in Fig. 16–2. The **intrinsic pathway** may be activated by surface contact with a foreign body or extravascular tissue, whereas the **extrinsic pathway** is activated by

a complex tissue factor. The pathways converge with the activation of **factor X,** which is the major rate-limiting step in the coagulation cascade. The activation of factor X leads to the formation of **thrombin,** and thrombin in turn catalyzes the conversion of **fibrinogen** to **fibrin.** The fibrin meshwork traps erythrocytes and platelets to complete the formation of a hemostatic thrombus (clot).

Pathologic Thrombus Formation

The processes leading to **thrombosis** and **embolism** are complex and not completely understood.

Atherosclerosis and other abnormalities affecting the vascular endothelium may serve as a stimulus for platelet aggregation and blood coagulation in arteries. Venous pooling, sluggish blood flow, and inflammation of veins may permit inappropriate platelet adhesion and coagulation in vessels. Platelet aggregation appears to have a larger role in the formation of **arterial thrombi (white thrombi),** whereas coagulation predominates in the formation of **venous thrombi (red thrombi).** However, platelet aggregation followed by coagulation occurs both in arteries and in veins, and the processes differ only in the degree of contribution by platelets or coagulation to the thrombus.

An arterial or venous thrombus may become dislodged from the vessel wall so as to form an **embolus** that travels through the circulation and eventually occludes a smaller vessel in the lungs or brain, thereby causing pulmonary embolism or a cerebrovascular accident, respectively.

ANTICOAGULANT DRUGS
Oral Anticoagulants

Anticoagulants are drugs that retard coagulation and thereby prevent the occurrence or enlargement of a thrombus. Table 16–2 compares the properties of oral anticoagulants with those of parenteral anticoagulants.

Drug Properties

Chemistry and Mechanisms. Coumarins were originally found in spoiled clover hay and identified

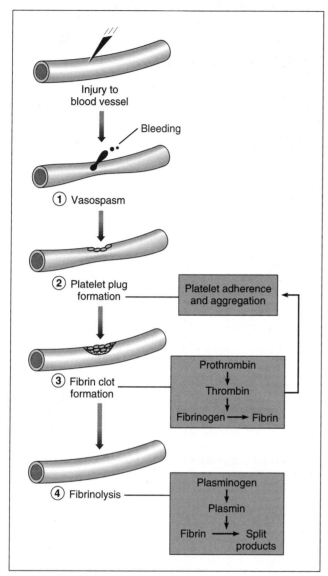

FIGURE 16–1. Normal hemostasis. (1) When a small blood vessel is injured, vasospasm reduces blood flow and facilitates platelet aggregation and coagulation. (2) The platelets adhere to extravascular collagen and are activated to release mediators that cause platelet aggregation and the formation of a platelet plug to arrest bleeding. (3) Exposure of the blood to tissue factors also activates coagulation and leads to the formation of a fibrin clot, which arrests bleeding until the vessel is repaired. (4) After the vessel is repaired, the clot is removed by the process of fibrinolysis.

as substances that caused hemorrhage in cattle. Coumarin derivatives, such as warfarin and dicumarol, were subsequently developed as anticoagulants. In addition to coumarin derivatives, the oral anticoagulants include indanediones such as anisindione.

Warfarin and other oral anticoagulants are structurally related to vitamin K (Fig. 16–3A and 16–3B). These drugs work by inhibiting the synthesis of clotting factors II (prothrombin), VII, IX, and X, whose carboxylation is dependent on a reduced form of vitamin K. As shown in Fig. 16–4, warfarin blocks the reduction of oxidized vitamin K and thereby prevents the posttranscriptional carboxylation of these four

TABLE 16–1. Coagulation Factors

Factor*	Common Synonym	Dependent on Vitamin K†
I	Fibrinogen	No
II	Prothrombin	Yes
III	Tissue thromboplastin	No
IV	Calcium	No
V	Proaccelerin	No
VII	Proconvertin	Yes
VIII	Antihemophilic factor	No
IX	Plasma thromboplastin component	Yes
X	Stuart factor	Yes
XI	Plasma thromboplastin antecedent	No
XII	Hageman factor	No
XIII	Fibrin stabilizing factor	No

*Factor VI is no longer considered to be a coagulation factor.
†Proteins C and S, which are endogenous anticoagulants that inactivate factors Va and VIIIa and promote fibrinolysis, are also dependent on vitamin K.

factors. Oral anticoagulants also work by inhibiting the synthesis of proteins C and S, which are endogenous anticoagulants that inactivate factors V and VIII and promote fibrinolysis. It is possible that the inhibition of proteins C and S contributes to a transient procoagulant effect of the oral anticoagulants when they are first administered.

Pharmacokinetic and Pharmacologic Effects. Oral anticoagulants are absorbed from the gut and

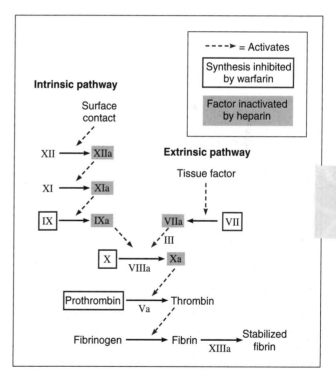

FIGURE 16–2. Blood coagulation and sites of drug action. Blood coagulation involves the sequential activation of proteolytic clotting factors. The intrinsic pathway may be activated by surface contact with a foreign body, whereas the extrinsic pathway is activated by tissue factor. The pathways converge with the activation of factor X, which leads to the formation of thrombin and fibrin. Warfarin and other oral anticoagulants inhibit the synthesis of the vitamin K–dependent clotting factors. Heparin inactivates various clotting factors.

TABLE 16–2. Comparison of the Pharmacologic Properties of Oral and Parenteral Anticoagulants

Property	Oral Anticoagulants	Parenteral Anticoagulants
Active in vitro	No	Yes
Onset of action	Delayed	Immediate
Mechanism of action	Inhibit synthesis of clotting factors	Inactivate clotting factors
Safe to take during pregnancy	No	Yes
Antidote	Phytonadione (vitamin K_1)	Protamine sulfate

are extensively metabolized before they are excreted in the urine. Unlike the parenteral anticoagulants, the oral anticoagulants cross the placenta and may cause fetal hemorrhage and malformations.

The oral anticoagulants have a delayed onset of action, owing to the time required to deplete the pool of circulating clotting factors after synthesis of new factors is inhibited. The half-life of circulating factors II, VII, IX, and X ranges from 6 hours (factor VII) to 50 hours (factor II). Therefore, the maximal effect of oral anticoagulants is not observed until 3–5 days after starting therapy with these drugs. Patients with acute thromboembolism are usually treated with heparin and an oral anticoagulant, and the heparin may be withdrawn after the oral anticoagulant becomes effective. A period of several days is also required for coagulation factor levels to return to normal after oral anticoagulants are discontinued. The recovery of clotting factors can be accelerated by administration of phytonadione (vitamin K_1), as described below.

Adverse Effects and Interactions. The most common adverse effect of oral anticoagulants is bleeding (Table 16–3), which may range in severity from mild nosebleed to life-threatening hemorrhage. Patients should be instructed to report any signs of bleeding, including hematuria and ecchymoses.

The oral anticoagulants are contraindicated in pregnancy because of their potential to cause fetal hemorrhage and various structural malformations that are collectively referred to as the fetal warfarin syndrome. These malformations are partly due to

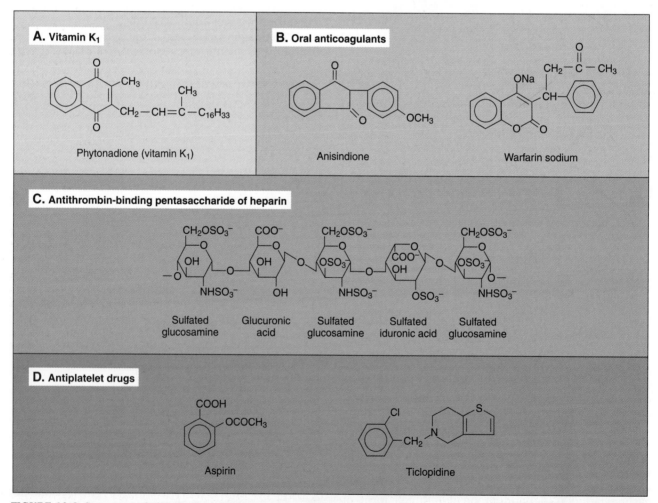

FIGURE 16–3. Structures of vitamin K_1 and selected anticoagulant and antiplatelet drugs. (A) If oral anticoagulants cause bleeding, phytonadione (vitamin K_1) can be given to accelerate the recovery of clotting factors. **(B)** Oral anticoagulants include anisindione and warfarin sodium, agents that are structurally related to vitamin K. **(C)** Parenteral anticoagulants include heparin, a naturally occurring mixture of sulfated mucopolysaccharides that bind to antithrombin. **(D)** Antiplatelet drugs include aspirin and ticlopidine.

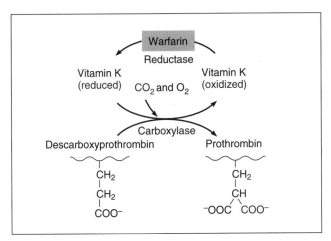

FIGURE 16–4. Mechanisms of action of warfarin and other oral anticoagulants. Oral anticoagulants block the reduction of oxidized vitamin K (vitamin K epoxide) and thereby prevent vitamin K–dependent carboxylation of clotting factors.

antagonism of vitamin K–dependent maturation of bone proteins during a process in which certain proteins undergo carboxylation in the same manner as the nascent clotting factors. Warfarin and other oral anticoagulants block the process and may cause chondrodysplasia punctata and various birth defects that are listed in Table 4–6.

Most drug interactions with oral anticoagulants are due to induction or inhibition of cytochrome P450 enzymes, but a few are due to the antagonism or potentiation of the anticoagulant effect. The most serious interactions are with drugs that increase the anticoagulant effect and place the patient at risk for hemorrhage. Because the number of drugs that interact with oral anticoagulants is large, patients who are taking anticoagulants should be instructed to consult their physician before starting or discontinuing any other medication.

Treatment with high doses of salicylates or with some third-generation cephalosporins has a direct hypoprothrombinemic effect and thereby increases the anticoagulant effect of warfarin and related drugs. In contrast, treatment with rifampin or barbiturates induces cytochrome P450 enzymes and thereby decreases the anticoagulant effect of warfarin. Cholestyramine inhibits the absorption of warfarin from the gut. Amiodarone, cimetidine, fluconazole, metronidazole, phenylbutazone, sulfinpyrazone, and trimethoprim-sulfamethoxazole all inhibit the metabolism of warfarin. In addition, phenylbutazone and sulfinpyrazone directly inhibit clot formation and platelet aggregation.

Phytonadione directly antagonizes the effect of oral anticoagulants on clotting factor synthesis and is used to treat hemorrhage caused by anticoagulant activity.

Indications. Oral anticoagulants are primarily used in the long-term management of patients who have a thromboembolic disorder such as **deep vein thrombosis** or **atrial fibrillation** and patients who have an **artificial heart valve** (Table 16–4). They are

also used in conjunction with heparin for the treatment of **myocardial infarction.** The goal of oral anticoagulant use is to inhibit embolization and thereby prevent the serious and potentially fatal sequelae of thrombosis. Oral anticoagulants can keep an established thrombus from extending, but they cannot dissolve one.

The dosage of oral anticoagulants to be given is based on the patient's **prothrombin time** (PT). This measurement is determined by drawing a blood sample, adding a tissue thromboplastin preparation to initiate coagulation in it, and comparing the in vitro clotting time in the sample with that in a standardized control preparation. As a general rule of thumb, the dosage of anticoagulant to be given should prolong the PT of the patient so that it is 1.3–1.5 times the PT of the control.

When the international reference thromboplastin preparation is used as the standardized control preparation, the ratio is expressed as the **international normalized ratio** (INR) and is calculated as follows:

$$INR = (PT_{observed} / PT_{control})^{ISI}$$

where the $PT_{observed}$ and $PT_{control}$ are the prothrombin times of the patient and control, respectively, and the ISI is the international sensitivity index of the thromboplastin reagent being used. For most indications, an INR of 2–3 is recommended. However, for patients with mechanical prosthetic heart valves and for those with recurrent systemic embolization, an INR of 3–4.5 is recommended.

The patient's PT should be monitored daily during the initiation of therapy and whenever another drug is added to or withdrawn from the treatment regimen. Concurrent heparin therapy may cause an increase of 10–20% in the patient's PT, so the target PT and INR levels should be increased by the same amount. Once the patient's PT has stabilized, it should be monitored every 4–6 weeks.

Treatment of Bleeding. If bleeding occurs, the oral anticoagulant should be withheld until the bleeding can be evaluated and the patient's PT can be determined. The treatment of bleeding may include a reduction in drug dosage and the administration of **phytonadione (vitamin K₁).** If bleeding is serious or if the INR is markedly elevated (>20), **fresh frozen plasma** or **factor IX concentrate** may be warmed and administered to rapidly replace clotting factors.

Coumarin Derivatives

Warfarin is completely absorbed after oral administration. About 99% of the drug is bound to plasma proteins, and it is almost completely metabolized by two cytochrome P450 enzymes (CYP1A2 and CYP2C). These excellent properties make warfarin the oral anticoagulant of choice for patients who require therapy for any of the indications discussed above. Other oral anticoagulants either have less favorable pharmacologic and pharmacokinetic prop-

TABLE 16-3. Adverse Effects, Contraindications, and Drug Interactions of Anticoagulant, Antiplatelet, and Fibrinolytic Drugs

Drug	Common Adverse Effects	Contraindications	Common Drug Interactions
Oral anticoagulants			
Anisindione	Agranulocytosis, birth defects, bleeding, and renal toxicity.	Bleeding, hypersensitivity, pregnancy, and recent surgery.	Unknown.
Dicumarol	Birth defects and bleeding.	Aneurysm, bleeding, hypersensitivity, pregnancy, and recent surgery.	Serum levels altered by drugs that induce or inhibit cytochrome P450, by drugs that inhibit gut absorption, and by drugs that directly increase or decrease the anticoagulant effect (see text).
Warfarin	Same as dicumarol.	Same as dicumarol.	Same as dicumarol.
Parenteral anticoagulants			
Dalteparin	Bleeding and thrombocytopenia.	Aneurysm, bleeding, hypersensitivity, and recent surgery.	Risk of bleeding increased by salicylates.
Enoxaparin	Same as dalteparin.	Same as dalteparin.	Same as dalteparin.
Heparin	Bleeding, hyperkalemia, and thrombocytopenia.	Same as dalteparin.	Same as dalteparin.
Hirudin and related drugs	Bleeding.	Same as dalteparin.	Same as dalteparin.
Antiplatelet drugs			
Abciximab	Bleeding, bradycardia, hypotension, and thrombocytopenia.	Aneurysm, bleeding, hypersensitivity, recent surgery, stroke, and thrombocytopenia.	Unknown.
Aspirin	Gastrointestinal irritation and bleeding, hypersensitivity reactions, and tinnitus.	Bleeding, hypersensitivity, and Reye's syndrome.	Increases hypoglycemic effect of sulfonylureas. Increases risk of gastrointestinal bleeding and ulceration associated with methotrexate, valproate, and other drugs. Inhibits uricosuric effect of probenecid.
Dipyridamole	Gastrointestinal distress, headache, mild and transient dizziness, and rash.	Hypersensitivity.	Decreases metabolism of adenosine. Increases risk of bradycardia associated with β-adrenergic receptor antagonists.
Ticlopidine	Bleeding, diarrhea, gastrointestinal pain, increased cholesterol and triglyceride levels, nausea, and neutropenia.	Bleeding, hematopoietic disorders, hemostatic disorders, hypersensitivity, and severe liver disease.	Increases levels of drugs metabolized by liver microsomal enzymes.
Fibrinolytic drugs	Bleeding, hypersensitivity reactions, and reperfusion arrhythmias.	Aneurysm, bleeding, brain tumor, hemorrhagic stroke, recent surgery, and severe hypertension.	Increases risk of bleeding associated with anticoagulant and antiplatelet drugs.

erties or are more toxic and should be used only in cases in which the patient is intolerant of warfarin.

Dicumarol is a coumarin derivative that is incompletely absorbed from the gut and may cause considerable gastrointestinal distress. For these reasons, it is seldom used.

Anisindione

Anisindione has pharmacologic properties that are similar to those of the coumarin anticoagulants, but it has greater toxicity. Like other indanediones, it may cause renal toxicity characterized by acute tubular necrosis or may cause agranulocytosis. Therefore, it is usually reserved for patients who are intolerant of or unresponsive to warfarin.

Parenteral Anticoagulants

The parenteral anticoagulants include heparin, hirudin, and the derivatives of these natural agents.

Heparin and Fractionated Heparin

In its natural form, **heparin** contains fractions with high molecular weights ranging from 5000 to

TABLE 16–4. Clinical Uses of Anticoagulant, Antiplatelet, and Fibrinolytic Drugs

Clinical Use	Primary Drug*	Secondary Drug*
Acute thrombotic stroke	Fibrinolytic drug	—
Artificial heart valve	Warfarin or aspirin	Dipyridamole
Atrial fibrillation	Heparin or warfarin	Aspirin
Deep vein thrombosis		
Treatment	Heparin or warfarin	—
Surgical prophylaxis	Dalteparin or enoxaparin	Heparin
Myocardial infarction	Fibrinolytic drug, heparin, aspirin, or warfarin	—
Percutaneous translu-minal coronary angioplasty	Abciximab, heparin, or aspirin	—
Pulmonary embolism	Fibrinolytic drug, heparin, or warfarin	—
Transient ischemic attacks	Aspirin	Warfarin
Unstable angina	Aspirin	—

*If aspirin is contraindicated or is not tolerated, ticlopidine may be used. If warfarin is contraindicated or is not tolerated, another oral anticoagulant may be used.

30,000 and fractions with low molecular weights ranging from 2000 to 9000. **Enoxaparin** and **dalteparin,** two low-molecular-weight forms of fractionated heparin, have recently been marketed, and several others are currently under investigation.

Chemistry and Mechanisms. Heparin is a naturally occurring mixture of sulfated mucopolysaccharides produced by mast cells and basophils. It can be obtained from porcine intestine or bovine lung.

As shown in Fig. 16–2, heparin inactivates clotting factors. The predominant effect of unfractionated heparin is to potentiate the activity of an endogenous anticoagulant called **antithrombin III** (AT-III). This substance then inactivates thrombin (factor IIa) and other clotting factors. The structure of the heparin pentasaccharide that binds to AT-III is shown in Fig. 16–3C.

Enoxaparin and dalteparin directly inactivate factor Xa and have less direct effect on thrombin via activation of AT-III.

Pharmacokinetic and Pharmacologic Effects. Heparin is not absorbed from the gut and must be given parenterally. It is usually administered by continuous intravenous infusion. It is removed from the circulation by the reticuloendothelial system, is eliminated from the body by renal and hepatic mechanisms, and has a half-life of about 90 minutes. The dosage of heparin is generally determined by monitoring the **activated partial thromboplastin time** (aPTT), but other laboratory measurements have also been used. The dosage is considered adequate when the aPTT is 1.5–2 times normal.

Enoxaparin and dalteparin are usually administered subcutaneously, and their maximal effect occurs from 3 to 5 hours after injection. When they are used, the aPTT does not need to be monitored.

Adverse Effects and Interactions. Adverse effects, contraindications, and drug interactions are listed in Table 16–3. The most common serious adverse effect of fractionated and unfractionated heparin is bleeding. Thrombocytopenia and hyperkalemia may also occur, with hyperkalemia usually due to the suppression of aldosterone secretion.

Indications. Heparin is indicated for the treatment of **acute thromboembolic disorders,** including peripheral and pulmonary embolism, venous thrombosis, and coagulopathies such as disseminated intravascular coagulation. It is used prophylactically to prevent clotting in **arterial and heart surgery,** during **blood transfusions,** and in **renal dialysis** and **blood sample collection.** Heparin is also used to prevent embolization of thrombi that may cause a cerebrovascular event in patients with **acute atrial fibrillation.** Low doses of heparin may be administered subcutaneously to prevent **deep vein thrombosis** and **pulmonary embolism** in high-risk patients.

Enoxaparin or dalteparin can be administered subcutaneously to prevent deep vein thrombosis following hip replacement surgery.

Treatment of Bleeding. The treatment of heparin-induced hemorrhage consists of administering **protamine sulfate,** which is a positively charged basic protein that physically combines with negatively charged heparin and thereby inactivates it. Protamine is administered intravenously for this purpose, and the dosage is based on the estimated amount of residual heparin in the body. Severe bleeding may require the administration of **fresh frozen plasma.**

Hirudin and Related Drugs

Hirudin is a natural anticoagulant obtained from *Hirudo medicinalis,* the medicinal leech. Hirudin and its analogues directly inhibit thrombin, without the need for AT-III. These drugs are currently undergoing clinical investigation for the treatment of **unstable angina** and **acute myocardial infarction.**

ANTIPLATELET DRUGS

The mechanisms of platelet aggregation and the sites of antiplatelet drug action are depicted in Fig. 16–5.

Platelets adhere to the damaged vascular endothelium via linkage of glycoprotein Ia receptors with exposed collagen and via linkage of Ib receptors with von Willebrand's factor, a circulating factor that is similar to clotting factor VIII. The adherence of platelets to vascular endothelium activates the platelets and leads to the synthesis and release (degranulation) of various mediators of platelet aggregation, including thromboxane A_2 (TXA_2), adenosine diphosphate (ADP), and 5-hydroxytryptamine (5-HT, or serotonin). These mediators increase the expression of glycoprotein IIb/IIIa receptors that bind to fibrinogen and thereby cause platelet aggregation. Aspirin and ticlopidine act by inhibiting the synthesis or activity of specific mediators of platelet aggregation,

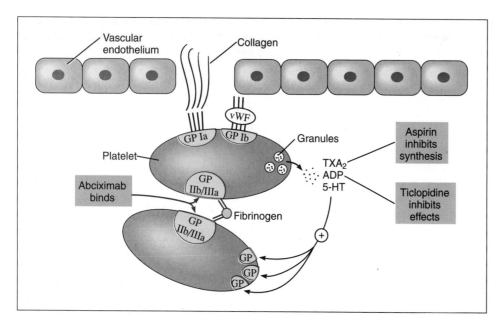

FIGURE 16–5. Platelet aggregation and sites of drug action. Platelets adhere to damaged endothelium via linkage of glycoprotein (GP) Ia receptors with exposed collagen and via linkage of GP Ib receptors with von Willebrand's factor (vWF). This activates the platelets and leads to the synthesis and release (degranulation) of various mediators of platelet aggregation, including thromboxane A_2 (TXA$_2$), adenosine diphosphate (ADP), and 5-hydroxytryptamine (5-HT, or serotonin). These mediators increase the expression of GP receptors and promote platelet aggregation via the binding of fibrinogen to GP IIb/IIIa receptors.

while abciximab acts by binding to glycoprotein IIb/IIIa receptors.

Aspirin

Aspirin is a nonsteroidal anti-inflammatory drug (NSAID) that has analgesic, antipyretic, and anti-inflammatory effects. It also inhibits platelet aggregation and is used in the prevention and treatment of arterial thromboembolic disorders.

Mechanisms and Pharmacologic Effects. Aspirin and most other NSAIDs inhibit the synthesis of prostaglandins from arachidonic acid, as described in greater detail in Chapter 30. The most important prostaglandins affecting platelet aggregation are prostacyclin (also called prostaglandin I_2, or PGI$_2$) and TXA$_2$. Prostacyclin is synthesized by vascular endothelial cells and inhibits platelet aggregation, whereas TXA$_2$ is synthesized by platelets and promotes platelet aggregation. Under normal conditions, prostacyclin serves to prevent platelet aggregation and thrombosis, whereas TXA$_2$ becomes predominant during thrombus formation.

Low doses of aspirin have been found to selectively inhibit the synthesis of TXA$_2$ without having much effect on prostacyclin, whereas higher doses inhibit the synthesis of both compounds. Hence, the dosage of aspirin used to inhibit platelet aggregation is sometimes lower than that used to produce other pharmacologic effects. Unlike other NSAIDs, aspirin irreversibly inhibits cyclooxygenase, the enzyme that catalyzes an early step in TXA$_2$ synthesis. For this reason, aspirin inhibits platelet aggregation for the life of the platelet and effectively reduces platelet aggregation when administered once a day or every other day.

Indications. Aspirin is primarily used to prevent arterial thrombosis in patients with **ischemic heart disease and stroke,** but it has many other indications as well. In patients with **unstable angina,** it is used to prevent myocardial infarction. In patients

with recent **myocardial infarction,** it is used to prevent enlargement of a coronary thrombus and potentially reduce the severity of cardiac damage. In patients with **transient ischemic attacks,** it can be used to prevent an initial or subsequent stroke. In patients who have **artificial heart valves** or are undergoing **percutaneous transluminal coronary angioplasty,** it is used to prevent thrombosis.

Adverse Effects and Interactions. Aspirin may cause bleeding, especially in the gastrointestinal tract, where it inhibits the synthesis of prostaglandins that promote secretion of bicarbonate and mucus. These substances protect the gastric mucosa from the potentially damaging effects of stomach acid and pepsin. High doses of aspirin and other salicylates have a direct hypoprothrombinemic effect that may increase the anticoagulant effect and thereby increase the likelihood of bleeding. Other adverse effects of aspirin are discussed in Chapter 30, and interactions are listed in Table 16–3.

Ticlopidine

Ticlopidine is a newer oral antiplatelet drug that is not an NSAID. Its structure is shown in Fig. 16–3D. Ticlopidine works by inhibiting ADP-induced expression of platelet glycoprotein receptors and thereby reducing fibrinogen binding and platelet aggregation. Like aspirin, it prolongs the bleeding time and irreversibly inhibits platelet function for the life of the platelet.

Ticlopidine is rapidly absorbed from the gut, is extensively metabolized before it is excreted in the urine and feces, and has a steady-state half-life of about 4.5 days. Because it can cause mild to severe neutropenia, patients who are treated with ticlopidine must have a complete blood count (CBC) with white cell differential every 2 weeks from the second week to the third month of treatment. After 3 months, a CBC is only required when patients exhibit signs or symptoms of an infection.

In patients who are intolerant of or unresponsive to aspirin, ticlopidine has been used to prevent **thrombotic stroke.** It is currently being studied as an antithrombotic drug for patients with intermittent claudication of blood vessels, chronic arterial occlusion, atrioventricular shunts or fistulas, open heart surgery, and sickle cell anemia.

Abciximab

Abciximab is a parenterally administered antiplatelet drug that consists of the Fab fragment of a chimeric human-murine monoclonal antibody called 7E3. The drug binds to platelet glycoprotein IIb/IIIa receptors and prevents binding by fibrinogen and other adhesive molecules.

Abciximab is used solely for the prevention of platelet aggregation and thrombosis in patients undergoing **percutaneous transluminal coronary angioplasty.** In this setting, it is administered in combination with aspirin and heparin.

The most common adverse effect of abciximab is bleeding. Other adverse reactions include thrombocytopenia, hypotension, and bradycardia.

Dipyridamole

Dipyridamole is a coronary vasodilator and a relatively weak antiplatelet drug.

As a vasodilator, dipyridamole is used during **myocardial perfusion imaging (thallium imaging)** to dilate and evaluate the arteries of patients with coronary artery disease.

As an antiplatelet drug, dipyridamole acts primarily by inhibiting platelet adhesion to the vessel wall when it is given in normal clinical doses. It also inhibits platelet aggregation by increasing the formation of cyclic adenosine monophosphate (cAMP) and lowering the level of platelet calcium when it is given in supraclinical doses. At the present time, dipyridamole is seldom used as an antiplatelet drug, except in combination with either aspirin or warfarin for the prevention of thrombi in patients with **artificial heart valves.** In clinical trials involving patients with thromboembolic disorders, investigators found no convincing evidence that taking a combination of dipyridamole and aspirin was more beneficial than taking aspirin alone. The efficacy of using dipyridamole alone has not been adequately studied in patients with thromboembolic disorders.

FIBRINOLYTIC DRUGS

The fibrinolytic drugs, or **thrombolytic drugs,** include **alteplase** and **reteplase,** which are recombinant forms of human tissue plasminogen activator (t-PA); **urokinase,** an enzyme obtained from human urine; **streptokinase,** a protein obtained from streptococci; and **anistreplase,** a preformed complex of streptokinase and plasminogen. Unlike the anticoagulant and antiplatelet drugs, these drugs can be used to dissolve an existing thrombus. They are primarily used to dissolve clots in patients undergoing **myocardial infarction, thrombotic stroke,** or **pulmonary embolism.** Moreover, recent studies suggest that their use in patients with acute ischemic (thrombotic) stroke may reduce the incidence of the neurologic sequelae of stroke.

Chemistry and Mechanisms. The fibrinolytic drugs are enzymes or large proteins that convert plasminogen to plasmin. Plasmin degrades fibrin and fibrinogen and thereby causes clot dissolution (Fig. 16–6). Urokinase and the recombinant forms of t-PA (alteplase and reteplase) directly convert plasminogen to plasmin. Streptokinase is not an enzyme, so it must combine with plasminogen to form an activator complex that converts inactive plasminogen to plasmin. In anistreplase, streptokinase and plasminogen are already formed into a complex (the anisoylated plasminogen streptokinase activator complex, or APSAC).

Pharmacokinetic and Pharmacologic Effects. The fibrinolytic drugs are administered parenterally to dissolve clots. In anistreplase, the anisoyl groups are bound to the catalytic site on plasminogen and serve to stabilize the complex until it is administered.

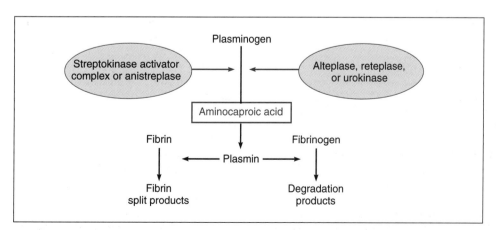

FIGURE 16–6. Fibrinolysis and sites of drug action. Alteplase, reteplase, or urokinase catalyzes the conversion of plasminogen to plasmin. Streptokinase combines with plasminogen to form an active catalyst (activator complex) that converts inactive plasminogen to plasmin. In anistreplase, streptokinase and plasminogen are already formed into a complex. Plasmin is a protease that breaks down fibrinogen and fibrin to degradation (split) products. Aminocaproic acid inhibits the conversion of plasminogen to plasmin.

Once injected, it is deacylated at a controlled rate. For this reason, anistreplase can be given as a single intravenous injection, and it might be preferred for prehospitalization fibrinolysis.

Adverse Effects and Interactions. Table 16–3 lists adverse effects and drug interactions. The most common adverse effect is hemorrhage. Fibrinolytic drugs create a general lytic state that may lyse both normal and pathologic thrombi. However, because t-PA selectively activates plasminogen that is bound to fibrin, the recombinant forms of t-PA may cause fewer cases of hemorrhage than streptokinase causes. Arrhythmias such as bradycardia and tachycardia have been reported in patients treated with fibrinolytic drugs and are believed to be caused by free radicals that are generated during the reperfusion of the coronary artery after fibrinolysis. The administration of streptokinase can cause various types of hypersensitivity reactions, including fatal anaphylactic shock. For this reason, it should not be used repeatedly in the same patient.

Treatment of Bleeding. By competitively blocking plasminogen activation (see Fig. 16–6), **aminocaproic acid** inhibits fibrinolysis. This drug is used to stop the bleeding caused by fibrinolytic drugs. It is also used to prevent bleeding in patients who have hemophilia, patients who are recovering from gastrointestinal or prostate surgery, and patients who have cancer and are undergoing radiation therapy or chemotherapy. Aminocaproic acid can be administered orally or intravenously and is excreted by the kidneys. Its adverse effects include thrombosis, hypotension, and arrhythmias.

Summary of Important Points

- When a small blood vessel is injured, hemorrhage is prevented by the processes involved in normal hemostasis: vasospasm, platelet plug formation, and fibrin clot formation. After the vessel is repaired, the clot is removed via the process of fibrinolysis.
- Oral anticoagulants, such as warfarin, inhibit vitamin K–dependent synthesis of clotting factors II, VII, IX, and X.

- Parenteral anticoagulants, such as heparin, inactivate clotting factors. Unfractionated heparin primarily inactivates thrombin by activating antithrombin III, while fractionated heparin primarily inactivates factor Xa.
- Oral antiplatelet drugs act by interfering with the synthesis or activity of mediators of platelet aggregation. Aspirin inhibits thromboxane A_2 synthesis, and ticlopidine inhibits adenosine diphosphate activity. Abciximab, a parenteral antiplatelet drug, prevents the binding of fibrinogen to glycoprotein receptors.
- Fibrinolytic drugs directly or indirectly convert plasminogen to plasmin and thereby stimulate fibrin degradation. These drugs are used to lyse clots in patients undergoing myocardial infarction, thrombotic stroke, or pulmonary embolism.
- Any of the anticoagulant, antiplatelet, or fibrinolytic drugs may cause bleeding. Phytonadione (vitamin K_1) is used to counteract bleeding caused by oral anticoagulants. Protamine sulfate is used to neutralize heparin, and aminocaproic acid is used to inhibit fibrinolysis.

Selected Readings

CARS Investigators. Randomised double-blind trial of fixed low-dose warfarin with aspirin after myocardial infarction. Lancet 350:389–396, 1997.

Chinese Acute Stroke Trial Cooperative Group (CAST). Randomised placebo-controlled trial of early aspirin use in 20,000 patients with acute ischaemic stroke. Lancet 349:1641–1649, 1997.

Fuster, V., et al. Aspirin as a therapeutic agent in cardiovascular disease. Circulation 87:659–675, 1993.

Hennekens, C. H. Aspirin in the treatment and prevention of cardiovascular disease. Annu Rev Public Health 18:37–49, 1997.

Lindley, R. I. Drug therapy for acute ischemic stroke: risks versus benefits. Drug Saf 19:373–382, 1998.

Maggioni, A. P., et al. Treatment of acute myocardial infarction today. Am Heart J 134:S9–S14, 1997.

Meijer, A., et al. Aspirin versus Coumadin in the prevention of reocclusion and recurrent ischemia after successful thrombolysis: results of the APRICOT study. Circulation 87:1524–1530, 1993.

O'Connor, R. E., et al. Thrombolytic therapy for acute ischemic stroke: why the majority of patients remain ineligible for treatment. Ann Emerg Med 33:9–14, 1999.

CHAPTER SEVENTEEN

HEMATOPOIETIC DRUGS

CLASSIFICATION OF HEMATOPOIETIC DRUGS

Minerals
- Ferrous sulfate and related compounds
- Iron dextran

Vitamins
- Folic acid
- Vitamin B_{12}

Hematopoietic growth factors
- Epoetin alfa
- Filgrastim
- Sargramostim

OVERVIEW

Mature blood cells are continuously formed in the bone marrow and are removed from the circulation by reticuloendothelial cells in the liver and spleen. The process by which blood cells are replaced is called **hematopoiesis.** This process requires **minerals** and **vitamins** and is regulated by **hematopoietic growth factors** that promote the differentiation and maturation of marrow progenitor cells to form leukocytes, erythrocytes, and platelets.

Anemia is defined as a subnormal concentration of erythrocytes or hemoglobin in the blood and may be due to inadequate erythropoiesis, blood loss, or accelerated hemolysis. Erythropoiesis can be impaired by the lack of essential nutrients or by the myelosuppressive effects of certain drugs or irradiation. Infection, cancer, endocrine deficiencies, and chronic inflammation can also cause anemia. **Iron, folic acid, and vitamin B_{12} deficiencies** are the most common causes of **nutritional anemia.**

This chapter describes the pharmacologic properties and uses of minerals, vitamins, and hematopoietic growth factors in the treatment of anemia and other blood cell deficiencies.

DRUGS
Minerals

Iron is an essential dietary mineral and serves as an important component of hemoglobin, myoglobin, and a number of enzymes. The average dietary intake of iron is 18–20 mg a day, but people with normal iron stores absorb only about 10% of this amount. Absorption is enhanced twofold or threefold when stored iron is depleted or when erythropoiesis occurs at an accelerated rate. The absorption of iron is regulated by the amount of iron that is stored in the intestinal mucosa.

Iron is absorbed from the intestines into the circulation, where it is bound to **transferrin** and transported to various tissues, including the bone marrow and liver. In these tissues, iron is stored as **ferritin** (Fig. 17–1). In the marrow, iron is incorporated into heme and packaged in new erythrocytes. The erythrocytes circulate in the blood for about 120 days and then are taken up and degraded by reticuloendothelial cells. These cells later return most of the iron to the plasma so that it can be utilized again in erythropoiesis. Iron is highly conserved by the body, and only small amounts of it are excreted via the intestinal tract.

The dietary iron requirement per kilogram of body weight is highest in infants and pregnant women, somewhat lower in children and nonpregnant women, and lowest in men. Pregnant women have the greatest need for routine **iron supplementation** because their dietary iron is often not able to meet the requirements for maternal and fetal erythropoiesis. Most multivitamin supplements contain iron, and many processed foods, including bread, are supplemented with iron.

If dietary iron intake is inadequate to support sufficient erythropoiesis and maintain a normal hemoglobin concentration in the blood, the body will utilize stored iron to maintain erythropoiesis until the stores are depleted. When iron stores are significantly depleted, the plasma iron level begins to fall and erythropoiesis is reduced. Over time, these changes lead to **hypochromic microcytic anemia,** a form of anemia in which the mean corpuscular hemoglobin concentration (MCHC) and the mean corpuscular volume (MCV) are decreased. The iron preparations described below are used to prevent and treat **iron deficiency anemia** in affected individuals.

Ferrous Sulfate and Related Compounds

Iron is administered orally in the form of **ferrous salts,** including **ferrous sulfate, ferrous gluconate,** and **ferrous fumarate.** Iron contained in these preparations is absorbed in the same manner as dietary iron. In patients with iron deficiency, the amount of iron absorbed increases progressively with larger

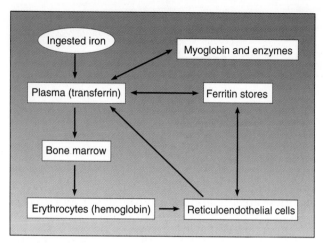

FIGURE 17–1. Iron metabolism. Ingested iron is absorbed from the intestinal mucosa into the circulation, where it is bound to transferrin. Iron is distributed to tissues for incorporation into hemoglobin, myoglobin, and enzymes, or it is stored as ferritin. After about 120 days, erythrocytes are degraded by reticuloendothelial cells, and the iron is returned to the plasma or stored.

doses, but the percentage absorbed decreases as the dosage increases. Food can retard iron absorption by 40–60%, but the gastric distress caused by iron often necessitates administering iron preparations with food. The percentage of iron absorbed from sustained-release preparations is lower than that absorbed from immediate-release preparations. This is because iron is primarily absorbed from the duodenum, and some of the sustained-release iron is transported to the lower intestinal tract before it is released for absorption.

In iron deficiency states, oral iron preparations are usually administered three times a day in doses that provide a total of 100–200 mg of elemental iron daily. The various iron salts contain different percentages of elemental iron. Ferrous sulfate contains about 20%, so that a 300-mg tablet contains approximately 60 mg of elemental iron. The duration of iron therapy depends on the cause and severity of the iron deficiency. In general, about 4–6 months of oral iron therapy is required to reverse uncomplicated iron deficiency anemia.

At therapeutic doses, iron salts have few adverse effects, but they sometimes cause epigastric pain, nausea, vomiting, diarrhea or constipation, and black stools. Liquid iron preparations can also stain the teeth. Bile acid–binding resins, such as cholestyramine, reduce the absorption of iron, whereas ascorbic acid increases iron absorption by maintaining iron in the reduced ferrous state. Ferrous iron is better absorbed than is ferric iron. Iron may reduce the absorption of tetracyclines, fluoroquinolones, levothyroxine, and vitamin E. The administration of these drugs should be separated from iron administration by at least 2 hours. The ingestion of large quantities of iron can cause serious and potentially lethal toxicity. Hence, iron preparations should be kept out of the reach of children.

Iron Dextran

Iron dextran is a mixture of ferric hydroxide and dextran. It is intended for intramuscular or intravenous treatment of iron deficiency anemia in patients who cannot tolerate oral iron preparations or fail to respond to oral iron therapy. The dosage of iron dextran required for each patient is calculated on the basis of the observed hemoglobin concentration and body weight. Dosage tables can be found in drug compendiums.

Following administration, the iron dextran complex is removed from the circulation by the reticuloendothelial system, and the iron is transferred to the plasma for distribution to the bone marrow and other tissues.

Because treatment with iron dextran has been associated with fatal anaphylactic reactions, it should be limited to the indications described above. Intramuscular administration of iron dextran may cause several adverse reactions at the injection site, including pain, inflammation, sterile abscesses, and brown discoloration of skin. For this reason, the iron preparation must be given by deep intramuscular injection into the outer quadrant of the buttock. A Z-track technique, in which the skin is displaced laterally prior to injection, is used to avoid leakage into the subcutaneous tissue. Intravenous administration may cause peripheral flushing and hypotensive reactions.

Vitamins

While many vitamins participate in the formation and function of erythrocytes, **folic acid** and **vitamin B$_{12}$** have a critical role in erythropoiesis, and a deficiency of either of them may cause **megaloblastic anemia.** The two vitamins serve as cofactors in biochemical reactions involving the addition of single-carbon units to various substrates, and the administration of one of the vitamins can partially compensate for a deficiency of the other. Therefore, it is critical that the specific vitamin deficiency be correctly identified before therapy is started.

Folic Acid

The structure of folic acid is shown in Fig. 17–2A. Active forms of this vitamin serve as enzyme cofactors that donate single-carbon atoms in the biosynthesis of amino acids and the purine and pyrimidine bases contained in DNA (Fig. 17–3A). Hence, folic acid plays a critical role in cell proliferation and erythropoiesis.

The requirement for folic acid increases markedly during pregnancy, and inadequate dietary intake of this vitamin is often responsible for **megaloblastic anemia in pregnant women.** Folic acid supplementation is especially important during pregnancy because it prevents anemia and reduces the incidence of neural tube birth defects such as spina bifida.

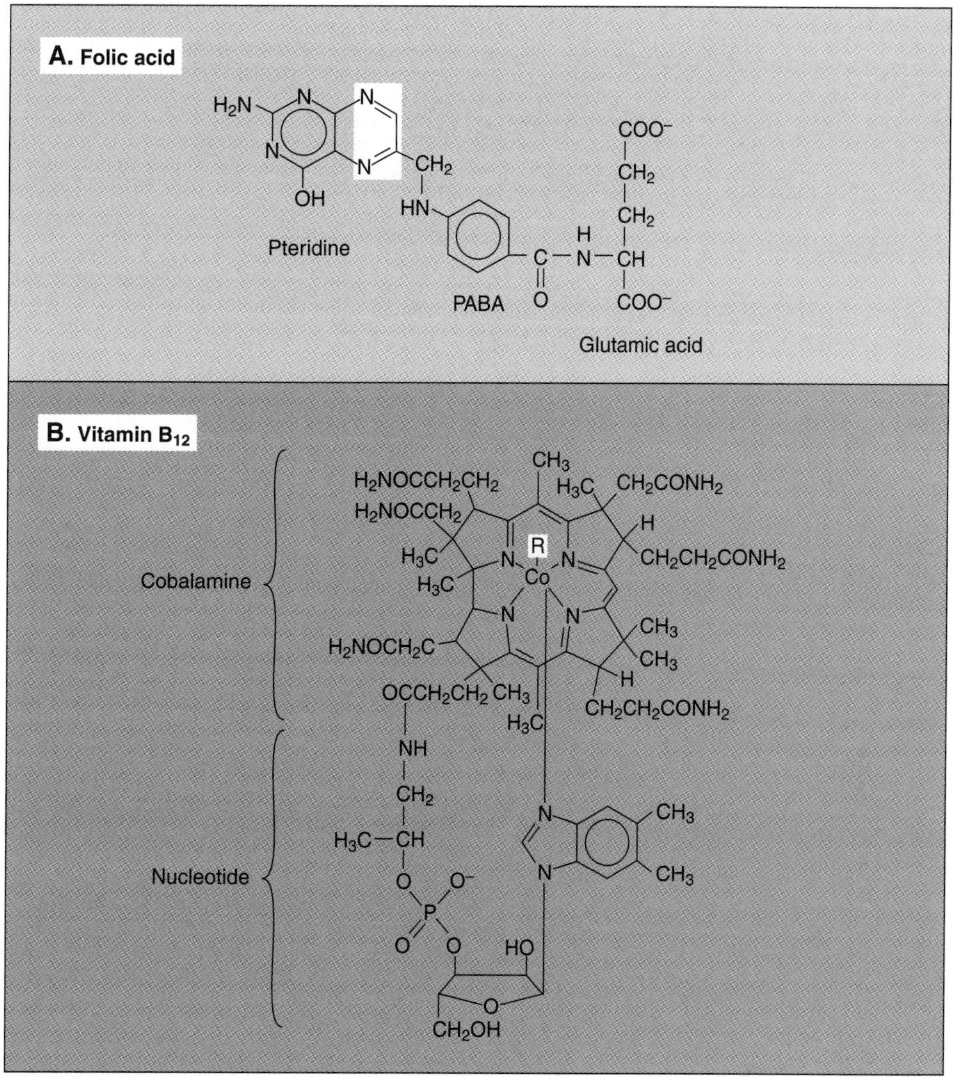

FIGURE 17–2. Structures of folic acid and vitamin B$_{12}$. **(A)** Folic acid consists of pteridine, *p*-aminobenzoic acid (PABA), and glutamic acid. The unshaded area shows the bonds that are reduced by folate reductase to form tetrahydrofolic acid. **(B)** Vitamin B$_{12}$ consists of a porphyrinlike ring with a central cobalt atom attached to a nucleotide. R = CN$^-$ (cyanocobalamin) or OH$^-$ (hydroxocobalamin).

Folic acid is well absorbed from the jejunum, and oral supplementation is effective both in preventing and treating megaloblastic anemia associated with **folic acid deficiency.** This disorder often results from insufficient folic acid intake in the diet, but it can also result from impaired folic acid absorption, such as that seen in patients with alcoholism and certain malabsorption syndromes. In patients with megaloblastic anemia, vitamin B$_{12}$ deficiency must be ruled out before treatment with folic acid is begun. This is because treatment with folic acid may partly correct the anemia caused by a vitamin B$_{12}$ deficiency but will not correct other problems associated with it. Irreversible neurologic damage may occur if a B$_{12}$ deficiency is incorrectly treated with folic acid.

Vitamin B$_{12}$

Vitamin B$_{12}$ consists of a porphyrinlike ring with a central cobalt atom attached to a nucleotide (see Fig. 17–2B). Exogenous vitamin B$_{12}$ is available as **cyanocobalamin** and **hydroxocobalamin.** In

the body, these forms of the vitamin are converted to methylcobalamin or deoxyadenosylcobalamin, which are cofactors for biochemical reactions. Vitamin B$_{12}$ serves as a cofactor for methylation reactions, including the conversion of homocysteine to methionine and the conversion of methylmalonyl CoA to succinyl CoA (see Fig. 17–3B).

Vitamin B$_{12}$ is essential for growth, cell replication, hematopoiesis, and myelin synthesis. It is obtained from dietary meats, dairy products, and eggs, and it is absorbed from the gut in the presence of **intrinsic factor** (a glycoprotein secreted by gastric parietal cells) and calcium. An inadequate secretion of intrinsic factor leads to **vitamin B$_{12}$ deficiency** and eventually results in **pernicious anemia.** Vitamin B$_{12}$ deficiency is also seen in patients who have malabsorption disorders, in individuals who have undergone gastrectomy, and in strict vegetarians who have a low dietary intake of the vitamin.

Since vitamin B$_{12}$ is not absorbed from the gut in the absence of intrinsic factor, the vitamin must be administered intramuscularly in the treatment of

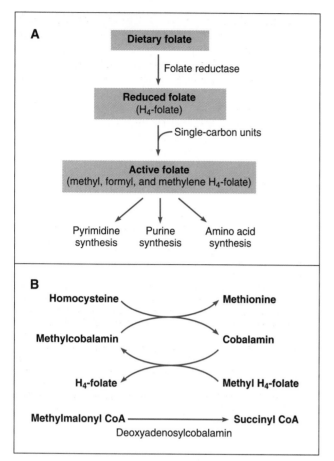

FIGURE 17–3. Biochemical reactions involving folic acid and vitamin B_{12}. **(A)** Dietary folate is reduced by folate reductase to tetrahydrofolate (H_4-folate). Single-carbon units are added to H_4-folate to form active folate, which donates single-carbon units in the synthesis of pyrimidine and purine bases and amino acids. **(B)** The two active forms of vitamin B_{12} are methylcobalamin and deoxyadenosylcobalamin. These forms are cofactors for methylation reactions, including the conversion of homocysteine to methionine and the conversion of methylmalonyl CoA to succinyl CoA. Methyl H_4-folate donates a methyl group to cobalamin to form methylcobalamin.

pernicious anemia, and treatment must be continued for life. At the start of therapy, injections are given daily for 5–10 days. Thereafter, maintenance doses are given once a month.

In patients with a dietary deficiency of vitamin B_{12}, treatment is given orally.

Hematopoietic Growth Factors

Colony-stimulating factors (CSF), **erythropoietin,** and other hematopoietic growth factors are endogenous glycoproteins that stimulate the differentiation and maturation of bone marrow progenitor cells. The growth factors bind to receptors on specific myeloid progenitor cells and thereby induce their differentiation and proliferation.

Some growth factors, including the three discussed below, have been manufactured by recombinant DNA technology, and these are administered parenterally to treat hematopoietic deficiencies.

Other growth factors, including several **interleukins,** are currently undergoing clinical trials or are in preclinical development.

Epoetin Alfa

Endogenous **erythropoietin** stimulates erythroid cell differentiation and proliferation and is secreted primarily by the kidney. Epoetin alfa, a form of erythropoietin produced by recombinant DNA technology, is used to treat anemia that is due to inadequate erythropoiesis. The most common indication for epoetin is **anemia due to chronic renal impairment or failure.** Other indications include **chemotherapy-induced anemia** in patients with cancer and **zidovudine-induced anemia** in individuals with human immunodeficiency virus (HIV) infection.

Epoetin is administered subcutaneously or intravenously three times a week. The dosage and duration of therapy are determined by the hematocrit response to epoetin treatment. The drug is usually well tolerated, and most of the adverse reactions that occur during therapy are attributable to the underlying disease state. However, the utilization of iron stores is increased in patients treated with epoetin. Therefore, patients should be given iron supplements to maintain transferrin saturation levels that will support epoetin-stimulated erythropoiesis.

Filgrastim and Sargramostim

Filgrastim is recombinant human **granulocyte CSF** (G-CSF), and sargramostim is recombinant human **granulocyte-macrophage CSF** (GM-CSF). The endogenous forms of these growth factors are produced by various leukocytes, fibroblasts, and endothelial cells. Because filgrastim is produced in *Escherichia coli* by recombinant DNA technology, it is not glycosylated and differs in this manner from G-CSF isolated from human cells.

Filgrastim and sargramostim are primarily used to treat **neutropenia associated with cancer chemotherapy and bone marrow transplantation.**

Filgrastim accelerates granulocyte recovery after myelosuppressive chemotherapy and thereby reduces the incidence of infections and shortens the period of hospitalization. Filgrastim is also used to mobilize hematopoietic progenitor cells into the peripheral blood when blood is being collected for leukapheresis. Studies indicate that filgrastim may be beneficial in the treatment of aplastic anemia, hairy cell leukemia, myelodysplasia, drug-induced and congenital agranulocytosis, and other forms of congenital or acquired neutropenia.

Sargramostim is used to accelerate myeloid cell recovery in patients who have lymphoma, acute lymphoblastic leukemia, or Hodgkin's disease and are undergoing autologous bone marrow transplantation or chemotherapy. It has also been used to reduce the incidence of fever and infections in patients with severe chronic neutropenia. Although endogenous

GM-CSF stimulates the production of several types of cells, sargramostim has little effect on erythrocytes or platelets in deficiency states and primarily serves to accelerate the development of neutrophils.

Filgrastim and sargramostim are usually administered subcutaneously or intravenously once a day for 2 weeks or until the absolute neutrophil count has reached 10,000/µL.

Summary of Important Points

- Iron deficiency causes hypochromic microcytic anemia, whereas folic acid or vitamin B_{12} deficiency causes megaloblastic anemia.
- Ferrous sulfate and other ferrous salts are administered orally for several months in the treatment of iron deficiency anemia.
- Folic acid supplementation is used during pregnancy to prevent anemia and birth defects.
- Folic acid treatment can partly mask the hematologic effect of vitamin B_{12} deficiency but does not prevent irreversible neurologic damage.
- Pernicious anemia is due to inadequate secretion of intrinsic factor and reduced vitamin B_{12} absorption. It is treated with intramuscular injections of cyanocobalamin or hydroxocobalamin.

- Epoetin alfa is recombinant human erythropoietin and is primarily used to treat anemia due to chronic renal failure.
- Filgrastim and sargramostim are recombinant forms of granulocyte colony-stimulating factor (G-CSF) and granulocyte-macrophage colony-stimulating factor (GM-CSF), respectively. They are used to treat neutropenia associated with cancer chemotherapy, bone marrow transplantation, and various disease states.

Selected Readings

Butterworth, C. E., and A. Bendich. Folic acid and the prevention of birth defects. Annu Rev Nutr 16:73–97, 1996.

McQuaker, I. G., et al. Low-dose filgrastim significantly enhances neutrophil recovery following autologous peripheral-blood stem-cell transplantation in patients with lymphoproliferative disorders: evidence for clinical and economic benefit. J Clin Oncol 15:451–457, 1997.

Messori, A., et al. G-CSF for the prophylaxis of neutropenic fever in patients with small cell lung cancer receiving myelosuppressive antineoplastic chemotherapy: meta-analysis and pharmacoeconomic evaluation. J Clin Pharm Ther 21:57–63, 1996.

Moore, J. O., et al. Granulocyte colony-stimulating factor (filgrastim) accelerates granulocyte recovery after intensive postremission chemotherapy for acute myeloid leukemia with aziridinyl benzoquinone and mitoxantrone. Blood 89:780–788, 1997.

Morstyn, G., et al. Clinical benefits of improving host defenses with rHuG-CSF. Ciba Found Symp 204:78–85, 1997.

SECTION IV

CENTRAL NERVOUS SYSTEM

PHARMACOLOGY

CHAPTER EIGHTEEN

INTRODUCTION TO CENTRAL NERVOUS

SYSTEM PHARMACOLOGY

OVERVIEW

The central nervous system (CNS) consists of the brain and spinal cord. When the brain receives sensory input, it processes and integrates the input by utilizing stored data (memory) and established patterns of information processing and then it generates cognitive, emotional, and motor responses. **Brain disorders** may result from structural or functional disturbances of these **sensory, integrative, or motor activities** of the CNS and are seen in association with a variety of disease processes, including degenerative, ischemic, and psychologic disturbances.

Drugs are used to relieve the symptoms of brain dysfunction, but they usually do not correct the underlying disorder. Although short-term drug treatment may be effective in relieving acute symptoms such as pain and insomnia, drug therapy for many brain disorders is a lifelong process.

After reviewing pertinent concepts of CNS function and neurotransmission, this chapter explains the general mechanisms by which drugs alter CNS activities and processes.

NEUROTRANSMISSION IN THE CENTRAL NERVOUS SYSTEM

Principles of Chemical Neurotransmission

Throughout the nervous system, chemical **neurotransmitters** serve as messengers that enable neurons to communicate with one another. Two basic **models of neuron communication** in the CNS have been postulated. According to the **"hard-wired" model,** neurotransmitters provide point-to-point communication between neurons in the same manner that wires are connected in an electronic device, with the result that one neurotransmitter communicates with only one neuron. According to the **"chemical soup" model,** neurotransmitters function more like hormones that diffuse from the original synapse and activate receptors on many neurons in their vicinity. In reality, both models are partly correct. Some neuronal systems behave as though they were hard-wired, while others are modulated by a chemical soup or milieu containing several neurotransmitters

and neuromodulators that are released from adjacent and more distal neurons. A **neuromodulator** is a substance that exerts a generalized and long-lasting effect on neurotransmission in a particular region of the brain.

The action of drugs on the CNS is similar to the chemical soup model of neurotransmission, because drug molecules are widely distributed throughout the brain and may simultaneously interact with receptors on neurons in several neuronal tracts. This lack of specificity may lead to therapeutic effects and adverse effects at the same time. For this reason, the development of agents that are more selective for specific receptor subtypes is a useful approach to improving the therapeutic index of CNS drugs.

Neurotransmitter Metabolism

Neurotransmitters are synthesized in neuronal cell bodies or terminals, and they are stored in neuronal vesicles until they are released into a synapse (Fig. 18–1). The release of neurotransmitters is activated by membrane depolarization and calcium influx into the cell. Calcium evokes the interaction of storage vesicle proteins (synaptobrevin and synaptotagmin) and membrane-docking proteins (syntaxin and neurexin) and leads to vesicle docking and exocytosis of the neurotransmitter.

Following exocytosis, the neurotransmitter may activate presynaptic and postsynaptic receptors. A neurotransmitter's action is then terminated either by its reuptake into the presynaptic neuron or by its degradation to inactive compounds, with degradation catalyzed by enzymes located in presynaptic and postsynaptic neuronal membranes or cytoplasm.

Neurotransmitters may also diffuse from the synapse of their origin to affect neurons in the surrounding vicinity. In this way, different neurotransmitters released from different types of neurons form a chemical soup or milieu, as described above. The net influence of the chemical soup on neurotransmission depends on the concentrations of the excitatory and inhibitory neurotransmitters acting at a particular synapse.

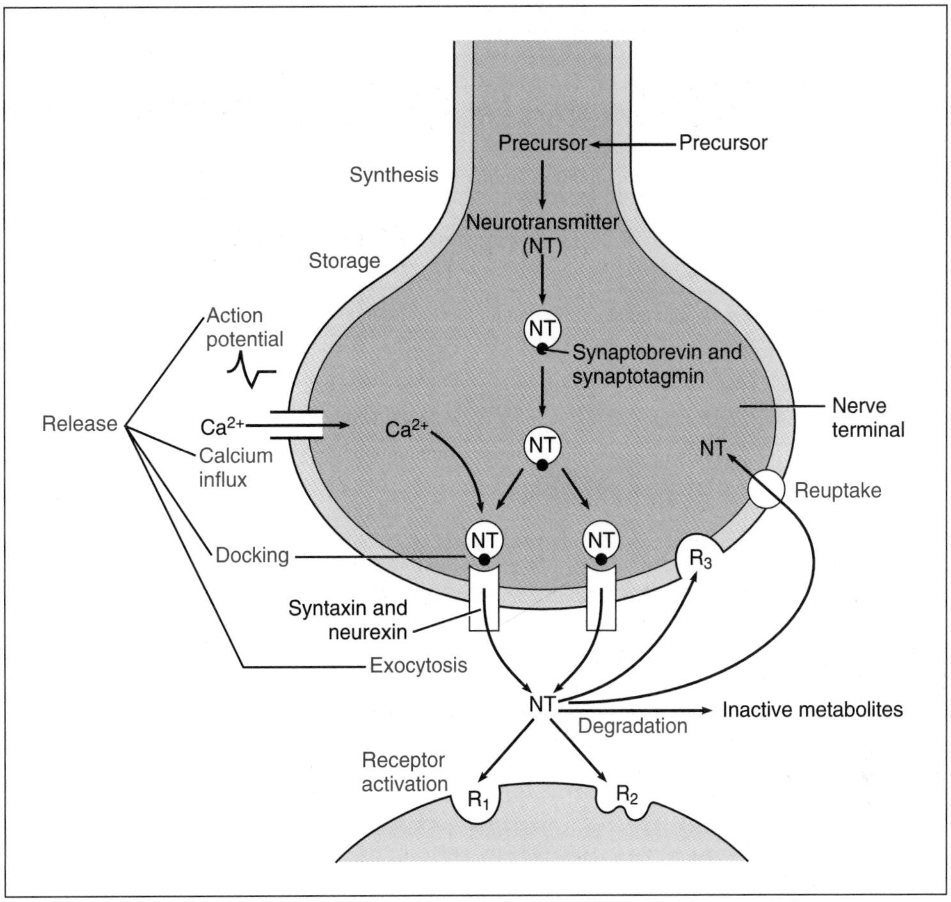

FIGURE 18–1. Central nervous system (CNS) neurotransmission and sites of drug action. CNS drugs act primarily by affecting the synthesis, storage, release, reuptake, or degradation of neurotransmitters (NT) or by activating receptors. NT are synthesized from precursors accumulated or synthesized in the neurons. The NT are stored in vesicles whose membranes contain proteins involved in NT release (synaptobrevin and synaptotagmin). The NT are released when an action potential–mediated calcium influx initiates interaction of synaptobrevin and synaptotagmin with neuronal membrane-docking proteins (syntaxin and neurexin). This leads to docking and exocytosis. Synaptic NT may activate presynaptic or postsynaptic receptors (R_1, R_2, and R_3). The action of NT is terminated by reuptake into the presynaptic neuron or by enzymatic degradation.

Excitatory and Inhibitory Neurotransmission

CNS neurotransmitters may evoke either an excitatory or an inhibitory synaptic membrane potential and trigger effects at presynaptic and postsynaptic sites on target neurons. If an **excitatory postsynaptic membrane potential** reaches threshold, it is conducted along the axonal membrane and may evoke the release of a neurotransmitter from the nerve terminal. An **inhibitory postsynaptic membrane potential** usually hyperpolarizes the cell membrane and inhibits action potential formation. Depending on whether a **presynaptic membrane potential** is excitatory or inhibitory, it will increase or decrease the release of a neurotransmitter from the neuron. Presynaptic receptors may also be coupled with cyclic adenosine monophosphate (cyclic AMP, or cAMP) and other second messengers that modulate neurotransmitter release.

As shown in Box 18–1, the interaction of multiple neurotransmitters at a particular site in a neuronal tract enables the complex interplay of various neuronal systems and contributes to the wide range of functional expression exhibited in the CNS. For example, inhibition of the release of an inhibitory neurotransmitter will actually increase neurotransmission in the target neuron. Similarly, drugs can act in complex ways to affect neurotransmission. Ethanol (ethyl alcohol), for instance, can diminish the inhibitory influence of the cerebral cortex on certain human behaviors and thereby facilitate these behaviors. This phenomenon is called **disinhibition** (removal of inhibition).

Fast Versus Slow Signals

Neurotransmitters in the CNS can be characterized as slow or fast, depending on the duration of the membrane potentials that they elicit. The best examples of **fast neurotransmitters** are gamma-aminobutyric acid (GABA) and glutamate, whose signal lasts for several milliseconds. Examples of **slow neurotransmitters** are norepinephrine and serotonin, whose signal may last from many milliseconds to as long as a second. A slow (long-acting) signal can influence the overall tone of a neuron because it may modulate the signals of several other fast neurotransmitters acting on the same neuron. For this reason, slow neurotransmitters are sometimes called **neuromodulators.**

Neurotransmitters and Receptors

Important neurotransmitters in the CNS include acetylcholine and several amino acids, biogenic amines, and peptides. Table 18–1 lists the names, receptors, mechanisms of signal transduction, neu-

---

BOX 18–1. **Patterns of Neurotransmission in the Central Nervous System**

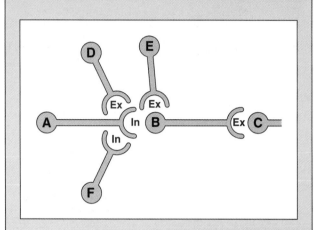

A, B, C, D, E, and F are neurons in a tract that projects from left to right. Neurons B, D, and E release excitatory neurotransmitters (Ex). Neurons A and F release inhibitory neurotransmitters (In). The net effect of neuronal interactions on neurotransmission from B to C is shown in the table below. Each interaction presupposes that the other neurons are quiescent at that time. Other, more complex interactions are possible.

Interaction	Effect on Neurotransmission (B → C)
A → B	Decreased
D → A → B	Greatly decreased
F → A → B	Increased
E → B	Increased

---

ronal tracts, and functions of the major neurotransmitters.

The receptors can be divided into two basic groups: **ionotropic receptors,** which are directly associated with ion channels, and **metabotropic receptors,** which are coupled with enzymes primarily via G proteins but sometimes via other intermediates. Although this terminology is most frequently applied to receptors for excitatory amino acids (aspartate and glutamate), it is equally appropriate for other neurotransmitter receptors.

The **mechanisms of signal transduction** (effector mechanisms) for neurotransmitters in the CNS are similar to those for neurotransmitters in the autonomic nervous system. The activation of ionotropic receptors alters chloride, sodium, potassium, or calcium influx and thereby evokes excitatory or inhibitory membrane potentials. The linkage of metabotropic receptors with some G proteins leads to activation or inhibition of adenylyl cyclase and the synthesis of cAMP, whereas the linkage with other G proteins leads to activation of phospholipase C and the formation of inositol triphosphate (IP_3) and di-

acylglycerol (DAG). The activation of metabotropic receptors may also increase ion channel activity via second messengers that activate kinases responsible for the phosphorylation of ion channels.

Acetylcholine

Acetylcholine is synthesized from acetyl CoA and choline, and it is degraded to acetate and choline by acetylcholinesterase (Fig. 18–2). Acetylcholine receptors are called **cholinergic receptors,** and there are two types: **muscarinic receptors** and **nicotinic receptors.** The properties and mechanisms of these receptors are compared in Table 6–1.

Drugs may affect acetylcholine neurotransmission by activating or blocking cholinergic receptors or by inhibiting cholinesterase. The general pharmacologic properties of cholinergic receptor agonists and antagonists are described in Chapters 6 and 7, respectively.

In the CNS, acetylcholine acts as an excitatory or inhibitory neurotransmitter in a number of neuronal tracts, including those which innervate the hippocampus, cerebral cortex, and basal ganglia. These tracts participate in memory, sensory processing, and motor coordination, respectively.

Amino Acids

Several amino acids are important neurotransmitters in the brain. Some of them, such as GABA and glycine, are inhibitory. Others, such as aspartate and glutamate, are excitatory.

Gamma-Aminobutyric Acid. GABA is synthesized from glutamic acid and is the most ubiquitous inhibitory neurotransmitter in the brain and spinal cord. Its receptors are designated as **$GABA_A$ receptors** and **$GABA_B$ receptors.** Drugs affect GABA neurotransmission primarily by activating or inhibiting the $GABA_A$–chloride ion channel complex. This ion channel complex contains receptors for several types of drugs, including the benzodiazepines (see Chapter 19). The functions of GABA include regulation of neuronal excitability throughout the CNS and motor coordination.

Glutamate and Aspartate. Glutamate and aspartate are acidic amino acids that function as excitatory neurotransmitters throughout the CNS. Their receptors are commonly described as **ionotropic receptors** or **metabotropic receptors,** based on the relative potency of their response to various experimental agonist drugs, one of which is *N*-methyl-D-aspartate (NMDA). The effector mechanisms of these receptors are listed in Table 18–1. Glutamate and aspartate participate in long-term potentiation of memory and have a role in neuronal toxicity and apoptosis evoked by trauma and ischemia. Antagonists of these neurotransmitters may find use in the treatment of stroke and other disorders that are characterized by loss of neuronal function.

TABLE 18–1. Major Neurotransmitters in the Central Nervous System*

Neurotransmitter	Receptors	Mechanisms of Signal Transduction	Neuronal Tracts	Functions
Acetylcholine	Muscarinic M_1, M_3, and M_5 M_2 and M_4 Nicotinic	$\uparrow IP_3$ and DAG. $\downarrow$cAMP; $\uparrow gK^+$. $\uparrow gCa^{2+}$, gK^+, and gNa^+.	Basal ganglia; basal nucleus of Meynert to cerebral cortex; septal area to hippocampus.	Excitatory (M_1, M_3, M_5, and nicotinic) or inhibitory (M_2 and M_4) NT; memory, motor coordination, and sensory processing.
Amino acids Gamma-aminobutyric acid (GABA)	$GABA_A$ $GABA_B$	$\downarrow$cAMP; $\uparrow gCl^-$. $\uparrow gCa^{2+}$ and gK^+.	Ubiquitous.	Major inhibitory NT in CNS; motor coordination and neuronal excitability.
Glutamate and aspartate	Ionotropic AMPA and KA NMDA Metabotropic	$\uparrow gK^+$ and gNa^+. $\uparrow gCa^{2+}$, gK^+, and gNa^+. $\downarrow$cAMP; $\uparrow IP_3$ and DAG.	Widely distributed throughout CNS.	Major excitatory NT in CNS; long-term potentiation (memory), neuronal toxicity and apoptosis, and pain processing.
Glycine	Strychnine-insensitive Strychnine-sensitive	$\uparrow gCl^-$. Modulate NMDA receptors.	Spinal cord; brain stem.	Major inhibitory NT in spinal cord; also found in brain stem; motor coordination and neuronal excitability.
Biogenic amines Dopamine	D_1 and D_5 D_2, D_3, and D_4	$\uparrow$cAMP. $\downarrow$cAMP.	Nigrostriatal, nucleus accumbens, mesolimbic, and tuberoinfundibular; chemoreceptor trigger zone.	Inhibitory NT; behavioral and drug reinforcement, emesis, hormone release, mood, motor coordination, and olfaction.
Histamine	H_1 H_2 H_3	$\uparrow IP_3$ and DAG. $\uparrow$cAMP. Unknown.	Hypothalamic tracts to entire CNS.	Excitatory NT; sedation, sleep, temperature regulation, and vasomotor function.
Norepinephrine	Adrenergic α_1 α_2 β_1 and β_2	$\uparrow IP_3$ and DAG. $\downarrow$cAMP. $\uparrow$cAMP.	Locus ceruleus (pons) to thalamus, cerebral cortex, cerebellum, and spinal cord; midbrain to hypothalamus.	Excitatory (α_1 and β_1) or inhibitory (α_2 and β_2) NT; anxiety, cerebellar function, learning, memory, mood, sensory processing, and sleep.
Serotonin (5-hydroxy-tryptamine, or 5-HT)	$5\text{-}HT_1$ $5\text{-}HT_2$ $5\text{-}HT_3$ $5\text{-}HT_4$	$\downarrow$cAMP; $\uparrow gK^+$. $\uparrow IP_3$ and DAG. $\uparrow gK^+$ and gNa^+. $\uparrow$cAMP.	Raphe nuclei (central brain stem) to forebrain and spinal cord.	Excitatory ($5\text{-}HT_2$, $5\text{-}HT_3$, and $5\text{-}HT_4$) or inhibitory ($5\text{-}HT_1$) NT; appetite, emotional processing, hallucinations, mood, pain processing, and sleep.
Peptides Opioid peptides	δ, κ, and μ	$\downarrow$cAMP and gCa^{2+}; $\uparrow gK^+$.	Widely distributed, especially in brain stem, spinal cord, and thalamus.	Inhibitory NT; emotions, hearing, motor coordination, neurohormone secretion, pain processing, taste, and vision.
Tachykinins Neurokinins Substance P	NK_1, NK_2, and NK_3 NK_1, NK_2, and NK_3	$\downarrow gK^+$; $\uparrow IP_3$ and DAG. $\downarrow gK^+$; $\uparrow IP_3$ and DAG.	Primary sensory neurons; cell bodies at all levels.	Excitatory NT; neuromodulation and pain processing.

*AMPA = α-amino-3-hydroxy-5-methyl-4-isoxazole propionic acid; cAMP = cyclic adenosine monophosphate; CNS = central nervous system; DAG = diacylglycerol, g = conductance; IP_3 = inositol triphosphate; KA = kainate; NK = neurokinin; NMDA = N-methyl-D-aspartate; and NT = neurotransmitter.

Glycine and Taurine. Glycine is an inhibitory transmitter in the spinal cord. Its **strychnine-insensitive receptors** are coupled with the chloride ion channel, and activation of these receptors leads to membrane hyperpolarization. Its **strychnine-sensitive receptors** are associated with the glutamate NMDA receptor and serve to modulate NMDA activity. Strychnine produces convulsive seizures by blocking the glycine site on the NMDA receptor.

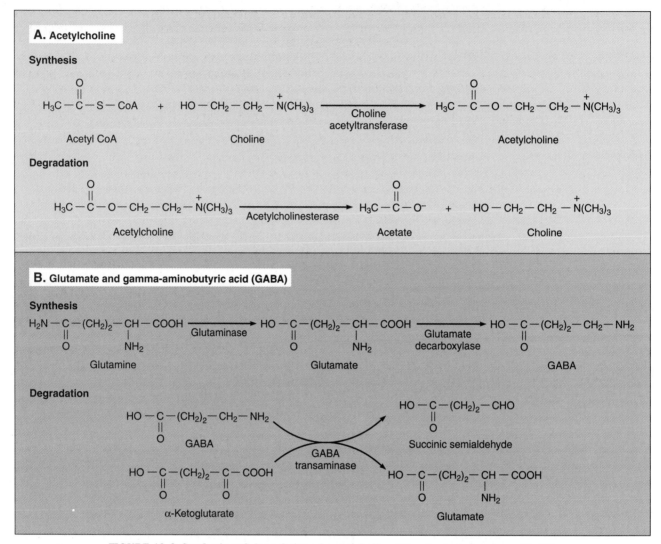

FIGURE 18–2. Synthesis and degradation of acetylcholine (A) and selected amino acids (B).

Taurine is a sulfur-containing amino acid that is postulated to act as a neurotransmitter or neuromodulator in the CNS. Taurine is believed to activate both strychnine-insensitive and strychnine-sensitive types of glycine receptors. Like glycine, taurine may serve to counteract the toxic effects of excessive glutamate on CNS neurons.

Biogenic Amines

Among the biogenic amines that function as CNS neurotransmitters are dopamine, norepinephrine, and serotonin. These neurotransmitters are formed by decarboxylation of amino acids, and they are catabolized in part by monoamine oxidase.

Dopamine. Dopamine is an inhibitory neurotransmitter that binds to five subtypes of **dopamine receptors.** The D_1 and D_5 **receptors** activate adenylyl cyclase and thereby increase cAMP levels. In contrast, the D_2, D_3, and D_4 **receptors** inhibit adenylyl cyclase and decrease cAMP levels. As shown in Table 18–2, amantadine, bromocriptine, clozapine, levodopa, and other drugs have effects on various steps in the synthesis and metabolism of dopamine. Dopamine is found in several neuronal tracts, plays a significant role in behavioral and drug reinforcement, and has an important effect on emesis, hormone (prolactin) release, mood, motor coordination, and olfaction. Its degradation results in the formation of **homovanillic acid** (HVA), a metabolite that is subsequently excreted in the urine (Fig. 18–3).

Norepinephrine. Norepinephrine is formed from dopamine and is degraded by monoamine oxidase and catechol-O-methyltransferase to a number of metabolites. The major metabolite excreted in the urine is **3-methoxy-4-hydroxymandelic acid,** or **vanillylmandelic acid** (VMA). The receptors for norepinephrine are classified as **α-adrenergic receptors** and **β-adrenergic receptors,** and their subtypes and properties are described in detail in Chapter 8. Norepinephrine is associated with several neuronal tracts projecting from the locus ceruleus in the pons to the thalamus, cerebral cortex, cerebellum, and spinal cord, and it is found in tracts projecting from the midbrain to the hypothalamus. This ubiquitous neurotransmitter participates in the regulation of anxiety, cerebellar function, learning, memory, mood, sensory processing (including pain), and sleep. Drugs may alter norepinephrine's neurotransmission by activating or blocking its receptors or by inhibiting its presynaptic neuronal uptake.

Serotonin.   Serotonin, or **5-hydroxytryptamine** (5-HT), is synthesized from tryptophan, is degraded to **5-hydroxyindoleacetic acid** (5-HIAA), and functions as an excitatory or inhibitory neurotransmitter. Serotonin is found in neuronal tracts projecting from the raphe nuclei in the central brain stem to many other parts of the brain. These tracts are involved in emotional processing and pain processing and have an effect on appetite, mood, sleep, and hallucinations. The subtypes and effector mechanisms of **serotonin receptors,** which are called **5-HT receptors,** are outlined in Table 18–1. In most areas of the brain, serotonin has an inhibitory effect mediated by the 5-HT_{1A} receptor. This type of receptor increases potassium conductance and decreases cAMP levels and thereby causes membrane hyperpolarization.

Drugs may affect serotonin function by stimulating or blocking 5-HT receptors or by blocking serotonin reuptake.

Histamine.   Histamine is an excitatory neurotransmitter found in hypothalamic tracts that project to many other parts of the brain. It is involved in sedation, sleep, temperature regulation, and vasomotor function. CNS **histamine receptors** are not currently considered a major site of therapeutic drug action. However, antagonism of these receptors is partly responsible for the drowsiness and sedation caused by some antihistamines.

Peptides

A number of peptides function as slow neurotransmitters and neuromodulators in the CNS. Unlike other neurotransmitters, peptides are synthesized in neuronal cell bodies and are then transported to nerve terminals for release. Once released, they are metabolized by various peptidases, but they do not undergo presynaptic reuptake. Some of the peptides are released as **cotransmitters** with other, nonpeptide neurotransmitters. The cotransmitters usually serve to amplify the effects of these other neurotransmitters.

TABLE 18–2.   Mechanisms of Drug Action in the Central Nervous System

Process	Drug Example	Mechanism	Major Uses
Neurotransmitter synthesis	Levodopa	Converted to dopamine; increases dopamine synthesis.	Parkinsonism.
Neurotransmitter storage	Reserpine	Blocks norepinephrine storage.	Hypertension.
Neurotransmitter release	Amantadine	Increases dopamine release.	Parkinsonism.
	Amphetamine	Increases norepinephrine release.	Attention deficit disorder and narcolepsy.
Neurotransmitter reuptake	Fluoxetine	Blocks serotonin reuptake.	Depression and obsessive-compulsive disorder.
Neurotransmitter degradation	Donepezil	Inhibits cholinesterase and acetylcholine catabolism.	Alzheimer's disease.
	Selegiline	Inhibits monoamine oxidase and dopamine catabolism.	Parkinson's disease.
	Tacrine	Inhibits cholinesterase and acetylcholine catabolism.	Alzheimer's disease.
Receptor activation	Bromocriptine	Activates dopamine receptors.	Parkinsonism.
	Buspirone	Activates serotonin receptors.	Anxiety and depression.
	Diazepam	Activates benzodiazepine receptors.	Anxiety.
	Morphine	Activates opioid receptors.	Analgesia.
Receptor blockade	Benztropine	Blocks cholinergic receptors.	Parkinsonism.
	Clozapine	Blocks dopamine and serotonin receptors.	Schizophrenia.
	Ondansetron	Blocks serotonin receptors.	Nausea and vomiting.
Signal transduction	Lithium	Inhibits second-messenger functions (G proteins and inositol phosphate metabolism).	Bipolar disorder.
Neuronal conduction	Carbamazepine	Blocks sodium channels.	Epilepsy.
	Lidocaine	Blocks sodium channels.	Local anesthesia.
	Phenytoin	Blocks sodium channels.	Epilepsy.
	Procaine	Blocks sodium channels.	Local anesthesia.
Neuronal membrane function	Halothane	Alters physicochemical properties of membranes.	General anesthesia.
	Nitrous oxide	Alters physicochemical properties of membranes.	General anesthesia.

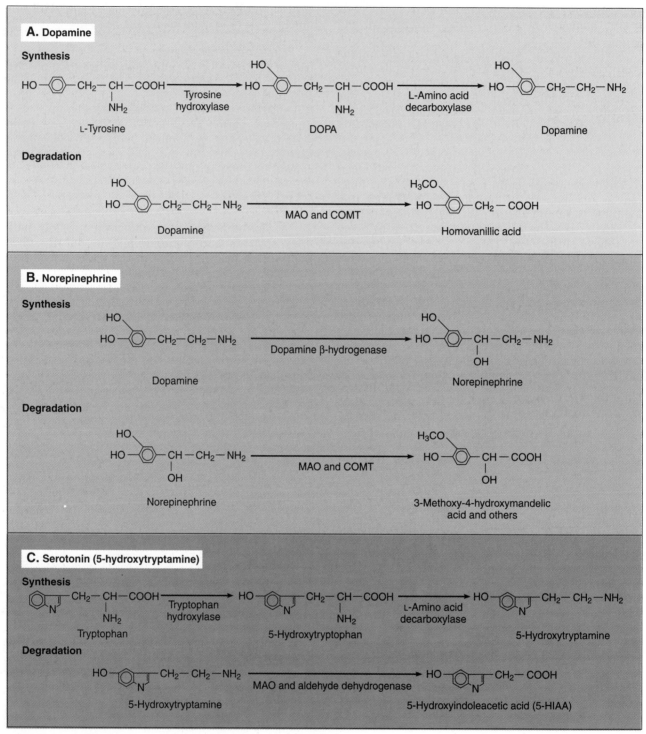

FIGURE 18–3. Synthesis and degradation of dopamine (A), norepinephrine (B), and serotonin (C). DOPA = dihydroxyphenylalanine; MAO = monoamine oxidase; and COMT = catechol-O-methyltransferase.

There are two groups of peptides that are known to function as neurotransmitters in the CNS. The first group consists of **opioid peptides** and includes **enkephalins.** The enkephalins inhibit pain neurotransmission in the spinal cord and midbrain. The second group consists of **tachykinins** and includes **neurokinins A and B** and **substance P.** Neurokinins modulate cardiovascular and behavioral responses to stress, and substance P participates in pain processing.

Other peptides that are thought to function as neuromodulators in the CNS include **cholecystokinin, gastrin, neuropeptide Y, somatostatin,** and **vasoactive intestinal polypeptide.**

Other Neurotransmitters

Several additional substances, including nitric oxide, carbon monoxide, proteins, and purines, may also serve as neurotransmitters or neuromodulators in the CNS.

Nitric oxide is a gas formed from arginine by calcium-calmodulin–stimulated nitric oxide synthase in CNS neurons. There is some evidence that nitric oxide acts as a **retrograde neurotransmitter** in that it can be released by a postsynaptic neuron and can diffuse to the presynaptic terminal, where it facilitates future neurotransmitter release by elevating levels of cyclic guanosine monophosphate (cyclic GMP, or cGMP). This action may contribute to long-term potentiation, which is involved in establishing memory. A similar function has been postulated for **carbon monoxide** in the CNS.

Several recently discovered **proteins** may function as neuromodulators or neurohormones in the CNS. These include **leptin** and **orexin**, which are formed in the lateral hypothalamus and are believed to play a role in regulating appetite, with leptin producing satiety and orexin producing hunger.

Purines that may serve as neurotransmitters include **adenosine** and **adenosine triphosphate** (ATP). Adenosine activates specific receptors identified as A_1, A_2, and A_3 **receptors.** Activation of A_1 and A_3 receptors increases cAMP formation, while activation of A_2 receptors inhibits cAMP formation. The physiologic role of adenosine has not been clearly established, but investigators believe that the inhibition of A_2 receptors by methylxanthines, such as caffeine, is responsible for the CNS stimulation produced by these drugs. Similarly, the role of ATP in neurotransmission is unclear, but there is some evidence indicating that ATP is a cotransmitter which is released with other neurotransmitters in the brain and which serves to augment the effects of these neurotransmitters.

MECHANISMS OF DRUG ACTION

Table 18–2 lists the many processes by which drugs affect the CNS and provides examples of agents acting via each process.

Drugs that alter CNS neurotransmitter function generally do so by altering the synthesis, storage, or release of a neurotransmitter; blocking the reuptake of a neurotransmitter; inhibiting the degradation of a neurotransmitter; or activating or blocking neurotransmitter receptors. A few CNS drugs act by directly blocking membrane ion channels or by altering the physiochemical properties of neuronal membranes so as to inhibit neurotransmission. While modulation of second-messenger signal transduction is an attractive target for novel pharmacologic agents, lithium is currently the only therapeutic drug that is believed to act by this mechanism.

Neurotransmitter Synthesis, Storage, and Release

Neurotransmitter synthesis can be increased by administering a precursor to a neurotransmitter, such as levodopa. Levodopa is then converted to dopamine by brain neurons. The vesicular storage of norepinephrine is blocked by reserpine, a plant alkaloid that may depress mood through this mechanism. Mood depression is a side effect of reserpine when it is used to treat hypertension. Drugs may cause nonexocytotic neurotransmitter release by interacting with the presynaptic neurotransmitter transporter. For example, amphetamine increases the release of norepinephrine by this mechanism, and amantadine increases the release of dopamine in patients with parkinsonism.

Neurotransmitter Reuptake and Degradation

Presynaptic reuptake and enzymatic degradation are the two primary mechanisms for terminating the action of most CNS neurotransmitters, and both of these processes are inhibited by drugs. Cocaine and many of the antidepressant drugs act by blocking the reuptake of dopamine, norepinephrine, or serotonin. Donepezil, selegiline, and tacrine are examples of agents that inhibit the degradation of acetylcholine or dopamine and thereby elevate the synaptic concentration of these neurotransmitters.

Receptor Activation or Blockade

Postsynaptic receptors are activated or blocked by several types of CNS drugs. For example, bromocriptine, a drug used in the treatment of parkinsonism, activates dopamine receptors, whereas antipsychotic drugs block dopamine and serotonin receptors.

Presynaptic receptors are involved in feedback inhibition of neurotransmitter release. They are called **autoreceptors** when they are activated by the same neurotransmitter that is released by the neuron, and they are called **heteroreceptors** when they are activated by a different neurotransmitter. Activation of presynaptic receptors decreases the concentration of the released neurotransmitter found in synapses, whereas blockade of these receptors increases the concentration. For example, activation of 5-HT_{1D} autoreceptors inhibits the release of serotonin and decreases its concentration in synapses.

Receptor Sensitization or Desensitization

Receptors undergo dynamic regulation in response to changes in synaptic neurotransmitter concentrations or in response to long-term drug administration. These stimuli may lead to **up-regulation** (sensitization) or to **down-regulation** (desensitization), which are characterized by an increase or a decrease, respectively, in the number of receptors (Fig. 18–4).

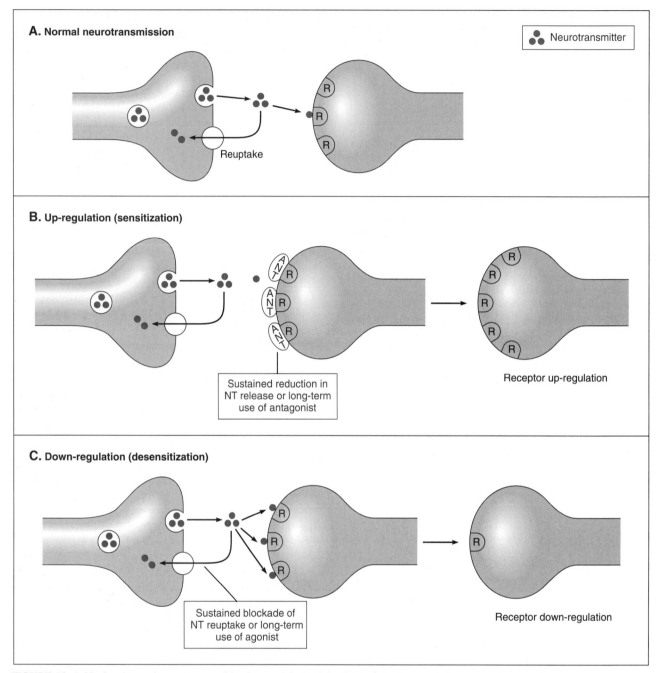

FIGURE 18–4. Mechanisms of receptor sensitization and desensitization. (A) Under normal circumstances, the neurotransmitter (NT) activates receptors and is removed from the synapse by neuronal reuptake. **(B)** The number of receptors may be increased (up-regulated) by a sustained reduction in NT release or by the long-term administration of a receptor antagonist (ANT). **(C)** The number of receptors may be decreased (down-regulated) by a sustained blockade of NT reuptake or by the long-term administration of a receptor agonist.

Receptor up-regulation is a compensatory reaction to a sustained decrease in neurotransmission, a condition that may be caused either by a sustained reduction in neurotransmitter release or by long-term receptor blockade. Receptor up-regulation leads to sensitization, so that a response can be elicited by lower concentrations of a neurotransmitter or a drug.

Receptor down-regulation may follow a sustained increase in neurotransmitter release, a sustained blockade of neurotransmitter reuptake, or long-term receptor activation by a drug. Down-regulation produces desensitization, so that higher concentrations of a neurotransmitter or drug are required to produce an effect. Desensitization is one of the primary mechanisms associated with **drug tolerance.**

NEURONAL SYSTEMS IN THE CENTRAL NERVOUS SYSTEM

Many CNS diseases and drug treatments affect cognitive processing, memory, motor coordination, and other complex brain functions discussed below. It is difficult to attribute these complex functions to specific neuronal tracts, because many of the functions are accomplished through the interaction of tracts that communicate with several brain regions and utilize various neurotransmitters.

Cognitive Processing

Cognitive processing occurs in **prefrontal cortical structures,** where sensory information is interpreted in a manner that stimulates the motor system and may result in action. The neuronal systems involved in cognitive processing include **association fibers** that arise from areas throughout the brain and converge on the anteromedial frontal, orbital frontal, and cingulate areas of the prefrontal cortex.

Cognitive processing utilizes memory and is influenced by emotions. At the same time, emotions are largely derived from cognition. Cognitive processing also encompasses abstract reasoning and forethought, which are processes that do not necessarily result in motor expression but may influence emotional processing and future acts.

Delirium is a general term that refers to disorders of cognitive processing, and one of manifestations of **schizophrenia** is impaired cognitive processing.

Drugs that affect cognitive processing include **antipsychotics, CNS stimulants, hallucinogens,** and **sedative-hypnotics.**

Memory

Memory is the ability to recall events and integrate them into cognitive processing, emotional processing, and ongoing motor activities. One form of memory, called **procedural memory,** is used to recall a set of practiced motor actions, such as riding a bicycle or typing on a keyboard, and it involves the interaction of **limbic structures,** the **cerebellum,** and the **basal ganglia.** Another form of memory, called **declarative memory,** involves thoughts and associations that may be used to determine future actions. For example, remembering that touching a hot stove is painful may keep a child from playing with matches in the future, and remembering that a family member's birthday is approaching may trigger activities such as planning a dinner. Declarative memory involves neuronal tracts in the **hippocampus, amygdala, thalamus,** and **cortical mantle.**

Dementia is a term used to describe a number of memory disorders, including **Alzheimer's disease.** The involvement of the basal ganglia in procedural memory may explain why some patients with **Parkinson's disease** have difficulties with practiced motor actions.

Drugs that affect memory include the **cholinesterase inhibitors** and **CNS depressants** such as the **benzodiazepines.**

Emotional Processing

Emotional processing is responsible for the generation of emotions such as anger, anxiety, fear, happiness, love, and sadness. These emotions represent the conscious perception of neuronal activity originating in **limbic structures,** including the hypothalamus, amygdala, septum, hippocampus, and mamillary bodies, as well as the cingulate and entorhinal portions of the frontal lobe cortex. The emotions contribute to a state of mental preparedness for anticipated future activities. For example, anxiety contributes to a state of heightened vigilance, which may amplify the response to a future stimulus or event.

Disorders in which emotional processing is defective include **anxiety states, mood disorders,** and **schizophrenia.**

Drugs that affect emotional processing in the limbic system include **antianxiety drugs, antidepressants, antipsychotics, CNS stimulants, opioids,** and **all drugs that produce drug dependence.** Hence, the majority of CNS drugs have some effect on emotional processing.

Sensory Processing

Sensory processing involves neuronal tracts that perceive external stimuli and transmit that information to the brain. These include the sensory systems responsible for vision, hearing, olfaction, touch, and pain.

The spinothalamic tracts relay touch and pain sensations to the **thalamus,** which projects this information to the **cortex.** The brain stem region known as the **reticular formation** plays a significant role in filtering sensory information before it is relayed to the thalamus and hypothalamus and eventually to the cortex. The reticular formation includes the **locus ceruleus** and **raphe nuclei,** whose neurons release norepinephrine and serotonin, respectively, and play an important role in determining the level of consciousness, sleep, and wakefulness. The cortex of the parietal and occipital lobes and part of the temporal lobe is involved in the recognition and integration of sensory perceptions.

Disorders in which sensory processing is defective include **sleep disorders, chronic pain syndromes,** and **sensory processing defects** (such as blindness, deafness, and taste dysfunction).

Among the drugs that affect sensory processing are **antidepressants, hallucinogens, local and general anesthetics, opioid analgesics,** and **sedative-hypnotics.**

Motor Processing

Motor processing refers to the neuronal activity that enables body movement. The structures involved in motor processing include the **cerebellum,** the motor strip of the **frontal lobe cortex,** the **basal ganglia,** and the suprasegmental nuclei that are found in the **brain stem** and are involved in the control of posture, such as the vestibular nuclei.

Disturbances in motor processing occur in **Parkinson's disease, Huntington's disease,** and a variety of **degenerative and demyelinating neuron disorders.**

Drugs that affect motor processing include **antiparkinsonian drugs, antispasmodics, CNS stimulants, muscle relaxants,** and **sedative-hypnotics.**

Autonomic Processing

Autonomic processing involves areas of the brain that integrate the activities of the **peripheral autonomic nervous system** (see Chapter 5). These areas include the **hypothalamus** and portions of the **brain stem,** such as the vasomotor center and the cranial nuclei of parasympathetic nerves.

Disorders of autonomic processing include **orthostatic hypotension** and **postural tachycardia syndrome.**

Some CNS drugs alter autonomic processing by affecting the actions of hypothalamic and brain stem nuclei, and others have a direct effect on peripheral autonomic neurotransmission. The drugs that affect autonomic processing include **antidepressants, antiparkinsonian drugs, antipsychotics,** and **drugs used to treat Alzheimer's disease.**

Summary of Important Points

- Central nervous system (CNS) drugs act primarily by affecting the synthesis, storage, release, reuptake, or degradation of neurotransmitters or by activating or blocking receptors.
- Long-term administration of drugs sometimes causes up-regulation (sensitization) or down-regulation (desensitization) of receptors. Up-regulation is evoked by receptor antagonists, while down-regulation is evoked by receptor agonists or reuptake inhibitors.
- Major CNS neurotransmitters include acetylcholine; amino acids (aspartate, gamma-aminobutyric acid [GABA], glutamate, and glycine); biogenic amines (dopamine, histamine, norepinephrine, and serotonin); and two groups of peptides (the opioid peptides, which include enkephalins, and the tachykinins, which include neurokinins and substance P).
- Some CNS neurotransmitters (such as aspartate, glutamate, histamine, and tachykinins) are excitatory; others (such as dopamine, GABA, glycine, and opioid peptides) are inhibitory; and still others (such as acetylcholine, norepinephrine, and serotonin) are both excitatory and inhibitory, with these actions exerted via different receptors.
- Neurotransmitters can be classified as fast or slow, depending on the duration of the neuronal signal that they evoke. GABA and glutamate are fast, while norepinephrine, the peptides, and serotonin are slow.
- Neurotransmitters that affect many neurons in a particular brain region are called neuromodulators.
- Receptors for CNS neurotransmitters can be classified as ionotropic (directly coupled with ion channels) or metabotropic (coupled with G proteins and second messengers).
- Many diseases of the CNS and the corresponding drugs used to treat these diseases have an effect on one or more of the following complex brain functions: cognitive processing, emotional processing, memory, motor processing, sensory processing, and autonomic processing.

Selected Readings

Carvey, P. M. Drug Action in the Central Nervous System. New York, Oxford University Press, 1998.

Keltner, N. L., and D. G. Folks, eds. Psychotropic Drugs, 2nd ed. St. Louis, Mosby, 1997.

Stahl, S. M. Essential Psychopharmacology: Neuroscientific Basis and Clinical Applications. Cambridge, Cambridge University Press, 1996.

CHAPTER NINETEEN

SEDATIVE-HYPNOTIC AND

ANXIOLYTIC DRUGS

CLASSIFICATION OF SEDATIVE-HYPNOTIC AND ANXIOLYTIC DRUGS

SEDATIVE-HYPNOTIC DRUGS
Benzodiazepines
- Alprazolam
- Chlordiazepoxide
- Clonazepam
- Diazepam
- Estazolam
- Flurazepam
- Lorazepam
- Midazolam
- Oxazepam
- Temazepam
- Triazolam

Barbiturates
- Amobarbital
- Pentobarbital
- Phenobarbital
- Thiopental

Antihistamines
- Diphenhydramine
- Hydroxyzine

Other sedative-hypnotic drugs
- Chloral hydrate
- Melatonin
- Zolpidem

NONSEDATING ANXIOLYTIC DRUGS
- Buspirone
- Propranolol

OVERVIEW

A **sedative** is a drug that reduces a person's response to external stimuli and causes drowsiness; a **hypnotic** is a drug that induces sleep; and a **sedative-hypnotic drug** is a sedative that induces sleep when administered in high doses. An **anxiolytic drug** is an agent that reduces anxiety and is also called an **antianxiety drug.** Most sedative-hypnotic drugs exert an anxiolytic effect, and a few nonsedating drugs have anxiolytic properties.

This chapter describes the pharmacologic properties of benzodiazepines, barbiturates, and other sedative-hypnotic and anxiolytic drugs that are used in the treatment of anxiety and sleep disorders. Although ethanol (ethyl alcohol) has sedative-hypnotic effects, it is not used therapeutically for these purposes, and its pharmacologic effects are described in Chapter 24.

Anxiety

Anxiety is normally an **adaptive response** that prepares a person to react appropriately to a threatening event, such as a hurricane or tornado. Anxiety is characterized by changes in mood (apprehension and fear), physiologic arousal, and increased perceptual acuity (hypervigilance). However, chronic anxiety is usually a **maladaptive response** to psychologic stress and may eventually impair a person's ability to perform activities of daily living. Moreover, chronic anxiety often contributes to visceral organ dysfunction and unpleasant symptoms. For example, patients with chronic anxiety may develop gastrointestinal, cardiovascular, and neurologic problems, including diarrhea, tachycardia, sweating, tremors, and dizziness. Ultimately, anxiety may contribute to heart disease and other disorders, including substance abuse.

Neurologic Basis of Anxiety

The neuronal pathways involved in anxiety disorders include the **sensory, cognitive, behavioral, motor, and autonomic pathways.** Sensory systems, cortical processing, and memory are involved in interpreting a stimulus to be dangerous and creating a state of heightened arousal. Motor systems and autonomic processing participate in the exaggerated responses to an anxiety state.

There is growing evidence that the **amygdala,** an almond-shaped structure in the temporal lobe, plays a central role in mediating most of the manifestations of anxiety, including the **conditioned avoidance reaction** (conditioned fear reaction) that underlies anxiety states. In experimental protocols, this reaction can be induced in animals by teaching them that a cue, such as a flashing light, will be followed by a noxious stimulus, such as a shock to the foot. During the anticipatory period, the animals conditioned in this manner will exhibit signs of anxiety, such as autonomic and behavioral arousal. Electrical stimulation of the amygdala will also induce feelings or signs of anxiety, whereas the presence of lesions in the amygdala or the administration of anxiolytic drugs will prevent the behavioral and physiologic manifestations of anxiety during the anticipatory period. It is believed that the amygdala participates in the long-term potentiation of the memory of adverse events that establishes anticipatory anxiety.

Classification and Management of Anxiety Disorders

The appropriate management of anxiety disorders requires an accurate diagnosis, may involve the use of pharmacologic agents, and usually includes individualized psychotherapy.

Acute Anxiety Disorders. Acute anxiety disorders, such as **adjustment disorder,** may result from illness, separation, or the anticipation of stressful events. Acute anxiety is often self-limiting and may resolve in a few weeks to a few months without drug treatment. A **benzodiazepine** may provide short-term relief from more severe acute anxiety conditions, and most patients benefit from counseling and psychotherapy. **Propranolol** is useful in the prevention of **stage fright,** or **acute situational or performance anxiety.**

Panic Disorder. Panic disorder is characterized by acute episodes of severe anxiety with marked psychologic and physiologic symptoms. During a panic attack, an individual may feel an impending sense of doom that is often accompanied by sweating, tachycardia, tremor, and other visceral symptoms. Patients with panic disorder often respond to a combination of psychotherapy and drug therapy with a **benzodiazepine** or an **antidepressant drug,** such as a **selective serotonin reuptake inhibitor** (SSRI). Benzodiazepines may provide immediate relief from panic attacks during the early phase of therapy, and **alprazolam** and **clonazepam** are benzodiazepines that have been particularly useful in this regard. The SSRIs, which are discussed in Chapter 22, may be the most effective agents for the long-term prevention and treatment of panic disorder. Behavioral therapy and cognitive therapy help enable the patient to identify situations that precipitate panic attacks and learn how to prevent these situations from causing a panic reaction.

Phobic Disorders. Phobias are conditions in which an individual is overly fearful about a particular condition, such as traveling in an airplane. **Agoraphobia,** which often coexists with panic disorder, is the fear of being in open or public places from which an escape might be difficult. Patients with phobic disorders often respond to a combination of psychotherapy and drug therapy. Like panic disorder, phobic disorders are treated with a **benzodiazepine** or an **antidepressant drug.** Benzodiazepines provide acute relief of symptoms and enable patients to more easily benefit from psychotherapy, whereas antidepressants are usually the most effective long-term

drug therapy for these disorders. Behavioral techniques may help patients confront the cause of their disorder and learn to avoid its anxiety-precipitating influence.

Obsessive-Compulsive Disorder. Obsessive-compulsive disorder has features similar to those of anxiety disorders and mood disorders. It is characterized by **obsessions** (recurring or persistent thoughts and impulses) and **compulsions** (repetitive behaviors in response to obsessions). Obsessive-compulsive disorder can be treated effectively with an **antidepressant drug** (see Chapter 22) and psychotherapy. Sedative-hypnotic drugs are usually not useful unless the patient concurrently suffers from another anxiety disorder.

Generalized Anxiety Disorder. Generalized anxiety disorder is usually defined as a persistent state of fear and apprehension concerning future events. Short-term therapy with a **benzodiazepine** may relieve acute symptoms and provide a useful bridge to psychotherapy. The severity of the disorder often fluctuates over time, and benzodiazepines may be effectively used on an intermittent basis to help patients deal with exacerbations of the disorder. **Buspirone** provides a useful alternative to benzodiazepines for the treatment of chronic anxiety states, because it produces little sedation and is not associated with tolerance or dependence. However, it must be taken for 3 or 4 weeks before its anxiolytic effects are felt.

Sleep

Sleep is a reversible state of reduced consciousness that is accompanied by characteristic changes in the electroencephalogram (EEG). As shown in Box 19–1, stages 1 through 4 of sleep are collectively called **non–rapid eye movement sleep** (NREM sleep), and stage 5 is called **rapid eye movement sleep** (REM sleep).

As an individual falls asleep, the high-frequency and low-amplitude activity of the alert state gradually diminishes during stages 1 and 2 and is replaced by lower-frequency and higher-amplitude signals during **slow-wave sleep** (stages 3 and 4). Over time, the individual returns to stage 1 and eventually to the REM stage. During REM sleep, the findings on EEG return to the alert pattern, with high-frequency and low-amplitude activity accompanied by random, jerky ocular movements. REM sleep is also known as **paradoxical sleep** because the pattern on EEG is characteristic of the awake state. A normal adult cycles through the sleep stages about every 90 minutes.

Sleep patterns change with age and are altered by sedative-hypnotic and other central nervous system (CNS) drugs.

Neurologic Basis of Sleep

The neuronal systems involved in sleep include the **basal forebrain nuclei** and the **reticular forma-**

BOX 19–1. Effect of Sedative-Hypnotic Drugs on Sleep Architecture

Terminology

Patterns on the electroencephalogram (EEG) vary with the stage of sleep. When a person falls asleep, the high-frequency and low-amplitude pattern of the **awake state** is gradually replaced by the progressively lower-frequency and higher-amplitude patterns of stages 1 through 4, which collectively are called **non–rapid eye movement sleep** (NREM sleep). Stages 3 and 4 are called **slow-wave sleep.** Stage 5 is called **rapid eye movement sleep** (REM sleep) because it is characterized by rapid, jerky eye movements. Stage 5 is also called **paradoxical sleep** because it is during stage 5 that the pattern on EEG returns to the pattern seen during the awake state.

Normal and Abnormal Sleep Patterns

The normal sleep pattern in adults consists of about five cycles, each of which lasts approximately 90 minutes. During each cycle, an individual progresses from stage 1 to stage 4 and then returns to stage 1, followed by a period of REM sleep. As the cycles progress through the night, they become shorter, and the amount of slow-wave sleep decreases.

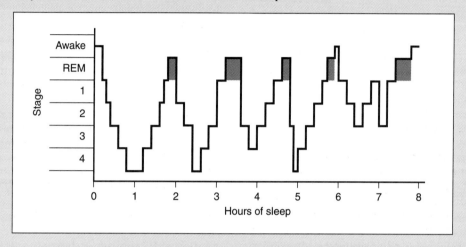

The sleep patterns of patients with insomnia vary widely but are often characterized by reduced amounts of slow-wave sleep and by one or more awakenings during the night. The time required to fall asleep (sleep latency) is usually prolonged, and the total sleep time is decreased in most patients with insomnia. Elderly adults often have a similar sleep pattern.

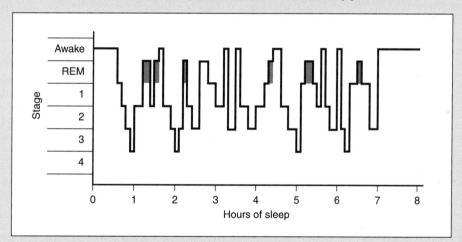

Effects of Drugs on Sleep Architecture

Benzodiazepines and most other hypnotics suppress stages 3, 4, and 5 of sleep (slow-wave and REM sleep). In contrast, zolpidem has little effect on sleep architecture. Therefore, use of zolpidem may restore the sleep pattern to normal.

State	Rapid Eye Movements	Pattern on EEG	Effect of Benzodiazepines	Effect of Zolpidem
Awake	No.	High-frequency, low-amplitude pattern.	Induce sleep.	Induces sleep.
Stages 1 and 2 sleep	No.	Lower-frequency, higher-amplitude pattern than awake state.	Increase length of stages.	Little change.
Stages 3 and 4 sleep	No.	Lower-frequency, higher-amplitude pattern than stages 1 and 2.	Decrease length of stages.	Little change.
Stage 5 sleep	Yes.	High-frequency, low-amplitude pattern.	Decrease length of stage.	Little change.

tion. Projecting from the basal forebrain to the cortex are cholinergic fibers that are believed to be involved in the induction of sleep. The basal forebrain is the only region of the brain that is active during slow-wave sleep and quiet at other times. The reticular formation serves to modify the sensory information that is relayed from the thalamus to the cortex in a way that permits the accurate transfer of information between these two structures. When reticular nuclei are quiescent, the thalamus does not transfer information to the cortex, and this facilitates the onset of sleep.

Drugs that block acetylcholine, including the **antihistamines,** probably induce drowsiness and sleep via their effects on the cholinergic projections of the reticular nuclei. In contrast, **caffeine** and related **methylxanthines** may increase arousal by blocking adenosine receptors and thereby increasing cholinergic activity in the reticular nuclei.

The **benzodiazepines** and **barbiturates** are believed to exert their effects on consciousness and sleep by facilitating the activity of **gamma-aminobutyric acid** (GABA) at various sites in the neuraxis. GABA is the most ubiquitous inhibitory neurotransmitter in the CNS and regulates the excitability of neurons in almost every neuronal tract. As shown in Fig. 19–1, the **GABA$_A$-chloride ionophore** has binding sites for benzodiazepines and barbiturates. Both types of drugs induce a conformational change in the chloride channel. The change induced by benzodiazepines increases the frequency with which the channel opens, while the change induced by barbiturates increases the length of time that the

channel remains open. By increasing chloride conductance, these drugs cause neuronal membrane hyperpolarization, and this in turn counteracts the depolarizing effect of excitatory neurotransmitters. Barbiturates also increase chloride conductance independent of GABA, which is probably why they are capable of causing greater toxicity than the benzodiazepines.

Classification and Management of Sleep Disorders

Insomnia. Some patients with insomnia find it difficult to go to sleep or to stay asleep during the night, while others awaken too early in the morning. In general, the management of insomnia depends on whether the sleep disorder is caused by physiologic, psychologic, or medical conditions.

Insomnia due to acute stress or a minor illness is usually self-limiting and may not require treatment. **Melatonin** is a useful drug for the treatment of mild insomnia, and it is available without a prescription. Melatonin is particularly useful in relieving **jet lag,** a form of acute insomnia caused by travel across several time zones.

Insomnia due to medical conditions whose symptoms interfere with sleep may be effectively treated with **benzodiazepines** or other **hypnotic drugs,** such as **zolpidem,** whereas insomnia due to psychologic and psychiatric disturbances is best managed with a combination of psychotherapy and **hypnotic drugs.** Benzodiazepines and most other hypnotic drugs decrease sleep latency (the time required to go to sleep) and increase sleep duration. Zolpidem, a newer drug, has the advantages of not affecting sleep architecture significantly, and it does not cause as much tolerance and dependence as do the older drugs. For these reasons, zolpidem has become the hypnotic drug of choice for treating most types of insomnia.

Other Sleep Disorders. Other sleep disorders include **hypersomnia** (difficulty in awakening), **narcolepsy** (sleep attacks), **enuresis** (bed-wetting during sleep), **somnambulism** (sleepwalking), **sleep apnea** (episodes of hypoventilation during sleep), and **nightmares** and **night terrors.** Most of these disorders are managed with a combination of psychotherapy and **antidepressant drugs** or **CNS stimulants.**

SEDATIVE-HYPNOTIC DRUGS

The sedative-hypnotic drugs include benzodiazepines, barbiturates, some antihistamines, and a few miscellaneous compounds, such as chloral hydrate and zolpidem. The properties of these drugs are summarized in Table 19–1, and their adverse effects, contraindications, and drug interactions are listed in Table 19–2.

Because the benzodiazepines have fewer adverse reactions and drug interactions and are safer in cases of overdose, they have largely replaced the barbiturates and other older drugs. Nevertheless, barbiturates are still used when benzodiazepines are ineffective or contraindicated. The sedating antihis-

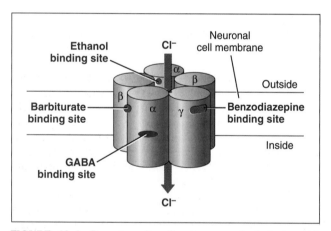

FIGURE 19–1. Receptor sites for gamma-aminobutyric acid (GABA), benzodiazepines, barbiturates, and ethanol on the GABA$_A$-chloride ionophore. The GABA$_A$-chloride ionophore is a glycoprotein pentamer that has varying combinations of α, β, and γ subunits. GABA binds to a site on the α or β subunit, and this causes conformational changes that open the chloride ion channel and lead to neuronal membrane hyperpolarization. Benzodiazepines bind to a site that is probably located on the γ subunit, and this facilitates GABA binding and increases the frequency of chloride channel opening. Barbiturates bind to another site and increase the duration of chloride channel opening, both in the presence and in the absence of GABA. Ethanol (ethyl alcohol) binds to a distinct site on the ionophore and enhances chloride influx. The ionophore also contains binding sites for steroids such as progesterone. These binding sites may mediate the behavioral effects of steroids.

TABLE 19–1. Pharmacokinetic Properties and Clinical Uses of Sedative-Hypnotic and Anxiolytic Drugs

Drug	Onset of Action*	Duration of Action*	Active Metabolites	Major Clinical Uses
Sedative-hypnotic drugs				
Benzodiazepines				
Alprazolam	Fast.	Medium.	Yes.	Anxiety, including panic disorder.
Chlordiazepoxide	Fast; very fast (IV).	Long.	Yes.	Alcohol detoxification; anxiety.
Clonazepam	Fast.	Medium.	No.	Anxiety, including panic disorder; seizure disorders.
Diazepam	Fast; very fast (IV).	Long.	Yes.	Alcohol detoxification; anxiety; muscle spasm; seizure disorders; spasticity.
Estazolam	Fast.	Medium.	Yes.	Insomnia.
Flurazepam	Fast.	Long.	Yes.	Insomnia.
Lorazepam	Fast; very fast (IV).	Medium.	No.	Anxiety; seizure disorders.
Midazolam	Very fast (IV).	Short (IV).	Yes.	Anesthesia.
Oxazepam	Fast.	Short.	No.	Anxiety.
Temazepam	Fast.	Medium.	No.	Insomnia.
Triazolam	Fast.	Short.	Yes.	Insomnia.
Barbiturates				
Amobarbital	Fast.	Medium.	No.	Insomnia.
Pentobarbital	Fast.	Short.	No.	Insomnia.
Phenobarbital	Slow.	Long.	No.	Seizure disorders.
Thiopental	Very fast (IV).	Short (IV).	No.	Induction of anesthesia.
Antihistamines				
Diphenhydramine	Fast.	Medium.	No.	Insomnia.
Hydroxyzine	Fast.	Long.	No.	Anxiety; sedation.
Other sedative-hypnotic drugs				
Chloral hydrate	Fast.	Medium.	Yes.	Insomnia; preanesthetic sedation.
Melatonin	Fast.	Medium.	No.	Insomnia, including jet lag.
Zolpidem	Fast.	Short.	No.	Insomnia.
Nonsedating anxiolytic drugs				
Buspirone	Very slow.	Long.	No.	Chronic anxiety.
Propranolol	Fast.	Medium.	Yes.	Situational or performance anxiety.

*Unless onset and duration of action are specifically indicated for intravenous (IV) administration, they are for oral administration. Very fast = <15 minutes; fast = 15–59 minutes; slow = 1–4 hours; very slow = 3–4 weeks; short = 1–6 hours; medium = 7–12 hours; and long = >12 hours.

tamines are occasionally used in the treatment of mild insomnia and anxiety and have less potential for abuse than do benzodiazepines and barbiturates.

Benzodiazepines

The benzodiazepines are a large group of drugs that have similar pharmacologic effects. The particular use of specific drugs is largely determined by their pharmacokinetic properties and route of administration. Some benzodiazepines have been developed and approved to treat anxiety, whereas others are approved for the management of insomnia or for other purposes.

Drug Properties

Chemistry. The benzodiazepine structure consists of a benzene ring fused to a seven-membered ring containing two nitrogen molecules (diazepine). Most benzodiazepines have a chlorine substitution on the fused benzene ring and another benzene moiety attached to the diazepine structure. Alprazolam and triazolam also have a triazole ring fused to the diazepine structure. The structures of representative benzodiazepines are shown in Fig. 19–2A.

Pharmacokinetics. The pharmacokinetic properties of various benzodiazepines are compared in Table 19–1.

The benzodiazepines are absorbed from the gut and distributed to the brain at rates that are proportional to their lipid solubility, which varies 50-fold among individual drugs in the class. As the plasma concentration of a benzodiazepine declines, the drug is redistributed from the brain to the blood, and this mechanism contributes significantly to the termination of its effects on the CNS.

All benzodiazepines are extensively metabolized in the liver. Some drugs are converted to active metabolites in phase I oxidative reactions catalyzed by cytochrome P450 enzymes. The active metabolites of chlordiazepoxide, diazepam, and flurazepam are long-acting and contribute to the long duration of action of these drugs. The active metabolites of alprazolam, estazolam, midazolam, and triazolam are shorter-acting. Each of these active metabolites is eventually conjugated with glucuronate to form an inactive metabolite that is excreted in the urine. Other drugs, such as lorazepam, oxazepam, and temazepam, bypass phase I oxidation and are metabolized only by phase II conjugation (Fig. 19–3). These three drugs may be safer for use by elderly patients, because the capacity to conjugate drugs does not

**TABLE 19–2.   Adverse Effects, Contraindications, and Drug Interactions
of Sedative-Hypnotic and Anxiolytic Drugs**

Drug	Common Adverse Effects	Contraindications	Common Drug Interactions
Sedative-hypnotic drugs			
Benzodiazepines			
Alprazolam	Arrhythmia; central nervous system (CNS) depression; drug dependence; hypotension; and mild respiratory depression.	Acute angle-closure glaucoma; hypersensitivity; and psychosis.	Alcohol and other CNS depressants potentiate effects. Fluoxetine and fluvoxamine increase serum levels and effects.
Chlordiazepoxide	Same as alprazolam.	Same as alprazolam.	Alcohol and other CNS depressants potentiate effects. Cimetidine increases and rifampin decreases serum levels.
Clonazepam	Same as alprazolam.	Acute angle-closure glaucoma; hypersensitivity; and severe liver disease.	Same as chlordiazepoxide.
Diazepam	Same as alprazolam.	Same as alprazolam.	Same as chlordiazepoxide.
Estazolam	Same as alprazolam.	Hypersensitivity and pregnancy.	Same as chlordiazepoxide.
Flurazepam	Same as alprazolam.	Hypersensitivity and pregnancy.	Same as chlordiazepoxide.
Lorazepam	Same as alprazolam.	Same as alprazolam.	Alcohol and other CNS depressants potentiate effects. Rifampin decreases serum levels.
Midazolam	Same as alprazolam.	Acute angle-closure glaucoma; coma; hypersensitivity; and shock.	Alcohol and other CNS depressants potentiate effects. Calcium channel blockers, erythromycin, and ketoconazole increase serum levels.
Oxazepam	Same as alprazolam.	Same as alprazolam.	Same as lorazepam.
Temazepam	Same as alprazolam.	Hypersensitivity and pregnancy.	Same as chlordiazepoxide.
Triazolam	Amnesia; confusion; and delirium. Other adverse effects same as alprazolam.	Acute angle-closure glaucoma; age <18 years; hypersensitivity; and psychosis.	Alcohol and other CNS depressants potentiate effects. Cimetidine, erythromycin, ketoconazole, and oral contraceptives increase serum levels.
Barbiturates			
Amobarbital	CNS depression; drug dependence; and respiratory depression.	Hypersensitivity; porphyria; respiratory depression; and severe liver disease.	Induces cytochrome P450 enzymes and increases metabolism of many drugs. Potentiates effects of other CNS depressants.
Pentobarbital	Same as amobarbital.	Same as amobarbital.	Same as amobarbital.
Phenobarbital	Same as amobarbital.	Same as amobarbital.	Same as amobarbital.
Thiopental	Same as amobarbital.	Same as amobarbital.	Same as amobarbital.
Antihistamines			
Diphenhydramine	Anticholinergic effects, such as blurred vision, dry mouth, and urinary retention; dizziness; and drowsiness.	Acute angle-closure glaucoma; hypersensitivity; and urinary obstruction.	Alcohol, barbiturates, and other CNS depressants potentiate CNS effects.
Hydroxyzine	Same as diphenhydramine.	Same as diphenhydramine.	Same as diphenhydramine.
Other sedative-hypnotic drugs			
Chloral hydrate	Severe cardiac, hepatic, or renal disease; and severe gastritis.	Hypersensitivity.	Alcohol and other CNS depressants potentiate effects.
Melatonin	Drowsiness; fatigue; and lethargy.	Hypersensitivity.	Alcohol and caffeine reduce melatonin secretion. Flumazenil and naloxone antagonize effects. Sedative-hypnotic drugs potentiate effects.
Zolpidem	Dizziness; drowsiness; and headache.	Hypersensitivity.	Alcohol and other CNS depressants potentiate effects.
Nonsedating anxiolytic drugs			
Buspirone	Dizziness; headache; and nervousness.	Hypersensitivity.	None.
Propranolol	Bradycardia; bronchoconstriction; depression; fatigue; hypersensitivity; hypotension; impaired glycogenolysis; and vivid dreams.	Asthma; atrioventricular block; bradycardia; hypersensitivity; and severe chronic obstructive pulmonary disease.	Cardiac depression increased by calcium channel blockers.

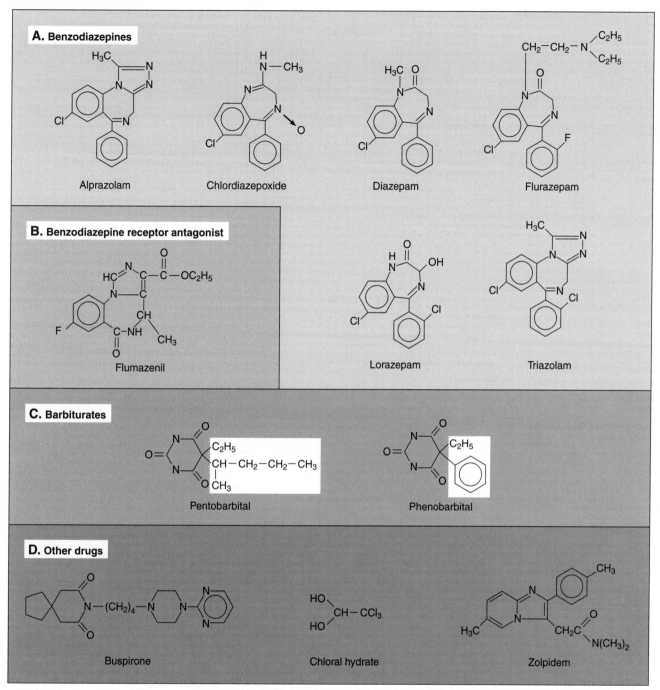

FIGURE 19–2. Structures of flumazenil and selected sedative-hypnotic and anxiolytic drugs. (A) Each benzodiazepine has a chlorobenzene moiety fused to a seven-membered diazepine ring. **(B)** Flumazenil, a benzodiazepine receptor antagonist, has a modified benzodiazepine structure. **(C)** Each barbiturate has a unique substitution at the 5 position. The substitutions are unshaded. **(D)** Buspirone is an azapirone that is a nonsedating anxiolytic drug. Chloral hydrate and zolpidem are both sedative-hypnotics; the former is a halogenated alcohol, while the latter is an imidazopyridine derivative.

decline with age as much as the capacity for oxidative biotransformation does. Hence, these three drugs are less likely to accumulate to toxic levels in elderly patients.

Benzodiazepines also undergo some degree of enterohepatic cycling that prolongs their duration of action. In fact, some patients who are taking a drug such as diazepam may notice an increased sedative effect after eating a fatty meal. The fatty meal causes the gallbladder to empty and thereby delivers bile containing diazepam to the intestines for reabsorption into the circulation.

Mechanisms. The benzodiazepines bind to receptors on the GABA$_A$-chloride ionophore (see Fig. 19–1). The **benzodiazepine receptors** are called **omega (ω) receptors,** and there are two types, designated ω_1 and ω_2. Benzodiazepines are believed to act as agonists at both the ω_1 and ω_2 receptor sites,

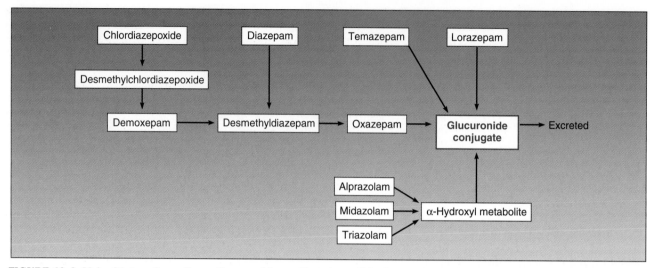

FIGURE 19–3. Major biotransformation pathways of benzodiazepines. Chlordiazepoxide and diazepam are converted to long-acting active metabolites. Alprazolam, midazolam, and triazolam are converted to a short-acting active metabolite. All benzodiazepines, including those with no active metabolites, are eventually converted to glucuronide compounds that are pharmacologically inactive and are excreted in the urine. The benzodiazepines that have no active metabolites include lorazepam, oxazepam, and temazepam, and these may be the safest benzodiazepines to use for the treatment of elderly patients.

whereas zolpidem (an imidazopyridine drug discussed below) is selective for the ω_1 receptor site. Activation of the ω receptors increases the affinity of the **GABA$_A$ receptor** for GABA. This increased affinity potentiates the effect of GABA by increasing the frequency with which the chloride channel opens in response to GABA. There appear to be subtle differences in the way that various benzodiazepines bind to the ω receptors, and this may contribute to slight differences in their pharmacologic effects.

In addition to their effects on GABA, benzodiazepines also inhibit the neuronal reuptake of **adenosine.** This action increases the inhibitory effect of adenosine on neurons that release acetylcholine from the pedunculopontine nucleus of the reticular formation, which is thought to be an important mediator of arousal. The effect of benzodiazepines on adenosine may also explain why these drugs dilate coronary arteries and decrease total peripheral resistance.

Pharmacologic Effects. The benzodiazepines produce a dose-dependent but limited depression of the CNS. Lower doses have a sedative and anxiolytic effect, whereas higher doses produce hypnosis (sleep) and anesthesia (Fig. 19–4). Benzodiazepines can relieve anxiety at doses that produce relatively little sedation. In contrast to the barbiturates, the orally administered benzodiazepines do not produce respiratory depression, coma, or death unless they are administered with another CNS depressant, such as alcohol. When benzodiazepines are given orally, their depressant effect on neurotransmission inhibits the further release of GABA before severe CNS depression occurs. Barbiturates do not exhibit this ceiling effect and may produce severe respiratory depression and death after administration of an excessive amount.

In addition to producing sedative-hypnotic and anxiolytic effects, benzodiazepines are able to produce **anterograde amnesia,** which means that an individual will not remember what happens from the time that the drug is administered to the time that the drug effects dissipate. This is in contrast to retrograde amnesia, in which a person cannot remember what happened before a certain point in time. The benzodiazepines produce anterograde amnesia because they interfere with the formation of new memory; they do not affect the ability to recall past events. The amnesic property of benzodiazepines is often useful when patients are undergoing stressful procedures, such as endoscopy or surgery. However, when these drugs are used on a long-term basis, such

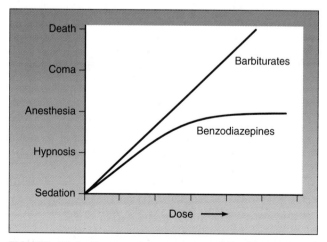

FIGURE 19–4. Dose-response curves of barbiturates and benzodiazepines. The barbiturates exhibit a linear dose-response effect, which progresses from sedation to respiratory depression, coma, and death. Benzodiazepines exhibit a ceiling effect, which precludes severe central nervous system depression following oral administration of these drugs. Intravenous administration of benzodiazepines may produce anesthesia and mild respiratory depression.

as in treating anxiety, the amnesic properties may have an adverse effect on the patient's ability to function. Triazolam, a widely used hypnotic, has been associated with problems caused by its amnesic effect.

The benzodiazepines have anticonvulsant effects and have been used in the treatment of seizure disorders (see Chapter 20). Even though benzodiazepines cause muscle relaxation only at doses that produce considerable sedation, they are occasionally used for the treatment of muscle spasm and spasticity. The muscle-relaxing effects of benzodiazepines are probably due to the fact that these drugs potentiate the effects of GABA on interneurons in the spinal cord.

Adverse Effects.   The adverse effects of benzodiazepines are largely due to CNS depression. The drugs frequently cause motor incoordination, dizziness, and excessive drowsiness. They impair cognitive processing and may affect concentration, judgment, and planning. They may also interfere with driving and other psychomotor skills. When longer-acting benzodiazepines, such as flurazepam, are used to treat insomnia, they may cause drowsiness and a drug hangover the next day. If this occurs, a shorter-acting drug, such as estazolam or zolpidem, should be substituted for the longer-acting drug.

Intravenous administration of benzodiazepines produces greater CNS depression than does oral administration, and intravenous administration may cause respiratory depression. The greater effect produced by intravenous administration is probably due to the more rapid uptake of the drug by brain tissue, which results in a greater potentiation of GABA before the self-limiting effect on GABA release has had time to develop.

The benzodiazepines have a mild euphoric effect and may reduce behavioral inhibitions in a manner similar to the disinhibitory effect of alcohol. The behavioral reinforcement produced by these drugs may contribute to their recreational abuse by polydrug abusers and to their inappropriate long-term use by patients. It appears that the reinforcing effects of benzodiazepines are less than the reinforcing effects of barbiturates but greater than the reinforcing effects of sedating antihistamines and possibly zolpidem.

Long-term use of the benzodiazepines may produce physical dependence, the severity of which is proportional to the dosage and duration of administration. After several months of continued use, most patients develop some degree of physical dependence. If their medication is abruptly discontinued, they will experience a withdrawal syndrome, characterized by rebound anxiety, insomnia, headache, irritability, and muscle twitches. The withdrawal syndrome is usually mild and not life-threatening. Nevertheless, to prevent its occurrence, the dosage of benzodiazepines should be gradually tapered over a period of several weeks. Because the various drugs in the benzodiazepine class exhibit cross-tolerance, any of them can be substituted for another one in order to prevent or counteract the withdrawal reaction.

Pharmacodynamic tolerance also occurs during long-term use of benzodiazepines. Unlike barbiturates, however, the benzodiazepines do not induce their own metabolism or cause pharmacokinetic tolerance.

Although the overall safety of the benzodiazepines is quite high, the use of benzodiazepines has been associated with hypotension, arrhythmia (tachycardia or bradycardia), and a number of other less common effects. Rarely, a massive overdose of a benzodiazepine has been fatal.

The incidence of fetal malformations in the offspring of women who take benzodiazepines during pregnancy is very low. Nevertheless, the benzodiazepine hypnotics are contraindicated during pregnancy and are included in pregnancy category X by the Food and Drug Administration. Zolpidem appears to be safer in pregnancy and is included in pregnancy category B.

Interactions and Treatment of Adverse Effects. Several drugs, including flumazenil and beta-carboline derivatives, interact with benzodiazepine receptors.

Flumazenil has been developed as a **benzodiazepine receptor antagonist** (see Fig. 19–2B). In addition to blocking the effects of agonists, such as diazepam, it blocks the effects of inverse agonists and has partial agonist properties (see Chapter 3) at the benzodiazepine receptor. Flumazenil can be used to counteract the adverse effects of benzodiazepines, such as respiratory depression resulting from intravenous administration of these drugs. Flumazenil is given intravenously, has a rapid onset of action, and has a short duration of action. Its potential adverse effects include seizures, arrhythmias, blurred vision, emotional lability, and dizziness.

The **beta-carboline derivatives** act as **inverse agonists.** An inverse agonist is a drug that decreases the response of an effector system below the basal level (see Chapter 3 and Fig. 3–3). The beta-carboline drugs act to decrease chloride conductance by the $GABA_A$-chloride ionophore, and this may cause anxiety and seizures. Some of the experimental inverse agonists enhance cognitive function and are being studied for the treatment of Alzheimer's disease.

Table 19–2 lists the individual benzodiazepines and outlines their interactions with various other drugs.

Indications.   The benzodiazepines are effective in the treatment of **anxiety disorders, insomnia, muscle spasm, seizure disorders,** and **spasticity.** When possible, the use of benzodiazepines should be limited to the short-term treatment of these conditions. If long-term use is medically justified, the physician should carefully monitor drug usage to prevent dosage escalation.

Alprazolam

Alprazolam is converted to a short-acting α-hydroxyl metabolite before undergoing glucuronide formation. Alprazolam has a medium duration of action and is primarily used in the management of

anxiety. Although it has special utility in the treatment of **panic disorder,** the larger doses usually required for controlling panic attacks may cause considerable sedation and contribute to drug dependence. Therefore, many patients with panic disorder are treated instead with antidepressants and behavioral therapy. Alprazolam may be useful as a short-term measure to relieve acute symptoms while other therapies are instituted.

Chlordiazepoxide and Diazepam

Chlordiazepoxide and diazepam are converted to long-acting metabolites, including desmethyldiazepam (also called nordiazepam or nordazepam). Desmethyldiazepam is eventually converted to oxazepam, which is excreted as a glucuronide conjugate (see Fig. 19–3).

Chlordiazepoxide and diazepam are effective in the treatment of **anxiety.** In patients undergoing **alcohol detoxification,** these drugs can be used to prevent seizures and other acute withdrawal reactions. The drug dosage is gradually tapered over several weeks.

Diazepam is also used to terminate **acute recurrent seizures** (see Chapter 20), to treat **severe muscle spasm,** and to treat **spasticity** associated with degenerative and demyelinating neurologic disorders.

Lorazepam, Oxazepam, and Temazepam

Because lorazepam, oxazepam, and temazepam do not form long-acting active metabolites, they have a short or medium duration of action. They are biotransformed to inactive glucuronide compounds. As mentioned earlier, they may be preferable for elderly patients because glucuronide conjugation does not decline significantly with aging.

Lorazepam may be administered orally or intravenously and is used for the treatment of **anxiety** and the control of **seizures.** Oxazepam is a short-acting drug that is administered orally to patients with **anxiety.** Temazepam is primarily used as a hypnotic for treating **insomnia.**

Estazolam, Flurazepam, and Triazolam

Estazolam, flurazepam, and triazolam have active metabolites with varying durations of action. Estazolam has a medium duration of action, while flurazepam has a longer one and triazolam has a shorter one.

All three drugs are used for the treatment of **insomnia.** A short- or medium-acting drug may be preferred for patients whose primary problem is getting to sleep, whereas a medium- or long- acting drug may be preferred for patients who complain of getting up too early.

The short-acting triazolam is more likely to cause rebound insomnia when it is discontinued. The long-acting flurazepam is less likely to cause rebound insomnia but is more likely to cause daytime drows-

iness. Triazolam has been associated with a higher incidence of amnesia, confusion, and delirium, especially in elderly patients. The dosage of triazolam in formulations marketed in the USA has been reduced by the Food and Drug Administration, and triazolam has been banned in the UK.

Other Benzodiazepines

Clonazepam is used for the treatment of **panic disorder** and **other anxiety disorders,** as well as for the treatment of **seizure disorders** (see Chapter 20).

Midazolam is used intravenously as an **anesthetic** for patients undergoing endoscopy, other diagnostic procedures, or minor surgery.

Barbiturates

The barbiturates include **amobarbital, pentobarbital, phenobarbital,** and **thiopental.** The properties, adverse effects, contraindications, and interactions of these drugs are outlined in Tables 19–1 and 19–2.

Drug Properties

Chemistry. The barbiturates are synthesized from urea and malonic acid, with each drug having a unique chemical group in the 5 position (see Fig. 19–2C).

Pharmacokinetics. The onset and duration of action of barbiturates are determined by their lipid solubility and rate of metabolic inactivation. Highly lipid-soluble drugs, such as amobarbital, pentobarbital, and thiopental, are rapidly absorbed from the gut, are rapidly redistributed from the brain to peripheral tissues as plasma concentrations fall, and are extensively metabolized to inactive compounds before they are excreted in the urine. Phenobarbital, a more polar drug, is more slowly absorbed from the gut and more slowly redistributed from the brain, and this contributes to its longer duration of action. Phenobarbital is partly converted to inactive metabolites, but a significant fraction of it is excreted unchanged in the urine.

Mechanisms and Effects. Barbiturates bind to a site on the $GABA_A$-chloride ionophore that is distinct from the site to which benzodiazepines bind (see Fig. 19–1). The barbiturates increase the affinity of the receptor for GABA and the duration of time that the chloride channel remains open. In contrast to the benzodiazepines, the barbiturates also act to directly increase chloride influx in the absence of GABA. For this reason, barbiturates do not exhibit a ceiling effect. As shown in Fig. 19–4, they have a linear dose-response curve. The higher doses progressively depress the CNS, causing respiratory depression, coma, and death. This accounts for the fact that the barbiturates have greater toxicity and a lower margin of safety than do the benzodiazepines.

Unlike the anxiolytic effect of benzodiazepines, that of barbiturates is associated with considerable sedation. When used for treating insomnia, the barbiturates may cause hangover and daytime sedation. Like the benzodiazepines, the barbiturates suppress slow-wave and REM sleep. Barbiturates may also cause tolerance and physical dependence during continuous use, and a withdrawal syndrome occurs if the drugs are abruptly discontinued. Short-acting barbiturates, such as pentobarbital, have been extensively abused.

Interactions. The barbiturates induce cytochrome P450 enzymes in the liver and thereby accelerate their own metabolism as well as that of other drugs metabolized by these enzymes. Maximal enzyme induction is obtained by the administration of phenobarbital, a long-acting drug, for several days. Barbiturates also induce the rate-limiting enzyme in porphyrin biosynthesis, δ-aminolevulinate synthase, and may thereby exacerbate porphyria, a condition in which a hereditary defect causes excessive porphyrin synthesis and excretion, with attendant neurologic and cutaneous manifestations.

Indications. The barbiturates were extensively used for the treatment of anxiety disorders and insomnia prior to the development of benzodiazepines, but they are seldom used for these purposes today. Unlike the benzodiazepines, the barbiturates do not produce significant muscle relaxation and are not used in treating muscle spasm or spasticity disorders.

Specific Drugs

Amobarbital and pentobarbital have been primarily used as hypnotics for the treatment of **insomnia.** Phenobarbital is used occasionally for the treatment of **seizure disorders,** and thiopental is administered intravenously to induce **anesthesia.** Thiopental has a high degree of lipid solubility and a very fast onset of action. It is also rapidly redistributed from the brain to other tissues (muscle and fat), which accounts for its short duration of action.

Antihistamines

Some of the **histamine antagonists** (antihistamines) cross the blood-brain barrier and produce varying degrees of sedation, and these drugs have been used in the treatment of **mild insomnia and anxiety disorders.** For example, **diphenhydramine** is the active ingredient in several nonprescription sleep preparations, and **hydroxyzine** has been used in the treatment of mild anxiety and is sometimes used as a **sedative** before surgery. The sedative action of these drugs is probably due to their ability to block acetylcholine released by neurons in the reticular formation.

Some tolerance may occur during the long-term use of antihistamines, but these drugs are not associated with physical dependence or significant drug abuse. The pharmacologic properties of antihistamines are discussed in detail in Chapter 26.

Other Sedative-Hypnotic Drugs
Chloral Hydrate

Chloral hydrate is an older hypnotic that is largely obsolete today. It is a prodrug that is converted to its active metabolite, trichloroethanol, by liver enzymes. Its effects are potentiated by alcohol, and the combination of alcohol and chloral hydrate gained fame under the monikers of "Mickey Finn" and "knock-out drops." Chloral hydrate is occasionally used for **preanesthetic sedation** in pediatric patients.

Melatonin

Melatonin is a neuroendocrine hormone synthesized in the pineal gland. The hormone interacts with specific receptors in the CNS and elsewhere, and it is believed to be the principal mediator of the biologic clock that determines circadian, seasonal, and reproductive rhythms in animal species. In humans, melatonin is released prior to the onset of sleep and produces drowsiness that facilitates sleep. Studies have shown that melatonin produces drowsiness even if administered during the daytime.

Melatonin is available without prescription and is sometimes effective in the treatment of **jet lag** in individuals who have rapidly traveled across several time zones and in the treatment of **insomnia in shift-change workers.** If melatonin is taken at bedtime for a few nights, it may accelerate the resetting of the biologic clock in these persons. Melatonin may also be effective in treating **insomnia in elderly patients** who do not secrete adequate melatonin, and it appears to be effective in treating **delayed sleep-phase syndrome** and **non–24-hour sleep-wake disorder.**

Melatonin has relatively few adverse effects when taken as a drug, but it may cause fatigue and lethargy. For this reason and also because some tolerance to its hypnotic effect may develop, the lowest effective dose should be used. Melatonin may potentiate the effects of benzodiazepines, and it has been used to prevent withdrawal syndrome in patients who are undergoing treatment for benzodiazepine dependence. The effects of melatonin may be partly antagonized by flumazenil (a benzodiazepine receptor antagonist) or by naloxone (an opioid receptor antagonist).

Zolpidem

Zolpidem is a unique imidazopyridine compound and is believed to selectively activate the ω_1 benzodiazepine receptor on the $GABA_A$-chloride ionophore. This selectivity may account for its relative lack of effects on normal sleep architecture, in that it does not significantly suppress REM or slow-wave sleep. Zolpidem appears to produce relatively little tolerance and dependence, and its short duration of action usually precludes daytime sedation and hangover. For these reasons, zolpidem has become the most widely used prescription drug for treating **insomnia.**

NONSEDATING ANXIOLYTIC DRUGS

Buspirone

Buspirone is a unique azapirone compound whose structure is depicted in Fig. 19–2D. The drug is used in the treatment of **chronic anxiety** and produces an anxiolytic effect without causing marked sedation, amnesia, tolerance, dependence, or muscle relaxation. In some patients, it may cause headache, dizziness, and nervousness, but these side effects are usually mild and temporary.

Buspirone is a partial agonist at serotonin 5-HT$_{1A}$ receptors and may exert its anxiolytic effect by activating feedback inhibition of serotonin release. By this action, it may cause up-regulation of postsynaptic serotonin receptors. This effect takes time to develop and would be consistent with the 3- to 4-week delay in the onset of the anxiolytic effect of buspirone.

Buspirone and other drugs affecting serotonin are discussed further in Chapter 26.

Propranolol

Propranolol, a β-adrenergic receptor antagonist (β-blocker), is sometimes used to prevent the physiologic manifestations of **stage fright,** or **acute situational or performance anxiety.** When taken an hour before the anticipated anxiety-provoking event, propranolol prevents tachycardia and other signs and symptoms of acute anxiety caused by sympathetic stimulation. The β-blockers also appear to have a role in preventing similar symptoms associated with other anxiety states, such as panic disorder.

The mechanisms and properties of β-blockers are discussed in detail in Chapter 9. Within the CNS, the drugs may act to block the effects of norepinephrine, but whether this action contributes to their anxiolytic effect is not certain.

Summary of Important Points

- Benzodiazepines are the most widely used sedative-hypnotic drugs and are indicated for the treatment of anxiety disorders, insomnia, muscle spasm, seizure disorders, and spasticity.
- Benzodiazepines bind to a receptor site on the GABA$_A$-chloride ionophore and thereby facilitate the binding of gamma-aminobutyric acid (GABA) and increase the frequency with which the chloride channel opens. Benzodiazepines also decrease the release of GABA, which limits the magnitude of central nervous system depression produced by these drugs.
- Some benzodiazepines (such as chlordiazepoxide and diazepam) have long-acting active metabolites. Others (such as alprazolam, midazolam, and triazolam) have shorter-acting active metabolites. All benzodiazepines, including those with no active metabolites, are eventually converted to inactive glucuronide compounds.

The benzodiazepines that have no active metabolites (such as lorazepam, oxazepam, and temazepam) may be the safest ones to use for the treatment of elderly patients.

- Benzodiazepines and other hypnotic drugs reduce the time required to fall asleep (sleep latency), reduce early awakenings, and increase total sleep time. Benzodiazepines and barbiturates reduce slow-wave sleep and rapid eye movement (REM) sleep.
- Pentobarbital, phenobarbital, and other barbiturates bind to the GABA$_A$-chloride ionophore but do not exhibit a ceiling effect and may cause respiratory depression, coma, and death.
- Unlike benzodiazepines, barbiturates induce their own metabolism as well as that of many other drugs metabolized by cytochrome P450 enzymes.
- Long-term administration of benzodiazepines and barbiturates may lead to tolerance and physical dependence, and abrupt discontinuation of their use will cause symptoms of withdrawal.
- Zolpidem is an effective short-acting hypnotic that has little effect on normal sleep architecture and produces few adverse effects.
- Sedating antihistamines (such as diphenhydramine and hydroxyzine) have been used to treat mild insomnia and anxiety. Older hypnotics, such as chloral hydrate, are largely obsolete but are occasionally used for preanesthetic sedation.
- Propranolol and other β-adrenergic receptor antagonists can be used to prevent the physiologic manifestations of situational or performance anxiety, including tachycardia.
- Flumazenil is a benzodiazepine receptor antagonist that may be used to counteract respiratory depression and other reactions that are usually caused by excessive doses of intravenously administered benzodiazepines.

Selected Readings

Chase, J. E., and B. E. Gidal. Melatonin: therapeutic use in sleep disorders. Ann Pharmacother 31:1218–1226, 1997.

Davidson, J. R. Use of benzodiazepines in panic disorder. J Clin Psychiatry 58(supplement 2):26–31, 1997.

Griffiths, R. R., and E. M. Weerts. Benzodiazepine self-administration in humans and laboratory animals: implications for problems of long-term use and abuse. Psychopharmacology (Berl) 134:1–37, 1997.

Kendler, B. S. Melatonin: media hype or therapeutic breakthrough? Nurse Pract 22:66–77, 1997.

Morgan, P. J., et al. Evaluation of zolpidem, triazolam, and placebo as hypnotic drugs the night before surgery. J Clin Anesth 9:97–102, 1997.

Roache, J. D., et al. Alprazolam reinforced medication use in outpatients with anxiety. Drug Alcohol Depend 45:143–155, 1997.

Robertson, J. M., and P. E. Tanguay. Case study: the use of melatonin in a boy with refractory bipolar disorder. J Am Acad Child Adolesc Psychiatry 36:822–825, 1997.

Ware, J. C., et al. Minimal rebound insomnia after treatment with 10-mg zolpidem. Clin Neuropharmacol 20:116–125, 1997.

CHAPTER TWENTY

ANTIEPILEPTIC DRUGS

CLASSIFICATION OF ANTIEPILEPTIC DRUGS*

Drugs for partial seizures and generalized tonic-clonic seizures
- Carbamazepine
- Phenobarbital
- Phenytoin
- Primidone
- Valproate

Adjunct drugs for partial seizures
- Clorazepate
- Felbamate
- Gabapentin
- Lamotrigine
- Topiramate

Drugs for generalized absence, myoclonic, or atonic seizures
- Clonazepam
- Ethosuximide
- Lamotrigine
- Valproate

Drugs for status epilepticus
- Diazepam
- Lorazepam
- Phenobarbital
- Phenytoin

*Note that some drugs are listed more than once.

OVERVIEW

Seizures are episodes of abnormal electrical activity in the brain that cause involuntary movements, sensations, or thoughts. Seizures may result from head trauma, stroke, brain tumors, hypoxia, hypoglycemia, fever, alcohol withdrawal, and other conditions that alter neuronal function. Recurrent seizures that cannot be attributed to any proximal cause are seen in patients with **epilepsy.** In some patients, epilepsy appears to have a genetic basis. Environmental perturbations, such as intrauterine or neonatal complications, have also been implicated in the development of epilepsy. In the USA, epilepsy affects 1–2% of the population and is the second most common neurologic disease (stroke is the most common).

Classification of Seizures

There are two main categories of seizures, **partial (focal) seizures** and **generalized seizures**

(Table 20–1). A partial seizure originates in one cerebral hemisphere, and the patient does not lose consciousness during the seizure. A generalized seizure arises in both cerebral hemispheres and involves loss of consciousness. Seizures are accompanied by characteristic changes in the electroencephalogram (EEG), as shown in Fig. 20–1. Most seizures are self-limited and last from about 10 seconds to 5 minutes. Some seizures are preceded by an **aura,** which is a sensation or mood that may help identify the anatomic location of the seizure focus.

About 60% of epileptic seizures are partial seizures. Electroencephalographic abnormalities are seen in one or more lobes of a cerebral hemisphere, and the patient may exhibit motor, sensory, and autonomic symptoms. In **simple partial seizures,** consciousness is not altered. However, in **complex partial seizures,** patients have an altered consciousness and exhibit repetitive behaviors (automatisms). Complex partial seizures often originate in the temporal lobe, in which case the disorder is called either **temporal lobe epilepsy** or **psychomotor epilepsy.** Some partial seizures progress along anatomic lines as the electrical discharges spread across the cortex. For example, the seizure first involves the fingers, then the hand, and finally the entire arm. This is characteristic of **jacksonian epilepsy,** or **jacksonian march.** Partial seizures may also evolve into generalized seizures.

The two main types of generalized seizures are **tonic-clonic seizures** and **absence seizures.** Generalized tonic-clonic seizures, which were formerly called **grand mal seizures,** begin with a brief tonic phase that is followed by a clonic phase with muscle spasms lasting 3–5 minutes, and they conclude with a postictal period of drowsiness, confusion, and a glazed look in the eyes. **Status epilepticus** is a condition in which patients experience recurrent episodes of tonic-clonic seizures without regaining consciousness or normal muscle movement between episodes. Generalized absence seizures, or **petit mal seizures,** are characterized by abrupt loss of consciousness and decreased muscle tone, and they may include a mild clonic component, automatisms, and autonomic effects. On the EEG, generalized absence seizures exhibit a synchronous 3-Hz (3 cycles per second) spike-and-wave pattern that usually lasts 10–15 seconds.

Less common types of generalized seizures include **myoclonic seizures** and **atonic seizures** (see Table 20–1).

TABLE 20–1. International Classification of Partial and Generalized Seizures

Classification	Characterization
Partial (focal) seizures	Arise in one cerebral hemisphere.
Simple partial seizure	No alteration of consciousness.
Complex partial seizure	Altered consciousness, automatisms, and behavioral changes.
Secondarily generalized seizure	Focal seizure becomes generalized and is accompanied by loss of consciousness.
Generalized seizures	Arise in both cerebral hemispheres and are accompanied by loss of consciousness.
Tonic-clonic (grand mal) seizure	Increased muscle tone is followed by spasms of muscle contraction and relaxation.
Tonic seizure	Increased muscle tone.
Clonic seizure	Spasms of muscle contraction and relaxation.
Myoclonic seizure	Rhythmic, jerking spasms.
Atonic seizure	Sudden loss of all muscle tone.
Absence (petit mal) seizure	Brief loss of consciousness, with minor muscle twitches and eye blinking.

Neurobiology of Seizures

Epileptic seizures are caused by synchronous neuronal discharges within a particular group of neurons, or **seizure focus,** which is often located in the cerebral cortex but may be found in other areas of the brain. Once initiated, the abnormal discharges spread to other parts of the brain and produce abnormal movements, sensations, or thoughts. The neuronal mechanisms that initiate a seizure are not fully understood, but there is growing evidence for the involvement of excessive excitatory neurotransmission mediated by **glutamate** (Fig. 20–2). Investigators believe that excessive activation of glutamate's N-methyl-D-aspartate receptors, or **NMDA receptors,** displaces Mg^{2+} ions from the **NMDA-calcium ionophore** and thereby facilitates calcium entry into neurons. **Calcium** is thought to contribute to the long-term potentiation of excitatory glutamate neurotransmission by activating the synthesis of nitric oxide.

Nitric oxide is a gas that may diffuse backward to the presynaptic neuron, where it facilitates glutamate release via stimulation of a G protein that activates the synthesis of cyclic guanosine monophosphate (cyclic GMP, or cGMP). These actions further increase NMDA receptor activation and calcium influx, which are believed to contribute to the **depolarization shift** that is observed in seizure foci. The depolarization shift consists of abnormally prolonged action potentials (depolarizations) that have spikelets. The shift recruits and synchronizes depolarizations by surrounding neurons and thereby initiates a seizure.

Several other mechanisms may be involved in seizures. One is the suppression of inhibitory neurotransmission of **gamma-aminobutyric acid** (GABA), and another is an increase in calcium influx via T-type calcium channels in thalamic neurons.

Mechanisms of Antiepileptic Drugs

Antiepileptic drugs are believed to suppress the formation or spread of abnormal electrical discharges in the brain. As shown in Table 20–2, the currently available drugs accomplish these actions via three mechanisms: (1) inhibition of the sodium or calcium influx responsible for neuronal depolarization, (2) augmentation of inhibitory GABA neurotransmission, and (3) inhibition of excitatory glutamate neurotransmission.

Effects on Ion Flux

Under normal circumstances, **voltage-sensitive (voltage-gated) sodium channels** are rapidly opened when the neuronal membrane potential (voltage) reaches its threshold. This causes rapid depolarization of the membrane and the conduction of an action potential along the neuronal axon. When the action potential reaches the nerve terminal, it evokes the release of a neurotransmitter. After the neuronal membrane is depolarized, the sodium channel is inactivated by closure of the channel's inactivation gate. The inactivation gate must be opened before the next action potential can occur.

Many antiepileptic drugs, including carbamazepine, lamotrigine, phenytoin, and topiramate, prolong the time that the sodium channel's inactivation gate remains closed, and this delays the formation of the next action potential. These drugs bind to the channel when it is opened. Since rapidly firing neurons are opened a greater percentage of the time than are slowly firing neurons, the drugs exhibit use-dependent blockade. For this reason, the drugs suppress abnormal repetitive depolarizations in a seizure focus more than they suppress normal neuronal activity. By these actions, carbamazepine and other drugs prevent the spread of abnormal discharges from a seizure focus to other neurons.

A few drugs, such as ethosuximide and valproate, block **T-type (low-threshold) calcium channels** that are located in thalamic neurons and participate in the initiation of generalized absence seizures.

Effects on Gamma-Aminobutyric Acid

Antiepileptic drugs facilitate GABA neurotransmission by various means. Benzodiazepines (such as clonazepam) and barbiturates (such as phenobarbital) enhance GABA activation of the **GABA-chloride ionophore** (see Chapter 19). Topiramate is believed to enhance activation of the **GABA_A receptor.** Gabapentin increases GABA release, whereas valproate inhibits GABA degradation. Drugs that augment GABA may serve to counteract the excessive excitatory neurotransmission responsible for initiating and spreading abnormal electrical discharges.

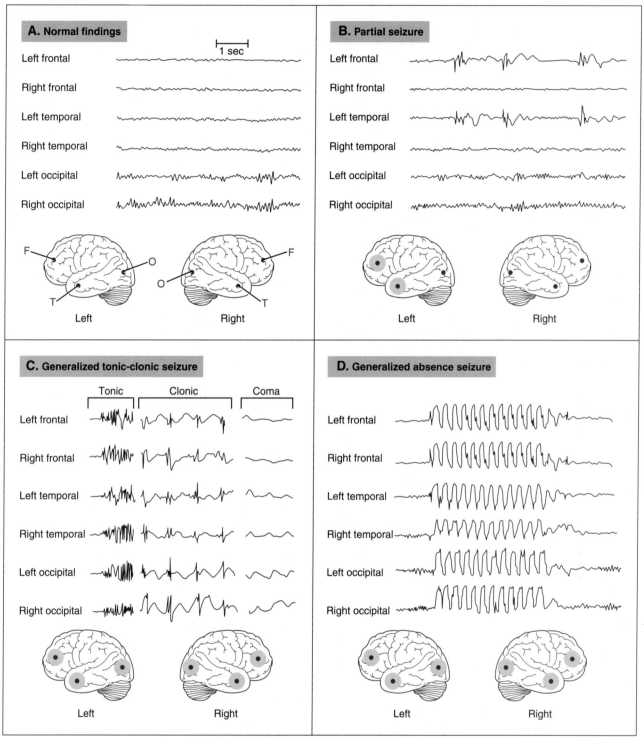

FIGURE 20–1. Patterns on electroencephalogram (EEG) in the normal state and during seizures. The locations of seizure foci are shown as shaded areas on the cerebral hemispheres. **(A)** In the normal state, the EEG shows asynchronous alpha (8–12 Hz) and beta (12–30 Hz) rhythms originating in the cortex of the frontal (F), temporal (T), and occipital (O) lobes. **(B)** During a partial seizure, synchronous discharges are observed in various areas of the brain. In this example, they are seen in the left frontal and left temporal lobes, but they are not seen in other lobes. **(C)** During a generalized tonic-clonic seizure, the tonic phase is characterized by low-frequency and high-amplitude waves, while the clonic phase shows synchronous oscillations. **(D)** During a generalized absence seizure, a synchronous 3-Hz spike-and-wave pattern is seen throughout the cortex.

Effects on Glutamate

A few antiepileptic drugs, including felbamate, topiramate, and valproate, inhibit glutamate neurotransmission, and other drugs that work via this mechanism are under development. This is an attractive mechanism of action because it may affect the formation of a seizure focus and thereby terminate a seizure at an early stage of its development.

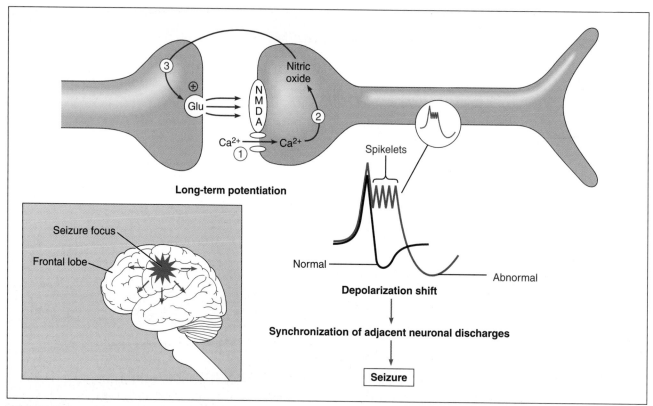

FIGURE 20–2. Neuronal mechanisms underlying seizures. In this example, a seizure is caused by the synchronous discharge of a group of neurons (focus) in the cortex. Activation of N-methyl-D-aspartate (NMDA) receptors increases calcium influx and nitric oxide synthesis. Nitric oxide then diffuses to the presynaptic neuron and increases the release of glutamate (Glu) via formation of cyclic guanosine monophosphate. Increased excitatory glutamate neurotransmission leads to long-term potentiation. Long-term potentiation is believed to facilitate a depolarization shift, characterized by prolonged depolarizations with spikelets. The depolarization shift may cause adjacent neurons to discharge synchronously and thereby precipitate a seizure.

TABLE 20–2. Mechanisms of Antiepileptic Drugs*

Drug	Effects on Ion Flux	Effects on GABA	Effects on Glutamate
Carbamazepine	Blocks voltage-sensitive sodium channels.	—	—
Clonazepam	—	Enhances GABA-mediated chloride flux.	—
Clorazepate	—	Enhances GABA-mediated chloride flux.	—
Diazepam	—	Enhances GABA-mediated chloride flux.	—
Ethosuximide	Blocks T-type calcium channels.	—	—
Felbamate	—	—	Blocks glycine activation of NMDA receptors.
Gabapentin	—	Increases GABA release.	—
Lamotrigine	Blocks voltage-sensitive sodium channels.	—	—
Lorazepam	—	Enhances GABA-mediated chloride flux.	—
Phenobarbital	—	Enhances GABA-mediated chloride flux.	—
Phenytoin	Blocks voltage-sensitive sodium channels.	—	—
Primidone	Possibly blocks voltage-sensitive sodium channels.	Enhances GABA-mediated chloride flux.	—
Topiramate	Blocks voltage-sensitive sodium channels.	Increases GABA activation of $GABA_A$ receptors.	Blocks kainate and AMPA receptors.
Valproate	Possibly blocks voltage-sensitive sodium channels and T-type calcium channels.	Increases GABA synthesis and inhibits GABA degradation.	Possibly decreases glutamate synthesis.

*AMPA = α-amino-3-hydroxy-5-methyl-4-isoxazole propionic acid; GABA = gamma-aminobutyric acid; and NMDA = N-methyl-D-aspartate.

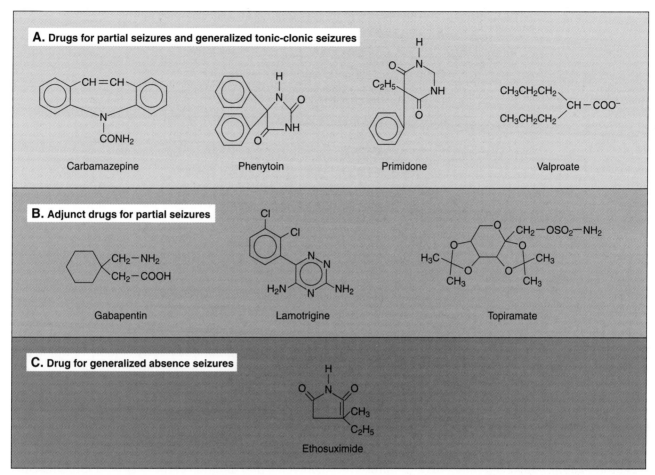

FIGURE 20–3. Structures of selected antiepileptic drugs. (A) Drugs for partial seizures and generalized tonic-clonic seizures include carbamazepine, which has a tricyclic structure that resembles the structure of tricyclic antidepressants such as imipramine; phenytoin, a hydantoin derivative; primidone, a barbiturate congener; and valproate, a low-molecular-weight, branched-chain fatty acid. **(B)** Adjunct drugs for partial seizures include gabapentin, a gamma-aminobutyric acid analogue; lamotrigine, a phenyltriazine; and topiramate, a monosaccharide derivative. **(C)** Ethosuximide is a succinimide derivative that is used to treat generalized absence seizures. Valproate and lamotrigine are also used for this purpose.

DRUGS

As indicated in the list at the beginning of this chapter, some drugs are active against only one or two types of seizures. In contrast, valproate has a broad spectrum of activity and is active against most types of seizures. Newer agents, such as lamotrigine and topiramate, are primarily used in combination with other drugs for the treatment of partial seizures. These newer agents are particularly useful because complex partial seizures are more resistant to treatment than are other types of seizures.

The pharmacologic properties of antiepileptic drugs are described below, while the chemical structures, pharmacokinetic properties, adverse effects, contraindications, and drug interactions are depicted in Fig. 20–3 and Tables 20–3, 20–4, and 20–5.

Drugs for Partial Seizures and Generalized Tonic-Clonic Seizures

The first-line drugs for partial seizures and generalized tonic-clonic seizures are carbamazepine,

phenytoin, and valproate. Carbamazepine and phenytoin have a similar mechanism of action and clinical effectiveness, and both drugs induce cytochrome P450 enzymes and increase drug metabolism. Valproate acts by a different mechanism and inhibits cytochrome P450 enzymes. Two other drugs that are effective against partial seizures as well as generalized tonic-clonic seizures are phenobarbital and primidone.

Carbamazepine

Chemistry and Pharmacokinetics. Carbamazepine has a tricyclic structure (see Fig. 20–3A) that resembles the structure of tricyclic antidepressants such as imipramine. Carbamazepine is adequately absorbed after oral administration, and it is biotransformed to an active metabolite, carbamazepine epoxide. Almost all of the drug is excreted as metabolites in the urine and feces.

Mechanisms and Effects. Carbamazepine blocks voltage-sensitive sodium channels in neuronal cell membranes. As described earlier, blockade of

TABLE 20-3. Pharmacokinetic Properties of Antiepileptic Drugs*

Drug	Oral Bioavailability	Time to Steady State	Elimination Half-Life and Route	Therapeutic Serum Concentration
Carbamazepine	80%	2–4 days	14 hours (M)	4–12 μg/mL
Clonazepam	95%	3–7 days	35 hours (M)	0.02–0.08 μg/mL
Clorazepate	95%	Not established	60 hours (M)	Not established
Diazepam	NA	NA	50 hours (M)	Not established
Ethosuximide	No data (well absorbed)	7–12 days	30 hours† (R and M)	40–100 μg/mL
Felbamate	90%	3–5 days	20 hours (R and M)	Not established
Gabapentin	60% (inversely related to dose)	1–2 days	5 hours (R)	Not established (probably >2 μg/mL)
Lamotrigine	98%	2–3 days	24 hours (R and M)	Not established (probably >3 μg/mL)
Lorazepam	NA	NA	15 hours (M)	Not established
Phenobarbital	95%	16–21 days	80 hours (M)	15–40 μg/mL
Phenytoin	Slow and variable	7–14 days (highly variable)	Dose-dependent (M)	10–20 μg/mL
Primidone	95%	1–5 days	10 hours (M)	5–12 μg/mL
Topiramate	80%	4–8 days	21 hours (R)	Not established
Valproate	93%	2–4 days	14 hours (M)	50–100 μg/mL

*Values shown are the mean of values reported in the literature. M = metabolic elimination; NA = not applicable (not administered orally); and R = renal elimination.
†The value shown is for children.

these channels inhibits the spread of abnormal electrical discharges from the seizure focus to other neurons by preventing the release of excitatory neurotransmitters from nerve terminals. Carbamazepine has additional mechanisms of action, but their contributions to its antiepileptic effects are unknown. For example, carbamazepine blocks adenosine receptors in a way that leads to up-regulation of these receptors, and it blocks norepinephrine reuptake in the same way that tricyclic antidepressants block it. The latter action is probably responsible for the mood-elevating effect of carbamazepine.

Carbamazepine may cause drowsiness, ataxia, and other symptoms of central nervous system (CNS) depression, as well as gastrointestinal reactions. Rarely, its use has been associated with aplastic anemia. In general, carbamazepine usually produces fewer adverse effects than does phenytoin.

Interactions. Carbamazepine is a potent inducer of cytochrome P450 enzymes that metabolize a wide range of drugs. Carbamazepine accelerates its own metabolism as well as that of many other drugs, including lamotrigine, phenytoin, topiramate, and valproate. For this reason, it decreases the serum level and effects of these drugs. Carbamazepine may also increase lithium toxicity.

Indications. In addition to its use in treating **partial seizures** and **generalized tonic-clonic seizures,** carbamazepine is the drug of choice for **trigeminal neuralgia** (tic douloureux), a condition that may cause chronic and intense pain on one or both sides of the face. Carbamazepine is also effective as an alternative to lithium in the treatment of **bipolar disorder,** a mood disorder discussed in Chapter 22.

Phenytoin

Chemistry and Pharmacokinetics. Phenytoin is a hydantoin derivative that was formerly called diphenylhydantoin. It is poorly soluble in water, and different pharmaceutical formulations of it may have different bioavailabilities. Hence, it is prudent to avoid switching from one formulation to another. If a switch must be made, serum drug levels should be monitored. A new formulation, called **fosphenytoin,** has become available for parenteral administration. Fosphenytoin is more soluble in water, and this prevents precipitation of the drug after intramuscular or intravenous administration.

Phenytoin is converted to an inactive hydroxylated metabolite by cytochrome P450 enzymes. The drug exhibits dose-dependent kinetics, whereby lower concentrations are eliminated by a first-order process but higher concentrations saturate biotransformation enzymes and exhibit zero-order kinetics. Phenytoin hydroxylation also exhibits genetic polymorphism. These factors are responsible for the considerable interpatient variation in the plasma drug concentrations produced by a given dose. Because of this variation, serum drug levels should be monitored at the start of therapy and whenever toxicity or therapeutic failure occurs.

Mechanisms and Effects. Like carbamazepine, phenytoin blocks voltage-sensitive sodium channels by prolonging the inactivation state of these channels. This enables phenytoin to inhibit the repetitive firing of neurons in a seizure focus.

Phenytoin may cause a number of adverse effects. The drug interferes with folate metabolism, and this may lead to megaloblastic anemia. Folate antagonism may also contribute to birth defects such as those seen in fetal hydantoin syndrome (a syndrome characterized by cardiac defects; malformation of ears, lips, palate, mouth, and nasal bridge; mental retardation; microcephaly; ptosis; strabismus; and other anomalies). By impairing cerebellar function, phenytoin may cause ataxia, diplopia, nystagmus, and slurred speech. By interfering with vitamin D metabolism and decreasing calcium absorption from the gut, phenytoin sometimes causes osteomalacia. Phenytoin adversely affects collagen metabolism and thereby contributes to gingival hyperplasia, a condition in which the gums may extend down over the teeth if good dental hygiene is not practiced. It may also cause hirsutism (excessive hair growth). Because of these effects, phenytoin use in children should generally be avoided.

Interactions. Phenytoin induces the CYP3A4 isozyme of cytochrome P450 and accelerates the metabolism of other antiepileptic agents, including felbamate, lamotrigine, topiramate, and valproate. It may also reduce levels of digoxin, steroids, vitamin K, and other drugs. In patients who are being treated with phenytoin, vitamin K supplements should be given to prevent hypoprothrombinemia and bleeding.

Carbamazepine induces the metabolism of phenytoin and decreases its serum levels, whereas cimetidine and other drugs inhibit the metabolism of phenytoin and increase its serum levels.

Indications. Despite its many adverse effects and drug interactions, phenytoin is widely used in the treatment of **partial seizures** and **generalized tonic-clonic seizures.** Like carbamazepine, it may worsen absence seizures and should not be used in patients with this type of seizures.

Phenobarbital and Primidone

Phenobarbital and primidone are both second-line drugs for **partial seizures** and **generalized tonic-clonic seizures.** Phenobarbital, a barbiturate, is the oldest of the currently used antiepileptic drugs.

TABLE 20–4. Adverse Effects, Contraindications, and Pregnancy Risk Data for Antiepileptic Drugs

Drug	Major Adverse Effects	Contraindications	Risk Category and Effects of Use During Pregnancy*
Carbamazepine	Aplastic anemia (rare); ataxia, drowsiness, and other symptoms of central nervous system (CNS) depression; gastrointestinal reactions; and nausea.	Hypersensitivity.	Category C; increased risk of birth defects; abnormal facial features; neural tube defects, such as spina bifida; reduced head size; and other anomalies.
Clonazepam	Arrhythmia; CNS depression; drug dependence; hypotension; and mild respiratory depression.	Acute angle-closure glaucoma; hypersensitivity; and severe liver disease.	Category C; apnea in newborn; increased risk of birth defects.
Clorazepate	Confusion; drowsiness; drug tolerance; and lethargy.	Hypersensitivity.	Category D; increased risk of birth defects.
Diazepam	Same as clonazepam.	Same as clonazepam.	Category D; increased risk of birth defects.
Ethosuximide	Dizziness; drowsiness; gastric distress; lethargy; and nausea.	Hypersensitivity.	Category C.
Felbamate	Aplastic anemia; fatigue; gastrointestinal reactions; headache; hepatic toxicity; and insomnia.	Bone marrow depression; hepatic disease; and hypersensitivity.	Category C.
Gabapentin	Ataxia; dizziness; drowsiness; nystagmus; and tremor.	Hypersensitivity.	Category C.
Lamotrigine	Ataxia; diplopia; dizziness; drowsiness; headache; nausea; rash; and Stevens-Johnson syndrome.	Hypersensitivity. Use cautiously in patients who are taking valproate or have hepatic or renal disease.	Category C; may reduce folate levels.
Lorazepam	Same as clonazepam.	Same as clonazepam.	Category D; increased risk of birth defects.
Phenobarbital	Ataxia; cognitive impairment; dizziness; drowsiness; drug dependence; rash; and respiratory depression.	Hypersensitivity; porphyria; respiratory depression; and severe liver disease.	Category D; bleeding at birth; minor congenital defects.
Phenytoin	Cerebellar symptoms; gastrointestinal disturbances; gingival hyperplasia; hirsutism; megaloblastic anemia and other blood cell deficiencies; osteomalacia; and psychiatric changes.	Bradycardia; hypersensitivity; and severe atrioventricular block or sinoatrial dysfunction.	Category D; may reduce folate levels; 2–3 times increased risk of birth defects; fetal hydantoin syndrome.
Primidone	Same as phenobarbital.	Hypersensitivity.	Category D.
Topiramate	Ataxia; dizziness; drowsiness; nystagmus; paresthesia; and psychomotor impairment.	Hypersensitivity. Use cautiously during pregnancy, during lactation, or in the presence of hepatic or renal disease.	Category C.
Valproate	Drowsiness; gastrointestinal disturbances; hepatic toxicity (rare); nausea; and weight gain.	Hepatic disease and hypersensitivity.	Category D; may reduce folate levels; teratogenic during the first trimester; neural tube defects, such as spina bifida.

*Pregnancy risk categories are defined by the Food and Drug Administration as follows: A = controlled studies show no risk; B = no evidence of risk in humans; C = risk cannot be ruled out; D = positive evidence of risk; and X = contraindicated in pregnancy.

TABLE 20–5. Interactions of Antiepileptic Drugs

Antiepileptic Drug	Interacting Drugs That Increase Serum Levels*	Interacting Drugs That Decrease Serum Levels†	Interactions That Cause Other Effects
Carbamazepine	Cimetidine, diltiazem, erythromycin, fluoxetine, isoniazid, and propoxyphene.	Carbamazepine.	Decreases serum levels of calcium channel blockers, clozapine, haloperidol, steroids, theophylline, thyroid, and warfarin. Increases lithium toxicity.
Clonazepam	Cimetidine and disulfiram.	Rifampin.	Increases central nervous system (CNS) depression if alcohol is ingested.
Clorazepate	Cimetidine and disulfiram.	Rifampin.	Increases CNS depression if alcohol is ingested.
Diazepam	Cimetidine.	Rifampin.	Increases CNS depression if alcohol is ingested.
Ethosuximide	Valproate.	—	May alter seizure pattern if taken in combination with haloperidol.
Felbamate	—	Carbamazepine and phenytoin.	Increases CNS depression if alcohol is ingested.
Gabapentin	—	Antacids.	—
Lamotrigine	Valproate.	Carbamazepine, phenobarbital, and phenytoin.	Decreases serum levels of valproate.
Lorazepam	—	Rifampin.	Increases CNS depression if alcohol is ingested.
Phenobarbital	Valproate.	Phenobarbital.	Decreases serum levels of many drugs. Increases meperidine toxicity.
Phenytoin	Chloramphenicol, cimetidine, isoniazid, and sulfonamides.	Carbamazepine.	Decreases serum levels of amiodarone, digoxin, quinidines, steroids, theophylline, vitamin K, and other agents.
Primidone	Valproate.	Phenobarbital.	—
Topiramate	—	Carbamazepine and phenytoin.	Decreases serum levels of oral contraceptives.
Valproate	Salicylates.	Carbamazepine, lamotrigine, and phenytoin.	May increase or decrease serum levels of carbamazepine and phenytoin.

*These drugs inhibit metabolism.
†Except for antacids (which reduce the absorption of gabapentin), these drugs induce metabolism.

Its pharmacologic properties are discussed in Chapter 19. Primidone has two active metabolites, phenobarbital and phenylethylmalonamide (PEMA), and the parent drug and its active metabolites probably all contribute to its antiepileptic effects.

Phenobarbital enhances the GABA-mediated chloride flux that causes membrane hyperpolarization. Primidone probably acts primarily by blocking sodium channels and preventing membrane depolarization. It may also potentiate GABA via formation of phenobarbital. Both primidone and phenobarbital are well absorbed from the gut, but primidone has a shorter half-life and therefore reaches steady-state levels more rapidly. Both drugs can cause ataxia, dizziness, drowsiness, and cognitive impairment. In excessive doses, they may depress respiration. Hypersensitivity to these drugs develops in a few patients and most frequently presents as a rash.

Valproate

Chemistry and Pharmacokinetics. Valproate is a low-molecular-weight, branched-chain fatty acid (see Fig. 20–3A). Several valproate formulations are available, including the free acid form (**valproic acid**), the sodium salt of valproic acid (**valproate sodium**), and a 1:1 mixture of valproic acid and valproate sodium (**divalproex sodium**). Divalproex sodium is absorbed more slowly than the other formulations, and it usually causes fewer adverse gastrointestinal and CNS side effects. Valproate is well absorbed from the gut and is metabolized to active metabolites and inactive conjugates before it is excreted.

Mechanisms and Effects. Valproate has several mechanisms of action that probably contribute to its broad spectrum of antiepileptic effects. It inhibits voltage-sensitive sodium channels and T-type calcium channels; it increases GABA synthesis and decreases GABA degradation; and it may decrease glutamate synthesis. By these actions, valproate inhibits the repetitive firing of neurons and the spread of epileptic seizures.

Valproate produces relatively little sedation or drowsiness, but it occasionally causes nausea, gastrointestinal complaints, and weight gain. Mild hepatic toxicity sometimes occurs and is usually reversible. Rarely, the drug has been associated with fatal hepatic toxicity. To prevent liver damage, the hepatic function of patients should be monitored when they begin therapy with valproate. Patients under 2 years of age are at the greatest risk of liver failure.

Valproate has been associated with an increased incidence of spina bifida and other birth defects in the offspring of women treated with the drug during pregnancy.

Interactions. Valproate inhibits the metabolism of other drugs and may increase the serum levels of lamotrigine, phenobarbital, and primidone. It may either increase or decrease the levels of carbamazepine and phenytoin, whereas these drugs decrease the levels of valproate. Because of these interactions, serum levels should always be monitored when another drug is added to or removed from the treatment regimen of a patient with seizure disorders. Patients should be warned that salicylates may increase the serum levels of valproate.

Indications. Of the various antiepileptic drugs, valproate has the broadest spectrum of activity. It is effective in the treatment of **partial seizures** and **all forms of generalized seizures,** and it may be given in combination with other drugs when a single drug does not adequately control seizures (see below). Valproate is also used as an alternative to lithium for the treatment of **bipolar disorder** (see Chapter 22).

Adjunct Drugs for Partial Seizures

The most difficult type of seizures to control with drug therapy are partial seizures and especially complex partial seizures. Therefore, efforts have focused on developing new drugs for these seizures. Unlike clorazepate, the other drugs discussed below have recently been introduced. Additional drugs are currently in development and include tiagabine, vigabatrin, and zonisamide.

Clorazepate

Clorazepate is a prodrug that is converted to diazepam in the body. Although it primarily has been used to treat patients with **anxiety disorders,** it also has been found useful as an adjunct drug for the treatment of **partial seizures.** It may cause drowsiness and lethargy, and tolerance may occur during long-term use of the drug.

Felbamate

Felbamate was a promising new drug for the treatment of partial seizures and other types of seizures until cases of fatal aplastic anemia and acute hepatic failure were reported. Since 1994, felbamate has been limited to the treatment of **partial seizures that are refractory to other drugs.** Felbamate has a unique mechanism of action in that it blocks glycine activation of NMDA receptors and may thereby inhibit processes responsible for the initiation of seizures. Efforts are under way to develop other drugs that act via this mechanism but exhibit less toxicity than felbamate.

Gabapentin

Gabapentin is a GABA analogue (see Fig. 20–3B) that appears to act by increasing the release of GABA from central neurons. It has no direct effect on GABA receptors itself. The absorption of gabapentin from the gut is inversely related to the dose. Because the drug has a relatively short half-life, it must be given several times a day. Gabapentin is effective when used in combination with other drugs to treat **all forms of partial seizures,** and studies indicate that for many patients it is also effective when used alone. Its adverse effects are minimal at usual therapeutic doses, but it may cause ataxia, dizziness, drowsiness, nystagmus, and tremor.

Lamotrigine

Lamotrigine blocks voltage-sensitive sodium channels and thereby interferes with neuronal membrane conduction and the release of excitatory neurotransmitters such as glutamate. It appears to be one of the more effective adjunct drugs for treating **partial seizures** in adults and children. It also appears to be useful in the treatment of **generalized tonic-clonic, atonic, and absence seizures** and in the treatment of **Lennox-Gastaut syndrome,** a syndrome characterized by multiple types of seizures in patients with mental retardation and other neurologic abnormalities.

Lamotrigine has excellent oral bioavailability. It is mostly conjugated with glucuronate in the liver and excreted by the kidneys. Serum levels of lamotrigine are decreased by carbamazepine and phenytoin and are increased by valproate. Serum levels of valproate are decreased by lamotrigine.

The primary side effects of lamotrigine include cerebellar dysfunction, drowsiness, and rash. Patients should be advised to report early signs of skin changes, because the rash may progress to Stevens-Johnson syndrome. This potentially fatal syndrome is a severe form of erythema multiforme and is characterized by mucocutaneous and systemic lesions, including ocular, gastrointestinal, cardiac, renal, and pulmonary inflammation and hemorrhage. The syndrome is more common in patients who are being treated with the combination of lamotrigine and valproate, possibly because valproate increases the serum level of lamotrigine. If children are treated with both drugs, the dosage of lamotrigine should be lower than that used in other patients. Dosage guidelines are provided in prescribing compendiums.

Topiramate

Topiramate is a monosaccharide derivative that has several mechanisms of action, including blockade of voltage-sensitive sodium channels; augmentation of GABA activation of $GABA_A$ receptors; and blockade of two types of glutamate receptors—namely, kainate receptors and α-amino-3-hydroxy-5-methyl-4-isoxazole propionic acid (AMPA) receptors.

Clinical studies indicate that about half of patients who have intractable partial seizures experience a 50% reduction in seizure frequency when topiramate is added to their treatment regimen. Therefore, topiramate is approved for adjunct use in the treatment of **partial seizures.** Because it has also demonstrated effectiveness as single-drug therapy (monotherapy) for partial seizures and as an adjunct in the treatment of generalized seizures, it may receive approval for these indications in the future.

Topiramate is adequately absorbed from the gut, is partly metabolized before excretion in the urine, and has a half-life of about 21 hours. Carbamazepine and phenytoin may induce the metabolism of topiramate and decrease its serum level. Topiramate may reduce the serum level of oral contraceptives. The side effects of topiramate include ataxia, dizziness, drowsiness, and other CNS effects listed in Table 20–4.

Drugs for Generalized Absence, Myoclonic, or Atonic Seizures

Ethosuximide

Chemistry and Pharmacokinetics. Ethosuximide, a drug whose structure is shown in Fig. 20–3C, is the most effective and least toxic of the several succinimide derivatives that have been used to treat epilepsy over the past 50 years. It is well absorbed from the gut, is widely distributed to tissues, and is metabolized to inactive compounds before it is excreted in the urine. Ethosuximide has a relatively long half-life of about 30 hours in children and 55 hours in adults.

Mechanisms and Effects. Ethosuximide inhibits T-type calcium channels in thalamic neurons. These low-threshold channels are believed to be responsible for the pacemaker current that generates the synchronous 3-Hz (3 cycles per second) spike-and-wave depolarizations observed in the EEG during absence seizures (see Fig. 20–1). Ethosuximide produces little toxicity, but it may cause dizziness, drowsiness, gastric distress, and nausea. These can usually be minimized by starting treatment with lower doses and then gradually increasing doses to the desired level.

Interactions. Valproate inhibits the metabolism of ethosuximide and increases its serum levels. Haloperidol (an antipsychotic drug) may alter the seizure pattern in patients treated with ethosuximide. No other important interactions have been identified.

Indications. Ethosuximide is safe and highly effective in the treatment of **generalized absence seizures in children** and is the drug of choice for this particular group of patients. However, ethosuximide is not very effective in the treatment of adults with absence seizures or of patients with other types of seizures, so valproate (discussed above) is usually used instead.

Clonazepam and Other Drugs

Clonazepam is a benzodiazepine that is used in the treatment of **absence, myoclonic, and atonic seizures.** However, it often produces more sedation than other antiepileptic drugs when used at doses that suppress seizures.

Because the efficacy of **valproate** is equal to or greater than that of clonazepam, it is frequently used instead to treat patients with **absence, myoclonic, and atonic seizures.**

Lamotrigine is sometimes used as an adjunct for the treatment of **absence and atonic seizures.**

The pharmacologic properties of valproate and lamotrigine are discussed earlier in this chapter, and those of clonazepam are discussed in Chapter 19.

Drugs for Status Epilepticus

Status epilepticus is a life-threatening emergency. Patients with this condition have recurrent episodes of tonic-clonic seizures without regaining consciousness or normal muscle movement between episodes. If their seizures are not controlled, prolonged hypoxia may lead to severe brain damage. Immediate attention must be given to cardiopulmonary support and to the administration of drugs that rapidly terminate the seizures. In fact, published reports indicate that seizures must be controlled within 60 minutes of the onset of an episode in order to have a favorable prognosis.

The drug of choice for status epilepticus is **diazepam** or **lorazepam.** Either drug is administered as a slow intravenous injection given every 10–15 minutes until seizures are controlled or a maximum dosage has been administered. The pharmacologic properties of these drugs are described in Chapter 19.

After diazepam or lorazepam is administered, **phenytoin** (or the newer form, fosphenytoin) is often administered intravenously in order to provide a longer duration of seizure control than is provided by a benzodiazepine. Large doses of **phenobarbital** may be effective if a benzodiazepine or phenytoin fails to control the seizures. In highly resistant cases, general anesthesia may be used to control the seizures.

THE MANAGEMENT OF SEIZURE DISORDERS

The effective management of patients with epilepsy requires an accurate diagnosis of the type of seizures that occur and also requires the rational selection and use of drugs.

Drugs of Choice

Table 20–6 lists the drugs of choice for treating the major types of seizures and also lists adjunct medications that may be employed in combination with a drug of choice in order to improve seizure control. The drugs of choice are based on clinical studies of their relative efficacy and safety.

For **partial seizures** and **generalized tonic-clonic seizures,** carbamazepine, phenytoin, and valproate are first-line drugs, and phenobarbital and primidone are second-line drugs. Carbamazepine generally causes fewer adverse effects than phenytoin, although phenytoin may be slightly less sedating

TABLE 20-6. Choice of Antiepileptic Drugs for Seizure Disorders*

| Drug | Partial Seizures | Generalized Seizures | | | | Status Epilepticus |
		Tonic-Clonic	Absence	Myoclonic	Atonic	
Carbamazepine	1	1	W	—	—	—
Clonazepam	—	W	3	2	1	—
Clorazepate	A	—	—	—	—	—
Diazepam	—	—	—	—	—	1
Ethosuximide	—	—	1†	—	—	—
Felbamate	A	—	—	—	—	—
Gabapentin	A	—	—	—	—	—
Lamotrigine	A	A	A	—	A	—
Lorazepam	—	—	—	—	—	1
Phenobarbital	2	2	—	—	—	3
Phenytoin	1	1	W	—	—	2
Primidone	2	2	—	—	—	—
Topiramate	A	—	—	—	—	—
Valproate	2	1	2†	1	1	—

*1 = drug of first choice; 2 = drug of second choice; 3 = drug of third choice; A = drug for adjunct use with other drugs; and W = drug may worsen the type of seizure shown.

†For absence seizures in children, ethosuximide is the drug of first choice and valproate is the drug of second choice. For absence seizures in adults, valproate is probably the drug of first choice.

than carbamazepine at equally effective doses. Of the several drugs that have been recently developed as adjunct medications for partial seizures, lamotrigine and topiramate appear particularly attractive at this time. However, the relative safety and efficacy of these drugs are still being evaluated.

For **generalized absence seizures,** ethosuximide is clearly the first choice in treating children with this condition, which usually has its onset during childhood and often remits during adolescence. Valproate is generally more effective in treating adults with absence seizures and in treating patients with multiple types of seizures.

For **generalized myoclonic and atonic seizures,** valproate is the drug of choice.

For **status epilepticus,** intravenous treatment with diazepam or lorazepam may be followed by intravenous treatment with phenytoin or phenobarbital.

Principles of Drug Use

In most cases, an attempt should be made to control seizures with single-drug therapy (monotherapy) because this will minimize side effects, reduce costs, and increase patient compliance.

Unless the patient is experiencing frequent seizures, it is usually best to start with a single drug and give it in a low dose (one-fourth to one-third of the therapeutic dose). The dose can be gradually increased until effective serum concentrations are achieved or intolerable adverse effects occur. The therapeutic serum concentrations of antiepileptic drugs and the time required to achieve steady-state levels after a change in dosage are shown in Table 20-3. Starting with a low dose enables the patient to develop tolerance to the CNS side effects of antiepileptic drugs and improves compliance.

If a single drug has significantly reduced the occurrence of seizures but has not eliminated them,

it is usually prudent to add another drug to the regimen, rather than switch to a new drug. Two drugs acting by different mechanisms may control seizures when a single drug is not adequate. The second drug should be given initially in a low dose, and the dosage should be gradually increased until therapeutic concentrations are reached or adverse effects occur. Because of the many interactions between antiepileptic drugs (see Table 20-5), the doses that are both safe and effective for combination therapy may differ from the doses that are safe and effective for monotherapy. For example, lamotrigine causes a much higher incidence of serious dermatologic toxicity in children who are concurrently taking valproate, and lamotrigine should be started at much lower doses in these patients.

Once a satisfactory drug regimen is achieved, the patient should be monitored periodically for drug toxicity and efficacy. Serum drug levels should be determined if there is evidence or suspicion of adverse effects, therapeutic failure, or patient noncompliance.

The appropriate duration of antiepileptic drug therapy is a topic of considerable controversy. If a patient who is undergoing drug therapy has not had a seizure for several years, it seems prudent to consider slowly withdrawing the medication, since this will minimize long-term side effects and offer life-style benefits and cost savings. However, about 25% of patients who withdraw from medication will relapse within 1 year. Factors that increase the likelihood of relapse include onset of seizures during adolescence, occurrence of complex partial seizures or generalized seizures, and abnormal interictal findings on EEG. If antiepileptic medication is to be discontinued, the dosage should be tapered slowly over several weeks, because abrupt withdrawal from medication is associated with a higher incidence of rebound seizures.

Summary of Important Points

- Seizures are caused by episodic, synchronous neuronal discharges in the cerebral cortex or elsewhere in the brain. They are classified as partial or generalized seizures on the basis of their clinical characteristics and electroencephalographic pattern.
- Some antiepileptic drugs work by blocking voltage-sensitive sodium channels or T-type calcium channels. Others augment inhibitory gamma-aminobutyric acid (GABA) neurotransmission or block excitatory glutamate neurotransmission.
- Carbamazepine, phenytoin, and valproate are the first-line drugs for partial seizures and generalized tonic-clonic seizures.
- Ethosuximide is the drug of choice for generalized absence seizures in children. Valproate and clonazepam are effective in absence, myoclonic, and atonic seizures.
- Gabapentin, lamotrigine, topiramate, and several other new drugs are used as adjuncts in the treatment of partial seizures, and some of these agents have activity against other types of seizures.
- Status epilepticus is a medical emergency that requires intravenous administration of diazepam or lorazepam, sometimes followed by intravenous use of phenytoin (fosphenytoin) or phenobarbital.
- Many antiepileptic drugs interact with other medications. Carbamazepine and phenytoin induce cytochrome P450 enzymes and decrease serum levels of the drugs with which they interact, whereas valproate inhibits the metabolism of the drugs with which it interacts.
- Antiepileptic drugs frequently produce central nervous system and gastrointestinal side effects, and some drugs cause infrequent but severe hematologic or hepatic toxicity. Valproate and phenytoin are known to cause birth defects, and both of these drugs may reduce folate levels.
- Except in urgent situations, antiepileptic therapy should begin with a low dose of a single drug, and the dosage should be increased until the desired serum concentration or full dosage is achieved. If a single drug is not effective, another drug may be added to the regimen or substituted. Drug use should be discontinued slowly. Serum levels should be monitored to verify adequate dosage and whenever toxicity, therapeutic failure, or noncompliance occurs or is suspected.

Selected Readings

Blum, D. E. New drugs for persons with epilepsy. *In* French, J. A., et al., eds. Antiepileptic Drug Development. Philadelphia, Lippincott-Raven, 1998.

Mattson, R. H. Antiepileptic drug monitoring: a reappraisal. Epilepsia 36(supplement 5):S22–S29, 1995.

Morris, H. H. New treatment options for epilepsy. Cleve Clin J Med 64:125–127, 1997.

Natsch, S., et al. Newer anticonvulsant drugs: role of pharmacology, drug interactions, and adverse reactions in drug choice. Drug Saf 17:228–240, 1997.

Patsalos, P. N., and J. S. Duncan. Antiepileptic drugs: a review of clinically significant drug interactions. Drug Saf 9:156–184, 1993.

Sirven, J. L., and J. D. Liporace. New antiepileptic drugs: overcoming the limitations of traditional therapy. Postgrad Med 102:147–160, 1997.

Willmore, L. J. Management of epilepsy in the elderly. Epilepsia 37(supplement 6):S23–S33, 1996.

Wilson, E. A., and M. J. Brodie. New antiepileptic drugs. Baillieres Clin Neurol 5:723–747, 1996.

Yerby, M. S. Contraception, pregnancy, and lactation in women with epilepsy. Baillieres Clin Neurol 5:887–908, 1996.

CHAPTER TWENTY-ONE

DRUGS FOR

NEURODEGENERATIVE DISEASES

CLASSIFICATION OF DRUGS FOR NEURODEGENERATIVE DISEASES*

DRUGS FOR PARKINSON'S DISEASE
  Drugs that increase dopamine levels
  • Amantadine
  • Carbidopa
  • Levodopa
  • Selegiline
  • Tolcapone
  Dopamine receptor agonists
  • Bromocriptine
  • Pergolide
  • Pramipexole
  • Ropinirole
  Acetylcholine receptor antagonists
  • Benztropine
  • Trihexyphenidyl

DRUGS FOR HUNTINGTON'S DISEASE
  • Diazepam
  • Haloperidol

DRUGS FOR ALZHEIMER'S DISEASE
  • Donepezil
  • Tacrine

DRUGS FOR MULTIPLE SCLEROSIS
  • Baclofen
  • Interferon beta-1b
  • Prednisone

DRUGS FOR AMYOTROPHIC LATERAL SCLEROSIS
  • Baclofen
  • Gabapentin
  • Riluzole

*Note that baclofen is listed more than once.

OVERVIEW

Parkinson's disease, Huntington's disease, Alzheimer's disease, multiple sclerosis, and **amyotrophic lateral sclerosis** are neurodegenerative diseases characterized by the irreversible loss of neuronal function in a particular part of the central nervous system (CNS). Although the etiology of these diseases in particular cases is usually unknown, there is evidence for the involvement of heredity, autoimmunity, and environmental factors. While substantial progress has been made in treating Parkinson's disease, drug therapy for the other neurodegenerative diseases has had only limited success. New information concerning the pathogenesis of these diseases may enable the development of more successful drugs in the near future.

PARKINSON'S DISEASE

Parkinson's disease, or **paralysis agitans,** is characterized by a **resting tremor** (involuntary trembling when a limb is at rest), **rigidity** (inability to initiate movements), and **bradykinesia** (slowness of movement). The disease results from the degeneration of **dopaminergic neurons** that arise in the substantia nigra and project to other structures in the basal ganglia.

Etiology and Pathogenesis

The causes of neuron degeneration in Parkinson's disease remain largely unknown. In most cases, heredity appears to have a limited role. However, scientists have identified a defective gene responsible for a rare condition called **autosomal recessive juvenile parkinsonism,** which begins to affect people in their teens and 20s.

One of the better-known theories for an environmental origin of Parkinson's disease is called the **oxidative stress theory.** According to this theory, oxidation of **dopamine** in the basal ganglia yields highly reactive **free radicals** that are toxic to dopaminergic neurons and lead to their degeneration. Free radicals are molecules that lack an electron in their outer orbits and are capable of extracting an electron from other biomolecules and thereby causing molecular and cellular damage.

The **basal ganglia** are a group of interconnected subcortical nuclei that include the striatum (caudate and putamen), substantia nigra, globus pallidus, and subthalamus. In healthy individuals, the basal ganglia receive input from the entire cerebral cortex, process this information, and send feedback to the motor area of the cortex in a way that leads to the smooth coordination of body movements. Even simple movements, such as walking, involve a complex sequence of motor acts whose smooth execution requires the continuous interplay of the cortex and basal ganglia. In patients with Parkinson's disease, neuron degeneration interrupts this interplay. Because the basal ganglia also participate in procedural memory and other cognitive functions, patients with Parkinson's disease may have difficulty remembering how to perform learned motor skills, such as driving a car.

The basal ganglia function via a series of reciprocal innervations among themselves and the cortex (Fig. 21–1). The striatum receives input from the cerebral cortex and substantia nigra, and it sends output to the thalamus via the globus pallidus. The thalamus then feeds information back to the motor area of the cortex. Two pathways connect the striatum and the thalamus: a **direct pathway,** which is excitatory, and an **indirect pathway,** which is inhibitory. In patients with Parkinson's disease, the degeneration of dopaminergic neurons results in decreased activity in the direct pathway and increased activity in the indirect pathway. As a result, thalamic feedback to the cortex is reduced, and patients exhibit bradykinesia and rigidity.

Excitatory **cholinergic neurons** also participate in the interconnections between structures in the basal ganglia. In Parkinson's disease, the degeneration of inhibitory dopaminergic neurons leads to excessive cholinergic activity in these pathways. For this reason, patients with Parkinson's disease can be treated effectively with drugs that inhibit cholinergic activity in the basal ganglia or with drugs that increase dopamine levels and dopaminergic activity in the basal ganglia.

Drugs That Increase Dopamine Levels

Dopamine levels in the basal ganglia can be increased by a variety of drugs in a variety of ways. Levodopa increases dopamine levels by increasing dopamine synthesis; selegiline does so by inhibiting dopamine breakdown; and amantadine does so by increasing dopamine release from neurons. Carbidopa and tolcapone increase the amount of levodopa that enters the brain and thereby enhance dopamine synthesis. The sites of action of these drugs are illustrated in Fig. 21–2.

Levodopa

Chemistry and Pharmacokinetics. Levodopa, also called L-**dopa** or **dihydroxyphenylalanine,** is the biosynthetic precursor of **dopamine.** Its structure is shown in Fig. 21–3A. Levodopa increases the concentration of dopamine in the brain and is the main treatment used to alleviate motor dysfunction in patients with Parkinson's disease. Dopamine itself is not effective in the treatment of Parkinson's disease when administered systemically, because it does not cross the blood-brain barrier.

Levodopa is absorbed from the proximal duodenum by the same process that absorbs large neutral

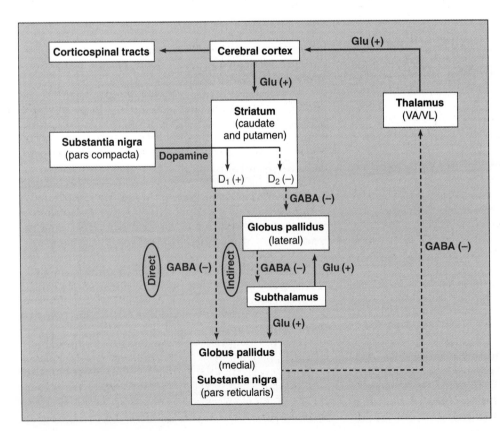

FIGURE 21–1. Pathophysiology of Parkinson's disease. The striatum receives input from the entire cerebral cortex and the substantia nigra and sends projections to the thalamus via direct and indirect pathways through the globus pallidus, substantia nigra, and subthalamus. Striatal dopamine D_1 receptors excite the direct pathway, whereas D_2 receptors inhibit the indirect pathway. In Parkinson's disease, the degeneration of dopaminergic neurons leads to decreased activity in the direct pathway and increased activity in the indirect pathway. As a result of these changes, thalamic input to the motor area of the cortex is reduced, and the patient exhibits rigidity and bradykinesia. GABA = gamma-aminobutyric acid; Glu = glutamate; VA/VL = ventral anterior and ventral lateral nuclei; (+) = excitatory; and (−) = inhibitory.

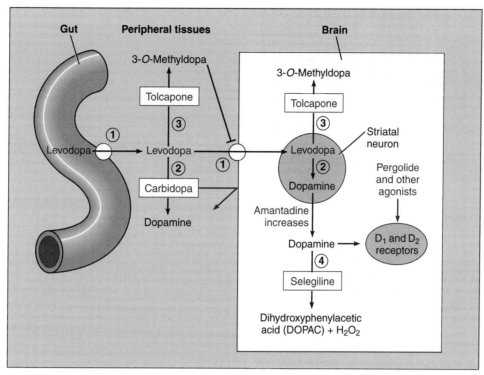

FIGURE 21–2. Mechanisms of dopaminergic drugs used in the treatment of Parkinson's disease. Levodopa is transported across the gut wall and the blood-brain barrier and is converted to dopamine in striatal neurons. Carbidopa inhibits the peripheral decarboxylation of levodopa and thereby increases the amount of levodopa that enters the brain. Carbidopa does not cross the blood-brain barrier and does not inhibit dopamine synthesis in the brain. Tolcapone inhibits the methylation of levodopa both in peripheral tissues and in the brain. Tolcapone increases levodopa bioavailability and increases brain uptake of levodopa. Selegiline inhibits the degradation of dopamine to dihydroxyphenylacetic acid (DOPAC) and hydrogen peroxide (H_2O_2). By this action, selegiline increases dopamine levels in the striatum, and it may reduce the formation of free radicals that are derived from H_2O_2. Amantadine increases the release of dopamine from striatal neurons. Pergolide and other dopamine receptor agonists activate dopamine receptors in the striatum. Numbered structures and enzymes are as follows: 1 = pump that transports large neutral amino acids; 2 = L-aromatic amino acid decarboxylase (LAAD); 3 = catechol-O-methyltransferase (COMT); and 4 = monoamine oxidase type B (MAO-B).

amino acids (see Fig. 21–2). **Dietary amino acids** compete with levodopa for transport into the circulation, and amino acids can also reduce the transport of levodopa into the brain. For these reasons, the ingestion of high-protein foods may decrease the effectiveness of levodopa, and a protein-restricted diet may improve the response to levodopa in some patients.

Levodopa is metabolized by two pathways in peripheral tissues. It is converted to **dopamine** by **L-aromatic amino acid decarboxylase** (LAAD), and it is metabolized to **3-O-methyldopa** (3OMD) by **catechol-O-methyltransferase** (COMT). A drug that inhibits LAAD (such as carbidopa) or inhibits COMT (such as tolcapone) is used in combination with levodopa to increase the amount of levodopa that enters brain tissue. LAAD requires **vitamin B$_6$ (pyridoxine)** as a cofactor. For this reason, vitamin B$_6$ supplements may enhance the peripheral decarboxylation of levodopa and should not be coadministered with levodopa.

Levodopa exhibits a large first-pass effect, and about 95% of an administered dose is metabolized in the gut wall and liver before it reaches the systemic circulation. Additional amounts of levodopa are converted to dopamine and 3OMD before

the drug enters the CNS. Therefore, only about 1% of the administered dose of levodopa reaches brain tissue.

Mechanisms and Pharmacologic Effects. In the brain, levodopa is taken up by dopaminergic neurons in the striatum and is converted to dopamine by LAAD. Levodopa thereby increases the amount of dopamine released by these neurons in patients with Parkinson's disease, and it serves as a form of replacement therapy. Levodopa can counteract all of the signs of parkinsonism, although the degree and duration of its effectiveness are usually not optimal. As the disease progresses and more dopaminergic neurons are lost, the conversion of levodopa to dopamine declines.

About 60–70% of nigrostriatal dopaminergic neurons are lost before the clinical symptoms of Parkinson's disease are first observed, and the degeneration of these neurons continues throughout the course of the disease. Over time, patients begin to experience two types of fluctuation in the effectiveness of levodopa, both of which are probably related to a reduced concentration of dopamine in the striatum. The first type, a **"wearing off" effect,** occurs toward the end of a dosage interval. The second type, the **"on-off" phenomenon,** is charac-

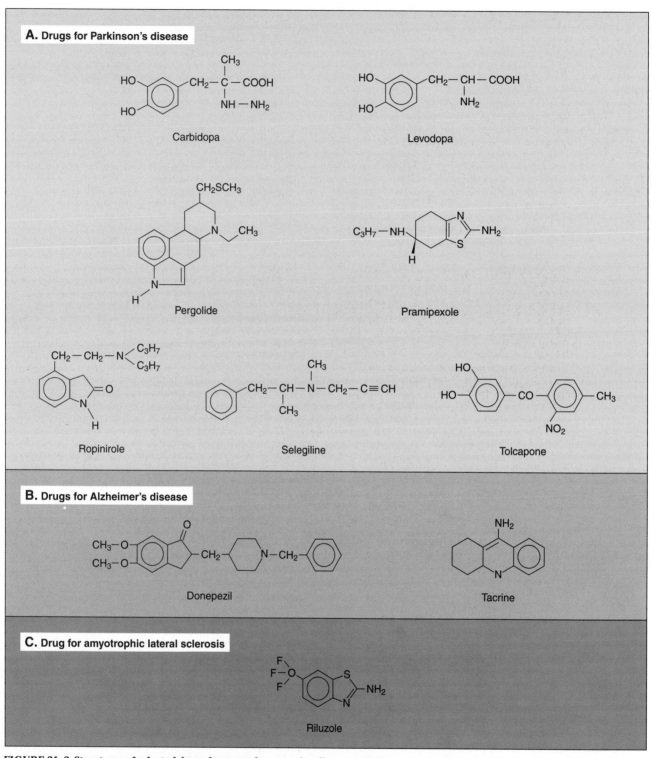

FIGURE 21–3. Structures of selected drugs for neurodegenerative diseases. (A) Numerous drugs for Parkinson's disease act by increasing dopamine levels. Examples include carbidopa, a decarboxylase inhibitor; levodopa, a dopamine precursor; selegiline, a monoamine oxidase type B (MAO-B) inhibitor; and tolcapone, a catechol-*O*-methyltransferase (COMT) inhibitor. Other drugs for Parkinson's disease serve as dopamine receptor agonists. Examples include pergolide, pramipexole, and ropinirole. **(B)** Drugs for Alzheimer's disease include donepezil and tacrine, both of which are cholinesterase inhibitors. **(C)** Riluzole, a glutamate inhibitor, was the first drug specifically approved for the treatment of amyotrophic lateral sclerosis.

terized by severe motor fluctuations that occur randomly.

Adverse Effects. When levodopa is used alone, nausea and vomiting occur in about 80% of patients, orthostatic hypotension is reported in 25%, and cardiac arrhythmias occur in 10%. These effects, which are attributed to the formation of dopamine in peripheral tissues, are substantially reduced when carbidopa is administered with levodopa to block the peripheral formation of dopamine.

About 30% of patients who are treated with levodopa on a long-term basis eventually develop involuntary movements, or dyskinesias, as a result of excessive dopamine concentrations in the striatum. Dyskinesias most often occur when levodopa concentrations are highest, in which case they are called **peak-dose dyskinesias.** The dyskinesias often involve the oral and facial musculature, and patients may appear as if they are chewing on large pieces of food while protruding their lips. Other common dyskinesias involve writhing and flinging movements of the arms and legs. Less commonly, levodopa causes psychotic effects, including hallucinations and distorted thinking, which are probably due to excessive dopamine concentrations in mesolimbic and mesocortical pathways that utilize dopamine as a neurotransmitter. Although dyskinesias and psychotic effects could be managed by reducing the levodopa dosage, the therapeutic efficacy of the drug would be reduced as well.

Some patients treated with levodopa complain of sedative effects, agitation, delirium, vivid dreams, or nightmares. However, others report a pleasant euphoria after taking the drug.

Interactions. Levodopa has important interactions with a number of medications. Drugs that delay gastric emptying, such as anticholinergic drugs, may slow levodopa absorption and reduce its peak serum concentration. Drugs that promote gastric emptying, such as antacids and cisapride, may increase levodopa bioavailability. Nonselective monoamine oxidase (MAO) inhibitors, such as phenelzine, inhibit the breakdown of dopamine and sometimes cause a hypertensive crisis in patients receiving levodopa. Antipsychotic drugs block dopamine receptors and may reduce the effectiveness of levodopa and exacerbate motor dysfunction. Because clozapine is much less likely to do this than other antipsychotic drugs, it is often used to manage psychotic reactions in patients receiving levodopa (see Chapter 22).

Indications. Levodopa is effective in the management of patients with **idiopathic Parkinson's disease** and in the treatment of patients with **postencephalitic parkinsonism** (a disorder portrayed in the movie *Awakenings*). It is also used to treat **parkinsonian symptoms caused by carbon monoxide poisoning, manganese intoxication, or cerebral arteriosclerosis.**

Carbidopa

Carbidopa, a structural analogue of levodopa, inhibits the conversion of levodopa to dopamine in peripheral tissues and thereby increases the amount of levodopa that enters the brain (see Fig. 21–2). Carbidopa is highly ionized at physiologic pH, and it does not cross the blood-brain barrier. For this reason, it does not inhibit the formation of dopamine in the CNS.

Carbidopa substantially reduces the gastrointestinal and cardiovascular side effects of levodopa, enabling about a 75% reduction in the dosage of levodopa. A **levodopa-carbidopa combination** is available in immediate-release and sustained-release formulations that contain different ratios of the two drugs. The sustained-release formulations are designed to reduce the "wearing off" effect described above.

Amantadine

Amantadine is an antiviral drug that is used in the prevention and treatment of influenza but also has a beneficial effect on Parkinson's disease. Amantadine probably works by increasing the release of dopamine from nigrostriatal neurons, but it may also inhibit the reuptake of dopamine by these neurons. Amantadine is generally better tolerated than levodopa or dopamine agonists, but it is also less effective.

Amantadine is used in the treatment of early or mild cases of Parkinson's disease and as an adjunct to levodopa. Its adverse effects include sedation, restlessness, vivid dreams, nausea, dry mouth, and hypotension. It may also cause livedo reticularis, which is a reddish-blue mottling of the skin with edema. CNS side effects are more likely to occur in the elderly because of their reduced capacity to excrete the drug by the kidneys.

Selegiline

Chemistry and Pharmacokinetics. Selegiline, also known as **deprenyl,** is a modified phenylethylamine compound whose structure is shown in Fig. 21–3A. The drug is well absorbed from the gut and is partly metabolized to amphetamine. Its pharmacokinetic properties are summarized in Table 21–1.

Mechanisms and Pharmacologic Effects. Selegiline inhibits monoamine oxidase type B (MAO-B) and thereby prevents the oxidation of dopamine to **dihydroxyphenylacetic acid** (DOPAC) and **hydrogen peroxide,** as shown in Fig. 21–2. By this action, selegiline increases dopamine levels in the basal ganglia and decreases the formation of hydrogen peroxide. In the presence of iron, hydrogen peroxide is converted to **hydroxyl and hydroxide radicals** that may participate in the degeneration of nigrostriatal neurons in patients with Parkinson's disease.

Some investigators believe that selegiline inhibits the progression of Parkinson's disease either by inhibiting the formation of free radicals or by inhibiting the formation of an active metabolite of an environmental toxin. The ability of selegiline to inhibit disease progression is controversial. It was initially suggested by studies showing that selegiline was able to prevent parkinsonism that is induced by **1-methyl-4-phenyl-1,2,3,6-tetrahydropyridine** (MPTP). MPTP is a toxic by-product of the synthesis of "designer" street drugs, and people who took drugs contaminated with MPTP in the 1980s developed classic signs of parkinsonism. MPTP must be converted to 1-methyl-4-phenylpyridium (MPP^+) by MAO-B before it can damage dopaminergic neurons, and studies demonstrated that selegiline blocked this reaction. The results of these studies have led some investigators

TABLE 21–1. Pharmacokinetic Properties of Drugs for Neurodegenerative Diseases*

Drug	Oral Bioavailability	Elimination Half-Life (Hours)	Route of Elimination
Drugs for Parkinson's disease			
Drugs that increase dopamine levels			
Amantadine	75%	24	R
Carbidopa	U	2	U
Levodopa-carbidopa	80%	3	M
Selegiline	70%	2	M
Tolcapone	U	2	M and R
Dopamine receptor agonists			
Bromocriptine	6%	6	M
Pergolide	70%	6	M
Pramipexole	90%	9	R
Ropinirole	55%	6	R and M
Acetylcholine receptor antagonists			
Benztropine	U	U	U
Trihexyphenidyl	≈100%	11	U
Drugs for Huntington's disease			
Diazepam	≈100%	60	M
Haloperidol	65%	24	M
Drugs for Alzheimer's disease			
Donepezil	≈100%	70	M, R, and F
Tacrine	17%	3	M
Drugs for multiple sclerosis			
Baclofen	≈100%	4	R and M
Interferon beta-1b	NA	U	M
Prednisone	80%	25	M and R
Drugs for amyotrophic lateral sclerosis			
Baclofen	≈100%	4	R and M
Gabapentin	60%	5	R
Riluzole	60%	20	M

*Values shown are the mean of values reported in the literature. F = fecal; M = metabolism; NA = not applicable (not administered orally); R = renal; and U = unknown. For drugs with more than one route of elimination, routes are listed in order of importance.

to postulate that idiopathic Parkinson's disease is caused by an environmental toxin whose action resembles that of MPTP.

Adverse Effects and Interactions. Adverse effects are listed in Table 21–2. Unlike the nonselective MAO inhibitors used in treating mood disorders, selegiline does not inhibit monoamine oxidase type A (MAO-A), an enzyme that catalyzes the degradation of catecholamines. For this reason, selegiline is much less likely to cause hypertension when it is administered in combination with sympathomimetic amines or when it is taken with foods that contain tyramine. However, the drug's selectivity for MAO-B is lost when it is given in higher doses, so the drug's potential for interactions of this type still exists. Selegiline can cause adverse effects if it is adminis-

tered with meperidine or with selective serotonin reuptake inhibitors such as fluoxetine.

Indications. Selegiline may be used as a single drug for the treatment of **early or mild Parkinson's disease,** and it is used as an adjunct with levodopa-carbidopa for **advanced disease.** Selegiline reduces the dosage requirement for levodopa, and it may improve motor function in patients who experience "wearing off" and "on-off" difficulties with levodopa.

The most controversial role of selegiline is its use as a **neuroprotective agent.** While some clinical studies have indicated that selegiline slows the progression of Parkinson's disease, others have indicated that it does not.

Tolcapone

Tolcapone is a new drug for enhancing the effectiveness of levodopa in the treatment of Parkinson's disease. It inhibits COMT, the enzyme that converts levodopa to 3OMD in the gut and liver. By this action, tolcapone produces a twofold increase in the oral bioavailability and half-life of levodopa. Because 3OMD competes with levodopa for transport into brain tissue, it may contribute to the "wearing off" and "on-off" effects that occur during long-term levodopa therapy. By inhibiting 3OMD formation, tolcapone may stabilize dopamine levels in the striatum and contribute to a more sustained improvement in motor function.

In clinical studies, tolcapone was found to increase the efficacy of levodopa while reducing the dosage requirement for levodopa. Tolcapone was well tolerated, and most of the side effects were similar in frequency to those reported with use of a placebo. Although tolcapone caused diarrhea and nausea in some patients, these side effects tended to decrease over time.

Dopamine Receptor Agonists

The dopamine receptor agonists directly activate dopamine receptors in the striatum. Because they do not require a functional dopaminergic neuron in order to produce their effects, they are sometimes helpful in advanced cases of Parkinson's disease, in which few dopaminergic neurons remain functional. The drugs work primarily by activating D_2 **receptors.** As shown in Fig. 21–1, activation of these receptors leads to inhibition of the indirect neuronal pathway from the striatum to the thalamus and increases thalamic stimulation of the motor area of the cortex.

Bromocriptine and Pergolide

Bromocriptine and pergolide are both **ergot alkaloids.** (Other ergot alkaloids are discussed in Chapter 29.) Bromocriptine is a D_2 receptor agonist and a D_1 receptor antagonist. In contrast, pergolide acts as both a D_1 and D_2 receptor agonist. Pergolide is much more potent than bromocriptine, has a higher affinity for D_2 receptors, and has a longer

TABLE 21–2. Adverse Effects, Contraindications, and Interactions of Drugs for Neurodegenerative Diseases

Drug	Major Adverse Effects	Contraindications	Major Drug Interactions
Drugs for Parkinson's disease Drugs that increase dopamine levels			
Amantadine	Dry mouth; hypotension; livedo reticularis; nausea; restlessness; sedation; and vivid dreams.	Age under 1 year and hypersensitivity to amantadine.	Benztropine and trihexyphenidyl potentiate central nervous system (CNS) side effects.
Levodopa-carbidopa	Agitation; arrhythmias; delirium; distorted thinking, hallucinations, and other psychotic effects; dyskinesias; hypotension; nausea and vomiting; nightmares or vivid dreams; and sedation.	Acute angle-closure glaucoma and hypersensitivity to carbidopa or levodopa.	Antacids and cisapride may increase bioavailability. Anticholinergic drugs may reduce peak serum level. Antipsychotic drugs, such as haloperidol, may decrease effects. Nonselective monoamine oxidase (MAO) inhibitors, such as phenelzine, may cause a hypertensive crisis.
Selegiline	Confusion; dyskinesias; hallucinations; hypotension; insomnia; and nausea.	Hypersensitivity to selegiline.	Severe reactions may result if taken with meperidine or with fluoxetine or other selective serotonin reuptake inhibitor (SSRI).
Tolcapone	Diarrhea and nausea.	Hypersensitivity to tolcapone.	Unknown.
Dopamine receptor agonists Bromocriptine	Confusion; decreased prolactin levels; dry mouth; dyskinesias; hallucinations; nausea; orthostatic hypotension; sedation; and vivid dreams.	Hypersensitivity to any ergot alkaloid; hypertension; peripheral vascular disease; and severe ischemic heart disease.	Dopamine antagonists may reduce effects.
Pergolide	Same as bromocriptine.	Same as bromocriptine.	Same as bromocriptine.
Pramipexole	Dizziness; hallucinations; insomnia; nausea and vomiting; and sedation.	Hypersensitivity to pramipexole.	Cimetidine inhibits renal excretion and increases serum levels.
Ropinirole	Same as pramipexole.	Hypersensitivity to ropinirole.	Ciprofloxacin increases serum levels.
Acetylcholine receptor antagonists Benztropine	Agitation; confusion; constipation; delirium; dry mouth; memory loss; urinary retention; and tachycardia.	Acute angle-closure glaucoma; gastrointestinal and genitourinary obstruction; hypersensitivity; myasthenia gravis; peptic ulcer; and prostatic hyperplasia.	Additive anticholinergic effect with antihistamines and phenothiazines.
Trihexyphenidyl	Same as benztropine.	Same as benztropine.	Same as benztropine.
Drugs for Huntington's disease Diazepam	Arrhythmias; CNS depression; drug dependence; hypotension; and mild respiratory depression.	Acute angle-closure glaucoma; hypersensitivity to diazepam; and psychosis.	Alcohol and other CNS depressants potentiate effects. Cimetidine increases and rifampin decreases serum levels.
Haloperidol	Extrapyramidal side effects and increased prolactin levels.	Hypersensitivity to haloperidol and severe CNS depression.	Barbiturates and carbamazepine decrease and quinidine increases serum levels.
Drugs for Alzheimer's disease Donepezil	Bradycardia; diarrhea; gastrointestinal bleeding; and nausea and vomiting.	Hypersensitivity to donepezil and sick sinus syndrome.	Anticholinergic drugs inhibit effects.
Tacrine	Bradycardia; diarrhea; gastrointestinal bleeding; hepatotoxicity; nausea and vomiting; and urinary incontinence.	Hepatitis; hypersensitivity to tacrine; and sick sinus syndrome.	Anticholinergic drugs inhibit effects. Cimetidine increases serum levels. Smoking decreases serum levels. Tacrine increases effects of succinylcholine and theophylline.

Continued

**TABLE 21-2. Adverse Effects, Contraindications, and Interactions
of Drugs for Neurodegenerative Diseases** *(Continued)*

Drug	Major Adverse Effects	Contraindications	Major Drug Interactions
Drugs for multiple sclerosis			
Baclofen	Dizziness; fatigue; and weakness.	Hypersensitivity to baclofen.	Unknown.
Interferon beta-1b	Chills; diarrhea; fever; headache; hypertension; myalgia; pain; and vomiting.	Hypersensitivity to albumen or interferon beta-1b.	Increases serum levels of zidovudine.
Prednisone	Aggravation of diabetes mellitus; gastrointestinal bleeding; mood changes; pancreatitis; and seizures.	Hypersensitivity to prednisone and systemic fungal infection.	Barbiturates, carbamazepine, phenytoin, and rifampin decrease serum levels.
Drugs for amyotrophic lateral sclerosis			
Baclofen	Dizziness; fatigue; and weakness.	Hypersensitivity to baclofen.	Unknown.
Gabapentin	Ataxia; dizziness; drowsiness; nystagmus; and tremor.	Hypersensitivity to gabapentin.	Antacids decrease serum levels.
Riluzole	Asthenia; diarrhea; dizziness; drowsiness; increased hepatic enzyme levels; nausea and vomiting; paresthesias; and vertigo.	Hepatitis and hypersensitivity to riluzole.	Quinolones and theophylline may increase serum levels. Omeprazole, rifampin, and smoking may decrease serum levels.

duration of action. Either drug may serve as a useful adjunct to levodopa in patients who have advanced Parkinson's disease and experience "wearing off" effects and "on-off" motor fluctuations.

Dopamine receptor agonists produce adverse effects that are similar to those of levodopa. Nausea may occur in as many as 50% of patients when they are first treated with a receptor agonist and is primarily due to stimulation of dopamine receptors in the vomiting center located in the medulla. Dose-related CNS effects of the receptor agonists include confusion, dyskinesias, sedation, vivid dreams, and hallucinations. Other adverse effects include orthostatic hypotension, dry mouth, and decreased prolactin levels. Nausea and many other adverse effects subside over time. To enable patients to develop tolerance to the effects, treatment should begin with a low dose, and the dosage should be increased gradually.

Pramipexole and Ropinirole

In contrast to the older dopamine receptor agonists, pramipexole and ropinirole are not ergot alkaloids. Both act as selective D_2 receptor agonists. In addition, pramipexole activates D_3 receptors, and this may contribute to its effectiveness in Parkinson's disease. The pharmacologic properties, adverse effects, and drug interactions of pramipexole and ropinirole are summarized in Tables 21-1 and 21-2.

Clinical studies have shown that pramipexole or ropinirole can delay the need for levodopa when used in early stages of Parkinson's disease. In advanced stages, pramipexole can reduce the "off" period and decrease the levodopa dosage requirement. Thus, while the older agonists (bromocriptine and pergolide) are primarily used as adjunct ther-

apy in advanced Parkinson's disease, the newer agonists may prove effective as monotherapy in both early and advanced disease. Further clinical studies are needed to determine the ultimate role of the newer drugs in treating patients with Parkinson's disease.

Acetylcholine Receptor Antagonists

Several centrally acting acetylcholine receptor antagonists, or **anticholinergic drugs,** are used in the management of Parkinson's disease. Two examples are **benztropine** and **trihexyphenidyl.** The anticholinergic drugs are generally less effective than the dopaminergic drugs, but they may be helpful as adjunct therapy in combination with levodopa and other drugs that augment dopaminergic activity. The anticholinergic drugs are more effective in reducing **tremor** than in reducing other manifestations of Parkinson's disease, although they may provide some reduction of bradykinesia and rigidity in patients with mild dysfunction. These drugs also inhibit the neuronal reuptake of dopamine by central dopaminergic neurons and may thereby prolong the action of dopamine.

In addition to being useful in the treatment of **early and advanced Parkinson's disease,** the anticholinergic drugs may also reduce **parkinsonian symptoms caused by dopamine receptor antagonists** such as haloperidol (see Chapter 22).

Treatment Considerations

Optimal management of Parkinson's disease requires that the disabilities of each patient be carefully assessed before drug treatment is recommended. Early disease of mild intensity may be best managed with exercise, nutrition, and education. Speech, occupational, and physical therapies may also be quite helpful.

For patients whose clinical manifestations are limited to mild tremor and slowness, anticholinergic drugs or amantadine may be helpful.

For patients with more severe functional disabilities, the dopaminergic drugs are the most effective treatment. Combination therapy with levodopa and carbidopa is usually prescribed for these patients, but monotherapy with a new dopamine receptor agonist, such as pramipexole or ropinirole, may provide an effective alternative for patients who have either early or advanced Parkinson's disease. Clinicians should remember that dopaminergic drugs have a delayed onset of action, so improvement in the patient's condition may not be noted until 2–3 weeks after therapy is started.

Tolcapone and selegiline inhibit the metabolism of levodopa and dopamine, respectively, and may be used to enhance the effectiveness of levodopa in patients with early or advanced disease. Some clinicians begin selegiline treatment early in the disease in an effort to retard disease progression.

For patients who have more advanced disease and begin to experience the "wearing off" and "on-off" fluctuations of levodopa-carbidopa, it is sometimes helpful to change the drug dosage or formulation. For example, the "wearing off" effect may be minimized by increasing the frequency of doses or using a combination of sustained-release and immediate-release formulations. Alternatively, an additional dopaminergic drug may be added to the treatment regimen. The addition of tolcapone, for example, may reduce motor fluctuations by increasing and stabilizing levodopa concentrations in the striatum. A reduction in dietary protein may also improve the response to levodopa in some patients.

HUNTINGTON'S DISEASE
Etiology and Pathogenesis

Huntington's disease, or **Huntington's chorea,** is an autosomal dominant hereditary disorder that is characterized by abnormally expansive or choreoathetoid movements (dance-like movements) of the limbs, rhythmic movements of the tongue and face, and mental deterioration that leads to personality disorders, psychosis, and dementia. Patients are usually in their late 30s when the disease begins, and progressive respiratory depression usually causes death in 10–15 years.

Huntington's disease is due to the degeneration of **gamma-aminobutyric acid (GABA) neurons** in the **striatum** and elsewhere in the brain. This degeneration may be caused by glutamate-induced neurotoxicity. The loss of GABA neurons that project from the striatum to the lateral globus pallidus leads to disinhibition of thalamic nuclei and to an increase in thalamic input to the motor area of the cortex (see Fig. 21–1).

Treatment

The symptoms of Huntington's disease are consistent with excessive dopaminergic activity in the basal ganglia. Therefore, drugs that block dopamine receptors, such as **haloperidol** and other antipsychotic drugs (see Chapter 22), produce some improvement in motor function and are also helpful in relieving the psychosis that accompanies the disease. **Diazepam** and other benzodiazepine drugs (see Chapter 19) potentiate GABA and may also reduce excess movements in patients with Huntington's disease. However, the efficacy of benzodiazepines declines significantly with disease progression.

In the future, new treatments may result from identification of the function of huntingtin, the abnormal gene product that is synthesized in Huntington's disease. Drugs that inhibit glutamate neurotoxicity might also prove useful in the treatment of this disease.

ALZHEIMER'S DISEASE
Etiology and Pathogenesis

Alzheimer's disease is a type of **progressive dementia** for which no cause is known and no cure has been found. In the USA, it accounts for about 60% of all cases of dementia in patients over 65 years of age and is associated with 100,000 deaths each year. The disease has a tremendous negative impact on patients and their families because of its devastating effects on the patient's cognitive, emotional, and physical function.

Alzheimer's disease results from the destruction of **cholinergic and other neurons** in the **cortex** and **limbic structures of the brain,** particularly the amygdala, basal forebrain, and hippocampus. Major changes in these structures include cortical atrophy, neurofibrillary tangles, and neuritic plaques containing β-amyloid protein. The cholinergic neurons destroyed in Alzheimer's disease include those which originate in Meynert's nucleus in the basal forebrain. These neurons project to the frontal cortex and hippocampus, and they have a critical role in memory and cognition.

Treatment

In patients with Alzheimer's disease, treatment with **donepezil** or **tacrine** has been administered in an effort to improve cholinergic neurotransmission in affected areas of the brain. Although these **centrally acting cholinesterase inhibitors** may slow the deterioration of cognitive function, they do not affect the underlying neurodegenerative process, so the disease is eventually fatal. The structures, properties, adverse effects, and drug interactions of donepezil and tacrine are outlined in Fig. 21–3B, Table 21–1, and Table 21–2.

Studies in patients with Alzheimer's disease have demonstrated that those treated with donepezil for 24 weeks had significantly better cognitive function than those treated with a placebo. Donepezil is a piperidine-type reversible cholinesterase inhibitor that selectively inhibits cholinesterase in the CNS and increases acetylcholine levels in the cerebral cortex. The drug is well absorbed after oral administration and crosses the blood-brain barrier. Because it has a long half-life of about 70 hours, it is usually administered once a day. The adverse effects of donepezil include diarrhea, nausea, and vomiting, but these are usually mild and transient. Unlike acridine drugs, such as tacrine, donepezil is not associated with hepatotoxicity.

Tacrine was the first centrally acting cholinesterase inhibitor approved for the treatment of Alzheimer's disease. It has a lower bioavailability and a shorter half-life than does donepezil, and it must be administered several times a day. Tacrine is an acridine compound and is associated with a significant incidence of hepatotoxicity and with peripheral cholinergic side effects such as diarrhea, nausea, and urinary incontinence. Because of these adverse effects, few patients can tolerate the higher doses required to demonstrate cognitive improvement in Alzheimer's disease.

MULTIPLE SCLEROSIS
Etiology and Pathogenesis

Multiple sclerosis is a chronic disease characterized by the **demyelination of neurons** in the CNS. Although its etiology is unknown, the disease is postulated to have an autoimmune or viral origin. Demyelination leads to disruption of nerve transmission and is accompanied by an inflammatory response and the formation of plaques in the brain and spinal cord. These plaques typically contain decreased numbers of **oligodendrocytes** (myelin-forming cells). The neurologic symptoms of multiple sclerosis depend on the area of the brain that is affected and may include pain, spasticity, weakness, ataxia, fatigue, and problems with speech, vision, gait, and bladder function. Many patients experience relapses and remissions, but some have a more severe and unremitting progression of disease.

Treatment

The goals of therapy are to reduce target organ and CNS dysfunction, decrease the severity of acute exacerbations, and reduce or prevent relapses and progression.

Spasticity is frequently treated with physical therapy, but **antispastic drugs,** such as **baclofen** (see Tables 21–1 and 21–2), may be useful in severe cases.

Acute exacerbations are treated with **adrenal corticosteroid drugs,** such as **prednisone.** These drugs have anti-inflammatory activity and are discussed in Chapter 33. In patients with multiple sclerosis, corticosteroids shorten the duration of exacerbations and ameliorate symptoms, possibly by decreasing edema. They are administered orally in milder cases and are given parenterally in high doses in more severe cases.

Interferon beta-1b is the first drug to demonstrate an ability to halt and even reverse the progression of multiple sclerosis. In clinical studies, the drug was found to reduce the frequency of relapses and the number of new lesions detected by magnetic resonance imaging in patients who were ambulatory, had a relapsing-remitting type of multiple sclerosis, and had experienced at least two exacerbations during the last 2 years. Interferon beta-1b is a synthetic analogue of a recombinant interferon-beta produced in *Escherichia coli.* Although the drug's exact mechanism of action is unknown, its effects in patients with multiple sclerosis may be due to its immunomodulating properties. Interferon beta-1b increases the cytotoxicity of natural killer cells and increases the phagocytic activity of macrophages. In addition, it reduces the amount of interferon-gamma secreted by activated lymphocytes. Because interferon-gamma has been shown to exacerbate the symptoms of multiple sclerosis, a reduction in its secretion may halt the disease. The pharmacologic effects and uses of various interferons are discussed more thoroughly in Chapter 45.

AMYOTROPHIC LATERAL SCLEROSIS
Etiology and Pathogenesis

Amyotrophic lateral sclerosis (ALS), also called **Lou Gehrig disease,** is a progressive disease of the **motor neurons.** It is characterized by muscle wasting, weakness, and respiratory failure leading to death in 2–5 years. The cause of ALS is unknown, but there is evidence for a defect in **superoxide dismutase,** an enzyme that scavenges superoxide radicals.

Treatment

The current treatment for ALS is largely symptomatic. Spasticity may be partly controlled with **baclofen,** a GABA$_B$ agonist whose properties are outlined in Tables 21–1 and 21–2. The decline in muscle strength may be slowed by **gabapentin,** an antiepileptic drug discussed in Chapter 20.

Although a large number of drugs have been studied for their potential to reduce the progression of ALS and prolong the length of survival, the first drug that has been specifically approved for use in the treatment of ALS is **riluzole** (see Fig. 21–3C). This drug has been shown to prolong the time before patients require a tracheostomy and also to prolong life by approximately 3 months. Riluzole is believed to protect motor neurons from the neurotoxic effects of excitatory amino acids such as glutamate and to prevent the anoxia-related death of cortical neurons. Its exact mechanism of action is unclear, but it may inhibit voltage-gated sodium channels that mediate the release of glutamate from neurons. Clinical studies in patients with ALS indicate that riluzole is more effective in those with bulbar-onset disease than in those with limb-onset disease.

Experimental studies with recombinant human **insulinlike growth factor** (ILGF) indicate that this compound may also retard the progression of ALS. ILGF is believed to exert a neuroprotective effect throughout the central and peripheral nervous system. ILGF and other experimental treatments may counteract pathophysiologic mechanisms of ALS and lead to improved symptomatic control and prolonged length of survival.

Summary of Important Points

- Parkinson's disease is a chronic disease caused by degeneration of dopaminergic neurons that arise in the substantia nigra. It is characterized by resting tremor, rigidity, and bradykinesia.
- Parkinson's disease is primarily treated with drugs that increase dopamine levels in the basal ganglia or activate dopamine receptors.
- Levodopa is converted to dopamine by L-aromatic amino acid decarboxylase (LAAD). It is often coadministered with carbidopa, which inhibits the peripheral decarboxylation of levodopa and increases its brain uptake.
- Other drugs that increase dopamine levels in the basal ganglia include tolcapone, which inhibits methylation of levodopa, and selegiline, which inhibits the breakdown of dopamine catalyzed by monoamine oxidase type B (MAO-B). Amantadine increases dopamine release and may inhibit its neuronal reuptake.
- Direct-acting dopamine receptor agonists include bromocriptine, pergolide, pramipexole, and ropinirole. These drugs are often used as adjuncts to levodopa in the treatment of patients whose response to levodopa is inadequate.
- Levodopa and other dopaminergic drugs may cause significant adverse effects, including nausea, dyskinesias, nightmares, and orthostatic hypotension.
- Acetylcholine receptor antagonists (anticholinergic drugs) can reduce the tremor seen in Parkinson's disease, but their effectiveness is limited.
- Huntington's disease is caused by degeneration of gamma-aminobutyric acid (GABA) neurons in the striatum and other parts of the brain. Degeneration of neurons leads to excessive dopamine neurotransmission and choreoathetoid movements. Dopamine receptor antagonists may provide some improvement in affected patients.
- Alzheimer's disease is a progressive dementia that is partly due to loss of cholinergic neurons in the cortex and limbic structures of the brain. Donepezil and tacrine, two centrally acting cholinesterase inhibitors, may produce some cognitive improvement in patients with this disease.
- Multiple sclerosis is a demyelinating disease whose exacerbations may be attenuated with corticosteroid drugs. Treatment with interferon beta-1b retards disease progression in some patients.
- Amyotrophic lateral sclerosis is a progressive disease of the motor neurons. Riluzole, the first drug approved for its treatment, has a limited effect on patient survival.

Selected Readings

Hingtgen, C. M., and E. Siemers. The treatment of Parkinson's disease: current concepts and rationale. Compr Ther 24:560–566, 1998.

Koller, W. C. Neuroprotection for Parkinson's disease. Ann Neurol 44(supplement 1):S155–S159, 1998.

Kurth, M. C., et al. Tolcapone improves motor function and reduces levodopa requirements in patients with Parkinson's disease experiencing motor fluctuations. Neurology 48:81–87, 1997.

Lang, A. E., and A. M. Lozano. Parkinson's disease. N Engl J Med 339:1130–1143, 1998.

Lange, K. W. Clinical pharmacology of dopamine agonists in Parkinson's disease. Drugs Aging 13:381–389, 1998.

Ruottinen, H. M., and U. K. Rinne. Catechol-O-methyltransferase inhibition in the treatment of Parkinson's disease. J Neurol 245(supplement 3):P25–P34, 1998.

Wagner, M. L., and B. E. Landis. Riluzole: a new agent for amyotrophic lateral sclerosis. Ann Pharmacother 31:738–744, 1997.

Waters, C. H. Managing the late complications of Parkinson's disease. Neurology 49:S49–S57, 1997.

Waters, C. H., et al. Tolcapone in stable Parkinson's disease: efficacy and safety of long-term treatment. Neurology 49:665–671, 1997.

Watts, R. L. The role of dopamine agonists in early Parkinson's disease. Neurology 49:S34–S48, 1997.

PSYCHOTHERAPEUTIC DRUGS

CLASSIFICATION OF PSYCHOTHERAPEUTIC DRUGS

ANTIPSYCHOTIC DRUGS
Phenothiazines
- Chlorpromazine
- Fluphenazine
- Thioridazine
- Trifluoperazine

Thioxanthenes
- Thiothixene

Butyrophenones
- Haloperidol

Azepines
- Clozapine
- Loxapine
- Olanzapine

Other antipsychotic drugs
- Molindone
- Risperidone

ANTIDEPRESSANT DRUGS
Tricyclic antidepressants
- Amitriptyline
- Clomipramine
- Desipramine
- Imipramine
- Nortriptyline

Selective serotonin reuptake inhibitors
- Fluoxetine
- Fluvoxamine
- Paroxetine
- Sertraline

Monoamine oxidase inhibitors
- Phenelzine
- Tranylcypromine

Other antidepressant drugs
- Bupropion
- Hypericum
- Mirtazapine
- Nefazodone
- Trazodone
- Venlafaxine

MOOD-STABILIZING DRUGS
- Carbamazepine
- Lithium
- Valproate

OVERVIEW

The major psychiatric disorders include psychoses, such as schizophrenia, and affective disorders, such as depression. **Psychoses** are disorders in which patients exhibit gross disturbances in their comprehension of reality, as evidenced by false perceptions (hallucinations) and false beliefs (delusions). In contrast, **affective disorders** are emotional disturbances in which the mood is excessively low (depression) or high (mania). During the past 50 years, tremendous advances have been made in the treatment of these disorders. The newer antipsychotic drugs used to treat schizophrenia and the newer antidepressant and mood-stabilizing drugs used to treat affective disorders appear to cause fewer adverse reactions and to be more effective than the older psychotherapeutic agents. Treatment-resistant disorders still pose a significant problem to clinicians, but some progress has been made in the treatment of refractory disease.

SCHIZOPHRENIA
Clinical Findings

Schizophrenia, the most common form of psychosis, affects about 1% of the world's population. Its hallmarks are delusions, hallucinations, disorganized thinking, and emotional abnormalities. Several forms of the disease, including paranoid, disorganized, and catatonic forms, are differentiated on the basis of symptomatology.

As shown in Table 22–1, the symptoms of schizophrenia can be divided into two groups. The so-called **positive symptoms,** which include delusions and hallucinations, probably result from excessive neuronal activity in mesolimbic neuronal pathways. These symptoms are usually the primary manifestations of acute psychotic episodes. The so-called **negative symptoms,** which include apathy, withdrawal, and lack of motivation and pleasure, probably result from insufficient activity in mesocortical neuronal pathways. The negative symptoms are generally more difficult to treat, often persist after positive symptoms resolve, and are associated with a poor prognosis.

Etiology and Pathogenesis

Schizophrenia is a complex and heterogeneous disease whose etiology and pathogenesis are incompletely understood.

TABLE 22-1.   Classification of Symptoms of Schizophrenia

Positive Symptoms	Negative Symptoms
Agitation	Apathy (avolition)
Delusions	Affective flattening
Disorganized speech	Lack of motivation
Disorganized thinking	Lack of pleasure (anhedonia)
Hallucinations	Poverty of speech (alogia)
Insomnia	Social isolation

Epidemiologic studies indicate that the children of two schizophrenic parents have about a 40% risk of developing the disease, so heredity appears to have a major role in determining susceptibility to schizophrenia. Adoption studies show that the risk is associated with the biologic parents and is not altered by the environment during childhood.

Some investigators believe that the maturation of neurons in genetically susceptible fetuses is impaired by a disturbance that occurs in utero via unknown mechanisms. The postulated in utero disturbance is thought to cause abnormal migration of neurons in the fetal brain during the second trimester of pregnancy. This leads to maldevelopment of the cortex and to formation of abnormal brain circuits. In most patients, the clinical manifestations of schizophrenia do not appear until adolescence, possibly because the neuron dysfunction is not expressed until brain maturation is completed.

Dopamine Hypothesis

According to the dopamine hypothesis, schizophrenia results from abnormalities in dopamine neurotransmission in mesolimbic and mesocortical neuronal pathways (Box 22–1). Because much of the evidence supporting this hypothesis is based on the effects of drugs that alter dopamine neurotransmission, the hypothesis has been called a **pharmacocentric hypothesis.**

Several observations support the dopamine hypothesis. First, most antipsychotic drugs block dopamine D_2 receptors, and there is an excellent correlation between the clinical potency of these drugs and their in vitro affinity for these receptors. Second, drugs that act by increasing the neuronal release of dopamine or by blocking the reuptake of dopamine (drugs such as amphetamines and cocaine) can induce psychotic behavior that resembles the behavior of schizophrenic patients.

Dopamine turnover in the brain, which reflects the neuronal release of dopamine, can be studied by measuring the concentration of the principal metabolite of dopamine, homovanillic acid, in the cerebrospinal fluid. While elevated levels of homovanillic acid are not found in patients with chronic schizophrenia, they are found in some schizophrenic patients undergoing acute psychotic episodes. There is also evidence for a dopamine receptor defect in schizophrenic patients. Positive emission tomography (PET) scanning using D_2 receptor ligands has revealed that schizophrenic patients have decreased D_2 receptor densities in the prefrontal lobe cortex (but increased D_2 receptor densities in the caudate nucleus). These findings lend support to the dopamine hypothesis and to another hypothesis called the hypofrontality hypothesis.

Hypofrontality Hypothesis

According to the hypofrontality hypothesis, schizophrenia is caused by abnormal neurotransmission in the prefrontal lobe cortex. Studies using computed electroencephalography (brain mapping) indicate that schizophrenic patients have increased slow-wave activity in the prefrontal lobe. This finding is thought to correlate with lack of volition (apathy), a core symptom of schizophrenia. Other studies show that the level of blood flow in the frontal lobe of schizophrenic patients is lower than that of normal subjects during tasks that involve the frontal lobe association areas.

Anatomic studies show that schizophrenic patients have lateral ventricular enlargement in association with neuronal loss in the parahippocampal cortex and other periventricular structures, such as the amygdala, hippocampus, and prefrontal association areas. Findings in these studies are consistent with other evidence that schizophrenia may result from abnormalities in the dorsolateral prefrontal lobe cortex secondary to underdevelopment of projections from the parahippocampal area.

Linked Hypotheses

In 1988, D. R. Weinberger offered an explanation that links the dopamine and hypofrontality hypotheses of schizophrenia. According to Weinberger, underdeveloped and dysfunctional mesocortical pathways account for the negative symptoms of schizophrenia. Because the prefrontal lobe cortex inhibits the nucleus accumbens, the loss of cortical inhibition of this structure (disinhibition) leads to increased dopamine neurotransmission in mesolimbic pathways (see Box 22–1). The resulting increased activity in these pathways is responsible for the positive symptoms of schizophrenia. This explanation is consistent with the observation that dopamine D_2 receptor antagonists can alleviate the positive symptoms of schizophrenia but have less effect on the negative symptoms. It is also consistent with the idea that drugs which block serotonin 5-HT$_2$ receptors may thereby increase dopamine release in the frontal lobe cortex (mesocortical pathways) and alleviate the negative symptoms of schizophrenia. Although the Weinberger explanation does not account for all of the known biologic abnormalities of schizophrenia, it provides a useful model for further research.

ANTIPSYCHOTIC DRUGS

Antipsychotic drugs are agents that reduce psychotic symptoms and improve the behavior of schizophrenic patients. Antipsychotic drugs are also

---

BOX 22–1. Neurobiology of Schizophrenia and Sites of Drug Action

---

Postulated Neuronal Dysfunction in Schizophrenia

As shown in the accompanying figure, there are numerous dopamine pathways in the brain.

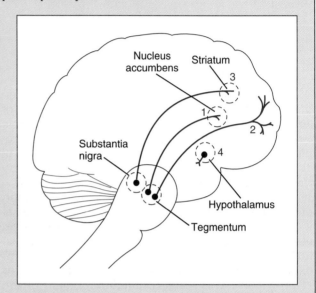

(1) Mesolimbic Pathway. Dopamine travels from the midbrain tegmental area to the nucleus accumbens. Increased activity in this pathway may cause delusions, hallucinations, and other so-called positive symptoms of schizophrenia.

(2) Mesocortical Pathways. There are several mesocortical pathways. Decreased activity in the pathway that goes from the midbrain to the prefrontal lobe cortex may cause apathy, withdrawal, lack of motivation and pleasure, and other so-called negative symptoms of schizophrenia. Mesocortical dysfunction also disinhibits the mesolimbic pathway.

(3) Nigrostriatal Pathway. The pathway from the substantia nigra to the striatum is involved in the coordination of body movements. Inhibition of this pathway causes the extrapyramidal side effects of antipsychotic drugs.

(4) Tuberoinfundibular Pathway. The pathway from the hypothalamus to the pituitary inhibits the release of prolactin. Inhibition of this pathway leads to elevated serum prolactin levels.

Sites of Drug Action

Some antipsychotic drugs (such as clozapine, olanzapine, and risperidone) block serotonin 5-HT$_2$ receptors in the mesocortical pathway to the prefrontal lobe cortex. This increases the release of dopamine (DA) and thereby alleviates the negative symptoms of schizophrenia. Most antipsychotic drugs (including those listed above) block dopamine D$_2$ receptors in the mesolimbic pathway to the nucleus accumbens, and this alleviates the positive symptoms of schizophrenia.

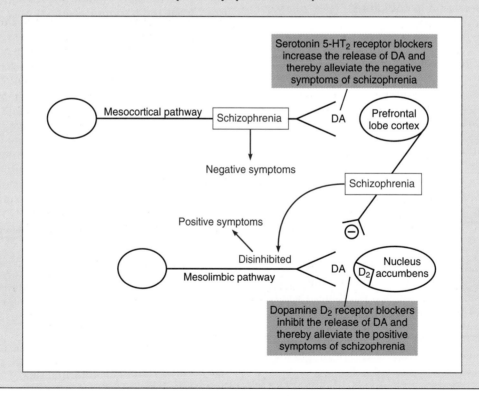

---

called **neuroleptic drugs** because they suppress motor activity and emotional expression. The accidental discovery of the antipsychotic properties of chlorpromazine in the early 1950s ushered in a new era in the treatment of schizophrenia and stimulated research concerning the neurobiology of mental illness and psychopharmacology. Nearly 40 years later, the introduction of clozapine had an equally important impact. Clozapine has been found to exhibit greater activity against the negative symptoms of schizophrenia and to produce significantly fewer extrapyramidal side effects than the previous antipsychotic drugs. For this reason, the discovery of clozapine has stimulated the development of new antipsychotic drugs with improved pharmacologic properties.

Mechanisms of Action

The antipsychotic drugs interact with multiple neurotransmitter systems. While the therapeutic effects of these drugs are believed to result from competitive blockade of **dopamine receptors** and **serotonin (5-hydroxytryptamine, or 5-HT) receptors,** the adverse effects are attributed to the blockade of a variety of receptors (Table 22–2).

Typical antipsychotic drugs have an equal or greater affinity for D_2 receptors than for $5-HT_2$ receptors. As shown in Fig. 22–1, there is an excellent correlation between the clinical potency of these drugs and their in vitro affinity for D_2 receptors. While antagonism of D_2 receptors in mesolimbic pathways is thought to repress the positive symptoms of schizophrenia, blockade of D_2 receptors in the basal ganglia is believed to be responsible for the parkinsonian and other extrapyramidal side effects that sometimes occur in patients taking antipsychotic drugs.

Atypical antipsychotic drugs, such as clozapine, have a greater affinity for $5-HT_2$ receptors than for D_2 receptors, and some atypical drugs have increased affinity for D_3 or D_4 receptors.

The mechanisms by which the blockade of dopamine and serotonin receptors alleviates the symptoms of schizophrenia are not completely understood. While these receptors are blocked immediately when antipsychotic drugs are first administered, the therapeutic effects of the drugs usually require several weeks to fully develop. This is because antipsychotic drugs produce three time-dependent changes in dopamine neurotransmission. When first administered, the drugs cause an increase in dopamine synthesis, release, and metabolism. This probably represents a compensatory response to the acute blockade of postsynaptic dopamine receptors produced by antipsychotic drugs. Over time, contin-

ued dopamine receptor blockade leads to inactivation of dopaminergic neurons and produces what has been called **depolarization blockade.** Depolarization blockade results in reduced dopamine release from mesolimbic and nigrostriatal neurons. This action is believed to alleviate the positive symptoms of schizophrenia while causing extrapyramidal side effects. Eventually, the reduction in dopamine release caused by depolarization blockade leads to dopamine receptor up-regulation and supersensitivity to dopamine agonists. This supersensitivity may contribute to the development of a delayed type of extrapyramidal side effect called tardive dyskinesia (see below).

In mesocortical and nigrostriatal pathways, $5-HT_2$ receptors mediate presynaptic inhibition of dopamine release. Blockade of these receptors by atypical antipsychotic drugs may increase dopamine release in these pathways. In the mesocortical pathway, this action may alleviate the negative symptoms of schizophrenia. In the nigrostriatal pathway, increased dopamine release counteracts the extrapyramidal side effects caused by D_2 receptor blockade.

In the peripheral autonomic nervous system, the antipsychotic drugs also block muscarinic receptors and α-adrenergic receptors, thereby causing adverse effects described in Tables 22–2 and 22–3.

Classification

Antipsychotic drugs are usually classified on the basis of their chemical structure, but they can also be classified according to whether they display typical or atypical pharmacologic properties. The **typical antipsychotic drugs** include the phenothiazines, the thioxanthenes, the butyrophenones, and some azepines (such as loxapine). The **atypical antipsychotic drugs** include other azepines (such as clozapine and olanzapine) and a benzisoxazole drug called risperidone.

Phenothiazines

Numerous phenothiazines are available for the treatment of schizophrenia and related conditions. The four representative examples discussed here are

TABLE 22–2. Mechanisms Responsible for the Therapeutic and Adverse Effects of Antipsychotic Drugs

Mechanism	Therapeutic Effects	Adverse Effects
Blockade of α_1-adrenergic receptors	—	Dizziness, orthostatic hypotension, and reflex tachycardia.
Blockade of dopamine D_2 receptors	Alleviation of positive symptoms of schizophrenia.	Extrapyramidal effects (akathisia, dystonia, and pseudoparkinsonism) and elevated serum prolactin levels.
Blockade of dopamine D_4 receptors	Alleviation of negative symptoms of schizophrenia and decrease in the incidence of extrapyramidal side effects.	—
Blockade of histamine H_1 receptors	—	Drowsiness and increase in appetite and weight.
Blockade of muscarinic receptors	—	Blurred vision, constipation, dry mouth, and urinary retention.
Blockade of serotonin $5-HT_2$ receptors	Alleviation of negative symptoms of schizophrenia and decrease in the incidence of extrapyramidal side effects.	Anxiety and insomnia.

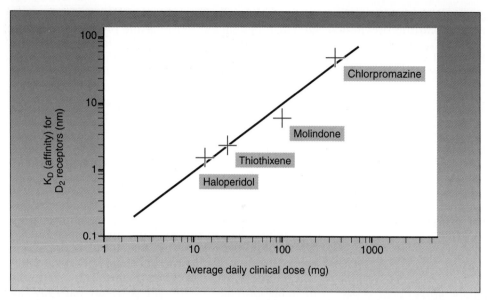

FIGURE 22–1. Correlation of antipsychotic drug potency and dopamine D_2 receptor binding. The clinical potency of the typical antipsychotic drugs is highly correlated with their in vitro affinity for D_2 (but not D_1) receptors.

chlorpromazine, fluphenazine, thioridazine, and trifluoperazine. These drugs have similar therapeutic effects but differ in their relative potency (Table 22–4) and in their side effect profiles (see Table 22–3).

Drug Properties

Chemistry and Pharmacokinetics. Each phenothiazine drug is a tricyclic compound that contains a thiazine group and two benzene rings (Fig. 22–2A). An aliphatic, piperidine, or piperazine group is attached to the nitrogen atom of the thiazine ring, and this group influences the relative potency and side effects of the various phenothiazine drugs. Drugs with an aliphatic group (such as chlorpromazine) or a piperidine group (such as thioridazine) have a lower potency than do drugs with a piperazine group (such as fluphenazine). Low-potency drugs cause more autonomic side effects but fewer extrapyramidal side effects than do high-potency drugs.

The phenothiazines are adequately absorbed from the gut after oral administration. Several phe-

TABLE 22–3. Adverse Effects of Antipsychotic Drugs*

Drug	Extrapyramidal Effects	Sedation	Anticholinergic Effects	Orthostatic Hypotension	Other Adverse Effects
Phenothiazines					
Chlorpromazine	+++	++++	+++	++++	Elevated serum prolactin levels and poikilothermy.
Fluphenazine	+++++	++	++	++	Same as chlorpromazine.
Thioridazine	++	++++	++++	++++	Cardiac arrhythmia, elevated serum prolactin levels, poikilothermy, and retinopathy.
Trifluoperazine	++++	++	++	++	Same as chlorpromazine.
Thioxanthenes					
Thiothixene	++++	++	++	++	Same as chlorpromazine.
Butyrophenones					
Haloperidol	+++++	+	+	+	Same as chlorpromazine.
Azepines					
Clozapine	+	+++++	+++++	++++	Agranulocytosis and cardiac arrhythmia.
Loxapine	++++	+++	++	+++	Same as chlorpromazine.
Olanzapine	+	++	+	+	Weight gain.
Other antipsychotic drugs					
Molindone	+++	+	++	++	Same as chlorpromazine.
Risperidone	++	+	+	++	Cardiac arrhythmia and elevated serum prolactin levels.

*Ratings range from extremely low (+) to extremely high (++++).

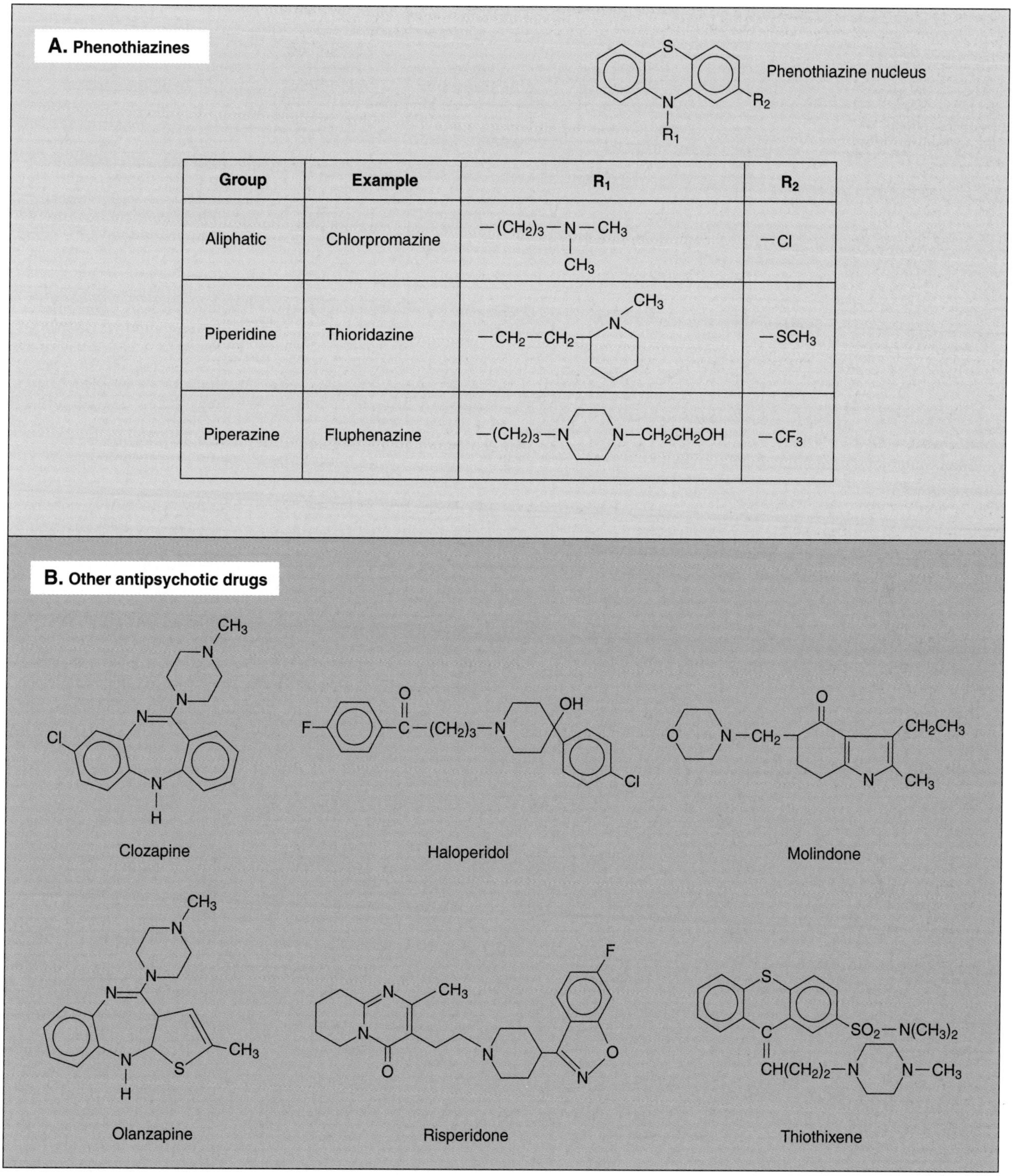

A. Phenothiazines

Phenothiazine nucleus

Group	Example	R₁	R₂
Aliphatic	Chlorpromazine	$-(CH_2)_3-N-CH_3$ with CH_3	$-Cl$
Piperidine	Thioridazine	$-CH_2-CH_2-$ (N-CH₃ piperidine)	$-SCH_3$
Piperazine	Fluphenazine	$-(CH_2)_3-N$ (piperazine) $N-CH_2CH_2OH$	$-CF_3$

B. Other antipsychotic drugs

Clozapine

Haloperidol

Molindone

Olanzapine

Risperidone

Thiothixene

FIGURE 22–2. Structures of selected antipsychotic drugs. (A) Each phenothiazine drug is a tricyclic compound that contains a thiazine group and two benzene rings. An aliphatic, piperidine, or piperazine group is attached to the nitrogen atom of the thiazine ring, and this group influences the relative potency and side effects of the various phenothiazine drugs. **(B)** Other antipsychotic drugs include clozapine and olanzapine, two examples of azepines; haloperidol, a butyrophenone; molindone, a dihydroindolone derivative; risperidone, a benzisoxazole; and thiothixene, a thioxanthene.

nothiazines are also administered parenterally. The drugs are extensively metabolized to a large number of active and inactive metabolites before they are excreted in the urine, and they have elimi-

nation half-lives ranging from 20 to 30 hours (see Table 22–4).

Mechanisms and Pharmacologic Effects. The phenothiazines are typical antipsychotic drugs

TABLE 22–4. Pharmacologic Properties of Antipsychotic Drugs*

Drug	Relative Potency†	Receptor Selectivity	Route of Administration	Elimination Half-Life and Route	Major Drug Interactions
Phenothiazines					
Chlorpromazine	Low	$D_2 > 5\text{-}HT_2$	Oral, IM, and IV	30 hours (M)	Additive effects with antiadrenergic, anticholinergic, and CNS depressants. Decreases serum levels of lithium. Concurrent use of a β-adrenergic receptor antagonist or an antidepressant may increase serum levels of both drugs.
Fluphenazine	High	$D_2 > 5\text{-}HT_2$	Oral and depot IM	20 hours (M)	Additive effects with anticholinergic and CNS depressants. Concurrent use of a β-adrenergic receptor antagonist or an antidepressant may increase serum levels of both drugs.
Thioridazine	Low	$D_2 > 5\text{-}HT_2$	Oral	30 hours (M)	Same as chlorpromazine.
Trifluoperazine	High	$D_2 > 5\text{-}HT_2$	Oral and IM	24 hours (M)	Same as chlorpromazine.
Thioxanthenes					
Thiothixene	High	$D_2 > 5\text{-}HT_2$	Oral and IM	35 hours (M)	Additive effects with anticholinergic and CNS depressants. Concurrent use of a β-adrenergic receptor antagonist may increase serum levels of both drugs.
Butyrophenones					
Haloperidol	High	$D_2 > 5\text{-}HT_2$	Oral and depot IM	24 hours (M)	Barbiturates and carbamazepine decrease serum levels. Quinidine increases serum levels.
Azepines					
Clozapine	Low	$5\text{-}HT_2 = D_4$ and $> D_2$	Oral	24 hours (M)	Not established; possible interaction with drugs that induce or inhibit cytochrome P450 isozyme CYP1A2.
Loxapine	Medium	$D_2 > 5\text{-}HT_2$	Oral and IM	20 hours (M)	Concurrent use of an antidepressant may increase serum levels of both drugs.
Olanzapine	High	$5\text{-}HT_2 > D_2$	Oral	30 hours (M)	Same as clozapine.
Other antipsychotic drugs					
Molindone	Medium	$D_2 > 5\text{-}HT_2$	Oral	2 hours (M)	Additive effects with anticholinergic and CNS depressants. Concurrent use of a β-adrenergic receptor antagonist or an antidepressant may increase serum levels of both drugs.
Risperidone	High	$5\text{-}HT_2 > D_2$	Oral	24 hours (M)	Not established; possible interaction with drugs that induce or inhibit cytochrome P450 isozyme CYP2D6.

*Values shown are the mean of values reported in the literature. D_2 = dopamine D_2 receptor; $5\text{-}HT_2$ = serotonin $5\text{-}HT_2$ receptor; IM = intramuscular; IV = intravenous; depot = long-acting form; M = metabolized; and CNS = central nervous system.
†Low = 50–2000 mg/d; medium = 20–250 mg/d; and high = 1–100 mg/d.

whose therapeutic effects appear to be primarily due to blockade of D_2 receptors. After therapy with a phenothiazine is initiated, the positive symptoms of schizophrenia usually subside in 1–3 weeks. Patients become less agitated and experience fewer auditory hallucinations. Grandiose or paranoid delusions subside and may disappear completely in some patients with continued treatment. At the same time, sleeping and eating patterns become normalized, and behavioral improvement occurs in the form of decreased hostility, combativeness, and aggression. Phenothiazines and other typical antipsychotic drugs may have some impact on negative symptoms, but it is usually less pronounced than the impact of atypical antipsychotic drugs.

Adverse Effects.   The most common adverse effects produced by phenothiazines and other antipsychotic drugs are shown in Table 22–3.

Blockade of dopamine receptors in the striatum may cause several forms of extrapyramidal side effects, including akathisia, pseudoparkinsonism, and dystonias. Patients with **akathisia,** or "motor restlessness," feel compelled to pace, shuffle their feet, or shift positions and are unable to sit quietly. **Pseudoparkinsonism** resembles idiopathic Parkinson's disease and is characterized by rigidity, bradykinesia, and tremor. **Dystonia** is a state of abnormal muscle tension that often affects the neck and facial muscles, including the tongue, pharynx, larynx, and eyes. Patients with dystonia may experience severe reactions, such as oculogyric crisis (a condition in which the eyeballs become fixed in one position, usually upward), glossospasm, tongue protrusion, and torticollis (a contracted state of the cervical muscles, producing twisting of the neck and an unnatural position of the head). Such reactions may be frightening and painful, and pharyngolaryngeal dystonias may even be life-threatening. Young males who are given large doses of high-potency drugs are at great risk of developing dystonias.

While akathisia, pseudoparkinsonism, and dystonias are acute extrapyramidal side effects that often occur early in the course of treatment with antipsychotic drugs, **tardive dyskinesia** (TD) is a disorder that usually develops after months or years of treatment. The disorder is characterized by abnormal oral and facial movements, such as tongue protrusion and lip smacking. In later stages, abnormal limb and truncal movements may also be observed. Investigators believe that TD results from supersensitivity to dopamine, which develops during long-term dopamine receptor blockade (see Chapter 18). This hypothesis is supported by the fact that the symptoms of TD temporarily subside if dopamine receptor blockade is increased by giving larger doses of an antipsychotic drug. However, this approach eventually leads to further receptor supersensitivity and worsening of the manifestations of TD.

Neuroleptic malignant syndrome is a severe form of drug toxicity that occurs in 0.5–1% of patients treated with antipsychotic drugs. It is a life-threatening condition characterized by muscle rigidity, elevated temperature (>38°C), altered consciousness, and autonomic dysfunction (tachycardia, diaphoresis, tachypnea, and urinary and fecal incontinence). The syndrome resembles malignant hyperthermia.

Phenothiazines may increase serum prolactin levels by blocking dopamine receptors in the tubero-infundibular pathway (see Box 22–1) and thereby cause gynecomastia in men and menstrual irregularities in women. Via their effects on the hypothalamus, antipsychotic drugs sometimes impair thermoregulation and cause poikilothermy, a condition in which the body temperature tends to approach the ambient temperature. This may lead to hyperthermia (including heat stroke) or hypothermia. In addition, high doses of thioridazine can cause pigmentary retinopathy and cardiac toxicity.

Treatment of Adverse Effects.   Acute extrapyramidal effects (akathisia, pseudoparkinsonism, and dystonias) that are caused by phenothiazines and other antipsychotic drugs can be managed by lowering the drug dosage, changing to an atypical antipsychotic drug, or administering an additional drug to counteract the adverse effects. Drugs that counteract the effects include **benztropine** (an anticholinergic drug), **diphenhydramine** (an antihistamine with significant anticholinergic activity), and **amantadine** (an agent that increases dopamine release in the basal ganglia and may be used in conjunction with an anticholinergic drug).

TD is not easily managed and does not necessarily subside if a causative drug is discontinued. Hence, prevention is important. To prevent TD, antipsychotic drugs should be used in the lowest doses for the shortest period of time required to control symptoms of schizophrenia. The drugs should be discontinued periodically in order to assess the need for continued treatment and possibly to reduce the development of dopamine supersensitivity. Patients should be evaluated regularly for early signs of TD, which are sometimes reversible. TD often becomes irreversible if it is not detected early or is allowed to persist.

Once detected, TD is best managed by reducing the dosage of antipsychotic medication. This results in significant improvement in many patients. There are no approved drugs for the treatment of TD, but some success has been reported with **amantadine, dopamine receptor agonists,** and **clozapine.** Other drugs that may be effective include **physostigmine** (a cholinergic agonist) and the **benzodiazepines.**

Neuroleptic malignant syndrome is managed by providing supportive care and immediately discontinuing treatment with the offending antipsychotic drug. A dopamine receptor agonist, such as **bromocriptine,** may significantly reduce rigidity, fever, and other manifestations of the syndrome. If future antipsychotic therapy is required in patients who have experienced this syndrome, an atypical drug should be used because the atypical drugs are associated with a lower incidence of neuroleptic malignant syndrome.

Interactions.   The major drug interactions of phenothiazines are listed in Table 22–4.

Indications.   Phenothiazines are primarily used to treat **schizophrenia** and other forms of psychosis, including **drug-induced psychosis** and psychosis associated with the manic phase of **bipolar disorder.** Phenothiazines are also used to treat severely agitated patients, including those with **dementia** and

severe mental retardation. Because the phenothiazines have antiemetic activity, some of them are used in the management of **nausea** and **vomiting** (see Chapter 28).

Chlorpromazine and Thioridazine

Chlorpromazine and thioridazine are low-potency phenothiazines with similar properties. Of the two agents, thioridazine produces greater anticholinergic effects, and this probably accounts for its tendency to cause fewer extrapyramidal side effects. High doses of thioridazine may cause pigmentary retinopathy and cardiac arrhythmia.

Fluphenazine and Trifluoperazine

Fluphenazine and trifluoperazine are high-potency phenothiazines that produce fewer autonomic side effects but more extrapyramidal side effects than do low-potency phenothiazines. Fluphenazine is available in a long-acting depot preparation that is intended for intramuscular injection every 1–3 weeks and is useful for treating patients who are not compliant with oral medication or are unable to take oral drugs.

Thioxanthenes

The chemical structure of the thioxanthenes is similar to that of the phenothiazines. In the thioxanthene structure, however, the nitrogen atom of the phenothiazine ring is replaced with a carbon atom (see Fig. 22–2B).

Thiothixene is one of the most widely used thioxanthenes, and it has pharmacologic properties that are similar to those of trifluoperazine (see Tables 22–3 and 22–4). Thiothixene is primarily used for the treatment of **schizophrenia.**

Butyrophenones

The most widely used butyrophenone is **haloperidol,** a drug whose chemical structure is shown in Fig. 22–2B. Haloperidol is a high-potency drug that has properties similar to those of fluphenazine and may cause significant extrapyramidal side effects (see Tables 22–3 and 22–4). Like fluphenazine, haloperidol is available in a long-acting depot preparation for intramuscular administration. Haloperidol is extensively metabolized in the liver, and its metabolites are excreted in the urine and bile.

In addition to its use in treating psychoses such as **schizophrenia,** haloperidol is employed in the treatment of **Tourette's syndrome** (Gilles de la Tourette's syndrome). This syndrome is characterized by facial and vocal tics, coprolalia (compulsive use of obscene words, particularly those related to feces), and echolalia (repetition of another person's words or phrases).

Azepines

Loxapine, clozapine, and olanzapine are azepine derivatives. While loxapine is a typical antipsychotic drug, clozapine and olanzapine are atypical drugs that produce fewer extrapyramidal side effects than do other antipsychotic drugs.

Loxapine

Loxapine is a dibenzoxazepine and a typical antipsychotic drug whose properties are similar to those of the phenothiazines.

Clozapine

Clozapine has a tricyclic dibenzodiazepine structure and a unique profile of pharmacologic and clinical effects. It is the first of a new generation of atypical antipsychotic drugs that cause significantly fewer extrapyramidal side effects while exhibiting greater activity against the negative symptoms of schizophrenia.

Because clozapine is a potent antagonist of a large number of receptors, it has been difficult to attribute its effects to a particular mechanism of action. It seems likely that its therapeutic effects result from blockade of D_4 receptors and $5-HT_2$ receptors. Both of these actions may contribute to its greater efficacy against the negative symptoms of schizophrenia and to its lower incidence of extrapyramidal side effects. The use of clozapine is associated with significant sedation and autonomic side effects. These adverse reactions are due to blockade of histamine, muscarinic, and α-adrenergic receptors. The use of clozapine is also associated with a 1.3% first-year incidence of potentially fatal agranulocytosis. For this reason, the Food and Drug Administration has required weekly monitoring of leukocyte counts during the first 6 months of therapy, the period during which the risk of agranulocytosis is greatest. After 6 months, biweekly monitoring of leukocyte counts is required.

Olanzapine

Olanzapine is a thienobenzodiazepine analogue of clozapine. Its pharmacologic properties are similar to those of clozapine, but it causes fewer autonomic side effects and has not been reported to cause agranulocytosis. Like clozapine, olanzapine causes minimal extrapyramidal side effects.

Olanzapine has about twice the affinity for $5-HT_2$ receptors as it does for D_2 receptors, and it is able to block dopamine D_3 and D_4 receptors. Although it also blocks histamine, muscarinic, and α-adrenergic receptors, it does so to a lesser extent than does clozapine.

Clinical trials indicate that olanzapine is as effective as haloperidol in alleviating the positive symptoms of schizophrenia, is superior to haloperidol in alleviating the negative symptoms, and produces significantly fewer extrapyramidal side effects. The most common adverse reactions to olanzapine have been sedation and weight gain. At higher doses, olanzapine may cause akathisia, pseudoparkinsonism, and dystonias.

Other Antipsychotic Drugs
Risperidone

Risperidone is a newer atypical antipsychotic drug that has a benzisoxazole structure. Its pharmacologic properties are similar to those of olanzapine, but it appears to cause less sedation, more orthostatic hypotension, and a higher incidence of extrapyramidal side effects than does olanzapine. In some patients, risperidone elevates levels of serum prolactin. It also lengthens the QT interval seen on the electrocardiogram and may predispose patients to cardiac arrhythmias, including torsade de pointes.

Molindone

Molindone is a dihydroindolone derivative with a unique spectrum of pharmacologic activities. Some authorities classify it as an atypical drug, but others do not. It appears to cause a relatively low incidence of autonomic side effects and sedation. Although its incidence of extrapyramidal side effects also appears to be relatively low, it is probably higher than that of the newer atypical antipsychotic agents when they are given in equivalent doses. Molindone has a relatively short half-life but is metabolized to active and inactive compounds that have a longer half-life. Molindone is sometimes effective in patients who do not tolerate or respond to other drugs.

Treatment Considerations

All typical antipsychotic drugs appear to be equally effective when used in equipotent doses for the treatment of schizophrenia. The highly sedating drugs are no more effective than the less-sedating drugs in calming agitated patients, and the less-sedating drugs are no more effective than the highly sedating drugs in treating withdrawn patients. Hence, the choice of drug is primarily based on the need to minimize autonomic or extrapyramidal side effects. Several controlled trials indicate that low-dose regimens are as effective as high-dose regimens and produce fewer side effects.

The atypical antipsychotic drugs represent an appealing choice for the treatment of schizophrenia, and some authorities believe that they will become the drugs of choice for treating most forms of psychosis. In comparison with the typical drugs, the atypical drugs produce a lower incidence of extrapyramidal side effects and appear to be more effective against the negative symptoms of schizophrenia. However, the long-term effectiveness of atypical drugs in patients with chronic schizophrenia has not yet been adequately studied.

During the first 2 weeks of treatment with an antipsychotic drug, many patients exhibit some alleviation of positive symptoms and an improvement in socialization, mood, and self-care habits. However, the maximal response to treatment generally requires 6 weeks or longer. After maximal improvement has been obtained, it may be possible to reduce the dosage during maintenance therapy. Antipsychotic medication is usually continued for at least 12 months after the remission of acute psychotic symptoms. At that time, a low-dose regimen or gradual withdrawal of medication should be considered in order to reduce the probability of developing TD. Antipsychotic drugs should be tapered slowly before discontinuation, since abrupt discontinuation may cause withdrawal symptoms such as insomnia, nightmares, nausea, vomiting, diarrhea, restlessness, salivation, and sweating.

AFFECTIVE DISORDERS

Affective disorders are also called **mood disorders.** The two most common affective disorders are major depressive disorder and bipolar disorder. The primary drugs used in their treatment are antidepressant drugs and mood-stabilizing drugs.

Clinical Findings
Major Depressive Disorder

Major depressive disorder (unipolar depression) is characterized by depressed mood, loss of interest or pleasure in life, sleep disturbances, feelings of worthlessness, diminished ability to think or concentrate, and recurrent thoughts of suicide. Depressed patients may also be irritable or anxious.

Bipolar Disorder

Bipolar disorder (previously called manic-depressive disorder) is characterized by recurrent fluctuations in mood, energy, and behavior that encompass the extremes of human experience. This disorder differs from major depression in that periods of mania alternate or occur simultaneously with depressive symptoms. The clinical presentation varies widely. The manic phase is characterized by elevated mood, inflated self-esteem (grandiosity), increased talking (pressure of speech), racing thoughts (flight of ideas), increased social or work activity, and decreased need for sleep. Manic patients may become hostile and uncooperative. As the manic phase intensifies, some patients experience psychotic symptoms such as delusions.

Typically, the manic phase occurs just before or just after a depressive episode. In many patients, depressive and manic episodes last several weeks or months. In some patients, however, the episodes change within hours or days (rapid cycling).

Etiology and Pathogenesis

According to the **biogenic amine hypothesis,** mood disorders result from abnormalities in serotonin, norepinephrine, or dopamine neurotransmission. Serotoninergic fibers projecting from the raphe nuclei in the midbrain to limbic structures are important in regulating mood, and these neuronal pathways are believed to be hypofunctional in depressed patients. The serotoninergic system is activated during behavioral arousal and increases cortical awareness of emotional reactions to environmental events. It is believed that impaired serotonin neurotransmission may decrease cortical responsiveness to emotional activation, leading to affective dysfunction and depression. Noradrenergic fibers that project from the locus ceruleus to the cerebral cortex may also play a role in depression, as may dopaminergic fibers innervating the nucleus accumbens.

There is evidence that links depression with abnormal circadian rhythms and melatonin regulation. Melatonin is the principal mediator of biologic rhythms and is known to suppress the activity of serotoninergic neurons. Investigators postulate that excess melatonin production contributes to the development of depression. This hypothesis is particularly relevant to seasonal affective disorder, which usually occurs during the winter months, when daylight is reduced and melatonin levels are increased. However, other types of depression may also be caused by abnormal melatonin regulation. Abnormalities in melatonin and serotonin metabolism may also contribute to the sleep disturbances seen in patients with affective disorders.

The biogenic amine hypothesis is supported by the fact that all antidepressant drugs act to increase serotonin, norepinephrine, or dopamine neurotransmission in the brain. Most antidepressant drugs increase the synaptic concentration of serotonin, and this leads to down-regulation of presynaptic autoreceptors. Investigators believe that the down-regulation in turn increases the firing rate of serotoninergic neurons and thereby produces the delayed therapeutic effect of antidepressant drugs. These mechanisms are depicted in Fig. 22–3.

ANTIDEPRESSANT DRUGS

Depression can be treated with tricyclic antidepressants, selective serotonin reuptake inhibitors, and a host of other antidepressants that have different structures and act by various mechanisms of action (Table 22–5). If patients fail to respond to these drugs, monoamine oxidase inhibitors may be used.

Because depressed patients may attempt suicide, the safety of an antidepressant in overdose is an important consideration when selecting a drug for a particular patient.

Tricyclic Antidepressants

The tricyclic antidepressants (TCAs) include **amitriptyline, clomipramine, desipramine, imipramine,** and **nortriptyline.** These agents are highly effective in the treatment of depression and several other disorders, but they are associated with a high incidence of adverse effects. They also cause severe toxicity when taken in excessive doses.

Drug Properties

Chemistry and Pharmacokinetics. Each TCA contains a three-ring nucleus with an aliphatic side chain attached to the central ring (Fig. 22–4A). The side chain terminates in either a secondary or

tertiary amine group. The type of amine group partly determines the drug's pharmacologic properties, as discussed below. The TCAs are incompletely absorbed after oral administration and are extensively metabolized to active and inactive metabolites in the liver. The tertiary amines are deaminated to pharmacologically active secondary amines, and several of these metabolites are available as drugs. For example, amitriptyline is converted to nortriptyline, and imipramine is converted to desipramine. The TCAs and their active metabolites have relatively long half-lives, ranging from 18 to 70 hours (Table 22–6).

Mechanisms and Pharmacologic Effects. All TCAs block the neuronal reuptake of norepinephrine and serotonin, but they do so to differing degrees (see Table 22–5). The blockade occurs as soon as drug administration begins and causes an immediate increase in the synaptic concentration of serotonin. The blockade is also believed to trigger a series of adaptive changes in norepinephrine and serotonin neurotransmission. These changes produce an antidepressant effect that becomes apparent about 2–4 weeks after drug therapy is started. Over time, the increased synaptic concentration of serotonin may cause down-regulation of presynaptic autoreceptors and thereby increase the firing rate of serotoninergic neurons. The short-term and long-term effects of TCAs and other reuptake inhibitors on serotonin neurotransmission are illustrated in Fig. 22–3.

Adverse Effects. Like many of the antipsychotic drugs, the TCAs produce autonomic side effects by blocking muscarinic and α-adrenergic receptors. Some of the TCAs also produce marked sedation (Table 22–7). In fact, TCAs are often administered at bedtime, when their sedative effects may have the added benefit of promoting sleep. The TCAs lower the seizure threshold and may induce seizures at therapeutic as well as toxic serum concentrations.

Taking an overdose of a TCA may cause life-threatening cardiac arrhythmia (which frequently presents as a wide QRS complex tachycardia); marked autonomic effects, including hypotension and sinus tachycardia; excessive sedation; and seizures.

Treatment of Adverse Effects. The type of arrhythmia that occurs with an overdose can be treated by the intravenous administration of **sodium bicarbonate.** Sodium bicarbonate increases the ratio of nonionized TCA to ionized TCA and thereby decreases the binding of the TCA to the sodium channel in cardiac membranes.

Interactions. Drug interactions are listed in Table 22–8.

Indications. TCAs have been used to treat all forms of **depression** and to treat several other conditions. The TCAs and other antidepressants are effective in the treatment of certain **anxiety disorders,** such as panic disorder, phobic disorders, and obsessive-compulsive disorder. Clomipramine is particularly effective in treating patients with obsessive-compulsive behavior. TCAs are beneficial in the

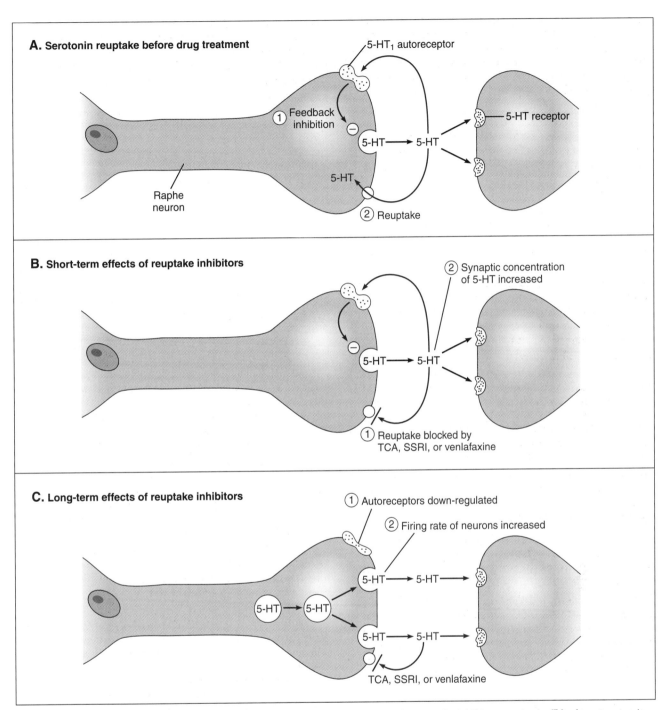

FIGURE 22–3. Mechanisms of neuronal reuptake inhibitors. (A) In the absence of a reuptake inhibitor, serotonin (5-hydroxytryptamine, or 5-HT) is released from raphe neurons that project to limbic structures. Serotonin activates postsynaptic and presynaptic 5-HT receptors and undergoes reuptake into the presynaptic neuron. **(B)** When a tricyclic antidepressant (TCA), a selective serotonin reuptake inhibitor (SSRI), or venlafaxine is initially given, the drug blocks the reuptake of 5-HT and increases its synaptic concentration. **(C)** With continued use of a TCA, SSRI, or venlafaxine, increased synaptic concentrations of 5-HT cause the down-regulation of presynaptic autoreceptors and an increase in the firing rate of raphe neurons.

management of certain **sleep disorders,** including somnambulism, night terrors, and enuresis. The TCAs repress abnormal rapid eye movement (REM) sleep and dreaming, which are conditions that contribute to somnambulism and night terrors. In patients with enuresis, TCAs appear to increase the awareness of the need to urinate and thereby facilitate waking up for this purpose. TCAs and other

antidepressants also have a role in the treatment of **chronic pain syndromes** because of their mood-elevating effect and analgesic activity.

Specific Drugs

Nortriptyline and desipramine are secondary amines formed by the demethylation of amitriptyline

TABLE 22–5. Mechanisms of Antidepressant Drugs*

Drug	Inhibition of Neuronal Reuptake of Norepinephrine	Inhibition of Neuronal Reuptake of Serotonin	Other Mechanisms
Tricyclic antidepressants			
Amitriptyline	++	++++	None.
Clomipramine	++	+++	None.
Desipramine	++++	+	None.
Imipramine	+++	+++	None.
Nortriptyline	+++	++	None.
Selective serotonin reuptake inhibitors			
Fluoxetine	0	+++	None.
Fluvoxamine	0	++++	None.
Paroxetine	0	++++	None.
Sertraline	0	++++	None.
Monoamine oxidase inhibitors			
Phenelzine	+	+	Inhibits monoamine oxidase.
Tranylcypromine	+	+	Inhibits monoamine oxidase.
Other antidepressant drugs			
Bupropion	+	+	Inhibits reuptake of dopamine.
Hypericum	++	++	Inhibits monoamine oxidase.
Mirtazapine	0	0	Increases release of serotonin and norepinephrine via blockade of α_2-adrenergic receptors.
Nefazodone	0/+	++	Blocks postsynaptic serotonin 5-HT$_2$ receptors.
Trazodone	0	+++	None.
Venlafaxine	+++	++++	None.

*Ratings range from none (0) to high (++++).

and imipramine, respectively. Secondary amines block norepinephrine uptake more than they block serotonin reuptake, and this is especially true of desipramine.

Amitriptyline, clomipramine, and imipramine are tertiary amines. They block serotonin reuptake to a greater extent than do secondary amines. They also produce more sedation and autonomic side effects than do secondary amines.

Studies have shown that all TCAs are equally effective in relieving depression, though some patients respond better to one drug than to another. The choice of a TCA is primarily based on the relative incidence of adverse effects produced by the different drugs. A drug that causes a higher degree of sedation may be chosen for highly agitated or anxious patients with depression, whereas a drug that causes a lower degree of sedation may be preferred for patients who are more apathetic or withdrawn.

Selective Serotonin Reuptake Inhibitors

The selective serotonin reuptake inhibitors (SSRIs) are a newer class of antidepressants that include fluoxetine, fluvoxamine, paroxetine, and sertraline. The SSRIs have become the most widely used drugs for the treatment of depression and certain anxiety disorders, such as panic disorder and obsessive-compulsive disorder. They are as effective as the TCAs but cause fewer autonomic side effects

and less sedation. They are also much safer than the TCAs following an overdose, in that the SSRIs seldom cause cardiac arrhythmia and are less likely to induce seizures.

Drug Properties

Chemistry and Pharmacokinetics. The SSRIs are a structurally heterogeneous group of compounds (see Fig. 22–4B). They are well absorbed from the gut after oral administration and are extensively metabolized by cytochrome P450 isozymes. Fluoxetine has a longer half-life than the other drugs in this class and is converted to an active metabolite that has an even longer half-life (see Table 22–6). The metabolites of other SSRIs have little or no pharmacologic activity.

Mechanisms and Pharmacologic Effects. The SSRIs selectively block the neuronal reuptake of serotonin and have much less effect on the reuptake of norepinephrine. Their efficacy in the treatment of depression supports the hypothesis that serotonin dysfunction plays a significant role in the pathophysiology of depression. The short-term and long-term effects of serotonin reuptake inhibition are illustrated in Fig. 22–3.

Adverse Effects. The SSRIs produce fewer sedative, autonomic, and cardiovascular side effects than do the TCAs. Unlike the TCAs, the SSRIs are usually administered in the morning, because they tend to increase alertness in patients. Their most

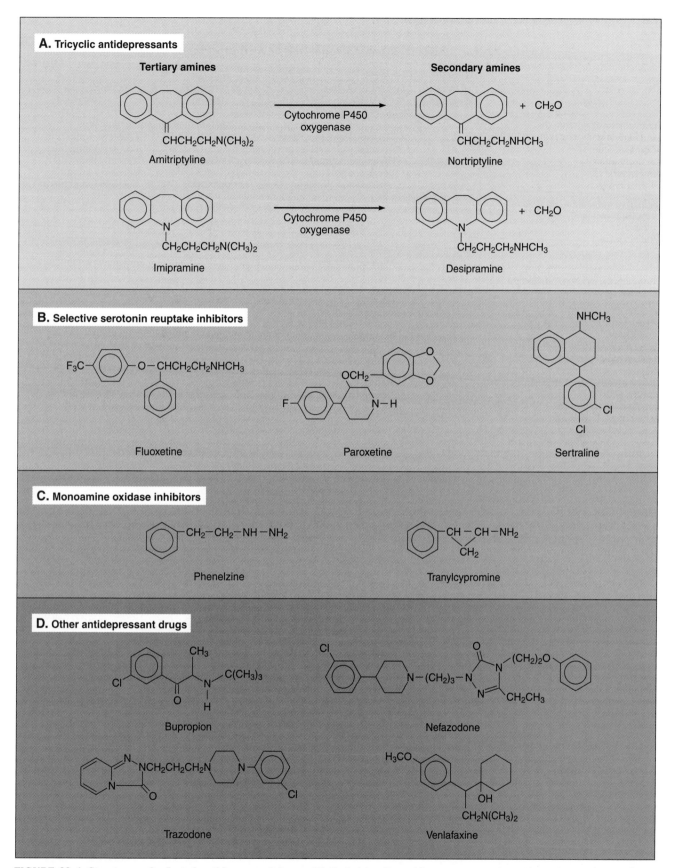

FIGURE 22–4. Structures of selected antidepressant drugs. (A) Each tricyclic antidepressant contains a three-ring nucleus with an aliphatic side chain attached to the central ring. The side chain terminates in either a secondary or tertiary amine group. Amitriptyline and imipramine are tertiary amines that are deaminated to nortriptyline and desipramine, respectively. All four of these substances are pharmacologically active. **(B)** The selective serotonin reuptake inhibitors include fluoxetine, paroxetine, and sertraline. **(C)** Phenelzine and tranylcypromine are first-generation monoamine oxidase (MAO) inhibitors that block both MAO-A and MAO-B. **(D)** Other antidepressant drugs include bupropion, an aminoketone; nefazodone and trazodone, two examples of triazolopyridine drugs; and venlafaxine, a phenylethylamine.

TABLE 22–6. Pharmacokinetic Properties of Antidepressant Drugs

Drug	Half-Life of Drug (Hours)	Active Metabolite	Half-Life of Metabolite (Hours)	Effect on Cytochrome P450 Isozymes
Tricyclic antidepressants				
Amitriptyline	40	Nortriptyline	35	Low-level inhibition
Clomipramine	30	Desmethylclomipramine	70	Low-level inhibition
Desipramine	18	Hydroxydesipramine	Unknown	Low-level inhibition
Imipramine	18	Desipramine	18	Low-level inhibition
Nortriptyline	35	Hydroxynortriptyline	Unknown	Low-level inhibition
Selective serotonin reuptake inhibitors				
Fluoxetine	60	Norfluoxetine	192	Very high level inhibition
Fluvoxamine	15	None	—	High-level inhibition
Paroxetine	21	None	—	High-level inhibition
Sertraline	26	Minimal activity	—	Low-level inhibition
Monoamine oxidase inhibitors				
Phenelzine	2	None	—	None
Tranylcypromine	3	None	—	None
Other antidepressant drugs				
Bupropion	15	Several	>15	Induction
Hypericum	30	Unknown	—	Unknown
Mirtazapine	30	Minimal activity	—	Low-level inhibition
Nefazodone	5	Hydroxynefazodone	3	Low-level inhibition
Trazodone	6	None	—	Low-level inhibition
Venlafaxine	5	Desmethylvenlafaxine	11	Low-level inhibition

common adverse effects are nervousness, dizziness, and insomnia. They occasionally cause male sexual dysfunction in the forms of priapism and impotence. Many of the side effects of SSRIs subside with continued use. The SSRIs should be used with caution in patients with seizure disorders, hepatic disorders, diabetes, or bipolar disorder.

Interactions. Because of their ability to inhibit cytochrome P450 isozymes, the SSRIs have significant interactions with a variety of drugs. Among the SSRIs, fluoxetine has the greatest effect on the CYP2D isozyme and sertraline has the least effect. Inhibition of CYP2D can increase the serum levels of antipsychotic drugs, TCAs, and dextromethorphan. Inhibi-

TABLE 22–7. Adverse Effects of Antidepressant Drugs*

Drug	Sedation	Anticholinergic Effects	Orthostatic Hypotension	Cardiac Conduction Disturbances
Tricyclic antidepressants				
Amitriptyline	++++	++++	+++	+++
Clomipramine	++++	++++	++	+++
Desipramine	++	++	++	++
Imipramine	+++	+++	+++	+++
Nortriptyline	++	++	++	++
Selective serotonin reuptake inhibitors				
Fluoxetine	0	0	0	0
Fluvoxamine	+	0	0	0
Paroxetine	+	+	0	0
Sertraline	0	0	0	0
Monoamine oxidase inhibitors				
Phenelzine	++	++	++	+
Tranylcypromine	+	++	++	+
Other antidepressant drugs				
Bupropion	+	+	0	+
Hypericum	0	0	0	0
Mirtazapine	+	+	++	+
Nefazodone	+++	0	+++	+
Trazodone	++++	0	+++	+
Venlafaxine	+	+	0	+

*Ratings range from none (0) to high (++++).

TABLE 22–8.   Interactions of Antidepressant Drugs and Lithium With Other Drugs

Tricyclic antidepressants (TCAs)
- Antipsychotic drugs, calcium channel blockers, cimetidine, methylphenidate, quinidine, and SSRIs increase serum levels of TCAs and may cause toxicity.
- Barbiturates, carbamazepine, ethanol (long-term), and phenytoin decrease serum levels of TCAs.
- TCAs decrease serum levels of levodopa.
- TCAs increase serum levels of phenytoin and oral anticoagulants.
- Concurrent use of a TCA and an MAO inhibitor may cause severe toxicity.
- TCAs should be used cautiously with sympathomimetic amines or quinidine-type drugs.

Selective serotonin reuptake inhibitors (SSRIs)
- SSRIs, especially fluoxetine, increase serum levels of many other drugs, including β-adrenergic receptor antagonists, alprazolam, antiepileptic drugs, antipsychotic drugs, carbamazepine, dextromethorphan, diazepam, methadone, phenytoin, TCAs, and theophylline.
- Concurrent use of an SSRI with an anticoagulant, lithium, or MAO inhibitor may result in increased pharmacologic effects or toxicity.

Monoamine oxidase (MAO) inhibitors
- MAO inhibitors block the metabolism of levodopa, sympathomimetic amines, and amines contained in certain foods. Concurrent use of an MAO inhibitor and these drugs or foods may cause severe hypertension.
- Concurrent use of an MAO inhibitor and another antidepressant may cause delirium, hypertensive crises, seizures, and serotonin syndrome. An MAO inhibitor should never be used concurrently with an SSRI. If an MAO inhibitor is used with a TCA or an atypical antidepressant, doses of both drugs must be significantly reduced.

Other antidepressant drugs
- Nefazodone may increase serum levels of alprazolam, digoxin, haloperidol, and possibly other drugs.
- Trazodone may increase the serum levels and the toxicity of carbamazepine and phenytoin and may have additive effects with these and other drugs that cause central nervous system depression or hypotension.

Lithium
- Diuretics and nonsteroidal anti-inflammatory drugs (except sulindac) decrease the clearance of lithium, increase the serum levels of lithium, and may cause lithium toxicity.
- Antipsychotic drugs increase the neurotoxicity of lithium.
- Sodium chloride increases the excretion of lithium and decreases the serum levels of lithium.

tion of CYP2C and CYP3A can increase serum levels of alprazolam, diazepam, carbamazepine, phenytoin, and other drugs (see Table 22–8). SSRIs may also increase the hypoprothrombinemic effect of warfarin.

The SSRIs should not be used concurrently with monoamine oxidase (MAO) inhibitors, because both types of drugs increase the serotonin levels in the brain and their concurrent use may precipitate the **serotonin syndrome.** This syndrome is characterized by agitation, restlessness, confusion, insomnia, seizures, severe hypertension, and gastrointestinal symptoms. At least 2 weeks should elapse between the discontinuation of treatment with either an MAO inhibitor or an SSRI and the start of treatment with the other drug. The exception is that 5 weeks must elapse between the discontinuation of fluoxetine and the administration of an MAO inhibitor.

Indications.   The SSRIs are used to treat **depression;** to treat **eating disorders,** such as bulimia nervosa and anorexia nervosa; and to treat **anxiety disorders,** such as panic disorder, phobic disorders, and obsessive-compulsive disorder. SSRIs may be effective in the management of other conditions, such as **fibromyalgia, autism,** and **premenstrual syndrome.**

Fluoxetine

Fluoxetine is the first drug approved for the treatment of bulimia nervosa and may be effective in the management of anorexia nervosa. The drug is well absorbed orally and is converted to an active metabolite, norfluoxetine. The parent compound has a half-life of 2.5 days, but its active metabolite has a half-life of about 8 days. This long duration of action may be a disadvantage if severe adverse effects occur.

Fluoxetine causes more drug interactions than do other SSRIs. It can impair the regulation of blood glucose levels in diabetic patients. It can also cause a syndrome of inappropriate antidiuretic hormone secretion (SIADH), characterized by persistent hyponatremia and elevated urine osmolality.

Paroxetine and Sertraline

Paroxetine and sertraline have half-lives of 21 hours and 26 hours, respectively. Paroxetine has a high bioavailability, whereas sertraline undergoes extensive first-pass elimination. Sertraline has relatively little effect on P450 isozymes and causes fewer drug interactions than does fluoxetine. Sertraline may be preferred in elderly patients because its elimination is not affected substantially by aging. Paroxetine is somewhat more sedating than fluoxetine and sertraline.

Fluvoxamine

Fluvoxamine is approved for the treatment of obsessive-compulsive disorder but has also been used to treat depression and panic disorder. Fluvoxamine has a half-life of about 15 hours and may be associated with sedative effects.

Monoamine Oxidase Inhibitors

Because the monoamine oxidase (MAO) inhibitors have many potentially serious interactions with other drugs and with food, they are not considered drugs of choice in the treatment of depression. They are generally used as alternative therapy when patients have failed to respond adequately to other drugs.

Classification

The MAO inhibitors are classified according to their selectivity for the two main types of MAO. Type A (MAO-A) preferentially oxidizes serotonin but will also metabolize norepinephrine and dopamine. Type B (MAO-B) preferentially metabolizes dopamine. MAO-A is found in higher concentrations in the gut and other peripheral tissues than is MAO-B, and the inhibition of MAO-A is believed to be responsible for the antidepressant effects of the MAO inhibitors.

The first-generation MAO inhibitors for treating depression include **phenelzine** and **tranylcypromine** and are irreversible inhibitors of both MAO-A and MAO-B. Their chemical structures are shown in Fig. 22–4C. The second-generation MAO inhibitors include **meclobemide** and are reversible inhibitors of MAO-A (RIMAs). The RIMAs are used in many countries for treating depression but are not yet available in the USA. **Selegiline** represents a third type of MAO inhibitor, which selectively inhibits MAO-B and is used in the treatment of Parkinson's disease (see Chapter 21).

Drug Properties

The first-generation MAO inhibitors, phenelzine and tranylcypromine, are adequately absorbed from the gut and have relatively short half-lives (see Table 22–6). However, they irreversibly bind to and inhibit MAO, and their pharmacologic effects persist for many hours after their serum levels have declined. Phenelzine and tranylcypromine may increase serotonin levels more than they do norepinephrine levels in the brain, and their antidepressant effects are probably caused by down-regulation of presynaptic autoreceptors and subsequent increased firing of serotoninergic neurons. As with other antidepressants, the clinical effects of MAO inhibitors are delayed for several weeks after therapy begins.

As shown in Table 22–8, the MAO inhibitors interact with SSRIs, TCAs, and other antidepressant drugs and have the potential to cause severe toxicity when administered with these drugs. Concurrent administration of MAO inhibitors and TCAs or other antidepressants requires dosage reduction and careful monitoring.

MAO inhibitors may cause severe hypertension when administered with sympathomimetic amines or with foods containing certain amines. These foods include many types of cheese (especially aged cheeses), beer, some wines (especially Chianti), some meats and fish (especially canned meat, liver, sardines, and herring), some fruits and vegetables (especially raisins, broad beans, avocados, and canned figs), and some products when consumed in large quantities (especially chocolate and coffee).

Other Antidepressant Drugs

Several other drugs with diverse chemical structures (see Fig. 22–4D) and diverse mechanisms of action are available for the treatment of depression.

Bupropion

Bupropion is an aminoketone whose mechanism of action is not well understood. It is a relatively weak inhibitor of the neuronal reuptake of dopamine, norepinephrine, and serotonin. Bupropion produces few anticholinergic side effects, causes very little sedation, and rarely produces cardiovascular effects or sexual dysfunction. It may cause agitation, insomnia, nausea, and weight loss. A formulation of bupropion has been developed as adjunct therapy for patients who are attempting to quit smoking cigarettes (see Chapter 24).

Hypericum

Extracts of the plant called St. John's wort (*Hypericum perforatum*) have been found to exhibit antidepressant activity, and products containing these extracts are available in health food stores. The extracts contain a substance called hypericin and several flavones. Some of these compounds inhibit MAO, while others appear to block the neuronal reuptake of serotonin. Hypericum appears to cause fewer adverse effects than do TCAs. Clinical studies are being conducted to evaluate the clinical efficacy and safety of hypericum.

Mirtazapine

Mirtazapine is a newer tetracyclic piperazinoazepine drug that is structurally different from other antidepressants and has both antidepressant and antianxiety effects. Mirtazapine blocks presynaptic α_2-adrenergic autoreceptors and heteroreceptors and thereby increases the neuronal release of norepinephrine and serotonin, respectively. It increases central norepinephrine concentrations to a greater degree than do the TCAs, and it is also a potent antagonist of 5-HT_2 and 5-HT_3 receptors. Mirtazapine is better tolerated and causes fewer adverse reactions than do the TCAs. However, it may significantly elevate hepatic enzyme levels, and it has been associated with a few cases of agranulocytosis.

Nefazodone and Trazodone

Nefazodone and trazodone are both triazolopyridine drugs.

Nefazodone acts primarily by inhibiting 5-HT_2 receptors. It has little or no anticholinergic, antiadrenergic, or antihistamine activity. It may cause sedation, dizziness, nausea, and visual changes, but it has not been associated with priapism or sexual dysfunction.

Trazodone selectively inhibits the neuronal reuptake of serotonin. It causes considerable sedation and orthostatic hypotension, but it does not produce anticholinergic side effects and has minimal effects on cardiac conduction.

Venlafaxine

Venlafaxine is a structurally unique antidepressant that strongly blocks the reuptake of both norepinephrine and serotonin (see Fig. 22–3). It has a side effect profile similar to that of the SSRIs. It does not inhibit muscarinic, adrenergic, or histamine receptors, and it produces few autonomic, sedative, or cardiovascular side effects.

Treatment Considerations

Depression is one of the most common mental illnesses. Because it tends to be underdiagnosed, it often goes untreated. The primary treatment for patients with depression is drug therapy, but psychotherapy enhances the response to pharmacologic treatment and increases patient compliance with medication. Electroconvulsive therapy is sometimes used as an alternative when antidepressants have been ineffective or are not tolerated. Over 80% of patients respond to treatment with drugs, psychotherapy, electroconvulsive therapy, or a combination of these modalities.

The initial drug used in the treatment of depression is usually either a TCA or an SSRI, depending on clinician preference. There is a growing body of evidence that SSRIs are better tolerated by patients, produce fewer adverse effects, and are safer in overdose than are TCAs. The disadvantages of SSRIs include their higher cost and the increased tendency of some SSRIs to cause drug interactions. Sertraline causes fewer drug interactions than do other SSRIs and may be preferred in the treatment of patients who are taking other drugs that may interact with SSRIs.

If TCAs or SSRIs are not effective or well tolerated, the clinician has a growing choice of other antidepressants, such as mirtazapine, nefazodone, and venlafaxine. Mirtazapine and venlafaxine are attractive because of their low incidence of sedation, autonomic side effects, and cardiac toxicity (see Table 22–7). In comparison with other antidepressants, nefazodone has demonstrated a lower incidence of activating side effects, such as nervousness, agitation, and insomnia, and it does not cause sexual dysfunction.

It usually takes 2–4 weeks for antidepressants to elevate the mood of depressed patients, and some patients do not respond until after 6 weeks or longer. Some authorities believe that many cases of treatment-resistant depression are due to inadequate drug dosage, inadequate duration of therapy, or patient noncompliance. Moreover, studies indicate that many patients who failed to respond to treatment in the past will respond to adequate doses of SSRIs or other new antidepressants.

To prevent relapse, antidepressants are usually continued for 4–9 months after remission of depressive symptoms.

MOOD-STABILIZING DRUGS
Lithium

Lithium is the lightest of the alkali metal elements and was accidentally discovered to have a calming effect in patients with mania. Lithium has been called a mood stabilizer because it reduces both manic and depressive symptoms and thereby tends to normalize the mood in patients with bipolar disorder. However, lithium has greater activity against manic symptoms than it does against depression, and it is primarily used to treat or prevent the manic phase of bipolar disorder.

Pharmacokinetics. Lithium is administered orally in the form of lithium carbonate or lithium citrate, and it is available in immediate-release and sustained-release preparations. About 95–100% of the administered dose is absorbed from the gut. Lithium is widely distributed throughout the body, with the highest concentrations found in the thyroid gland, bone, and some areas of the brain. The drug is not metabolized. It has a half-life of about 24 hours and is excreted in the urine. Lithium is extensively reabsorbed from the renal tubules, and the renal clearance of lithium is about 20% of the glomerular filtration rate. Lithium clearance increases during pregnancy. Sodium competes with lithium for renal tubular reabsorption and may thereby increase the excretion of lithium.

Mechanisms and Pharmacologic Effects. The mechanisms by which lithium produces its mood-stabilizing effects are not well understood. The drug appears to act by suppressing the formation of second messengers involved in neurotransmitter signal transduction, but the relationship between this action and the drug's clinical effect is unclear. Lithium reduces the formation of inositol triphosphate (IP_3) by inhibiting *myo*-inositol-1-phosphatase, an enzyme in the inositol phosphate pathway. This enzyme participates in the regeneration of inositol and the inositol phosphate precursors to IP_3. By reducing IP_3 formation, lithium reduces the neuronal response to serotonin and norepinephrine, whose effects are partly mediated by IP_3 (see Table 18–1). Lithium also interferes with the formation of cyclic adenosine monophosphate.

Lithium produces a calming effect in manic patients, but the maximal response to lithium often requires several days or weeks of treatment. For this reason, other drugs may need to be employed during the early phase of treatment while awaiting the full response to lithium (see below). The serum concentration of lithium should be monitored after initiating therapy and at periodic intervals thereafter. While the concentration should be between 0.6 and 1.2 mEq/L, a concentration of 0.8–1.0 mEq/L is considered optimal for most patients. Monitoring the concentration serves to verify the adequacy of dosage and may warn of potential toxicity.

Adverse Effects. Lithium has a relatively low margin of safety. Elevated lithium levels may cause neurotoxicity and cardiac toxicity leading to arrhythmia. Nausea with vomiting may be one of the earliest signs of lithium overdose. It is important for the clinician and patient to distinguish the signs of lithium toxicity from the adverse effects of lithium that often occur with therapeutic serum levels.

Lithium is fairly well tolerated by most patients, but it produces a number of unpleasant side effects that decrease patient compliance. Common side effects include drowsiness, weight gain, a fine hand tremor, and polyuria. The hand tremor can usually be controlled by the administration of a β-adrenergic receptor antagonist. Lithium causes polyuria because it interferes with the action of antidiuretic hormone and thereby inhibits the kidney's ability to concentrate the urine. In some patients, lithium causes hypothyroidism by blocking thyroid hormone synthesis and release.

Interactions. Nonsteroidal anti-inflammatory drugs (NSAIDs) and diuretics decrease lithium clearance by about 25% and increase lithium levels. Other drugs may increase lithium neurotoxicity. The most important drug interactions of lithium are listed in Table 22–8.

Other Mood-Stabilizing Drugs

Although lithium is the primary drug used to treat and prevent manic symptoms in bipolar disorder, other drugs have been found to have equal or greater efficacy and may be better tolerated by some patients. These include **carbamazepine** and **valproate,** antiepileptic drugs whose pharmacologic properties are described in Chapter 20.

Treatment Considerations

The treatment of bipolar disorder must be individualized on the basis of symptoms, response to drug therapy and other treatment modalities, and the minimization of adverse effects. Drug treatment with **lithium** is often the cornerstone of therapy, since lithium may abort an acute manic episode, may prevent future manic episodes, and also appears to exert a mild antidepressive effect. Because of the dynamic nature of the disorder, however, therapy must be frequently reevaluated and modified.

Lithium usually controls an acute manic episode within 1 or 2 weeks after initiating therapy. Other drugs may be required to control acute symptoms while awaiting the full effect of lithium to develop. **Benzodiazepines** may relieve manic symptoms and promote sleep. An antipsychotic drug may be required to suppress delusions and other psychotic symptoms accompanying mania. **Risperidone** and **olanzapine** are effective in patients with bipolar

disorder and cause fewer adverse effects than do typical antipsychotic drugs, such as haloperidol.

Lithium is usually continued for 9–12 months after the initial manic episode, and then its use may be slowly tapered, with continued monitoring of symptoms. Many patients experience hypomanic symptoms for several days or longer before developing a full manic episode, and lithium therapy may be reinstituted in these patients in an attempt to abort a full manic episode. Long-term prophylactic therapy may be given to patients who have had two or three episodes and to those whose symptoms develop rapidly. However, long-term patient compliance with lithium is often poor.

Depression that persists after lithium therapy is instituted may respond to **antidepressant drugs.** The use of antidepressants in patients who have bipolar disorder and are not taking lithium or another mood-stabilizing drug will evoke a manic response (switch phenomenon) in many patients.

There is a growing list of alternatives to lithium for bipolar disorder. This list includes several antiepileptic drugs. **Carbamazepine** exhibits antimanic, antidepressant, and prophylactic effects that are equivalent to those of lithium, and it causes fewer adverse effects in many patients. Moreover, about 60% of manic patients who do not respond to lithium will respond to carbamazepine within the first several days of treatment. There is also evidence that lithium and carbamazepine may be synergistic in their antimanic activity in patients with refractory bipolar disorder. **Valproate** is another drug that is approved for the treatment of mania in bipolar disorder. It appears to be especially useful in patients with rapid cycling of manic and depressive episodes and in patients with coexisting substance abuse. Other antiepileptic drugs have demonstrated antimanic activity in clinical studies and may be approved for treating bipolar disorder in the future.

Summary of Important Points

- Schizophrenia may result from abnormal neuronal migration that occurs in utero in genetically susceptible fetuses. According to the dopamine and hypofrontality hypotheses, this abnormality leads to dysfunctional dopamine neurotransmission in the prefrontal lobe cortex.
- Delusions, hallucinations, and other so-called positive symptoms of schizophrenia may result from excessive dopamine neurotransmission in mesolimbic pathways. Apathy, withdrawal, lack of motivation and pleasure, and other so-called negative symptoms may result from impaired dopamine neurotransmission in mesocortical pathways.
- The typical antipsychotic drugs include phenothiazines, thioxanthenes, butyrophenones, and some azepines (such as loxapine). The atypical antipsychotic drugs include other azepines (such as clozapine and olanzapine) and a benzisoxazole drug called risperidone.

- Typical antipsychotic drugs are believed to act by blocking dopamine D_2 receptors in mesolimbic pathways. Atypical antipsychotic drugs act by blocking serotonin 5-HT$_2$ and D_2 receptors. Both classes of drugs alleviate the positive symptoms of schizophrenia, but the typical drugs cause a higher incidence of extrapyramidal side effects (akathisia, pseudoparkinsonism, dystonia, and tardive dyskinesia) and are less effective against the negative symptoms of schizophrenia.

- Low-potency antipsychotics (chlorpromazine and thioridazine) produce more autonomic side effects and sedation than do high-potency drugs (fluphenazine and haloperidol), but the high-potency drugs cause more extrapyramidal side effects. Clozapine sometimes causes agranulocytosis, so leukocyte counts must be monitored.

- Depression is believed to result from inadequate serotonin neurotransmission in limbic structures, and most antidepressant drugs increase serotonin neurotransmission in the brain.

- The tricyclic antidepressants (TCAs) block serotonin and norepinephrine reuptake. They effectively treat depression, but they have significant autonomic and cardiovascular side effects. When taken in an overdose, they may cause seizures and cardiac arrhythmia.

- The selective serotonin reuptake inhibitors (SSRIs) are antidepressants that have fewer autonomic and cardiovascular side effects and cause less sedation than do the TCAs. In comparison with other SSRIs, fluoxetine has a longer half-life and causes more drug interactions. Sertraline causes fewer drug interactions.

- Other antidepressants, such as bupropion, mirtazapine, nefazodone, trazodone, and venlafaxine, have different mechanisms of action that lead to increased serotonin neurotransmission in the brain.

- The nonselective monoamine oxidase (MAO) inhibitors, such as phenelzine and tranylcypromine, bind to and inhibit MAO type A and type B. These drugs prevent the breakdown of serotonin, norepinephrine, sympathomimetic drugs, and amines contained in certain foods. To prevent a hypertensive crisis in patients who are taking MAO inhibitors, the use of interacting drugs and foods must be avoided.

- Lithium is a mood-stabilizing drug that is primarily used to treat and prevent the manic phase of bipolar disorder. It has a narrow therapeutic range, so its serum concentrations must be carefully monitored. Overdose may result in neurotoxicity and cardiac toxicity. Lithium produces many side effects, including tremor, weight gain, and polyuria. Alternatives to lithium include carbamazepine and valproate.

Selected Readings

Arnt, J., and T. Skarsfeldt. Do novel antipsychotics have similar pharmacologic characteristics? A review of the evidence. Neuropsychopharmacology 18:63–101, 1998.

Blacker, D. Maintenance treatment of major depression: a review of the literature. Harv Rev Psychiatry 4:1–9, 1996.

Davis, R., et al. Nefazodone: a review of its pharmacology and clinical efficacy in the management of major depression. Drugs 53:608–636, 1997.

Dykstra, T. J., and M. J. Menolasino. Neuroleptic malignant syndrome: case report and review. JAOA 97:355–357, 1997.

Graeff, F. G., et al. Role of 5-HT in stress, anxiety, and depression. Pharmacol Biochem Behav 54:129–141, 1996.

Kando, J. C., et al. Olanzapine: a new antipsychotic agent with efficacy in the management of schizophrenia. Ann Pharmacother 31:1325–1334, 1997.

Lejoyeux, M., and J. Ades. Antidepressant discontinuation: a review of the literature. J Clin Psychiatry 58(supplement 7):11–16, 1997.

Lenox, R. H., and D. G. Watson. Lithium and the brain: a psychopharmacologic strategy to a molecular basis for manic-depressive illness. Clin Chem 40:309–314, 1994.

Lieberman, J. A. Atypical antipsychotic drugs as a first-line treatment of schizophrenia. J Clin Psychiatry 57(supplement 11):68–71, 1996.

Linde, K., et al. St John's wort for depression: an overview and meta-analysis of randomised clinical trials. BMJ 313:253–258, 1996.

Tollefson, G. D., et al. Olanzapine versus haloperidol in the treatment of schizophrenia and schizoaffective and schizophreniform disorders. Am J Psychiatry 154:457–465, 1997.

Tran, P. V., et al. Double-blind comparison of olanzapine versus risperidone in the treatment of schizophrenia and other psychotic disorders. J Clin Psychopharmacol 17:407–418, 1997.

Ware, M. R. Fluvoxamine: a review of the controlled trials in depression. J Clin Psychiatry 58(supplement 5):15–23, 1997.

Weinberger, D. R. Schizophrenia and the frontal lobe. Trends Neurosci 11:367–370, 1988.

Winn, P. Schizophrenia research moves to the prefrontal cortex. Trends Neurosci 17:265–268, 1994.

CHAPTER TWENTY-THREE

OPIOID ANALGESICS AND ANTAGONISTS

CLASSIFICATION OF OPIOID ANALGESICS AND ANTAGONISTS

Strong opioid agonists
- Fentanyl
- Meperidine
- Methadone
- Morphine
- Oxycodone
- Sufentanil

Moderate opioid agonists
- Codeine
- Hydrocodone
- Propoxyphene

Other opioid agonists
- Dextromethorphan
- Diphenoxylate
- Loperamide
- Tramadol

Mixed opioid agonist-antagonists
- Buprenorphine
- Butorphanol
- Nalbuphine
- Pentazocine

Opioid antagonists
- Naloxone
- Naltrexone

OVERVIEW

Pain and Pain Relievers

Pain is an unpleasant sensory and emotional experience that normally serves to alert an individual to actual or potential tissue damage. This damage may be caused by exposure to noxious chemical, mechanical, or thermal stimuli (such as acids, pressure, percussion, and extreme heat) or by the presence of a pathologic process (such as a tumor, muscle spasm, inflammation, nerve damage, organ distention, or other mechanism that activates nociceptors on sensory neurons). While pathologic pain may serve a protective function by alerting a person to the presence of a health problem, its unbridled expression often leads to considerable morbidity and suffering. For this reason, drugs that relieve pain have been employed as symptomatic therapy for a wide variety of disease states, ranging from acute and chronic physical injuries to terminal cancer.

Three general categories of drugs can be given to relieve or prevent pain. **Analgesics** are usually ad-ministered orally or parenterally and are capable of relieving pain without causing the loss of consciousness. **General anesthetics** are agents that are administered by inhalation or parenterally to cause the loss of consciousness and prevent the awareness of pain during surgery. **Local anesthetics** are applied topically or injected at the site where the pain originates, and they prevent transmission of pain impulses to the spinal cord and brain. The anesthetic drugs are discussed in Chapter 25.

Based on their mechanisms of action, analgesics may be classified as **opioid analgesics** or **nonopioid analgesics.** Opioid analgesics act primarily in the spinal cord and brain to inhibit the neurotransmission of pain. In contrast, nonopioid analgesics act primarily in peripheral tissues to inhibit the formation of pain impulses by nociceptive stimuli, and they exert their effects via the inhibition of prostaglandin synthesis. In addition to relieving pain, most of the nonopioid drugs also exhibit significant anti-inflammatory and antipyretic activity, in which case they are called **nonsteroidal anti-inflammatory drugs** (NSAIDs). The NSAIDs are described in greater detail in Chapter 30.

To facilitate the selection of an appropriate analgesic or anesthetic medication, patients are usually asked to describe their pain in terms of its intensity, duration, and location. In some cases, patients complain of an **intense, sharp, stinging pain.** In other cases, they describe a **dull, burning, aching pain.** These two types of pain are transmitted predominantly by different types of neurons (Box 23–1). Pain can be further distinguished on the basis of whether it is somatic, visceral, or neuropathic in origin. **Somatic pain** is often well localized to specific dermal, subcutaneous, or musculoskeletal tissue. **Visceral pain** originating in thoracic or abdominal structures is often poorly localized and may be referred to somatic structures. For example, cardiac pain is often referred to the chin, neck, shoulder, or arm. **Neuropathic pain** is usually caused by nerve damage, such as that resulting from nerve compression or inflammation. Neuropathic pain is characteristic, for example, of trigeminal neuralgia (tic douloureux), postherpetic neuralgia, and certain types of back and limb injuries.

Pain Pathways

Exposure to a noxious stimulus activates **primary afferent neurons** and evokes action potentials

BOX 23–1. Pain Pathways and Sites of Drug Action

Pain activates primary afferent neurons that enter the spinal cord, where they synapse with interneurons that stimulate spinothalamic fibers. The neospinothalamic tract projects to the primary sensory cortex, which alerts the individual to the presence and location of pain. The paleospinothalamic tract projects to limbic structures, which mediate the emotional response to pain. Descending neuronal tracts from the periaqueductal gray matter activate neurons that release norepinephrine (NE), serotonin (5-hydroxytryptamine, or 5-HT), and enkephalin (Enk) in the spinal cord and thereby block ascending pain transmission. Opioid analgesics activate the descending pathways and directly activate opioid receptors on afferent nerve terminals in the spinal cord. Nonopioid analgesics reduce the activation of primary afferent neurons via inhibition of prostaglandin synthesis. NMR = nucleus magnus raphae; LC = locus ceruleus; SP = substance P; and Glu = glutamate.

Primary Afferent Neuron	Ascending Pathway	Projections	Type of Pain	Functions
Aδ (fast)	Neospinothalamic.	Reticular formation, thalamus, and sensory cortex.	Intense, sharp, stinging pain.	Pain localization and withdrawal reflexes.
C (slow)	Paleospinothalamic.	Thalamus, periaqueductal gray matter, and limbic structures.	Dull, burning, aching pain.	Autonomic reflexes, pain memory, and pain discomfort.

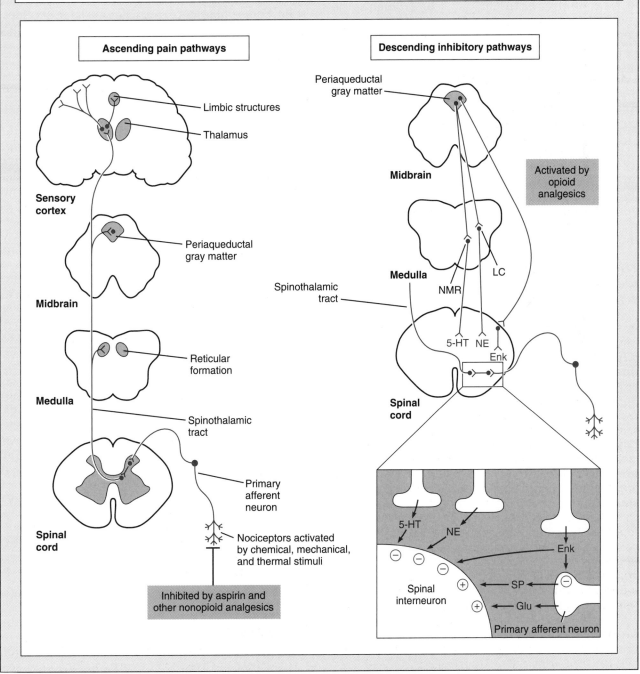

that are conducted into the dorsal horn of the spinal cord, where the neurons release substance P, glutamate, and other excitatory neurotransmitters. This stimulates interneurons, which in turn activate contralateral spinothalamic neurons that transmit pain impulses via **ascending pain pathways** to the medulla, midbrain, thalamus, limbic structures, and cortex.

As shown in Box 23–1, the primary afferent neurons consist mostly of **Aδ fibers** and **C fibers,** which are responsible for sharp pain and dull pain, respectively. Spinal reflexes activated by these fibers can lead to withdrawal from a noxious stimulus before pain is recognized by higher structures. Projections to the sensory cortex alert an individual to the presence and anatomic location of pain, whereas projections to limbic structures (such as the amygdala) enable the individual to experience discomfort, suffering, and other emotional reactions to pain.

The activation of spinothalamic neurons in the spinal cord can be blocked by **descending inhibitory pathways** from the midbrain and by sensory **Aβ fibers** arising in peripheral tissues. These two systems constitute the neurologic basis of a hypothesis of pain called the **gate hypothesis.** According to this hypothesis, pain transmission by spinothalamic neurons can be modulated, or gated, by the activity of other neurons and their neurotransmitters. This hypothesis triggered the search for endogenous opioid substances and eventually led to the discovery of the **enkephalins** and other opioid peptides and their receptors.

The descending inhibitory pathways arise in the periaqueductal gray matter (PAGM) in the midbrain, and they project to medullary nuclei that transmit impulses to the spinal cord (see Box 23–1). The medullary neurons include serotoninergic nerves arising in the nucleus magnus raphae (NMR) and noradrenergic nerves arising in the locus ceruleus (LC). When these nerves release **serotonin** and **norepinephrine** in the spinal cord, they inhibit spinal interneurons that would otherwise transmit pain impulses to the spinothalamic tracts. Nerve fibers from the PAGM also activate spinal neurons that release enkephalins. The enkephalins act presynaptically and postsynaptically to block pain transmission by primary afferent neurons. Opioid analgesics activate the descending PAGM, NMR, and LC neurons, and they also directly activate opioid receptors in the spinal cord.

The activation of spinothalamic neurons is also inhibited by peripheral Aβ sensory fibers that stimulate the release of enkephalins from spinal cord neurons. The Aβ neurons appear to mediate the analgesic effect produced by several types of tissue stimulation, including acupuncture and transcutaneous electrical nerve stimulation (TENS). This mechanism also explains the pain relief that may be produced by simply rubbing or massaging an injured tissue.

Opioid Peptides and Receptors

It has been known for centuries that extracts of the **opium poppy** can be used to relieve pain and treat diarrhea. During the 19th century, **morphine** was isolated from opium, and its pharmacologic effects were characterized and quantified. Later, opioid receptors were identified as specific sites to which morphine and other opioid agonists bind in order to elicit their pharmacologic effects. The presence of stereoselective receptors for morphine in brain tissue indicated the likelihood of an endogenous ligand for these receptors, and this eventually led to the discovery of the three major families of opioid peptides: **enkephalins, endorphins,** and **dynorphins.**

The opioid peptides are derived from larger precursor proteins that are widely distributed in the brain. Endorphins and dynorphins are large peptides, whereas enkephalins are small peptides containing five amino acids. In each enkephalin, four of the five amino acids are the same, and the fifth one is either methionine or leucine. Hence, the two types of enkephalins are called **met-enkephalin** and **leu-enkephalin.**

The enkephalins are released from neurons throughout the pain axis, including those in the PAGM, medulla, and spinal cord. Enkephalins activate opioid receptors in these areas and thereby block the transmission of pain impulses. The enkephalins appear to act as neuromodulators in that they exert a long-acting inhibitory effect on the release of excitatory neurotransmitters by several neurons.

The opioid receptors are members of the G protein–coupled receptor family. Activation of opioid receptors leads to inhibition of adenylyl cyclase, a decrease in the concentration of cyclic adenosine monophosphate (cAMP), and an increase in the conductance of potassium in affected neurons (Fig. 23–1). These actions cause presynaptic inhibition of neurotransmitter release and cause postsynaptic inhibition of membrane depolarization.

The opioid receptors have been classified as **mu (μ) receptors, delta (δ) receptors,** or **kappa (κ) receptors,** based on the relative affinity that they show for experimental opioid receptor ligands. However, most of the clinically useful opioid analgesics have limited selectivity for opioid receptor subtypes. The μ receptors appear to mediate most of the pharmacologic effects of morphine and other strong opioid agonists, whereas the κ receptors are activated by most of the mixed opioid agonist-antagonists (Table 23–1).

OPIOID DRUGS
Classification

The opioid drugs can be classified as full agonists, mixed agonist-antagonists, or pure antagonists.

Based on their maximal clinical effectiveness, the **full agonists** can be characterized as strong or moderate agonists. In experimental pain models, all

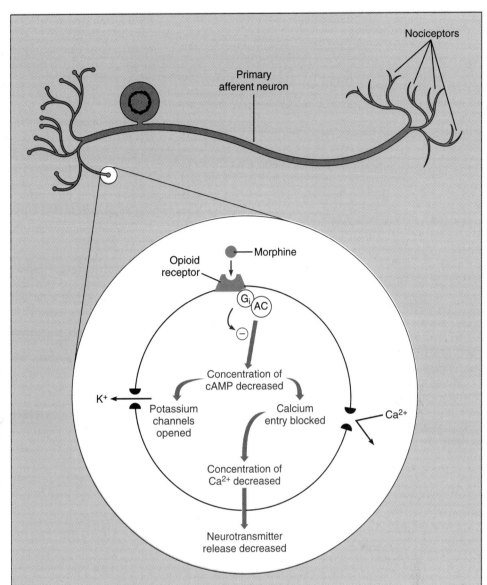

FIGURE 23–1. Mechanisms of opioid action in the spinal cord. Morphine and other opioid agonists activate presynaptic μ, δ, and κ opioid receptors on primary afferent neurons. These receptors are coupled negatively to adenylyl cyclase (AC) via G proteins (G_i). Inhibition of cyclic adenosine monophosphate (cAMP) formation leads to opening of potassium channels and closing of calcium channels. Potassium efflux causes membrane hyperpolarization. The closing of calcium channels inhibits the release of neurotransmitters, such as substance P.

of the full agonists exert the same maximal analgesic effect. In humans, the **strong opioid agonists** are tolerated when they are given in a dosage sufficient to relieve severe pain. However, the **moderate opioid agonists** will cause intolerable side effects if they are given in a dosage sufficient to alleviate pain that is severe. For this reason, the moderate agonists are administered in submaximal doses for the treatment of moderate to mild pain, and they are usually given in combination with nonopioid analgesics to enhance their clinical effectiveness.

The **mixed opioid agonist-antagonists** are analgesic drugs that have varying combinations of agonist, partial agonist, and antagonist activity and varying degrees of affinity for the different opioid receptor subtypes (see Table 23–1).

The **pure antagonists** have no analgesic effects. They are used to counteract the adverse effects of opioids taken in overdose.

Strong Opioid Agonists

The strong opioid agonists include naturally occurring drugs, such as morphine, and a number of synthetic drugs, including fentanyl, meperidine, and methadone. These drugs have equivalent analgesic effects but differ in their pharmacokinetic properties (Table 23–2), adverse effects, and uses.

Morphine

Chemistry and Pharmacokinetics. The isolation of morphine from opium is illustrated in Fig. 1–2, and the structure of morphine is shown in Fig. 23–2A. Morphine is the principal alkaloid of the opium poppy, *Papaver somniferum*. It is a phenanthrene alkaloid and constitutes about 10% of dried opium. Opium also contains papaverine and other benzylisoquinoline alkaloids that do not have analgesic properties.

TABLE 23–1. Opioid Receptor Selectivity of Enkephalins and Representative Opioid Drugs*

Agent	Receptor Subtype		
	Mu (μ)	Delta (δ)	Kappa (κ)
Enkephalins	Ag++	Ag+++	
Opioid agonists			
Fentanyl	Ag+++		
Methadone	Ag+++		
Morphine	Ag+++		Ag+
Mixed opioid agonist-antagonists			
Buprenorphine	P		Ant
Butorphanol	P		Ag+++
Nalbuphine	Ant		Ag++
Pentazocine	P		Ag++
Opioid antagonists			
Naloxone	Ant	Ant	Ant
Naltrexone	Ant	Ant	Ant

*Activity is indicated as follows: Ag+ to Ag+++ = low to high agonist activity; P = partial agonist activity; and Ant = antagonist activity.

The diacetic acid ester of morphine is heroin, a drug that is frequently abused (see Chapter 24).

Morphine is well absorbed from the gut, but it undergoes considerable first-pass metabolism in the liver, where a significant fraction of the drug is converted to glucuronides. For this reason, larger doses are required when the drug is administered orally than when it is administered parenterally. The principal metabolite of morphine is the 3-glucuronide, which is pharmacologically inactive. A significant amount of the 6-glucuronide is also formed. The 6-glucuronide is more active than morphine and has a longer half-life. Hence, the 6-glucuronide contributes significantly to the analgesic effectiveness of morphine. Morphine is primarily excreted in the urine in the form of glucuronides. A small amount is excreted in the bile and undergoes enterohepatic cycling.

Mechanisms and Effects. Morphine is a potent agonist, and μ receptors are responsible for most of its pharmacologic effects (see Table 23–1).

(1) Central Nervous System Effects. Morphine acts in the central nervous system to produce analgesia, sedation, euphoria or dysphoria, miosis, nausea, vomiting, respiratory depression, and inhibition of the cough reflex (Table 23–3).

Analgesia is produced by activation of opioid receptors in the spinal cord and at several supraspinal levels, as illustrated in Box 23–1. Sedation and euphoria may be caused by effects on midbrain dopaminergic, serotoninergic, and noradrenergic nuclei. Miosis is produced by the direct stimulation of the Edinger-Westphal nucleus of the oculomotor nerve (cranial nerve III), which activates parasympathetic stimulation of the iris sphincter muscle.

The major adverse effect of morphine and other opioids is respiratory depression, which is usually the cause of death in severe overdoses. Opioids re-

TABLE 23–2. Pharmacokinetic Properties of Opioid Drugs*

Drug	Route of Administration	Duration of Action (Hours)	Elimination Half-Life (Hours)	Active Metabolite
Strong opioid agonists				
Fentanyl	Parenteral, transdermal, and transmucosal†	1	4	No
Meperidine	Oral and parenteral	3	3	Yes
Methadone	Oral and parenteral	8	24	No
Morphine	Oral and parenteral	4	3	Yes
Oxycodone	Oral	4	Unknown	No
Sufentanil	Parenteral	1	2	No
Moderate opioid agonists				
Codeine	Oral	4	3	Yes
Hydrocodone	Oral	4	4	No
Propoxyphene	Oral	4	9	Yes
Other opioid agonists				
Dextromethorphan	Oral	6	11	No
Diphenoxylate	Oral	6	12	Yes
Loperamide	Oral	6	10	No
Tramadol	Oral	4	6	Yes
Mixed opioid agonist-antagonists				
Buprenorphine	Parenteral	5	5	No
Butorphanol	Intranasal and parenteral	3	3	No
Nalbuphine	Parenteral	4	5	No
Pentazocine	Oral and parenteral	4	4	No
Opioid antagonists				
Naloxone	Parenteral	2	4	No
Naltrexone	Oral	24	12	Yes

*Values shown are the mean of values reported in the literature.
†Fentanyl lozenges are available for pediatric preanesthetic use.

A. Morphine and its derivatives

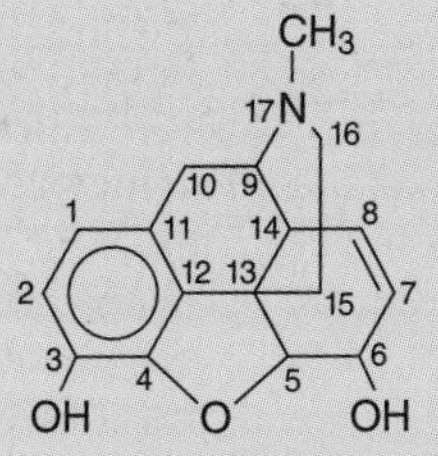

Substitution on Morphine Structure

Drug	3 Position	6 Position	17 Position	Other Changes*
Agonists				
Morphine	—OH	—OH	—CH₃	–
Codeine	—OCH₃	—OH	—CH₃	–
Heroin	—OCOCH₃	—OCOCH₃	—CH₃	–
Hydrocodone	—OCH₃	=O	—CH₃	(1)
Oxycodone	—OCH₃	=O	—CH₃	(1), (2)
Agonist-antagonists				
Butorphanol	—OH	—H	—CH₂—◇	(2), (3)
Nalbuphine	—OH	—OH	—CH₂—◇	(1), (2)
Antagonists				
Naloxone	—OH	=O	—CH₂CH=CH₂	(1), (2)
Naltrexone	—OH	=O	—CH₂—◁	(1), (2)

*Other changes in the morphine molecule are as follows: (1) Single bond between C7 and C8. (2) OH added to C14. (3) No oxygen between C4 and C5.

B. Other opioid drugs

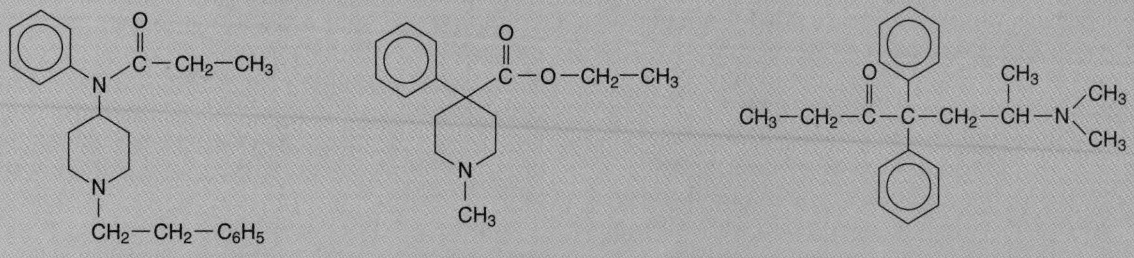

Fentanyl　Meperidine　Methadone

FIGURE 23–2. Structures of morphine and its derivatives (A) and of other selected opioid drugs (B).

duce the hypercapnic drive (the stimulation of respiratory centers by increased carbon dioxide levels) while producing relatively little effect on the hypoxic drive. Opioids reduce the respiratory tidal volume and rate, causing the rate to fall to 3 or 4 breaths per minute after an opioid overdose. These effects are rapidly reversed by the intravenous administration of an opioid antagonist such as naloxone (see below).

Morphine and other opioids inhibit the cough reflex at sites in the medulla where this reflex is integrated. The antitussive actions of opioids are discussed in greater detail in Chapter 27.

(2) Cardiovascular Effects. The most prominent cardiovascular effect of morphine and many other opioids is vasodilation, which is partly due to histamine release from mast cells in peripheral tissues. Morphine may cause orthostatic hypotension owing to decreased peripheral resistance and a

TABLE 23–3. Major Pharmacologic Effects of Opioid Agonists

Central nervous system (CNS) effects
Analgesia
Dysphoria or euphoria
Inhibition of cough reflex
Miosis
Physical dependence
Respiratory depression
Sedation

Cardiovascular effects
Decreased myocardial oxygen demand
Vasodilation and hypotension

Gastrointestinal and biliary effects
Constipation (increased intestinal smooth muscle tone)
Increased biliary sphincter tone and pressure
Nausea and vomiting (via CNS action)

Genitourinary effects
Increased bladder sphincter tone
Prolongation of labor
Urinary retention

Neuroendocrine system effects
Inhibition of release of luteinizing hormone
Stimulation of release of antidiuretic hormone and prolactin

Immune system effects
Suppression of function of natural killer cells

Dermal effects
Flushing
Pruritus
Urticaria (hives) or other rash

reduction in baroreceptor reflex activity. In patients with coronary artery disease, the decreased peripheral resistance leads to a reduction of cardiac work and myocardial oxygen demand.

(3) Gastrointestinal, Biliary, and Genitourinary Effects. Morphine and most other opioids act to increase smooth muscle tone in the gastrointestinal, biliary, and genitourinary systems.

In the gastrointestinal tract, increased muscle tone leads to inhibition of peristalsis and causes constipation. For this reason, the opioids are the oldest and most widely used medication for the treatment of diarrhea (see Chapter 28). By stimulating the chemoreceptor trigger zone in the medulla, the opioids also cause nausea and vomiting.

When morphine and other opioids increase the tone of the biliary sphincter (sphincter of Oddi), this increases the biliary pressure and may cause an exacerbation of pain in patients with biliary dysfunction. Opioids also increase the tone of the bladder sphincter and may cause urinary retention in some patients.

Therapeutic doses of morphine may prolong labor. For this reason, butorphanol, meperidine, or nalbuphine is usually employed for obstetric analgesia.

(4) Other Effects. Opioids have an effect on neuroendocrine and immunologic function. In the hypothalamus, they stimulate the release of antidiuretic hormone and prolactin and inhibit the release of luteinizing hormone. Opioids also sup-

press the activity of certain types of lymphocytes, including natural killer cells, and this action may contribute to the high rate of infectious diseases in heroin addicts.

Allergic reactions to opioid analgesics are not uncommon. In most cases, however, a patient who is allergic to a particular opioid will be able to use an opioid from a different chemical class. For example, someone who is allergic to codeine will probably not be allergic to propoxyphene or fentanyl.

Tolerance and Physical Dependence. Repeated administration of an opioid agonist will lead to pharmacodynamic tolerance not only of the administered drug but also of other opioid agonists. Tolerance is primarily due to down-regulation of opioid receptors. The degree of tolerance depends on the potency and dosage of the drug being administered. Significant tolerance develops after repeated administration of morphine, whereas relatively little tolerance occurs with long-term administration of a weaker opioid agonist, such as propoxyphene.

Drug tolerance is usually accompanied by a similar degree of physical dependence. Physical dependence is defined as a physiologic state in which a person's continued use of a drug is required for his or her well-being. Tolerance and physical dependence appear to represent the establishment of a new equilibrium between the neuron and its environment, wherein the neuron becomes less responsive to the opioid while requiring continued opioid inhibition to maintain cellular homeostasis. If the opioid drug is abruptly withdrawn, the equilibrium is disturbed and a rebound hyperexcitability occurs owing to the loss of the inhibitory influence of the drug. This produces a withdrawal reaction, the manifestations of which depend on the particular type of drug (see Chapter 24).

Because opioids demonstrate cross-tolerance, one opioid drug can substitute for another opioid drug and prevent symptoms of withdrawal in a physically dependent person. Tolerance develops to most of the effects of opioids but not to miosis and constipation. Although considerable tolerance to respiratory depression occurs, a sufficiently high dose of an opioid can still be fatal to highly tolerant individuals.

Indications. Morphine remains the standard of comparison for analgesic drugs. It is primarily used to treat **severe pain associated with trauma, myocardial infarction, and cancer.** In patients with myocardial infarction, it relieves pain and anxiety while also dilating coronary arteries and reducing the myocardial oxygen demand. Morphine is available in both parenteral and oral formulations, including a long-acting oral formulation that is useful in patients with severe chronic pain.

Fentanyl and Its Derivatives

Fentanyl is a synthetic opioid agonist whose structure is shown in Fig. 23–2B. Fentanyl and its derivatives, including **sufentanil,** are the most potent opioid agonists available. Because of its high potency and lipid solubility, fentanyl has been formulated in a long-acting transdermal skin patch to provide continuous pain relief for patients with **severe pain.** It is also available for parenteral administration preoperatively and postoperatively and as an **adjunct to general anesthesia.** Fentanyl produces less nausea than does morphine.

Meperidine

Meperidine is a synthetic opioid agonist with an unusual profile of pharmacologic properties (Table 23–4). It has no antitussive activity and has variable effects on pupil size. Because its effect on gastrointestinal, biliary, and uterine smooth muscle is less pronounced than that of morphine, it is less likely than morphine to cause constipation or an increase in biliary pressure. Meperidine does not prolong labor as much as morphine does, so it can be used for analgesia in obstetrics.

The parenteral formulation of meperidine is often used as an **obstetric or postsurgical analgesic.** The oral formulation is used to treat **moderate to severe pain** in the outpatient setting. The drug is converted to a toxic metabolite, normeperidine, which may cause central nervous system excitation, convulsions, and tremors when meperidine is administered in large doses or for a prolonged period.

Hence, the drug is usually employed for the **short-term treatment of acute pain syndromes.**

Methadone

Methadone is a long-acting synthetic opioid agonist. Although it is available in parenteral formulations, it is most often administered orally to ambulatory patients for the treatment of **opioid addiction** or **pain.** Use of the oral formulation by opioid-dependent patients can prevent their craving for heroin or other opioids, but it does not cause significant euphoria or other reinforcing effects. Because of its long duration of action, it can be administered once a day for this purpose. The treatment for opioid-dependent patients is called a **methadone maintenance program.**

Oxycodone

Oxycodone is one of several semisynthetic morphine derivatives (see Fig. 23–2A) that are available as analgesics. Oxycodone is usually administered orally in combination with a nonopioid analgesic, such as acetaminophen, for the treatment of **moderate or severe pain.**

Moderate Opioid Agonists

The moderate opioid agonists are less potent than the strong opioid agonists. Because they do not

TABLE 23–4. Comparison of the Properties of Opioid Drugs*

Drug	Analgesia	Respiratory Depression	Antitussive Effect	Constipation	Dependence Liability
Strong opioid agonists					
Fentanyl	++++	+++	+++	+++	+++
Meperidine	++++	+++	0	+	+++
Methadone	++++	+++	+++	+++	+++
Morphine	++++	+++	+++	++++	+++
Oxycodone	+++ to ++++	+++	+++	+++	+++
Sufentanil	++++	+++	+++	+++	+++
Moderate opioid agonists					
Codeine	+++	++	+++	++	++
Hydrocodone	+++	++	+++	++	++
Propoxyphene	++	+	0 to +	+	++
Other opioid agonists					
Dextromethorphan	0	+	+++	0	+
Diphenoxylate	0	+	0	+++	+
Loperamide	0	+	0	+++	+
Tramadol	+++	+	+	+	+
Mixed opioid agonist-antagonists					
Buprenorphine	+++	++	+	++	+
Butorphanol	+++	++	0	+	+
Nalbuphine	+++	++	0	+	+
Pentazocine	+++	++	0	+	+
Opioid antagonists					
Naloxone	0	0	0	0	0
Naltrexone	0	0	0	0	0

*Ratings range from none (0) to high (++++).

produce maximal analgesia at doses that are well tolerated by patients, the moderate agonists are employed at submaximal doses, almost always in combination with a nonopioid analgesic. Fixed-dose combination products containing one of the moderate opioid agonists and **acetaminophen, aspirin,** or **ibuprofen** are available for the treatment of moderate pain.

Codeine and Hydrocodone

Codeine is a naturally occurring opioid obtained from the opium poppy. Structurally, it is the 3-O-methyl derivative of morphine. Codeine is converted to morphine by cytochrome P450 isozyme CYP2D6, and persons lacking this isozyme obtain little pain relief from the drug.

Codeine is a less potent analgesic than morphine, and the doses required to obtain maximal analgesia produce intolerable side effects, such as constipation. For this reason, codeine is usually given in lower doses in combination with a nonopioid analgesic for the treatment of **mild to moderate pain.** Codeine also produces a significant antitussive effect and is included in many cough syrups to alleviate or prevent **coughing.**

The properties and uses of hydrocodone are similar to those of codeine.

Propoxyphene

Propoxyphene is a chemical analogue of methadone but has much weaker opioid agonist properties. Propoxyphene has about half the analgesic activity of codeine when administered in usual therapeutic doses. It is most frequently used in combination with acetaminophen for the treatment of **mild to moderate somatic and visceral pain.** Propoxyphene is usually well tolerated, but prolonged administration may lead to the accumulation of a toxic metabolite.

Other Opioid Agonists

Tramadol is a dual-action analgesic. It not only activates μ receptors but also inhibits the neuronal reuptake of serotonin and norepinephrine. The relationship between neuronal reuptake inhibition and analgesia is not certain. However, reuptake inhibition may potentiate the inhibitory effects of serotonin and norepinephrine on pain transmission in the spinal cord (see Box 23–1). Tricyclic antidepressants and other neuronal reuptake inhibitors also have analgesic effects, and the antidepressants have been used to treat chronic pain syndromes. For this reason, investigators believe that neuronal reuptake inhibition by tramadol contributes to the drug's analgesic activity. The analgesic effect of tramadol is only partly inhibited by opioid antagonists such as naloxone.

Tramadol is administered orally for the treatment of **moderate pain.** It has a definite but limited drug dependence liability. Nevertheless, it has been employed successfully in the treatment of **chronic pain syndromes** and produces minimal cardiovascular and respiratory depression. The drug lowers the seizure threshold, and the risk of seizures is increased if tramadol is used concurrently with antidepressants.

Several other opioid agonists are available but have little analgesic activity. These include **dextromethorphan,** which has significant antitussive activity and is used in the treatment of **cough** (see Chapter 27), and **diphenoxylate** and **loperamide,** which activate opioid receptors in gastrointestinal smooth muscle and are used in the treatment of **diarrhea** (see Chapter 28).

Mixed Opioid Agonist-Antagonists

The mixed opioid agonist-antagonists are drugs that exhibit partial agonist or antagonist activity at μ receptors and show agonist or antagonist activity at κ receptors. Examples are **buprenorphine, butorphanol, nalbuphine,** and **pentazocine.**

Drug Properties

Chemistry and Pharmacokinetics. The opioid agonist-antagonists have a large chemical substituent on the nitrogen atom (see Fig. 23–2A), which is probably responsible for their partial agonist or antagonist activity at μ receptors. Their pharmacokinetic and pharmacologic properties are shown in Tables 23–2 and 23–4. All of the agonist-antagonists can be given parenterally. In addition, pentazocine is available for oral use and butorphanol is available as a nasal spray. Butorphanol is rapidly absorbed from the nasal mucosa, which thereby enables the use of the drug on an outpatient basis.

Mechanisms and Effects. The selectivity of agonist-antagonists for opioid receptor subtypes is shown in Table 23–1. The most important pharmacologic property of these drugs with respect to their clinical activity is the lack of full agonist effects at μ receptors.

The opioid agonist-antagonists produce less respiratory depression as the doses are increased than do strong opioid agonists such as morphine. Hence, the agonist-antagonists are safer in overdose. They also appear to have a lower liability for drug dependence and abuse than do full opioid agonists. Both of these advantages probably result from the lack of full agonist activity at μ receptors. The agonist-antagonists produce less constipation than do most of the full agonists. However, the agonist-antagonists sometimes cause anxiety, nightmares, and psychotomimetic effects, including hallucinations, as a result of the activation of κ receptors. They may also precipitate withdrawal in a person dependent on a full opioid agonist.

Indications. The parenterally administered agonist-antagonist drugs are primarily used for **preoperative and postoperative analgesia** and for **obstetric analgesia during labor and delivery.** The orally and nasally administered drugs are used for the alleviation of **moderate to severe pain.**

Specific Drugs

Buprenorphine is a partial agonist at μ receptors and an antagonist at κ receptors. It is somewhat longer-acting than most parenterally administered opioid analgesics and may be administered intramuscularly or intravenously.

Butorphanol and nalbuphine are κ receptor agonists and have partial agonist or antagonist activity at μ receptors. Both drugs are administered parenterally, and butorphanol is also available as a nasal spray.

Pentazocine is a κ receptor agonist with partial agonist activity at μ receptors. It is available for parenteral and oral use. The parenteral formulation is primarily used as a preanesthetic medication and as a supplement to surgical anesthesia. The oral formulations are used to treat moderate to severe pain, and one of them contains naloxone (an antagonist) to discourage parenteral abuse of the drug. Parenteral use of an oral pentazocine formulation may cause severe cardiopulmonary reactions. Pentazocine is also available in combination with aspirin or acetaminophen for oral administration.

Opioid Antagonists

Naloxone and **naltrexone** are competitive opioid receptor antagonists that can rapidly reverse the effects of morphine and other opioid agonists. The antagonists have two primary clinical uses: the treatment of opioid overdose and the prevention and treatment of opioid dependence and addiction. Naltrexone has also been useful in the treatment of alcohol dependence.

Naloxone and naltrexone are chemical analogues of morphine. They have a large structural substitution on the nitrogen atom (see Fig. 23–2B), and this substitution prevents the formation of bonds between the drug and receptor that are required for agonist activity.

In cases of **opioid overdose,** naloxone is administered intravenously to rapidly terminate respiratory depression and other toxic effects of opioid agonists. Because naloxone has a relatively short half-life (see Table 23–2), repeated doses of the drug may be needed to counteract the effects of the longer-lasting opioid agonists. As described earlier, naloxone is included in an orally administered formulation of pentazocine in order to discourage parenteral use of this preparation by drug addicts. Because naloxone has low oral bioavailability and is not effective when given orally, it does not block the effects of pentazocine when it is administered correctly.

Naltrexone is used to prevent and treat **opioid dependence and addiction.** In contrast to naloxone, naltrexone has high oral bioavailability and can be used on a long-term basis by opioid addicts who have undergone detoxification and are no longer using opioids.

THE MANAGEMENT OF PAIN
Factors Affecting the Choice of Treatment

The location, cause, and severity of pain and the risk of producing drug dependence are all factors that influence the way in which pain is managed.

Acute pain due to trauma, surgery, or short-term medical conditions may be effectively managed with an analgesic and appropriate treatment of the underlying condition. In patients with acute pain, the risk of producing drug dependence is extremely low. Hence, physicians and other health care professionals should not hesitate to administer adequate doses of a sufficiently strong analgesic to control pain.

Pain associated with arthritis, neuropathy, and other chronic but nonterminal conditions is more difficult to treat and is often managed with a combination of analgesics, coanalgesics, psychotherapy, physical therapy, and other treatment modalities. Use of opioid analgesics in the treatment of chronic pain is associated with a risk of opioid tolerance and physical dependence, so care must be exercised to prevent dosage escalation, drug dependence, and drug abuse. Strict guidelines for prescription refills should be in place, and a prescription refill flowchart may be used to monitor drug usage and prevent dosage escalation. In some clinics, patients are asked to sign an "opioid contract" in which they agree to procedures that will ensure proper utilization of opioid drugs, including random drug testing.

Patients with terminal illnesses, such as cancer, should receive sufficient doses of analgesics to control their pain, irrespective of the development of tolerance and dependence.

As a general rule, patients with acute or chronic pain should be treated with the least potent analgesic that will control their pain. Mild pain usually responds to a nonopioid analgesic. Moderate to severe pain is often treated with **codeine, hydrocodone, or oxycodone** in combination with a nonopioid analgesic. Severe pain usually requires the use of a strong opioid agonist, such as **fentanyl, meperidine, methadone,** or **morphine.** Although meperidine may be used for acute postsurgical pain and in other situations in which the duration of treatment is limited to a few days, it should not be used for longer durations, because of the possible accumulation of a toxic metabolite (normeperidine).

Acute Pain

Giving analgesics on an as-needed basis will sometimes produce wide swings in pain and sedation during the early phase of treatment. Therefore, in the initial stages of acute pain, analgesics should be given around the clock at regular intervals. The dosage should be titrated to control pain while minimizing sedation and other side effects. As the pain subsides over time and the need for analgesia decreases, the patient can be transferred to an as-needed schedule of medication.

Patient-controlled analgesia is a method of intravenous administration that permits the patient to self-administer preset amounts of an analgesic such as fentanyl via a syringe pump that is interfaced with a timing device. The method enables the patient to balance pain control with sedation. Its use depends on the patient's ability to activate the device, so it may not be suitable for elderly patients or immediately after surgery or trauma.

Chronic Pain

The treatment of chronic pain varies greatly with the underlying cause. While the discussion of specific chronic pain syndromes is beyond the scope of this text, a few general guidelines and comments will be offered.

Both **opioid analgesics** and **nonopioid analgesics** are useful in the management of chronic pain syndromes. If pain is associated with inflammation, nonopioid drugs with anti-inflammatory activity may be especially useful. If pain is associated with peripheral nerve or nerve root sensitization, treatment with **transcutaneous nerve stimulation** (TENS) or a **local anesthetic** may help. In some cases, cream containing **capsaicin** is effective. Capsaicin activates peripheral nociceptors on primary sensory neurons, thereby leading to increased release of substance P and eventually to the depletion of substance P in the central nervous system. Capsaicin produces a burning sensation for the first few days of application, but this is gradually replaced by an analgesic effect.

Chronic pain is frequently seen in association with systemic disorders such as diabetes. When pain has been present for a period of time, the responsiveness of dynamic wide-range nociceptive neurons in the spinal cord increases in a way that increases pain perception and memory. As these neurons become "wound up," their receptive fields increase so that pain is felt over a larger area. These changes appear to contribute to the maintenance of chronic neuropathic pain. Patients with this type of pain may benefit from a combination of nonpharmacologic therapies (such as TENS, acupuncture, and physical therapy), analgesic medications, and coanalgesic drugs. The most widely used **coanalgesics** are the **antiepileptic drugs** and the **antidepressant drugs.** These drugs provide pain relief in chronic pain syndromes and may potentiate the effects of opioid and nonopioid analgesics.

Antiepileptic drugs, such as **carbamazepine, gabapentin, phenytoin,** and **valproate,** are particularly effective in treating pain syndromes with an intermittent lancinating quality, such as trigeminal neuralgia and postherpetic neuralgia. However, they are also useful in syndromes characterized by continuous, burning neuropathic pain. They probably act by inhibiting the conduction of pain impulses in the central nervous system, but their exact mechanism is unknown. The general properties of these drugs are described in Chapter 20.

The **tricyclic antidepressants** (TCAs) are the most widely used antidepressants for the treatment of chronic pain, and they may be more effective than the selective serotonin reuptake inhibitors (SSRIs) in this respect. TCAs such as **amitriptyline** and **desipramine** are particularly effective in the management of postherpetic neuralgia, diabetic neuropathy, migraine headache, and neuropathic pain syndromes. They may also be beneficial in the management of pain associated with chronic fatigue syndrome. The properties of these drugs are described in Chapter 22.

Tramadol is a dual-action analgesic that combines opioid receptor activation with inhibition of neuronal reuptake of neurotransmitters in a manner similar to TCAs. As discussed earlier in this chapter, tramadol is effective in many chronic pain syndromes and causes little constipation, respiratory depression, or drug dependence.

Pain in Oncology Patients

Pain is the most common symptom of cancer, and it may be acute, chronic, or intermittent. Unfortunately, cancer-related pain is frequently undertreated. Most patients can be managed with oral medications, including opioid and nonopioid analgesics, antidepressant drugs, and antiepileptic drugs. Acupuncture, TENS, and other modalities are also useful. Severe cancer pain usually requires the administration of a strong opioid agonist, such as fentanyl, methadone, or morphine. To maintain stable serum drug levels and prevent breakthrough pain, it may be helpful to use a long-acting preparation, such as sustained-release morphine tablets or transdermal fentanyl skin patches, either alone or in combination with a rapid-acting preparation, such as morphine oral solution.

Summary of Important Points

- Pain impulses are transmitted by primary afferent neurons to the spinal cord, where interneurons activate contralateral spinothalamic tracts that project to limbic structures and the cortex.
- Descending inhibitory fibers from the periaqueductal gray matter activate midbrain and spinal cord neurons that release enkephalins, serotonin, and norepinephrine. Opioids activate these pathways and thereby inhibit ascending pain impulses.
- Opioid drugs include strong and moderate agonists, mixed agonist-antagonists, and pure antagonists.
- In addition to analgesia, opioid agonists can cause sedation, euphoria, miosis, respiratory depression, peripheral vasodilation, constipation, and drug dependence.
- Opioid receptors can be divided into μ, δ, and κ subtypes. All subtypes mediate analgesia, but μ

receptors are primarily responsible for respiratory depression and drug dependence.

- The strong agonists produce maximal analgesia at doses that can be tolerated by patients. They include morphine, fentanyl, meperidine, and methadone, and they primarily activate μ receptors. The first three of these agents are used to alleviate severe or moderate pain. Methadone is usually used in the treatment of opioid addiction (methadone maintenance programs).
- The moderate agonists produce maximal analgesia at doses that cannot be tolerated, so they are usually combined with a nonopioid analgesic. The moderate agonists include codeine, hydrocodone, and propoxyphene and are used for the treatment of moderate or mild pain.
- Other agonists include tramadol, a dual-action analgesic that activates opioid receptors and blocks neuronal reuptake of serotonin and norepinephrine.
- Buprenorphine, butorphanol, nalbuphine, and pentazocine are mixed opioid agonist-antagonists. These drugs exhibit partial agonist or antagonist activity at μ receptors and exhibit agonist or antagonist activity at κ receptors. They produce less respiratory depression and are associated with a lower risk of drug dependence than are opioid agonists.
- Naloxone and naltrexone are opioid antagonists. The antagonists are used to counteract the adverse effects of opioids in overdose or to prevent and treat opioid dependence.

Selected Readings

Diamond, A. W., and S. W. Coniam. The Management of Chronic Pain, 2nd ed. New York, Oxford University Press, 1997.

Irving, G. A., and M. S. Wallace. Pain Management for the Practicing Physician. New York, Churchill Livingstone, 1997.

Jeal, W., and P. Benfield. Transdermal fentanyl: a review of its pharmacologic properties and therapeutic efficacy in pain control. Drugs 53:109–138, 1997.

Katz, W. A. Pharmacology and clinical experience with tramadol in osteoarthritis. Drugs 52(supplement 3):39–47, 1996.

Rushton, A. R., and J. R. Sneyd. Opioid analgesics. Br J Hosp Med 57:105–106, 1997.

CHAPTER TWENTY-FOUR

DRUGS OF ABUSE

CLASSIFICATION OF DRUGS OF ABUSE

CENTRAL NERVOUS SYSTEM DEPRESSANTS
Alcohols and glycols
- Ethanol
- Ethylene glycol
- Isopropyl alcohol
- Methanol

Barbiturates and benzodiazepines
- Flunitrazepam
- Pentobarbital

Opioids
- Heroin

CENTRAL NERVOUS SYSTEM STIMULANTS
Amphetamine and its derivatives
- Amphetamine
- Fenfluramine
- Methamphetamine
- 3,4-Methylenedioxy-methamphetamine (MDMA)
- Methylphenidate
- Phentermine

Other stimulants
- Caffeine
- Cocaine
- Nicotine

OTHER PSYCHOACTIVE DRUGS
Cannabis and its derivatives
- Dronabinol
- Marijuana

Hallucinogens
- Lysergic acid diethylamide (LSD)
- Mescaline

Phencyclidine (PCP)

OVERVIEW
Drug Abuse

Humans have used drugs for mind-altering purposes for millennia. Every society has sanctioned the use of some drugs while banning the use of others. In many Western cultures, for example, products containing ethanol, nicotine, or caffeine have been socially acceptable to the majority of the population while the use of opioids, cocaine, marijuana, hallucinogens, and other psychoactive drugs has been illegal. Hence, what constitutes drug abuse is highly dependent on cultural attitudes.

From a medical and psychologic perspective, drug abuse can be defined as the use of a drug in a manner that is detrimental to the health or well-being of the drug user, other individuals, or society as a whole. Drug abuse is not restricted to the use of illegal drugs, as the cumulative health and social effects caused by the use of alcoholic beverages and tobacco products probably outweigh the negative effects of illicit drug use.

Drug Dependence

Drug dependence is a condition in which an individual feels compelled to repeatedly administer a psychoactive drug. Repeated drug use appears to be a learned behavior that is reinforced both by the pleasurable effects of the drug and by the negative effects of drug abstinence (withdrawal). These effects are the basis of drug craving in drug-dependent individuals. **Psychologic dependence** is due to the positive reinforcement of drug use that results from the activation of neurons located in the nucleus accumbens. **Physical dependence** is a state in which continued drug use is required to prevent an unpleasant **withdrawal syndrome.** Hence, physical dependence leads to negative reinforcement of drug use. Both psychologic and physical dependence appear to result from **neuronal adaptation** to the presence of the drug, albeit in different areas of the brain.

Psychologic Dependence

The craving for **alcohol, barbiturates, caffeine, cocaine, opioids,** and **phencyclidine** is remarkably similar, despite the varied behavioral and physiologic effects that these drugs produce. This similarity supports the hypothesis that psychologic dependence is mediated by a common neuronal pathway that leads to **behavioral reinforcement** of drug use. Psychoactive drugs that evoke behavioral reinforcement of their use appear to sensitize dopaminergic neurons that project from the ventral tegmental area to the nucleus accumbens. Other psychoactive drugs that are used for their mind-altering effects, including **lysergic acid diethylamide** (LSD) and **marijuana,** have a much smaller effect on this pathway and cause little or no psychologic dependence.

There is evidence that **dopamine** mediates drug reinforcement by activating protein kinases that are dependent on cyclic adenosine monophosphate (cAMP) and regulate the expression of transcription factors in the nucleus accumbens. The transcription factors, which include cAMP–response element binding protein, increase the synthesis of G proteins, cAMP-dependent protein kinases, and other cellular response elements that amplify the future response to dopamine. These mechanisms lead to sensitization to dopamine, a phenomenon that is believed to underlie behavioral reinforcement of drug use.

Investigators have observed that the peak of craving for a drug occurs at the time of the drug's peak effect on the central nervous system (CNS). They have also found that the degree of short-term reinforcement of drug use is linked to the rate of increase of dopamine levels in the nucleus accumbens. This relationship appears to account for the propensity of some drugs to produce drug dependence. It also appears to explain the difference in reinforcement effects produced by different routes of administration of a particular drug. For example, the oral administration of an opioid or cocaine causes less reinforcement and psychologic dependence than does the intravenous administration or inhalation of an equivalent dose of the same drug. The differences in effect are determined by the rate at which the drug is distributed to the brain and the rate at which dopamine levels in the nucleus accumbens are increased.

Physical Dependence

Physical dependence appears to result from the adaptation of specific areas of the brain to the continued presence of a drug. Physical dependence is associated with drug tolerance and with the development of a drug-specific withdrawal syndrome if the drug is discontinued. For this reason, physical dependence contributes to the continued use of a drug. The negative effects of nicotine withdrawal, for example, appear to be responsible for the strong craving for cigarettes by people who are dependent on nicotine.

Drug Addiction

Drug addiction usually refers to an extreme pattern of drug abuse in which an individual is continuously preoccupied with drug procurement and use and thus neglects other responsibilities and personal relationships. Addiction is usually associated with a high level of drug dependence.

Classification of Drugs of Abuse

The psychoactive drugs that are used by some individuals for nonmedicinal purposes can be classified as CNS depressants, CNS stimulants, and miscellaneous agents, with the latter group including marijuana, hallucinogens, and phencyclidine. After describing the pharmacologic effects of these drugs and any clinical use that they may have, this chapter discusses the management of drug abuse. Tables 24–1 through 24–4 provide information about the manifestations and treatment of drug intoxication, withdrawal, and dependence.

CENTRAL NERVOUS SYSTEM DEPRESSANTS
Alcohols and Glycols

In North America, about 12 million individuals have one or more symptoms of alcoholism, making **alcohol abuse** the number one drug abuse problem. In the USA alone, the annual cost of health care, lost work hours, criminal activity, and other problems related to alcohol use is roughly $90 billion.

The alcohols and glycols most commonly ingested are ethanol, methanol, and ethylene glycol. While ethanol selectively produces CNS depression, methanol and ethylene glycol affect multiple organ systems and can produce severe or life-threatening toxicity, even when ingested in relatively small doses.

Ethanol

Ethanol, or **ethyl alcohol,** is classified as a CNS depressant and has pharmacologic effects similar to those of the barbiturates and benzodiazepines.

Pharmacokinetics. Ethanol has sufficient lipid solubility to enable rapid and almost complete absorption from the gut. It is more rapidly absorbed from the duodenum than from the stomach, and food slows its absorption by slowing the rate of gastric emptying. Ethanol is widely distributed throughout the body and has a volume of distribution that is roughly equivalent to the total body water, or about 38 L per 70 kg of body weight.

As shown in Fig. 24–1, ethanol is primarily oxidized by **alcohol dehydrogenase** to form acetaldehyde and is then oxidized by **acetaldehyde dehydrogenase** to form acetate. The acetate derived from ethanol enters the citric acid cycle for further oxidation to carbon dioxide and water. The oxidation of ethanol utilizes significant quantities of nicotinamide adenine dinucleotide (NAD), and the depletion of NAD is responsible for some of the metabolic effects of ethanol that are described below. Ethanol also undergoes oxidation by **cytochrome P450 enzymes.** Unlike alcohol dehydrogenase metabolism, P450 enzyme metabolism is induced by long-term alcohol use. Therefore, P450 induction contributes to alcohol tolerance in heavy drinkers.

About 2% of ethanol is excreted unchanged by the kidneys and lungs. The concentration of ethanol in alveolar air is about 0.05% of that in the blood, and this relationship is used to estimate the **blood alcohol concentration** (BAC) in exhaled air when the **breathalyzer test** is administered. Because ethanol can markedly impair the psychomotor skills required to safely drive a vehicle, most states prohibit the operation of motor vehicles if the BAC exceeds 0.1% (100 mg/dL). A few states have lowered the legal limit to 0.08%.

TABLE 24–1. Common Signs and Symptoms of Drug Intoxication

Drug	Motor and Speech Impairment	Emotional and Perceptual Manifestations	Cardiovascular Manifestations	Other Manifestations
Alcohol	Ataxia, incoordination, loquacity, and slurred speech.	Euphoria, impaired attention, irritability, mood changes, and sedation.	Flushed face.	Nystagmus.
Amphetamines	Agitation and loquacity.	Decreased fatigue, euphoria, grandiosity, hypervigilance, and paranoia.	Hypertension or hypotension and tachycardia.	Chills, mydriasis, nausea, nystagmus, sweating, and vomiting.
Barbiturates	Same as alcohol.	Same as alcohol.	Hypotension.	Nystagmus.
Benzodiazepines	Same as alcohol.	Same as alcohol.	Hypotension.	Nystagmus.
Cocaine	Same as amphetamines.	Altered tactile sensation ("cocaine bugs"), decreased fatigue, euphoria, grandiosity, hypervigilance, and paranoia.	Same as amphetamines.	Same as amphetamines.
Hallucinogens	Dizziness, incoordination, tremor, and weakness.	Depersonalization, derealization, hallucinations, illusions, and synesthesia.	Tachycardia.	Blurred vision, mydriasis, and sweating.
Marijuana	Loquacity and rapid speech.	Euphoria, hallucinations (with high doses), jocularity, and sensory intensification.	Hypertension and tachycardia.	Conjunctivitis, dry mouth, increased appetite, and tightness in chest.
Opioids	Motor slowness and slurred speech.	Apathy, euphoria or dysphoria, impaired attention, and sedation.	None.	Miosis.
Phencyclidine	Agitation, ataxia, muscle rigidity, and slurred speech.	Anxiety, delusions, emotional lability, euphoria, and hallucinations.	Hypertension and tachycardia.	Hostility, miosis, nystagmus, and violent behavior.

TABLE 24–2. Emergency Treatment of Drug Intoxication

Drug	Pharmacologic Treatment	Nonpharmacologic Treatment
Alcohol	None.	Support vital functions.
Amphetamines	Lorazepam for agitation and haloperidol for psychosis.	Monitor and support cardiac function.
Barbiturates	None.	Support vital functions.
Benzodiazepines	Flumazenil.	Support vital functions.
Cocaine	Lorazepam for agitation or seizures.	Support vital functions.
Hallucinogens	Lorazepam for agitation.	Give reassurance and support vital functions.
Marijuana	Lorazepam for agitation.	Give reassurance and support vital functions.
Opioids	Naloxone.	Support vital functions.
Phencyclidine	Lorazepam for agitation and haloperidol for psychosis.	Minimize sensory input.

The capacity of alcohol dehydrogenase to metabolize ethanol is limited because the enzyme is saturated at relatively low ethanol concentrations. Hence, ethanol metabolism exhibits **zero-order kinetics** except when serum concentrations of ethanol are very low. For this reason, the BAC is largely determined by the rate of ethanol ingestion. An adult weighing 70 kg usually metabolizes only about 10 mL of absolute ethanol per hour, which is roughly equivalent to the amount of ethanol contained in one alcoholic drink. A BAC of 0.08–0.1% in most cases is reached after an adult consumes from two to four drinks (bottles of beer, glasses of wine, or ounces of distilled liquor) within an hour.

CNS Effects, Mechanisms, and Interactions. Ethanol potentiates the actions of gamma-aminobutyric acid (GABA) in a manner similar to that of benzodiazepines and barbiturates (see Chapter 19). It thereby produces sedative-hypnotic, anxiolytic, amnesic, and anticonvulsant effects. However, long-term ethanol use or ethanol withdrawal may lower the seizure threshold and thereby cause seizures. Predictably, ethanol potentiates the effects of benzodiazepines and barbiturates, so the combination of any of these drugs with ethanol can produce fatal CNS depression.

TABLE 24–3. Common Signs and Symptoms of Drug Withdrawal

Drug	Central Nervous System Manifestations	Musculoskeletal Manifestations	Cardiovascular Manifestations	Other Manifestations
Alcohol	Altered perceptions, insomnia, irritability, and seizures.	Tremor.	Hypertension and tachycardia.	Delirium tremens, nausea, and sweating.
Amphetamines	Depression, drowsiness, dysphoria, fatigue, increased appetite, and sleepiness.	None.	Bradycardia.	None.
Barbiturates	Anxiety, insomnia, irritability, and seizures.	Muscle twitches.	Hypertension and tachycardia.	None.
Benzodiazepines	Agitation, anxiety, dizziness, and insomnia.	Muscle cramps and myoclonic contractions.	Hypertension and tachycardia.	None.
Cocaine	Same as amphetamines.	None.	Bradycardia.	None.
Marijuana	Irritability, mild agitation, and sleep disturbances.	None.	None.	Nausea and stomach cramps.
Nicotine	Anxiety, dysphoria, hostility, impatience, irritability, and restlessness.	None.	Decreased heart rate.	Increased appetite.
Opioids	Anxiety, dysphoria, irritability, restlessness, and sleep disturbances.	Muscle aches.	Hypertension and tachycardia.	Diarrhea, fever, mydriasis, piloerection,* sweating, vomiting, and yawning.

*Because piloerection causes "goose bumps" or "gooseflesh," patients withdrawing from opioids are sometimes described as "going cold turkey."

Ethanol produces disinhibition and mild euphoria, which facilitate social interactions by reducing behavioral inhibitions and self-consciousness. These reinforcing effects are related to the rate at which the BAC is rising, which probably determines the rate at which dopamine and norepinephrine are released from neurons, both centrally and peripherally, and the rate at which dopamine concentrations increase in the nucleus accumbens. In many individuals, behavioral reinforcement leads to the continued consumption of alcoholic beverages and to ethanol intoxication. This problem is exacerbated by the limited rate at which ethanol can be eliminated from the body.

Ethanol has opioidlike effects that are partly mediated by the direct interaction of ethanol with δ opioid receptors. This interaction probably contributes to the analgesic, euphoric, and sedative effects of ethanol. Ethanol also interacts with catecholamines to form condensation products that possess opioidlike properties which can be reversed by naloxone. These condensation products, called hydroisoquinolines, may be responsible for some of the neurodegenerative effects of long-term ethanol abuse, including the impairment of memory and motor function and the loss of neuronal tissue.

Ethanol inhibits the release of acetylcholine from CNS neurons, and this action may contribute to the sedation and delirium that occur during alcohol intoxication. Ethanol also inhibits the release of antidiuretic hormone from the pituitary gland and thereby produces a diuretic effect. This diuretic effect is augmented by the consumption of large quantities of alcoholic beverages, such as beer.

Ethanol produces vasodilation and increases heat loss from the body, partly by interfering with temperature regulation by the hypothalamus. Hence, alcohol consumption may contribute to hypothermia during cold weather.

TABLE 24–4. Management of Drug Withdrawal and Dependence

Drug	Withdrawal	Dependence
Alcohol	Chlordiazepoxide, lorazepam, or clonidine;* multivitamins; and supplements of thiamine and magnesium.	Behavioral therapy and disulfiram.
Amphetamines	Bromocriptine.*	Behavioral therapy.
Barbiturates	Barbiturates.	Behavioral therapy and gradual dosage reduction.
Benzodiazepines	Benzodiazepines.	Behavioral therapy and gradual dosage reduction.
Cocaine	Bromocriptine.*	Behavioral therapy.
Marijuana	None.	None.
Nicotine	Nicotine chewing gum, nicotine skin patches, bupropion, or clonidine.*	Behavioral therapy and clonidine.*
Opioids	Methadone or clonidine.*	Behavioral therapy and naltrexone or clonidine.*

*The roles of clonidine and bromocriptine have not been firmly established.

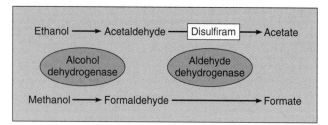

FIGURE 24–1. Metabolism of ethanol and methanol. Alcohols are oxidized to aldehydes by alcohol dehydrogenase. The aldehydes are oxidized to acetate or formate by aldehyde dehydrogenase. Disulfiram inhibits aldehyde dehydrogenase and leads to the accumulation of acetaldehyde during ethanol ingestion.

Other Effects, Mechanisms, and Interactions. In addition to producing CNS effects, ethanol ingestion produces a variety of short-term and long-term cardiovascular and autonomic effects.

Blood pressure fluctuations are due to the combination of peripheral vasodilation, depression of regulatory centers in the medulla, and the release of norepinephrine from sympathetic neurons. Consumption of large amounts of ethanol on a long-term basis may eventually lead to alcoholic cardiomyopathy and cardiac arrhythmias.

In alcoholic patients, thiamine deficiency secondary to a poor diet is commonly observed and leads to nerve demyelination. This in turn causes peripheral neuropathies, characterized by paresthesias and reduced sensory acuity. Thiamine deficiency may also cause Wernicke-Korsakoff syndrome, a behavioral disorder characterized by confusion, severe anterograde and retrograde amnesia, ataxia, nystagmus, and ophthalmoplegia. The administration of thiamine substantially reverses all but the amnesic effects seen in patients with this syndrome.

Alcoholic patients may also develop several metabolic disorders. The depletion of NAD (described above) causes several citric acid cycle metabolites and lactate to accumulate and eventually contributes to liver degeneration and impaired glycogenolysis. The resulting hypoglycemia exacerbates the effects of ethanol on the CNS. A dietary deficiency of folate can lead to megaloblastic anemia, while a deficiency of other vitamins and antioxidants contributes to the overall tissue damage observed in alcoholism.

The consumption of significant quantities of ethanol during pregnancy is responsible for the occurrence of the fetal alcohol syndrome, which is characterized by low birth weight, microcephaly, facial abnormalities (flattening), mental retardation, heart defects, and other abnormalities.

Ethanol interacts with drugs that are metabolized by cytochrome P450 enzymes. It also interacts with **disulfiram,** a drug that inhibits acetaldehyde dehydrogenase. When this drug is administered concurrently with ethanol, it leads to the accumulation of acetaldehyde and causes nausea, profuse vomiting, sweating, flushing, palpitations, and dyspnea. Because of its ability to cause these extremely unpleasant symptoms, disulfiram is sometimes pre-

scribed to encourage alcoholic patients to abstain from ethanol use. Other drugs that may cause disulfiramlike effects when administered concurrently with ethanol include metronidazole (a drug used in the treatment of protozoal infections) and some of the third-generation cephalosporin antibiotics.

Other Alcohols and Glycols

Methanol, also called **methyl alcohol** or **wood alcohol,** is a highly toxic form of alcohol that can cause profound anion gap metabolic acidosis and severe damage to the eyes. As shown in Fig. 24–1, methanol is converted to formaldehyde and then to formate. Formate is primarily responsible for optic nerve damage, which can result in visual field impairment or permanent blindness. In cases of methanol poisoning, patients are treated with ethanol, which serves to saturate alcohol dehydrogenase and thereby prevent the formation of formaldehyde and formate. Ethanol has a greater affinity for alcohol dehydrogenase than does methanol. Hemodialysis is also used to reduce methanol levels in severe intoxication.

Isopropyl alcohol is contained in many formulations of rubbing alcohol and produces more CNS depression than does ethanol or methanol. Isopropyl alcohol is converted to acetone, a substance that can be smelled on the breath. The treatment of intoxication is largely supportive.

Ethylene glycol is contained in antifreeze, and its ingestion can cause anion gap metabolic acidosis and serious toxicity to the kidneys, lungs, and CNS. Ethylene glycol is metabolized to oxalic acid, and calcium oxalate crystals may be found in the urine of patients after ethylene glycol ingestion. Treatment consists of supporting vital functions, giving ethanol, managing acidosis, and performing hemodialysis.

Barbiturates and Benzodiazepines

The pharmacologic properties of barbiturates and benzodiazepines are discussed in Chapter 19. These drugs are sedative-hypnotic agents that are prescribed for the treatment of anxiety disorders, insomnia, and other conditions. They are used recreationally for their euphoric and anxiolytic effects, and some polydrug users employ them to reduce the irritability and anxiety associated with cocaine or amphetamine use.

The short-acting barbiturates, such as **pentobarbital,** are the most widely abused sedative-hypnotic drugs. Several benzodiazepines have also been used illicitly, including **flunitrazepam.** Although this drug is not approved for use in the USA, it is employed throughout much of the world as an anxiolytic or hypnotic drug. In the USA, it is widely available on the streets and is sometimes referred to as **"roofies."** Flunitrazepam has gained fame as a party drug, a club drug, and a drug that contributes to date rape. It is an extremely potent benzodiazepine that is tasteless when dissolved in a beverage. Flunitrazepam produces drowsiness, impaired motor skills, and anterograde amnesia. Hence, victims do not recall events that happened the night before. Despite its street reputation, most studies have found that flunitrazepam is no more likely to cause toxicity or dependence than are other benzodiazepines.

The long-term use of barbiturate or benzodiazepine drugs may lead to psychologic and physical dependence, and their abrupt withdrawal produces symptoms that are similar to those caused by alcohol withdrawal (see Table 24–3).

Opioids

The most commonly abused opioid drug and one of the most widely used street drugs is **heroin.** This drug is prepared from morphine after its extraction from raw opium and is also called **diacetylmorphine.** It is highly potent and can be easily dissolved in water and injected intravenously. Because it is also highly lipid-soluble and rapidly enters the CNS following injection, heroin may produce an intense euphoric sensation called a "rush." Long-term heroin users develop considerable drug tolerance and physical dependence, and they undergo a wide variety of withdrawal symptoms (see Table 24–3) if they abruptly discontinue their use of the drug.

Other opioids produce effects similar to those of heroin, but usually to a lesser degree. These effects vary with the potency and pharmacokinetic properties of the opioid and with the route of administration. Opioids administered orally tend to produce less euphoria and dependence than do opioids administered by other routes. For this reason, an orally administered drug such as methadone (see Chapter 23) can be used to prevent the craving for heroin as well as the opioid withdrawal reaction without causing significant reinforcement or exacerbating drug dependence.

CENTRAL NERVOUS SYSTEM STIMULANTS

The CNS stimulants include amphetamine, amphetamine derivatives, cocaine, caffeine, and nicotine. The amphetamine compounds and cocaine increase the synaptic concentration of norepinephrine and dopamine and exert sympathomimetic effects.

Amphetamine and Its Derivatives

Amphetamine and its derivatives (Fig. 24–2A) increase the synaptic concentration of norepinephrine and dopamine by causing a calcium-independent release of these neurotransmitters from the nerve terminal and also by competitively inhibiting monoamine oxidase.

The use of amphetamines produces a constellation of central and peripheral effects, including euphoria, insomnia, psychomotor stimulation, anxiety, loss of appetite, increased concentration, decreased fatigue, respiratory stimulation, and hyper

thermia. It also produces sympathomimetic effects such as mydriasis, tachycardia, and hypertension. The euphoria and other reinforcing effects are due to increased dopamine levels in the nucleus accumbens, while the jittery and anxious feelings produced by amphetamines are primarily due to enhanced release of norepinephrine in the central and peripheral nervous systems.

The amphetamines have a few legitimate medical indications. First, amphetamines or antidepressant drugs can be used to treat **narcolepsy,** a condition characterized by sleep attacks, in which the patient suddenly falls asleep during normal daytime activities. Second, amphetamines can be used to treat **attention deficit disorder** (ADD), a disorder characterized by hyperactivity and the inability to focus attention or concentrate on a task. Amphetamine-type drugs are the most effective treatment for the majority of patients with ADD, and methylphenidate is widely used for this purpose. Third, amphetamine derivatives, such as phentermine, can be used as adjuncts in the treatment of **obesity.**

Methamphetamine

Amphetamine and methamphetamine are closely related sympathomimetic amines, and both are drugs of abuse. Of the two, methamphetamine is often preferred by abusers because it causes less norepinephrine to be released and can be more easily pyrolyzed (burned) and smoked. When methamphetamine free base is extracted by ether, pyrolyzed, and smoked, it is called **"ice."** The euphoria produced by smoking "ice" is much greater than that produced by taking methamphetamine orally, probably because of the faster rate at which dopamine levels are increased by inhaling the drug.

Methylphenidate

Methylphenidate is an amphetamine derivative that usually causes less irritability, anxiety, and anorexia than does amphetamine. When it is used to treat children with ADD, it is administered in the morning and at noontime, with the last dose preferably given no later than 3:00 PM in order to avoid insomnia. The drug may reduce the appetite and may temporarily slow the growth of children slightly, but it usually does not have a long-term effect on growth or development.

Methylphenidate is not associated with significant dependence when it is used for the treatment of ADD, but it is abused on the street.

Phentermine and Fenfluramine

Phentermine and fenfluramine are amphetamine derivatives that have been used as appetite suppressants in the treatment of obesity. The drugs act by stimulating the satiety center in the hypothalamus. In comparison with amphetamine, they produce less CNS stimulation and have a lower dependence liabil

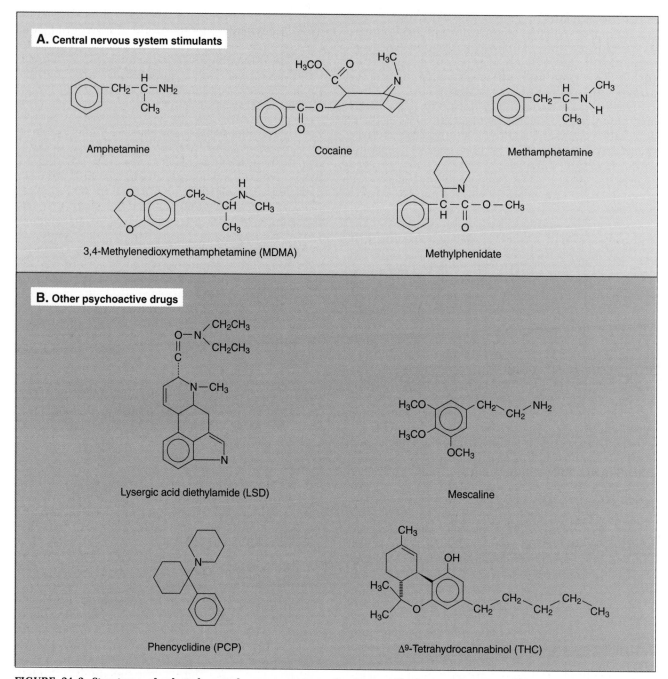

FIGURE 24–2. Structures of selected central nervous system stimulants and other psychoactive drugs. (A) Methamphetamine, 3,4-methylenedioxymethamphetamine (MDMA), and methylphenidate are all derivatives of amphetamine. Cocaine is an alkaloid derived from the leaves of *Erythroxylon coca*. **(B)** Lysergic acid diethylamide (LSD) and mescaline are hallucinogens. Phencyclidine (PCP) was originally developed as a dissociative anesthetic but was withdrawn from the market because it produces hallucinations and delirium, sometimes with hostility and violent behavior. Δ^9-Tetrahydrocannabinol (THC) is the primary cannabinoid in marijuana.

ity. However, fenfluramine and its active stereoisomer, dexfenfluramine, were withdrawn from the US market in 1997 after they were found to cause valvular heart disease and pulmonary hypertension.

Phentermine and other amphetamine derivatives are still available as an adjunct to dietary restrictions in the treatment of obesity. Tolerance often develops to the anorectic effects of these drugs after a few weeks to a few months of use.

Other Amphetamine Derivatives

Several other amphetamine derivatives have been clandestinely synthesized and sold as **"designer drugs"** on the street. These include **3,4-methylenedioxymethamphetamine** (MDMA), a drug that is sometimes called **"ecstasy"** and produces both psychostimulant and psychotomimetic effects by increasing dopamine and serotonin levels in the brain.

Users of MDMA report that the drug causes euphoria, increases empathy, enhances pleasure, heightens sexuality, and expands consciousness without loss of control. However, MDMA has a small margin of safety, and excessive doses may cause various unpleasant effects, such as nausea, anorexia, and anxiety, or may be life-threatening. In MDMA users, a number of deaths have resulted from cardiac arrhythmias, hyperthermia, rhabdomyolysis, and disseminated intravascular coagulation. Long-term use leads to degeneration of serotoninergic neurons, which may contribute to some of the associated psychiatric complications, including panic reactions, psychosis, depression, and suicide.

Other Stimulants

Cocaine

Cocaine produces both psychostimulant and local anesthetic activity and has limited clinical use as a local anesthetic (see Chapter 25). The stimulant effects are due to inhibition of the neuronal reuptake of norepinephrine and dopamine. Cocaine binds to the neurotransmitter transport proteins and causes them to undergo a conformational change that reduces their capacity to transport dopamine or norepinephrine. By this mechanism, cocaine increases the synaptic concentration of these neurotransmitters.

Cocaine is an alkaloid derived from the leaves of a plant indigenous to South America, *Erythroxylon coca*. When native South Americans chew the leaves to relieve fatigue, there are relatively few adverse effects. However, the use of purified forms of cocaine is associated with significant drug dependence, as well as cardiovascular, pulmonary, and neurologic toxicity.

In the past, many cocaine users took powdered cocaine hydrochloride by snorting it. Cocaine taken in this manner is absorbed across the nasal mucosa and into the circulation. More recently, cocaine free base became available in the form of pellets or rocks and was called **"crack"** because the user would crack off a dose of the substance. Unlike cocaine hydrochloride, crack cocaine can be smoked. Crack cocaine becomes aerosolized when it is heated, and inhaling the substance into the lungs causes it to be rapidly absorbed into the circulation. Inhalation of crack cocaine produces serum levels that are comparable to those obtained by intravenous administration of the drug. For this reason, crack cocaine produces a euphoric effect that is more intense than that obtained by snorting cocaine. The higher serum levels achieved with crack cocaine also increase the potential for overdose toxicity, particularly during repeated administration.

The common signs and symptoms of cocaine intoxication are listed in Table 24–1. Unlike other drugs of abuse, cocaine has the ability to alter tactile sensation, causing its users to feel as if insects are crawling under their skin (the sensation of "cocaine bugs") and causing them to scratch and produce self-inflicted skin lesions. Cocaine often stimulates respiration at lower doses, and high doses may produce irregular breathing and apnea (Cheyne-Stokes respiration). The local anesthetic actions of cocaine probably contribute to the drug's cardiac toxicity when high doses are administered.

With frank overdoses, the potential for neurotoxicity and cardiac toxicity increases. Cocaine overdose victims often suffer from delirium and may become aggressive and violent. The pulse may become rapid, weak, and irregular. In some cases, cocaine overdose causes tonic-clonic seizures (including status epilepticus), malignant encephalopathy, high-output cardiac failure, or myocardial infarction. When fatalities occur, they typically result from ventricular fibrillation or cardiac arrest. For this reason, the management of cocaine overdose must include cardiovascular and pulmonary support, as well as the administration of a benzodiazepine, such as lorazepam, to control agitation or seizures.

Cocaine withdrawal produces fatigue, depression, nightmares or other sleep disturbances, and increased appetite. The management of cocaine withdrawal is largely supportive. Bromocriptine, a dopamine receptor agonist, has been used to reduce craving for the drug, but the effectiveness of this treatment for withdrawal has not been firmly established.

Nicotine

Nicotine is the principal alkaloid of plants of the genus *Nicotiana* and is widely available in the form of various tobacco products that may be chewed or smoked.

Nicotine is a lipid-soluble tertiary amine. It is rapidly absorbed into the circulation from the mouth or the respiratory tract and is then quickly distributed to the brain. The drug's CNS effects are rapidly terminated by redistribution from the brain to the peripheral tissues. Although nicotine has a half-life of about 30 minutes, it is metabolized to cotinine, which has a half-life of about 2 hours. The induction of cytochrome P450 enzymes by tars contained in cigarette smoke accelerates the metabolism of nicotine, and this leads to the development of pharmacokinetic tolerance to the drug. Because the use of cigarettes accelerates the metabolism of β-adrenergic receptor antagonists, benzodiazepines, opioids, and theophylline, cigarette smokers may require higher doses of these drugs to maintain therapeutic serum levels.

Nicotine activates cholinergic nicotinic receptors in the central and peripheral nervous systems and produces a complex constellation of subjective and physiologic effects. The CNS effects of nicotine are similar to those of the psychostimulants and include mild euphoria, increased arousal and concentration, improved memory, and appetite suppression. In addition to activating cholinergic receptors, nicotine inhibits monoamine oxidase. The drug's ability to inhibit this enzyme may partly explain its ability to activate dopaminergic neurotransmission and its dependence liability. However, the monoamine oxidase inhibitors used in treating depression do not cause significant drug dependence or the intense drug craving associated with nicotine use. Hence, other mechanisms must contribute to the reinforcement of nicotine use and to nicotine addiction.

Caffeine

Caffeine citrate is occasionally administered intravenously to treat **apnea in neonates.** It is also available in nonprescription tablets for the prevention of **fatigue.**

Caffeine is a methylxanthine that produces mild stimulation by blocking adenosine receptors on neurons throughout the CNS. Because adenosine inhibits dopamine release, caffeine indirectly enhances dopamine neurotransmission. This action is probably responsible for the drug's stimulant effects and dependence liability.

Caffeine is the most widely ingested drug, as it is contained in coffee, cola beverages, teas, and other products that are used throughout the world. Caffeine use decreases the desire to sleep, elevates the mood, and causes an increase in alertness, concentration, motivation, and talkativeness. By arousing the sympathetic system, it causes a mild stimulation of heart rate and blood pressure. Caffeine also relaxes most smooth muscles and causes diuresis by increasing renal blood flow.

Because caffeine increases the secretion of gastric acid and pepsin, it may contribute to gastritis and peptic ulcers. High doses of caffeine produce nausea, vomiting, increased muscle tone, and tremors. Although extremely high doses of caffeine may cause delirium, seizures, and even death, these doses are almost impossible to reach by ingesting caffeinated beverages such as coffee. They can be reached by ingesting caffeine tablets, but abuse of caffeine tablets is limited by the fact that large doses of them produce such unpleasant symptoms.

The manifestations of caffeine withdrawal are relatively mild but include headache, impaired concentration, irritability, depression, anxiety, flu-like symptoms, and blurred vision. The withdrawal symptoms may be lessened by reducing caffeine consumption gradually over a period of several weeks.

OTHER PSYCHOACTIVE DRUGS
Cannabis and Its Derivatives

In the USA, a synthetic cannabis derivative called **dronabinol** has been approved for the **treatment of nausea** caused by cancer chemotherapy and for the **stimulation of appetite** in patients who have acquired immunodeficiency syndrome (AIDS) and are suffering from anorexia. The drug is administered orally for these purposes.

The most well-known form of cannabis is **marijuana,** which consists of the dried flowers and leaves of *Cannabis sativa* and is considered a drug of abuse. The primary cannabinoid in marijuana is Δ^9-**tetrahydrocannabinol** (THC), a drug whose structure is shown in Fig. 24–2B. When cannabis is inhaled, about 20% of the THC is absorbed into the circulation. In contrast, when cannabis is ingested orally, only about 6% of the THC is absorbed from the gut, owing to the extensive first-pass metabolism. THC has multiple effects on neuronal function. It binds stereospecifically to protein receptors in cell membranes, and this action is linked with inhibition of adenylyl cyclase and cAMP production. It also inhibits voltage-gated calcium channels that regulate neurotransmitter release. Through these and other actions, THC appears to modulate the activity of acetylcholine, dopamine, and serotonin.

When marijuana is smoked, pyrolysis releases THC and other substances. The plasma level of THC peaks within several minutes. Then it falls rapidly during the first hour, as the drug is redistributed to adipose tissue. Thereafter, it declines slowly, owing to metabolism and excretion in the urine and feces. Because of its high lipophilicity, THC is stored in fat, and the drug and its metabolites can be detected in the body for weeks.

Marijuana use initially causes mild stimulation followed by a depressive phase. The stimulant phase is described as a dreamlike euphoric state characterized by an altered sense of time, increased visual acuity, difficulty in concentrating, and impaired short-term memory. The depressive phase is characterized by drowsiness, lethargy, and increased appetite. The psychoactive effects of marijuana depend somewhat on the environment and the extent of prior use of the drug. For example, first-time users are more likely to experience anxiety than are habitual users.

Marijuana has been implicated as the cause of an amotivational syndrome that is characterized by a lack of desire to work or excel in any part of life. It has also been described as a "gateway drug" whose initial use leads to the subsequent use of drugs such as cocaine or heroin. There is little scientific evidence to support either of these claims. Contrary to reports in the popular press, marijuana causes only minor changes in the levels of testosterone and other hormones, and these changes are reversible. Studies in humans have consistently demonstrated that marijuana reduces aggressive behavior, even though animals injected with THC may show aggression.

Experimental studies have demonstrated that cannabinoids are effective in the treatment of asthma, glaucoma, and vomiting. This is because their use causes bronchodilation, decreased intraocular pressure, and inhibition of nausea. Their use can also cause tachycardia.

The common signs and symptoms of marijuana intoxication and withdrawal are listed in Tables 24–1 and 24–3.

Hallucinogens

Prescription drugs, fever, and disorders such as schizophrenia are all capable of causing hallucinations, which are false perceptions that result from abnormal sensory processing. Unlike prescription drugs, however, drugs such as **lysergic acid diethylamide** (LSD) and **mescaline** are able to produce hallucinations without causing delirium. These street drugs are taken orally and usually begin to produce hallucinations within an hour. The effects of LSD may last as long as 12 hours, whereas the effects of mescaline last about 6 hours. The mechanisms responsible for the effects are incompletely understood. There is some evidence that LSD selectively activates certain subtypes of serotonin (5-hydroxytryptamine, or 5-HT) receptors in the neocortex, limbic system, and brain stem. According to one hypothesis, the activation of $5-HT_2$ receptors in the reticular formation leads to the generalization of sensory stimuli so as to evoke hallucinations.

Although the use of LSD or mescaline usually causes visual hallucinations, it can also cause auditory, tactile, olfactory, gustatory, kinesthetic, and synesthetic hallucinations. Visual hallucinations often follow a temporal pattern in which amorphous bursts of light are followed by geometric forms and then by faces or scenes. Some users also report the occurrence of synesthesia, a condition in which one sensory modality assumes the characteristics of another. In a synesthetic hallucination, for example, sounds may be seen or colors may be heard.

The hallucinogens have little effect on cognitive function or arousal. If mood changes occur, they are generally an exaggeration of the predrug mood and are highly context-dependent. They are usually pleasant, but they may be terrifying and cause enough anxiety to resemble a panic attack. Mood changes are accompanied by somatic signs of sympathetic activation, including increased heart rate, increased blood pressure, and dilated pupils. Nausea and vomiting may occur, particularly with mescaline.

Overdoses are rarely serious, but the occasional panic attack ("bad trip") may require intervention that consists of removing the patient to a quiet room and having someone remain with the patient for reassurance.

Phencyclidine

Phencyclidine (PCP) is still a widely used street drug, despite its reputation for causing dangerous side effects and despite efforts to reduce its supply by limiting the sale of chemicals used in its synthesis. PCP was originally developed as a dissociative anesthetic similar to ketamine, but the occurrence of a high incidence of postanesthetic hallucinations and delirium forced its removal from the market.

PCP is sometimes called **"angel dust"** and can be taken via various routes. The drug is incompletely and erratically absorbed from the gut, so it is usually smoked. In some cases, it is sprinkled on tobacco or marijuana and then smoked. In other cases, it is combined with cocaine and heroin before it is used.

PCP produces a unique spectrum of effects that are probably due to blockade of glutamate N-methyl-D-aspartate (NMDA) receptors. As shown in Table 24–1, these effects include euphoria, hallucinations, and psychotomimetic activity, sometimes accompanied by hostility and violent behavior. PCP causes little tolerance, physical dependence, or withdrawal effects.

THE MANAGEMENT OF DRUG ABUSE

The use of psychoactive drugs may cause several distinct clinical problems, including drug intoxication or overdose, drug withdrawal, and drug dependence. The severity of these problems varies markedly among different classes of drugs and patterns of drug use. A diagnosis of drug intoxication or dependence in a particular individual is primarily based on the history, psychologic assessment, physical examination, and laboratory findings.

Drug Intoxication and Withdrawal

The initial treatment of drug intoxication or overdose consists of supporting cardiovascular and pulmonary functions. **Naloxone** or **flumazenil** may be administered to counteract the acute CNS depression caused by toxic doses of an opioid or a benzodiazepine, respectively (see Table 24–2). **Lorazepam** may be used to control agitation, and an antipsychotic drug such as **haloperidol** may be administered for psychosis. However, haloperidol should not be used in cases of cocaine overdose, because it lowers the seizure threshold and can exacerbate or precipitate seizures.

The next stage of treatment is the management of withdrawal reactions that occur as the drug is eliminated from the body (see Table 24–4). The pharmacologic treatment of withdrawal consists primarily of substitution therapy.

A benzodiazepine, such as **lorazepam** or **chlordiazepoxide,** can be administered to suppress the acute manifestations of withdrawal from alcohol, including delusions, hallucinations, a coarse tremor, and agitation **(delirium tremens).** The benzodiazepine is then gradually withdrawn over several weeks.

Methadone is usually employed to suppress withdrawal reactions in opioid users because it is long-acting and orally effective. Methadone is also given on a long-term basis in the treatment of heroin addiction.

Nicotine chewing gum and skin patches have been developed to mitigate nicotine withdrawal reactions in persons who are trying to quit smoking. Another drug used to treat nicotine withdrawal is the antidepressant **bupropion,** which is now available in a long-acting formulation for this purpose. The ability of bupropion to block the reuptake of dopamine may contribute to its effectiveness in treating drug dependence. The combined use of bupropion and nicotine patches is currently being investigated.

Clonidine, an α_2-adrenergic receptor agonist, is effective in reducing the sympathetic nervous system symptoms of alcohol, opioid, or nicotine withdrawal, and it may facilitate continued abstinence in persons who are dependent on these drugs.

Clinical studies have shown that **bromocriptine,** a dopamine receptor agonist, can lessen the symptoms of cocaine withdrawal, but its role has not been firmly established.

Drug Dependence

After treatment of drug intoxication and withdrawal, attention may be directed to the more difficult problem of treating drug dependence. In this endeavor, behavioral therapy and personal motivation are more important than pharmacologic treatments. Patients are rarely cured, and most clinicians view treatment as a lifelong process in which patients are continually recovering. Twelve-step groups, such as Alcoholics Anonymous and Narcotics Anonymous, have been successful in reducing recidivism, partly because they recognize that the individual is always in a state of remission from drug or alcohol dependence and that there is an ever-present possibility of slipping into drug use again.

Pharmacologic agents may be of limited use in treating drug dependence. **Disulfiram** is occasionally employed to sustain abstinence in alcoholics. The drug inhibits acetaldehyde metabolism and causes unpleasant symptoms when alcohol is ingested concurrently. **Naltrexone** prevents the euphoric and other effects obtained with opioid administration and has been used to treat opioid dependence. **Clonidine** has also been used to facilitate abstinence from opioids and nicotine.

Summary of Important Points

- Drug dependence is a condition in which an individual feels compelled to repeatedly administer a psychoactive drug. The condition is due to positive reinforcement (psychologic depen-

dence) and negative reinforcement (physical dependence) of continued drug use.
- Reinforcement of drug use results from increased levels of dopamine in the nucleus accumbens and from dopamine sensitization.
- Physical dependence results from neuronal adaptation to the continued presence of a drug and is usually associated with drug tolerance. Physical dependence results in a characteristic withdrawal syndrome when drug use is discontinued.
- Alcohol and other central nervous system (CNS) depressants produce motor and cognitive impairment, sedation, euphoria, and behavioral disinhibition.
- Amphetamines, cocaine, and other CNS stimulants produce euphoria, agitation, hypervigilance, mydriasis, and sympathetic nervous system arousal. Cocaine also produces altered tactile sensation, and cocaine overdose may cause severe cardiovascular and neurologic toxicity.
- Marijuana and cannabis derivatives produce a mild euphoria, talkativeness, conjunctivitis, and increased appetite.
- Lysergic acid diethylamide (LSD) and other hallucinogens cause hallucinations without producing delirium.
- The treatment of drug dependence and withdrawal may include some type of substitution therapy: a benzodiazepine substituted for alcohol; methadone substituted for an opioid; and nicotine chewing gum or skin patches substituted for cigarettes.

Selected Readings

Boghdadi, M. S., and R. J. Henning. Cocaine: pathophysiology and clinical toxicology. Heart Lung 26:466–485, 1997.

Cohen, R. S., and J. Cocores. Neuropsychiatric manifestations following the use of 3,4-methylenedioxymethamphetamine (MDMA, or "ecstasy"). Prog Neuropsychopharm Biol Psychiatry 21:727–734, 1997.

Karch, S. B. The Pathology of Drug Abuse, 2nd ed. Boca Raton, Fla., CRC Press, 1996.

Simmons, M. M., and M. J. Cupp. Use and abuse of flunitrazepam. Ann Pharmacother 32:117–119, 1998.

CHAPTER TWENTY-FIVE

LOCAL AND GENERAL ANESTHETICS

OVERVIEW

Anesthesia is a condition in which a person does not perceive pain. Drugs that block the conduction of pain impulses to the spinal cord are called **local anesthetics,** whereas drugs that interfere with sensory processing and prevent the perception of pain by the sensory cortex are called **general anesthetics.**

Local anesthetics are used to anesthetize a particular part of the body and can be given to patients undergoing surgery on the skin and subcutaneous tissues, ears, eyes, joints, or pelvis. They are also used for anesthesia during labor and delivery and for diagnostic procedures such as gastrointestinal endoscopy. Occasionally, local anesthetics are used to relieve pain associated with pathologic conditions.

General anesthetics are primarily used to prevent pain during major surgical procedures, including those involving thoracic, abdominal, and other internal organs. Unlike local anesthetics, general anesthetics usually produce loss of consciousness and amnesia and thereby prevent the anesthetized patient from recalling the surgical procedure.

LOCAL ANESTHETICS

Classification

Based on their chemical structure, the local anesthetics can be divided into ester-type drugs and amide-type drugs.

Drug Properties

Chemistry and Pharmacokinetics. Each local anesthetic has a lipophilic (hydrophobic) portion and a hydrophilic portion (Fig. 25–1). The hydrophilic portion is an amine that is a weak base and exists in both ionized and nonionized forms. The ionized and protonated form predominates at lower pH levels, and the nonionized form predominates at higher pH levels. Only the nonionized form can penetrate neuronal membranes to reach receptor sites on the internal surface of sodium channels. Conditions such as inflammation and acidosis decrease the pH of tissues and increase the ionization of local anesthetics. For this reason, local anesthetics are less effective in the presence of these conditions, and larger doses may be required to anesthetize inflamed or acidotic tissue.

Local anesthetics are usually formulated as the hydrochloride salt at a pH less than 7, because this formulation is more soluble and stable than the free base formulation. Once injected, the local anesthetic solution is quickly buffered to the pH of the tissue.

The duration of action of local anesthetics may be short, medium, or long (Table 25–1). Because local anesthetics act directly at the site of application, their duration of action is primarily determined by their rate of diffusion and absorption at the site of administration. Diffusion and absorption in turn depend on the chemical properties of the anesthetics and on such factors as local pH and blood flow. In some cases, epinephrine may be added to prolong a local anesthetic's duration of action by producing vasoconstriction and slowing its rate of absorption. However, because of the risk of ischemia and necrosis, epinephrine should not be used to anesthetize

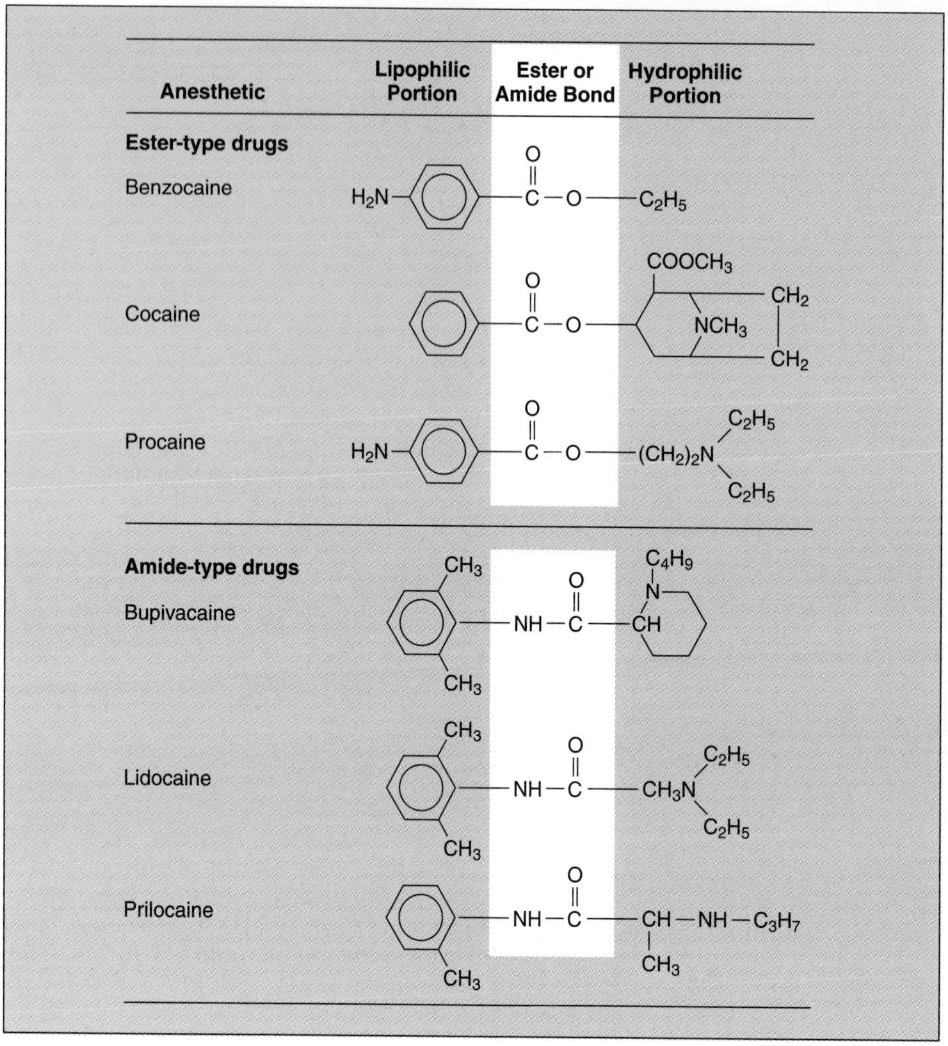

FIGURE 25–1. Structures of selected local anesthetics.

TABLE 25–1. Properties of Local Anesthetics

Drug	Potency	Duration of Action*	Parenteral Uses	Topical Uses
Ester-type drugs				
Benzocaine	Low.	Medium.	None.	Dermal, laryngeal, and oral.
Chloroprocaine	Low.	Short.	Epidural, infiltration, and nerve block anesthesia.	None.
Cocaine	Low.	Medium.	None.	Laryngeal, nasal, and urogenital.
Procaine	Low.	Short.	Infiltration, nerve block, and spinal anesthesia.	None.
Amide-type drugs				
Bupivacaine	High.	Medium.	Epidural, infiltration, nerve block, and spinal anesthesia.	None.
Etidocaine	Intermediate.	Long.	Infiltration and nerve block anesthesia.	None.
Lidocaine	Intermediate.	Short.	Epidural, infiltration, nerve block, and spinal anesthesia.	Dermal, laryngeal, and oral.
Mepivacaine	Intermediate.	Short.	Epidural, infiltration, nerve block, and spinal anesthesia.	None.
Prilocaine	Intermediate.	Short.	Infiltration anesthesia.	Dermal.
Ropivacaine	High.	Long.	Epidural, infiltration, and nerve block anesthesia.	None.

*The duration varies with the dose and route of administration. Short = 0.25–1.5 hours; medium = >1.5–5 hours; and long = >5 hours.

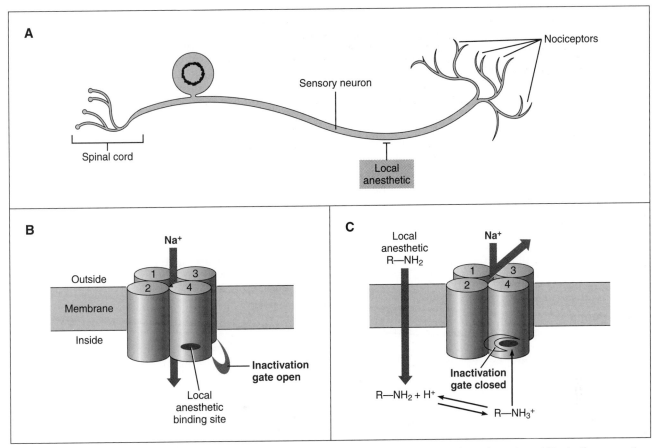

FIGURE 25–2. Mechanisms of action of local anesthetics. (A) The local anesthetic binds to sodium channels and blocks the generation and conduction of action potentials in peripheral neurons. **(B)** The sodium channel includes four transmembrane domains. The inactivation gate is a short intracellular loop between domains 3 and 4. The local anesthetic binds to amino acid residues located on domain 4. **(C)** The nonionized form of the local anesthetic ($R–NH_2$) penetrates the axonal membrane and is then converted to the ionized form ($R–NH_3^+$). The ionized form binds to the sodium channel in the open state, and this prolongs the sodium channel inactivation state. Sodium entry is blocked during the inactivation state.

tissues with end arteries, such as tissues of the fingers, toes, ears, nose, and penis.

Following systemic absorption, local anesthetics are primarily metabolized by hydrolytic enzymes (esterases and amidases), and the metabolites are excreted in the urine.

Mechanisms and Pharmacologic Effects. Local anesthetics are able to cause a reversible inhibition of axonal nerve conduction by binding to the sodium channel and decreasing the nerve membrane permeability to sodium. The anesthetics bind to the sodium channel at a site on the internal side of the plasma membrane and in a manner that prolongs the inactivation state of the channel (Fig. 25–2). The ionized and cationic form of local anesthetics has a greater affinity for the sodium channel than does the nonionized form.

Suppression of sodium influx prevents neuronal depolarization and blocks the conduction of nerve impulses. Local anesthetics have a greater affinity for sodium channels that are in the depolarized (open) configuration than for channels that are closed. Therefore, the degree of blockade increases as the frequency of nerve firing increases. The use-dependent blockade causes a greater inhibition of neurons that are depolarized more frequently by painful stimuli than of neurons that are firing less often. The degree of blockade of different neurons depends on the concentration and potency of the local anesthetic and on the size and myelination of the nerve. Small unmyelinated C fibers are more easily anesthetized than are large myelinated neurons. Autonomic and sensory nerves are blocked more easily than are motor neurons. Pain, temperature, touch, and sympathetic vasomotor activity are inhibited before proprioception, muscle tone, and somatic motor activity. Nerves recover from blockade in the reverse order.

Adverse Effects and Interactions. The adverse effects of local anesthetics are primarily due to their absorption into the systemic circulation and subsequent alteration of central nervous system (CNS), cardiovascular, and other organ system functions.

Local anesthetics often produce CNS stimulation (restlessness, tremor, and euphoria) followed by inhibition (drowsiness and sedation). Other symptoms of local anesthetic toxicity include headache, paresthesias, and nausea. Higher concentrations may cause seizures followed by coma. Death is usually due to respiratory failure.

Adverse cardiovascular effects include hypotension and cardiac depression. Most local anesthetics are vasodilators, and they also block vasoconstriction induced by the sympathetic nervous system. The majority of local anesthetics have antiarrhythmic activity, but toxic levels of local anesthetics suppress cardiac conduction and may cause tachyarrhythmia characterized by a wide QRS complex.

Local anesthetic blockade of autonomic ganglia and neuromuscular transmission may lead to loss of visceral and skeletal muscle tone. For this reason, local anesthetics potentiate the effect of neuromuscular blocking drugs such as tubocurarine, and local anesthetics must be used with great caution in patients with myasthenia gravis.

Allergic reactions to local anesthetics are fairly common. Repeated application of topical anesthetics is particularly prone to cause sensitization. The ester-type anesthetics cause hypersensitivity reactions more frequently than do the amide-type anesthetics. This is partly because ester-type anesthetics, such as procaine, are metabolized to p-aminobenzoic acid (PABA), which may be allergenic. PABA is an ingredient in some sunscreen products, and patients may acquire sensitivity by repeatedly using these products. Patients who are allergic to an ester-type anesthetic will usually tolerate an amide-type anesthetic. Allergy to a particular amide-type anesthetic does not necessary indicate cross-sensitivity to other amide-type anesthetics, and intradermal skin testing can be used to determine which anesthetics are tolerated.

Indications. Local anesthetics are usually administered parenterally but are sometimes applied topically. The route of administration depends on factors such as the site of anesthesia.

(1) Topical Anesthesia. The topical application of local anesthetics is used for anesthetization of the skin, mucous membranes, or cornea. A local anesthetic can be applied to the skin for the treatment of pruritus (itching) caused by poison ivy, insect bites, eczema, or cutaneous manifestations of systemic diseases such as chickenpox (varicella). A eutectic mixture of local anesthetics (EMLA), consisting of two or more solid compounds that form a liquid when they are combined, is sometimes used to anesthetize the skin prior to venipuncture or minor surgery. The topical application of a local anesthetic to mucous membranes can relieve pain caused by oral, nasal, laryngeal, or rectal disorders or surgery. For example, an anesthetic ointment is used to relieve the discomfort of hemorrhoids. A topically applied anesthetic may also be used to relieve itching or pain associated with genitourinary procedures or disorders. The topical ocular administration of local anesthetics is used to anesthetize the cornea prior to diagnostic or surgical procedures, such as radial keratotomy, the removal of foreign bodies, and cataract surgery.

(2) Infiltration Anesthesia. Infiltration is probably the most common route used to administer local anesthetics. The process involves injecting an anesthetic directly into a subcutaneous or other superficial tissue. Infiltration is primarily used for minor surgical procedures, such as the removal of foreign bodies. It is also frequently used for dental procedures. When a local anesthetic is to be administered by infiltration, epinephrine may be added to it to decrease its dosage and prolong its duration of action. However, as mentioned earlier, epinephrine should not be used to anesthetize fingers, toes, and other tissues with end arteries.

(3) Iontophoresis. Local anesthetics are occasionally administered by iontophoresis. This technique uses a small electric current to force molecules of the anesthetic into a tissue. Iontophoresis is primarily employed in dentistry. It eliminates the need to inject the anesthetic and is preferred by some patients for this reason.

(4) Nerve Block and Field Block Anesthesia. Nerve block and field block anesthesia are forms of **regional anesthesia,** the goal of which is to anesthetize an area of the body by blocking the conductivity of sensory nerves from that area. In nerve block anesthesia, a local anesthetic is injected into or adjacent to a peripheral nerve or nerve plexus. For example, a radial nerve block may be used to anesthetize the structures innervated by the radial nerve, including portions of the forearm and hand. Intraorbital block is often used for ocular surgery. Other examples of nerve block anesthesia are brachial plexus and cervical plexus blocks. In field block anesthesia, a local anesthetic is administered in a series of injections to form a wall of anesthesia encircling the operative field.

(5) Spinal Anesthesia. Spinal anesthesia is used to block somatic sensory and motor fibers during procedures such as surgery on the lower limb or pelvic structures. A local anesthetic is injected into the subarachnoid space below the level at which the spinal cord terminates. The spread of the anesthetic in the cerebrospinal fluid is controlled by the horizontal tilt of the patient and by the specific gravity (baricity) of the local anesthetic solution. Hyperbaric solutions of local anesthetics are available for this purpose, and these spread along the neuraxis for about 15 minutes. By this time, they have mixed with cerebrospinal fluid so as to become isobaric and are said to be "fixed" at a certain level of the spinal cord. Spinal anesthesia may cause headaches associated with lumbar puncture, and respiratory depression may occur if the anesthetic ascends too high up the spinal cord.

(6) Epidural Anesthesia. Epidural anesthesia is produced by injecting a local anesthetic into the lumbar or caudal epidural (extradural) space. A local anesthetic such as bupivacaine is often administered by this route to provide anesthesia during labor and delivery. After epidural administration, the local anesthetic is absorbed into the systemic circulation. Therefore, doses must be carefully monitored to prevent cardiac depression and neurotoxicity in the mother and neonate.

Ester-Type Drugs

Cocaine

Cocaine is a naturally occurring plant alkaloid and was the first local anesthetic to be discovered. It has both local anesthetic and CNS stimulant properties, and it is the only local anesthetic that causes significant vasoconstriction as a result of its sympathomimetic effect. Because of its CNS effects and potential for abuse (see Chapter 24), cocaine is seldom used as a local anesthetic. However, it is occasionally used to anesthetize the internal structures of the nose, where its vasoconstrictive action helps prevent bleeding after nasal surgery. A cocaine solution is applied to gauze and inserted into the nose for this purpose.

Procaine and Chloroprocaine

Procaine was the first synthetic local anesthetic drug to be prepared after the discovery of cocaine, and it became the standard of comparison for many years. Procaine and chloroprocaine have a low potency and a relatively short duration of action. They are not effective after topical administration and must be administered parenterally. Both drugs are metabolized to PABA. For this reason, they are more likely to cause allergic reactions than are the amide-type local anesthetics.

Benzocaine

Benzocaine is a frequently used topical anesthetic and is available in a number of nonprescription products for the treatment of sunburn, pruritus, and other skin conditions. In some patients, the drug causes hypersensitivity reactions, which may exacerbate preexisting dermatitis. Benzocaine is also used to anesthetize mucous membranes and is available in cough lozenges and sprays for the relief of coughing.

Amide-Type Drugs

Lidocaine and Etidocaine

Lidocaine produces local anesthesia after topical or parenteral administration. It is the most widely used local anesthetic and is available in a number of formulations. These include topical solutions and ointments, oral sprays, viscous gels for oral and laryngeal application, and various parenteral formulations. A eutectic mixture of lidocaine and prilocaine is available as a cream for anesthetizing intact skin to a depth of 5 mm. In pediatric patients, this EMLA has been used for local anesthesia prior to venipuncture, intravenous cannulation, or circumcision. Lidocaine is also employed for infiltration, nerve block, epidural, and spinal anesthesia.

Etidocaine has properties similar to those of lidocaine, but its duration of action is considerably longer. It is primarily used for infiltration and nerve block anesthesia.

Bupivacaine, Mepivacaine, and Ropivacaine

Bupivacaine, mepivacaine, and ropivacaine have similar clinical uses but differ in their duration of action, as shown in Table 25–1. Bupivacaine has been the most widely used local anesthetic for obstetrical anesthesia, but it causes cardiac depression more frequently than do many other local anesthetics. Ropivacaine is a newer drug that may cause fewer cases of cardiac toxicity.

Prilocaine

Prilocaine is a congener of lidocaine. It is converted to O-toluidine, a toxic metabolite that may cause methemoglobinemia if it is allowed to accumulate. For this reason, the use of prilocaine is limited to topical and infiltration anesthesia. Prilocaine combines with lidocaine to form a eutectic mixture, and this combination is used for topical anesthesia, as described above.

GENERAL ANESTHETICS

The first demonstration of general anesthesia for surgery was performed by William Morton at the Massachusetts General Hospital in 1846. The anesthetic that Morton used was diethyl ether, and his demonstration had a profound impact on the field of surgery. Prior to that time, surgery was limited to rapid procedures such as limb amputations. General anesthesia and the subsequent development of aseptic techniques permitted the evolution of surgical procedures to the sophisticated level that has been achieved today.

Diethyl ether is no longer used in developed countries, because it has a slow rate of induction, causes considerable postoperative nausea and vomiting, and is highly flammable. Use of another anesthetic gas, cyclopropane, has also been abandoned, because of its explosive nature and its tendency to cause cardiac arrhythmias. However, a variety of anesthetics are currently available for inhalational use. These include nitrous oxide and a growing number of halogenated hydrocarbons. The pharmacologic properties and adverse effects of these drugs are listed in Tables 25–2 and 25–3, respectively.

Inhalational Anesthetics

Classification

The inhalational anesthetics can be divided into nonhalogenated drugs and halogenated drugs.

Drug Properties

Chemistry and Pharmacokinetics. Structures of selected inhalational anesthetics are shown in Fig. 25–3A. These anesthetics are either gases or volatile liquids whose gaseous phase can be inhaled.

The **potency** of inhalational anesthetics is ex-

TABLE 25–2.   Properties of Inhalational Anesthetics

Drug	Minimum Alveolar Concentration (% vol/vol)*	Blood:Gas Partition Coefficient	Rate of Induction	Amount Metabolized	Amount of Skeletal Muscle Relaxation
Nonhalogenated drugs					
Nitrous oxide	>100	0.47	Fast	0%	None
Halogenated drugs					
Desflurane	6.0	0.42	Fast	<2%	Medium
Enflurane	1.7	1.9	Medium	5% (fluoride)	Medium
Halothane	0.75	2.3	Slow	20%	Low
Isoflurane	1.2	1.4	Medium	<2% (fluoride)	Medium
Sevoflurane	1.9	0.63	Fast	<2%	Medium

*The minimum alveolar concentration (MAC) is the concentration needed to produce anesthesia in half of the subjects.

pressed in terms of the inspired concentration of the anesthetic required to produce anesthesia in half of the subjects. This is called the **minimum alveolar concentration** (MAC). The MAC value is equivalent to the median effective dose (ED_{50}) of solid drugs.

The pharmacokinetics of inhalational anesthetics differ from those of solid drugs because the gaseous anesthetics enter and exit from the body through the same organ, the lungs. Moreover, the movement of anesthetic molecules between the lungs and other tissues is determined by the partial pressure of the anesthetic, rather than by the dissolved concentration of the anesthetic in tissue fluid. As the anesthetic's partial pressure in the blood increases, molecules of the anesthetic move into the brain and produce anesthesia.

The **rate of induction** of anesthesia is determined by three primary factors: (1) the alveolar concentration, or alveolar partial pressure, of the anesthetic; (2) the ventilation rate; and (3) the rate at which the anesthetic's partial pressure in the blood increases as the anesthetic is administered. This third factor is in turn influenced by the **blood:gas partition coefficient** (Box 25–1).

Because anesthetic molecules move from an area of higher partial pressure to an area of lower partial pressure, both the rate of induction and the depth of anesthesia can be rapidly adjusted by increasing or decreasing the partial pressure of the anesthetic in the patient's inspired air. After the concentration in inspired air is increased or decreased, the concentration in the blood and brain will increase or decrease. The ability to rapidly control the depth of anesthesia increases the safety of the inhalational anesthetics.

Mechanisms and Pharmacologic Effects.   The specific mechanism of action of inhalational anesthetics is unknown, but recent studies suggest that these agents interact stereoselectively with hydrophobic regions of proteins embedded in the lipid bilayer of neuronal membranes. The anesthetics are believed to reach their receptor sites by dissolving in neuronal membrane lipids, and there is a strong correlation between anesthetic potency and lipid solubility, as determined by the **oil:gas partition coefficient** (Box 25–2).

The inhalational anesthetics appear to increase chloride influx and potassium efflux from neurons. Both of these actions cause hyperpolarization of neuronal membranes and reduce membrane excitability. The effect of the anesthetics on chloride flux appears to be due to potentiation of the action of gamma-aminobutyric acid (GABA) at the GABA$_A$ chloride ionophore. Inhalational anesthetics also reduce sodium and calcium influx, and this prevents nerve firing and the release of neurotransmitters.

Adverse Effects.   Table 25–3 compares the adverse effects of nonhalogenated and halogenated anesthetics.

TABLE 25–3.   Adverse Effects of Inhalational Anesthetics

Drug	Airway Irritation	Respiratory Depression	Broncho-dilation	Hypotensive Effect	Arrhythmia Potential*
Nonhalogenated drugs					
Nitrous oxide	Low	None	None	None	None
Halogenated drugs					
Desflurane	Moderate	Low	None	Reduced systemic vascular resistance	Low
Enflurane	Low	Moderate	Moderate	Reduced cardiac output	Low
Halothane	Moderate	Low	Moderate	Reduced cardiac output	Moderate
Isoflurane	Moderate	Moderate	Moderate	Reduced systemic vascular resistance	Low
Sevoflurane	Low	Low	None	Reduced systemic vascular resistance	Low

*Anesthetics that sensitize the heart to catecholamines have the potential to cause epinephrine-induced arrhythmias.

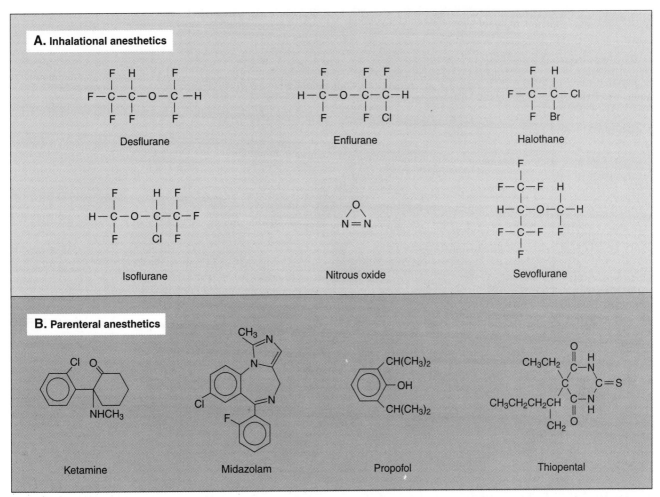

FIGURE 25–3. Structures of selected general anesthetics. (A) Inhalational anesthetics include nitrous oxide, which is a nonhalogenated gas; halothane, which is a halogenated hydrocarbon; and desflurane, enflurane, isoflurane, and sevoflurane, all of which are halogenated ethers. **(B)** Parenteral anesthetics include fentanyl (shown in Fig. 23–2B), ketamine, midazolam, propofol, and thiopental.

Nonhalogenated Drugs

Nitrous oxide is the only anesthetic gas used today. It is the least potent of the inhalational anesthetics, and it does not reduce consciousness to the extent required for major surgical procedures. However, nitrous oxide produces more analgesia than do the other inhalational anesthetics, and it is often used for minor surgery and dental procedures that do not require loss of consciousness. Nitrous oxide is frequently used as a component of **balanced anesthesia** in combination with another anesthetic agent and other drugs (see below). The nitrous oxide in balanced anesthesia provides analgesia and enables the use of a lower concentration of the other anesthetic agent.

Because nitrous oxide has a low blood:gas partition coefficient, induction and recovery are rapid when it is used. The anesthetic produces virtually no cardiovascular or respiratory depression, and it is generally considered quite safe. However, it oxidizes the cobalt moiety of vitamin B_{12} and thereby inhibits methylation of nucleic acids and proteins. Although these effects are minimal during acute exposure, chronic exposure to nitrous oxide may cause megaloblastic anemia.

Nitrous oxide, which is also called **"laughing gas,"** often produces mild euphoria when it is administered. For this reason, some recreational use of the drug has occurred.

Halogenated Drugs

In most areas of the world, the halogenated anesthetics have replaced older anesthetics, such as diethyl ether, because they have several advantages. The halogenated drugs have a more rapid rate of induction and recovery, cause a much lower incidence of postoperative nausea and vomiting, and are not flammable. However, they produce dose-dependent respiratory and cardiovascular depression. For this reason, respiratory and cardiovascular function must be carefully monitored during the use of halogenated anesthetics, and artificial ventilation and circulatory support may be required. The halogenated anesthetics cause uterine relaxation, which usually limits their use in obstetrics to women undergoing cesarian section. Because halogenated

BOX 25–1.   Pharmacokinetics of Inhalational Anesthetics

Rate of Induction of Anesthesia

The rate of induction of anesthesia is determined by three primary factors: (1) the alveolar concentration, or alveolar partial pressure, of the anesthetic; (2) the ventilation rate; and (3) the rate at which the anesthetic's partial pressure in the blood increases as the anesthetic is administered. This third factor is in turn influenced by the blood:gas partition coefficient.

The blood:gas partition coefficient is a measure of the anesthetic's solubility in the blood. In the example shown here, the coefficient of nitrous oxide is 0.47, whereas that of halothane is 2.3.

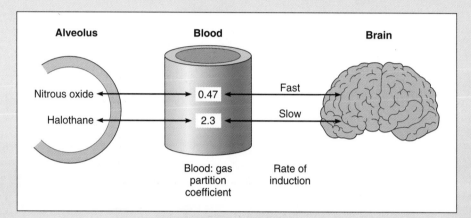

A high blood:gas partition coefficient corresponds with a high degree of solubility in the blood and with a low rate of rise in the anesthetic's partial pressure in the blood during induction. Anesthetics with a low coefficient, such as nitrous oxide, have a fast rate of induction because they saturate the blood quickly and their partial pressure rises quickly. Anesthetics with a higher coefficient, such as halothane, have a slow rate of induction because they dissolve slowly in the blood and it takes a long time for their partial pressure in the blood to rise.

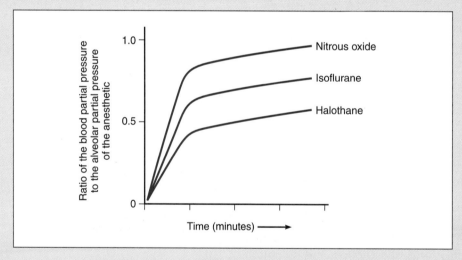

Adjusting the Rate or Depth of Anesthesia

The anesthetic's alveolar concentration and the ventilation rate can be altered by the anesthesiologist to accelerate or slow the rate of induction or recovery, to adjust the depth of anesthesia during surgery, or to maintain tissue oxygenation and eliminate carbon dioxide.

The anesthetic's alveolar concentration after induction is usually about half as high as during induction. In patients undergoing mechanical ventilation, the rate of induction or depth of anesthesia can be adjusted by changing the respiratory rate or tidal volume.

---

anesthetics produce relatively little analgesia or skeletal muscle relaxation, they are often given in combination with nitrous oxide, opioids, muscle relaxants, and other drugs in what is called **balanced anesthesia.**

Halothane is the prototypical halogenated anesthetic, and **desflurane, enflurane, isoflurane,** and **sevoflurane** are newer halogenated anesthetics.

Halothane is the most potent inhalational agent, but it has several disadvantages. Because of its relatively high blood:gas partition coefficient, its rate of induction and recovery is slower than that of other halogenated anesthetics. Because it sensitizes the heart to catecholamines more than other anesthetics do, it places patients at greater risk for cardiac arrhythmias. Hence, the utilization of epinephrine

BOX 25–2. Mechanisms of Action of Inhalational Anesthetics

The potency of an inhalational anesthetic, expressed in terms of the minimum alveolar concentration (MAC), is highly correlated with the lipid solubility (oil:gas partition coefficient) of the anesthetic. This correlation suggests that anesthetics interact with a hydrophobic component of neuronal membranes.

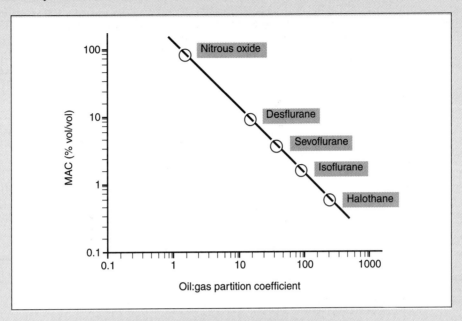

Inhalational anesthetics are believed to bind stereoselectively to hydrophobic regions of neuronal membrane proteins that interface with membrane lipids. The anesthetics potentiate gamma-aminobutyric acid (GABA) activity at the $GABA_A$ chloride ionophore and thereby increase chloride flux through the ionophore. They may also inhibit sodium and calcium influx through membrane channels. These actions hyperpolarize the neuronal membrane and inhibit neuron firing and the release of neurotransmitters.

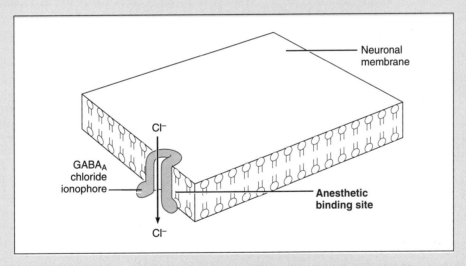

Because of their effects on neuronal membrane proteins, anesthetics disrupt neuronal firing and sensory processing in the thalamus and thereby cause loss of consciousness and analgesia. Anesthetics also inhibit neuronal output from layer V (the internal pyramidal layer) of the cortex, and this reduces motor activity.

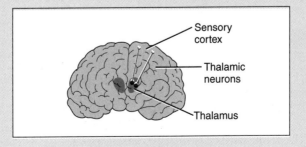

for hemostasis must be strictly limited in patients receiving halothane. Halothane undergoes appreciable metabolism and is converted to substances that may produce a hypersensitivity reaction and hepatitis. For this reason, a patient who is anesthetized with halothane should not be reexposed to it for 6–12 months.

Enflurane and isoflurane exhibit more rapid induction and recovery than halothane exhibits. They undergo less metabolic degradation and produce little cardiac arrhythmia. Enflurane and isoflurane produce more muscle relaxation, so this reduces the need for muscle relaxants during surgery. However, they cause more respiratory depression than the other halogenated drugs cause. At high concentrations, enflurane may produce CNS excitation, leading to seizures.

Desflurane and sevoflurane have a more rapid rate of induction and recovery than other halogenated anesthetics do, but desflurane is irritating to the respiratory tract, so this limits the concentrations of this agent that can be administered during induction. Sevoflurane is close to an ideal anesthetic. It exhibits a rapid and smooth induction and recovery, and it causes little cardiovascular or other organ system toxicity.

Parenteral Anesthetics

The parenteral anesthetics include barbiturates, benzodiazepines, opioids, and other compounds such as propofol. These drugs are used for a variety of purposes, including preanesthetic sedation, induction of anesthesia, perioperative analgesia, and anesthesia for minor surgical and diagnostic procedures. The structures and properties of several parenteral anesthetics are shown in Fig. 25–3B and Table 25–4.

Fentanyl

Fentanyl is a strong opioid agonist that is used for the treatment of moderate to severe pain (see Chapter 23). Because of its potent analgesic properties, it is also administered intravenously or epidurally in combination with other drugs for surgical or

obstetric analgesia and anesthesia. For example, it is frequently used to provide anesthesia during cardiac surgery, such as coronary artery bypass grafting, because it does not tend to cause cardiovascular toxicity. Fentanyl does not produce amnesia or complete loss of consciousness, so it is often combined with a benzodiazepine, such as **diazepam,** to produce amnesia and increased sedation.

Fentanyl has been used in combination with **droperidol,** a neuroleptic drug, to produce a condition called **neuroleptanesthesia.** Droperidol is a butyrophenone compound whose properties are similar to those of haloperidol (see Chapter 22). The advantage of neuroleptanesthesia is that it provides adequate analgesia and sedation during surgery while maintaining a sufficient level of consciousness to permit the patient to respond to questions during the surgical procedure. The disadvantages of neuroleptanesthesia include chest wall rigidity, which is due to the effects of fentanyl and droperidol on the basal ganglia. Fentanyl has a much shorter half-life than does droperidol, and supplemental doses of fentanyl may be needed during long surgical procedures.

Ketamine

Ketamine is chemically and pharmacologically related to phencyclidine (PCP), a street drug that is abused because of its pronounced effects on sensory perception (see Chapter 24). Both ketamine and PCP are thought to act by blocking the N-methyl-D-aspartate (NMDA) receptor for excitatory amino acids such as glutamate. Ketamine produces less sensory distortion and euphoria than does PCP and is therefore more suitable for use as an anesthetic.

When administered intravenously, ketamine produces **dissociative anesthesia,** a mental state in which the individual appears to be dissociated from the environment without complete loss of consciousness. This type of anesthesia is characterized by analgesia, reduced sensory perception, immobility, and amnesia. Unlike many inhalational anesthetics, ketamine usually increases blood pressure, and it has little effect on respiration with typical doses. The main drawback of ketamine is its tendency to cause

TABLE 25–4. Properties of Parenteral Anesthetics*

Drug	Duration of Action (Minutes)	Analgesia	Muscle Relaxation	Other Effects
Fentanyl	5–10 for IV 30–60 for IM	++++	0	Respiratory depression
Ketamine	5–10 for IV 12–25 for IM	+++	0	Postanesthetic delirium and hallucinations
Midazolam	5–20 for IV 20–40 for IM	0	+++	Amnesia
Propofol	5–10 for IV	0	0	Respiratory depression
Thiopental	5–10 for IV	0	0	Respiratory depression

*Values shown are the mean of values reported in the literature. IV = intravenous; and IM = intramuscular. Ratings range from none (0) to high (++++).

unpleasant effects during recovery, including delirium, hallucinations, and irrational behavior. Because children are less likely than adults to experience these adverse effects, ketamine is most often used in pediatric patients and is given in combination with a benzodiazepine for anesthesia during minor surgical or diagnostic procedures.

Midazolam

Midazolam is a short-acting benzodiazepine that is used for preoperative sedation as well as for endoscopy and other diagnostic procedures that do not require a high level of analgesia. Although its onset of action is slower than that of thiopental or propofol, it has the advantage of causing little cardiovascular or respiratory depression. If an overdose of midazolam occurs, the effects of the drug can be reversed by administration of flumazenil, a benzodiazepine antagonist.

Propofol and Thiopental

Propofol is a diisopropyl phenol compound, whereas thiopental is a thiobarbiturate. These drugs potentiate GABA activity at the GABA$_A$ chloride ionophore, and they are primarily used for induction of anesthesia. Their use is followed by the administration of an inhalational anesthetic for maintenance of anesthesia. Both drugs have a rapid onset of action, causing unconsciousness in about 20 seconds. Their duration of action is short (5–10 minutes) because they are redistributed from the brain to the peripheral tissues as their blood concentrations fall. Propofol has the advantages of being rapidly metabolized and eliminated from the body and causing little hangover. Thiopental is accumulated in fat and muscle. It is more slowly eliminated from the body, and some hangover may occur. Either drug may depress cardiovascular and respiratory function.

Summary of Important Points

- Local anesthetics produce use-dependent blockade of nerve conduction and thereby prevent pain associated with surgical and diagnostic procedures. Autonomic and sensory nerves are blocked more easily than are nerves affecting proprioception, muscle tone, and somatic motor activity.
- Local anesthetics are weak bases. The nonionized form permeates neuronal membranes, and the ionized form binds to the internal surface of sodium channels.
- Ester-type anesthetics, such as procaine and chloroprocaine, are converted to *p*-aminobenzoic acid (PABA) and may elicit hypersensitivity reactions.
- Amide-type anesthetics, such as lidocaine and mepivacaine, produce fewer allergic reactions than do ester-type anesthetics.
- All local anesthetics may cause central nervous system and cardiac toxicity, including seizures and cardiac arrhythmias.
- General anesthetics include inhalational agents, such as nitrous oxide and halothane, and parenteral agents, such as ketamine and propofol.
- The potency of inhalational anesthetics is expressed as the minimum alveolar concentration (MAC) required to produce anesthesia. The potency is proportional to the oil:gas partition coefficient.
- The rate of induction of inhalational anesthetics is determined in part by the blood:gas partition coefficient. Nitrous oxide has a low coefficient and a rapid rate of induction. Halothane has a higher coefficient and a slower rate of induction.
- All inhalational anesthetics except nitrous oxide suppress respiratory function and decrease blood pressure in a dose-dependent manner.
- Parenteral anesthetics are used to induce anesthesia and to provide anesthesia during minor surgical and diagnostic procedures. They are also used in combination with other anesthetics during major surgical procedures.

Selected Readings

Boldt, J., et al. Economic considerations of the use of new anesthetics: a comparison of propofol, sevoflurane, desflurane, and isoflurane. Anesth Analg 86:504–509, 1998.

Fee, J. P. Comparative tolerability profiles of the inhaled anesthetics. Drug Saf 16:157–170, 1997.

Gaiser, R. R., et al. Comparison of 0.25% ropivacaine and bupivacaine for epidural analgesia for labor and vaginal delivery. J Clin Anesth 9:564–568, 1997.

Kharasch, E. D. Metabolism and toxicity of the new anesthetic agents. Acta Anaesthesiol Belg 47:7–14, 1996.

Lener, E. V., et al. Topical anesthetic agents in dermatologic surgery: a review. Dermatol Surg 23:673–683, 1997.

Markham, A., and D. Faulds. Ropivacaine: a review of its pharmacology and therapeutic use in regional anesthesia. Drugs 52:429–449, 1996.

Parker, R. I., et al. Efficacy and safety of intravenous midazolam and ketamine as sedation for therapeutic and diagnostic procedures in children. Pediatrics 99:427–431, 1997.

Reinhart, D. J., et al. Outpatient general anesthesia: a comparison of a combination of midazolam plus propofol and propofol alone. J Clin Anesth 9:130–137, 1997.

PHARMACOLOGY OF THE

RESPIRATORY,

GASTROINTESTINAL, AND

OTHER ORGAN SYSTEMS

CHAPTER TWENTY-SIX

AUTACOID DRUGS

CLASSIFICATION OF AUTACOID DRUGS

Histamine H₁ receptor antagonists

First-generation antihistamines
- Chlorpheniramine
- Dimenhydrinate
- Diphenhydramine
- Hydroxyzine
- Meclizine
- Promethazine

Second-generation antihistamines
- Cetirizine
- Fexofenadine
- Loratadine

Intranasal antihistamines
- Azelastine

Serotonin agonists
- Buspirone
- Cisapride
- Sumatriptan

Serotonin antagonists
- Clozapine
- Cyproheptadine
- Methysergide
- Ondansetron

Prostaglandin drugs
- Alprostadil
- Carboprost tromethamine
- Dinoprostone
- Epoprostenol
- Latanoprost
- Misoprostol

OVERVIEW

Autacoids (sometimes called autocoids) are substances that are produced by tissues throughout the body and act locally to modulate the activity of smooth muscles, nerves, glands, platelets, and other tissues (Table 26–1). Several autacoids also serve as neurotransmitters in the central nervous system or enteric nervous system.

Autacoids regulate certain aspects of **gastrointestinal, uterine, and renal function,** and they participate in the development of **pain, fever, inflammation, allergic reactions, asthma, thromboembolic disorders,** and **other pathologic conditions.** Drugs that inhibit autacoid synthesis or block autacoid receptors are helpful in treating these conditions,

while drugs that activate autacoid receptors are useful for inducing labor, alleviating migraine headaches, counteracting drug-induced peptic ulcers, and other purposes.

Autacoids include monoamines, such as **histamine** and **serotonin,** as well as fatty acid derivatives, such as **prostaglandins** and **leukotrienes.** Autacoids activate specific receptors in target tissues. Their effects are usually restricted to the tissue in which they are formed, but extraordinarily large amounts of them may be released into the circulation in certain disorders, such as carcinoid tumor and anaphylactic shock, and thereby exert a systemic effect. Most autacoids are rapidly metabolized to inactive compounds, and some autacoids undergo tissue reuptake.

The purpose of this chapter is to provide basic information about autacoids and review the many types of drugs that influence their effects. Readers are referred to other chapters for more details about these drugs.

HISTAMINE AND RELATED DRUGS
Histamine

Histamine is produced primarily by mast cells and basophils, which are particularly abundant in the skin, gastrointestinal tract, and respiratory tract. Histamine is also produced by paracrine cells in the gastric fundus, where it stimulates acid secretion by parietal cells. Histamine functions as a neurotransmitter in the central nervous system.

Histamine Biosynthesis and Release

Histamine is formed when the amino acid **histidine** is decarboxylated in a reaction catalyzed by L-histidine decarboxylase. Histamine is stored in granules (vesicles) in mast cells and basophils until it is released. It is released from mast cells when membrane-bound **immunoglobulin E (IgE)** interacts with an IgE antigen to cause mast cell degranulation. This process can be blocked by **cromolyn sodium** and related drugs, as described in Chapter 27.

Mast cell degranulation can be triggered by bacterial toxins and by drugs such as **morphine** and **tubocurarine.** These stimuli activate receptors that are coupled with the formation of inositol triphosphate (IP₃) and diacylglycerol (DAG). This causes the release of intracellular calcium and the fusion of

TABLE 26–1. Effects of Autacoids

Autacoid	Effects on Vascular Smooth Muscle (VSM)	Effects on Nonvascular Smooth Muscle (NVSM)	Other Effects
Histamine	Vasodilation and edema.	Contraction of bronchial and other NVSM.	Itching; increase in gastric acid secretion.
Serotonin	Vasoconstriction in most vascular beds.	Contraction of gastrointestinal and other NVSM.	Central nervous system neurotransmission; stimulation of platelet aggregation.
Eicosanoids			
Leukotrienes	Vasoconstriction or vasodilation.	Contraction of bronchial and other NVSM.	Inflammatory effects; increase in vascular permeability.
Prostaglandin E	Vasodilation.	Relaxation of bronchial muscle and contraction of uterine muscle.	Inhibition of gastric acid secretion.
Prostaglandin F	Vasoconstriction in most vascular beds.	Contraction of bronchial and uterine muscle.	Increase in aqueous humor outflow.
Prostaglandin I	Vasodilation.	Contraction.	Inhibition of platelet aggregation.
Thromboxane A_2	Vasoconstriction.	Contraction.	Stimulation of platelet aggregation.

granule membranes with the plasma membrane, thereby releasing histamine and other compounds.

Histamine is inactivated by methylation and oxidation reactions that are catalyzed by a methyltransferase enzyme and diamine oxidase, respectively.

Histamine Receptors and Effects

Histamine receptors have been classified as H_1, H_2, and H_3.

H_1 receptors are involved in allergic reactions that cause **dermatitis, rhinitis, conjunctivitis,** and **other forms of allergy.** Activation of H_1 receptors in the skin and mucous membranes causes vasodilation, increases vascular permeability, and leads to erythema, congestion, edema, and inflammation. Stimulation of H_1 receptors on mucocutaneous nerve endings may cause pruritus (itching) and initiate the cough reflex. If sufficient histamine is released into the circulation, it may reduce blood pressure and lead to **anaphylactic shock.** Activation of H_1 receptors also causes bronchoconstriction and contraction of most gastrointestinal smooth muscles.

H_2 receptors are primarily concerned with **gastric acid secretion,** but they are also involved in **allergic reactions.** For this reason, H_2 receptor antagonists are sometimes used in combination with H_1 receptor antagonists in the treatment of allergy. Activation of H_2 receptors in the heart increases the heart rate and contractility, but the cardiac effects of histamine are not prominent under most conditions.

H_3 receptors are presynaptic receptors located on nerve terminals. Activation of these receptors inhibits the release of histamine and other neurotransmitters.

Antihistamines

Antihistamines, or **histamine receptor antagonists,** have been categorized on the basis of their receptor selectivity as H_1 receptor antagonists and H_2 receptor antagonists.

Histamine H_1 Receptor Antagonists

Classification. The following discussion focuses on the properties and uses of three groups of H_1 receptor antagonists. **Chlorpheniramine, dimenhydrinate, diphenhydramine, hydroxyzine, meclizine,** and **promethazine** are examples of first-generation drugs. **Astemizole, cetirizine, fexofenadine, loratadine,** and **terfenadine** are examples of second-generation drugs.* Drugs in these two groups are administered orally or parenterally. A major difference in the two groups is that the **first-generation antihistamines** are distributed to the central nervous system and may cause sedation, whereas the **second-generation antihistamines** do not cross the blood-brain barrier significantly. **Azelastine** is an example of an **intranasal antihistamine.**

Chemistry, Mechanisms, and Pharmacokinetics. The H_1 antihistamines contain an alkylamine group that resembles the side chain of histamine and permits them to bind to the H_1 receptor and act as competitive receptor antagonists. The drugs are able to block most of the effects of histamine on vascular smooth muscle and nerves and thereby prevent or counteract allergic reactions.

The structures of selected first- and second-generation drugs are shown in Fig. 26–1. When drugs in these groups are administered orally, they are rapidly absorbed and are widely distributed to tissues. Many of them are extensively metabolized in the liver by cytochrome P450 enzymes. Hydroxyzine and terfenadine have active metabolites that are themselves available as drugs (as cetirizine and fexofenadine, respectively), and these two drugs are excreted unchanged in the urine and feces.

Azelastine is a phthalazinone H_1 antihistamine that is marketed as a nasal spray for the treatment of allergic rhinitis. It blocks H_1 receptors and inhibits the release of histamine from mast cells, and it is

---

* Astemizole and terfenadine were withdrawn from the market in mid-1999. Their adverse effects and interactions are discussed in the text.

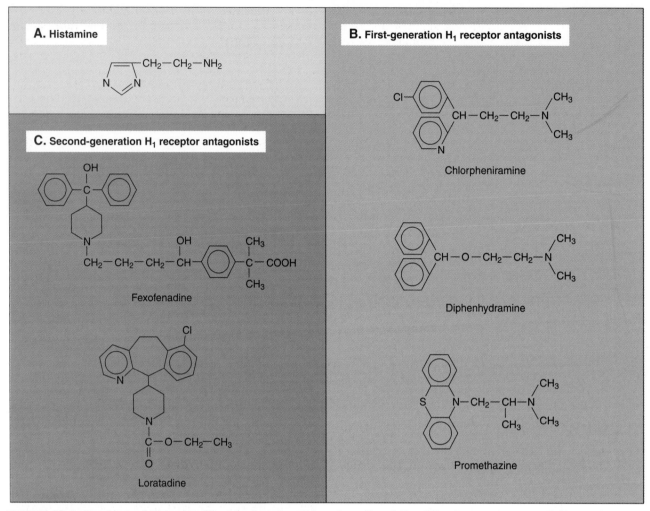

FIGURE 26–1. Structures of histamine (A) and selected antihistamines (B and C). Chlorpheniramine is an alkylamine derivative, diphenhydramine is an ethanolamine derivative, and promethazine is a phenothiazine derivative. Fexofenadine and loratadine are both piperidine derivatives.

much more potent than either sodium cromoglycate or theophylline in its inhibiting effect. The systemic bioavailability of azelastine following intranasal administration is about 40%, and the plasma half-life is about 22 hours. Azelastine is metabolized by cytochrome P450 enzymes to desmethylazelastine, a substance whose plasma concentrations are 20–30% of azelastine concentrations. Azelastine and its principal metabolite both act as antagonists at H_1 receptors. The unchanged drug and its active metabolite are primarily excreted in the feces.

Pharmacologic Effects and Indications. The H_1 antihistamines are all equally effective in treating **allergies,** but they differ markedly in their sedative, antiemetic, and anticholinergic properties (Table 26–2). The second-generation antihistamines cause little or no sedation, so they are often preferred for the treatment of allergies. Antihistamines are usually more effective when administered before exposure to an allergen than afterward. Hence, persons with seasonal allergies, such as allergic rhinitis (see Chapter 27), should take them on a regular basis throughout the period of risk.

(1) First-Generation Antihistamines. Because the first-generation antihistamines have sedative effects, they are occasionally used to produce **sedation.** They are also used to treat **nausea and vomiting,** to prevent **motion sickness** in persons traveling by plane or boat, or to treat **vertigo** (an illusory sense that the environment or one's own body is revolving).

The most sedating drugs are diphenhydramine, hydroxyzine, and promethazine. These drugs have been used for inducing sleep or for preoperative sedation. Their sedating properties may also be useful in relieving distress caused by the severe pruritus associated with some allergic reactions. Persons taking these drugs should be cautioned against driving or operating dangerous machinery.

Pheniramine drugs, such as chlorpheniramine, are less sedating than other first-generation drugs and are primarily used in the treatment of allergic reactions to pollen, mold spores, and other environmental allergens.

Meclizine, diphenhydramine, hydroxyzine, and promethazine have higher antiemetic activity than other antihistamines. Meclizine is somewhat less sedating than hydroxyzine and promethazine, so it is frequently used to prevent motion sickness or treat vertigo. Dimenhydrinate, which is a mixture of diphenhydramine and 8-chlorotheophylline, is also used for these purposes. Promethazine suppositories are often used to relieve nausea and vomiting associated with various conditions (see Chapter 28).

(2) Second-Generation Antihistamines. The second-generation drugs lack antiemetic activity, so their use is limited to the treatment of **allergies.** None of these drugs causes substantial sedation; however, cetirizine is more likely than astemizole, fexofenadine, or loratadine to cause some sedation. Because fexofenadine has a shorter half-life, it must be taken twice a day, whereas the other second-generation drugs are taken once a day. Fexofenadine and cetirizine are eliminated primarily as the unchanged drug in the feces and urine, respectively. Loratadine is metabolized to an active metabolite, which is excreted in the urine and feces.

(3) Intranasal Antihistamines. Azelastine is indicated for the treatment of symptoms of **allergic rhinitis,** including sneezing, nasal itching, and nasal discharge. It is administered as two sprays per nostril twice daily. The drug can cause drowsiness so should be used cautiously when patients are driving or operating dangerous machinery.

Adverse Effects and Interactions. The H_1 antihistamines produce few serious side effects.

(1) First-Generation Antihistamines. Sedation is the most common side effect of the first-generation antihistamines. Paradoxically, however, the drugs can produce excitement in infants and children and should be used with caution in these patients.

Diphenhydramine and promethazine have the highest anticholinergic activity (see Table 26–2), but other first-generation drugs also block cholinergic muscarinic receptors. As a result, the drugs may cause dry mouth, blurred vision, tachycardia, urinary retention, and other atropine-like side effects.

Anticholinergic toxicity is the principal manifestation of an overdose of first-generation antihistamines. Administration of physostigmine, a cholinesterase inhibitor that crosses the blood-brain barrier, may be required to counteract the anticholinergic effects of antihistamines in the central nervous system.

(2) Second-Generation Antihistamines. Two of the second-generation drugs, astemizole and terfenadine, may prolong the QT interval on the electrocardiogram and thereby precipitate a cardiac arrhythmia called torsade de pointes. Drugs that inhibit terfenadine metabolism, such as erythromycin and itraconazole, may elevate terfenadine levels and thereby precipitate this arrhythmia. Fexofenadine, the active metabolite of terfenadine, does not affect cardiac electrophysiology or cause arrhythmia. For this reason, it has largely replaced terfenadine in clinical use. Cetirizine and loratadine also lack cardiac effects.

(3) Intranasal Antihistamines. Adverse effects of azelastine include dizziness, fatigue, headache, nasal irritation, dry mouth, and weight gain.

Histamine H_2 Receptor Antagonists

Chapter 28 outlines the properties of H_2 receptor antagonists, which are primarily used to treat **peptic ulcer disease.**

SEROTONIN AND RELATED DRUGS
Serotonin

Serotonin, or **5-hydroxytryptamine** (5-HT), is an autacoid and neurotransmitter that is produced primarily by platelets, enterochromaffin cells in the gut, and neurons. As illustrated in Fig. 18–3C, serotonin is synthesized from the amino acid **tryptophan** and is converted to **5-hydroxyindoleacetic acid** (5-HIAA) by monoamine oxidase and aldehyde dehydrogenase. 5-HIAA is then excreted in the urine.

In the peripheral tissues, the physiologic effects of serotonin include platelet aggregation, stimulation of gastrointestinal motility, and modulation of vascu-

TABLE 26–2. **Pharmacologic Properties of Histamine H_1 Receptor Antagonists**

Drug	Duration of Action (Hours)	Sedative Effects	Antiemetic Effects	Anticholinergic Effects
First-generation antihistamines				
Chlorpheniramine	6	Medium	None	Medium
Dimenhydrinate	8	High	Medium	High
Diphenhydramine	8	High	Medium	High
Hydroxyzine	6	High	High	Medium
Meclizine	12	Medium	High	Medium
Promethazine	12	High	High	High
Second-generation antihistamines				
Cetirizine	24	Low	None	Very low
Fexofenadine	12	Very low	None	Very low
Loratadine	24	Very low	None	Very low
Intranasal antihistamines				
Azelastine	12	Low	None	Very low

lar smooth muscle contraction. Serotonin causes vasoconstriction in most vascular beds and contraction of most smooth muscles. In the central nervous system, serotonin is involved in the regulation of mood, appetite, sleep, emotional processing, and pain processing (see Chapter 18).

The four main types of **serotonin receptors** are designated as 5-HT$_1$ through 5-HT$_4$. The 5-HT$_1$ and 5-HT$_2$ receptors have several subtypes that are designated by letters (for example, 5-HT$_{1A}$ and 5-HT$_{1D}$). Although most serotonin receptors are G protein–coupled receptors, the 5-HT$_3$ receptor is a ligand-gated cation channel. The mechanisms of signal transduction for serotonin receptors are outlined in Table 18–1.

Drugs that affect serotonin activity are classified as serotonin agonists, serotonin antagonists, and serotonin reuptake inhibitors. Examples are mentioned below and discussed in detail in other chapters.

Serotonin Agonists

Serotonin agonists have been developed for use in the management of several specific disorders (Table 26–3). **Buspirone** is a partial agonist that acts at the 5-HT$_{1A}$ receptor and is used to treat **anxiety** and **depression** (see Chapter 19). **Cisapride** is a 5-HT$_4$ receptor agonist. Because it increases gastrointestinal muscle tone and motility, it can be used to treat **gastroesophageal reflux disease** and **gastrointestinal hypomotility** (see Chapter 28). **Sumatriptan** and related compounds, as well as several ergot alkaloids, are 5-HT$_{1D/1B}$ receptor agonists that are used to treat **migraine headaches** (see Chapter 29).

Serotonin Antagonists

Examples of serotonin antagonists include clozapine, cyproheptadine, methysergide, and ondansetron (see Table 26–3).

Clozapine is an atypical antipsychotic drug that acts partly by blocking 5-HT$_2$ receptors in the central nervous system. It is used in the treatment of **schizophrenia** (see Chapter 22).

Cyproheptadine is a 5-HT$_2$ receptor antagonist that also has H$_1$ antihistamine activity. This makes it useful in managing **urticaria** (hives) and other allergic reactions in which **pruritus** is a prominent feature. Cyproheptadine is administered orally every 8–12 hours and may cause slight to moderate drowsiness.

Methysergide is a 5-HT$_2$ receptor antagonist that is used to prevent **migraine headaches** (see Chapter 29).

Cyproheptadine and **methysergide** are both useful in the care of patients with **carcinoid tumor.** This tumor can produce huge quantities of serotonin, histamine, and other vasoactive substances that cause a constellation of clinical effects called the **carcinoid syndrome.** Affected patients suffer from malabsorption, violent attacks of watery diarrhea and cramping, and paroxysmal vasomotor attacks characterized by sudden red to purple flushing of the face and neck. The malabsorption and diarrhea can

TABLE 26–3. Serotonin (5-Hydroxytryptamine, or 5-HT) Receptors and Clinical Uses of Serotonin Agonists and Antagonists

Drug	5-HT Receptor	Clinical Use
Serotonin agonists		
Buspirone	5-HT$_{1A}$	Anxiety; depression.
Cisapride	5-HT$_4$	Gastroesophageal reflux disease; gastrointestinal hypomotility.
Sumatriptan	5-HT$_{1D/1B}$	Migraine headaches.
Serotonin antagonists		
Clozapine	5-HT$_2$	Schizophrenia.
Cyproheptadine	5-HT$_2$	Carcinoid syndrome; pruritus; urticaria.
Methysergide	5-HT$_2$	Carcinoid syndrome; migraine headaches.
Ondansetron	5-HT$_3$	Nausea and vomiting.

be managed by giving cyproheptadine or methysergide in combination with opioid antidiarrheal drugs.

Ondansetron and closely related compounds are selective 5-HT$_3$ receptor antagonists that are used as antiemetics. They prevent **nausea and vomiting** by blocking the effects of serotonin in the chemoreceptor trigger zone and in vagal afferent nerves in the gastrointestinal tract (see Chapter 28).

Serotonin Reuptake Inhibitors

Serotonin reuptake inhibitors are used in the treatment of **depression** and **other central nervous system disorders** (see Chapter 22).

EICOSANOIDS AND RELATED DRUGS
Eicosanoids

Eicosanoids are autacoids derived from arachidonic acid (eicosatetraenoic acid) and other 20-carbon fatty acids. These fatty acids are released from cell membrane phospholipids by **phospholipase A$_2$,** an enzyme that can be activated by chemical stimuli and by physical stimuli such as injuries.

Eicosanoid Biosynthesis and Classification

The two main groups of eicosanoids are the **prostaglandins** and the **leukotrienes,** whose formation begins with reactions catalyzed by **cyclooxygenase** and **5-lipoxygenase,** respectively. As shown in Fig. 26–2, subsequent reactions convert the products of these reactions to specific prostaglandins and leukotrienes.

Each prostaglandin and each leukotriene is assigned a letter and subscript number (for example, E$_1$). The letter refers to the specific ring structure of the substance, and the subscript number indicates the number of double bonds in the side chains.

Prostaglandins derived from arachidonic acid, an **omega-6 fatty acid,** have two double bonds; this is the case with prostaglandin E$_2$ (PGE$_2$) and prostaglandin I_2 (PGI$_2$, or prostacyclin). Prostaglandins derived from an **omega-3 fatty acid** have either 1 or 3 double bonds; this is the case with homo-γ-linolenic acid and eicosapentaenoic acid, which have 1 bond and 3 bonds, respectively. Prostaglandins derived from omega-6 fatty acids have different vasoactive and platelet-aggregating properties than do prostaglandins derived from omega-3 fatty acids.

Eicosanoid Receptors and Effects

Prostaglandins exert their effects on smooth muscle, platelet aggregation, neurotransmission, glandular secretion, and other biologic activities by activating specific receptors in target tissues. **Thromboxanes,** which are substances derived from prostaglandins (see Fig. 26–2), also act on smooth muscle and platelet aggregation. Different types of thromboxanes and prostaglandins have different physiologic effects.

While **platelet aggregation** is stimulated by thromboxane A$_2$ (TXA$_2$), it is inhibited by PGI$_2$. This particular prostaglandin is released primarily from vascular endothelial cells and serves to prevent platelet aggregation under normal conditions. In contrast, TXA$_2$ is produced and released only when a blood vessel is injured, at which time the adherence of platelets to vascular endothelium activates the platelets and leads to the synthesis and release of TXA$_2$ (see Chapter 16 and Fig. 16–5).

In some cases, the fatty acid precursor of a prostaglandin or thromboxane has a major impact on its biologic activity. For example, thromboxane A$_3$ (TXA$_3$), which is synthesized from eicosapentaenoic acid and other omega-3 fatty acids obtained from fish oils, produces relatively little platelet aggregation or vasoconstriction in comparison with TXA$_2$. This difference may partly explain the benefits of increased fish oil consumption on the incidence of thrombotic events in patients with certain diseases.

PGE$_2$ and PGI$_2$ both cause **vasodilation** in several vascular beds. These prostaglandins appear to play a role in maintaining **pulmonary blood flow,** and they also serve to maintain the **patency of the ductus arteriosus** until it is time for its closure. In the kidneys, PGE$_2$ and PGI$_2$ produce vasodilation and have important roles in modulating **renal blood flow** and **glomerular filtration.** These actions are particularly important in persons with renal insufficiency and in the elderly. The renal actions of prostaglandins also appear to exert an **antihypertensive effect,** partly by increasing water and sodium excretion. Because nonsteroidal anti-inflammatory drugs (NSAIDs) inhibit prostaglandin synthesis, their use can cause or exacerbate renal disorders and may counteract the antihypertensive effect of antihypertensive medications taken concurrently.

Many prostaglandins, including PGE$_2$ and prostaglandin F$_{2\alpha}$ (PGF$_{2\alpha}$), stimulate **uterine contractions** and increase **gastrointestinal motility.** Their uterine activity is the basis for several therapeutic applications, whereas their gastrointestinal actions may lead to adverse effects such as diarrhea and intestinal cramping. Several prostaglandins also produce a **cytoprotective effect on the gastrointestinal mucosa.**

The leukotrienes are produced primarily in inflammatory cells, including mast cells, basophils, eosinophils, macrophages, and polymorphonuclear leukocytes. Leukotrienes C$_4$ and D$_4$ (LTC$_4$ and LTD$_4$) are the main components of the **slow-reacting sub-**

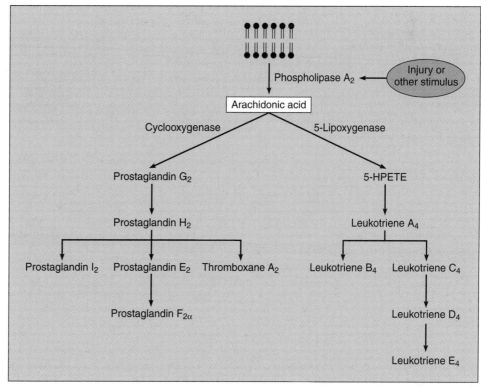

FIGURE 26–2. Synthesis of eicosanoids. When phospholipase A$_2$ is activated by an injury or other stimulus, it catalyzes the hydrolysis of arachidonic acid and other 20-carbon fatty acids from cell membrane phospholipids. Arachidonic acid is converted to prostaglandins and leukotrienes by cyclooxygenase and 5-lipoxygenase, respectively. Other enzymes complete the synthesis of specific eicosanoids. 5-HPETE = 5-hydroperoxyeicosatetraenoic acid.

stance of anaphylaxis (SRS-A). These two leukotrienes are secreted in the presence of asthma and anaphylaxis and play a major role in bronchospastic disease.

Prostaglandin Drugs

The effects and clinical uses of prostaglandin drugs are outlined in Table 26–4.

Prostaglandin E₁ Derivatives

Alprostadil is identical to PGE_1 and is available in several formulations for specific clinical uses.

Alprostadil is given by continuous intravenous infusion for maintenance of the **patency of the ductus arteriosus** in neonates who are awaiting surgery for some types of congenital heart diseases. These include cyanotic heart defects (pulmonary atresia or stenosis, tricuspid atresia, tetralogy of Fallot, and transposition of the great vessels) and acyanotic heart defects (coarctation of the aorta and hypoplastic left ventricle).

Alprostadil is available in injectable and pellet formulations for the treatment of **erectile dysfunction** in men. For this purpose, the drug is injected into the penis or pellets are implanted in the urethra. Adverse effects in men treated with alprostadil include penile pain, penile fibrosis, flushing, diarrhea, headache, and fever.

Misoprostol is a PGE_1 analogue that is available in an orally administered formulation for the prevention of NSAID-induced **gastric ulcers** and **duodenal ulcers** (see Chapter 28). Misoprostol treatment is particularly useful in patients who take NSAIDs on a long-term basis to alleviate the symptoms of arthritis and other inflammatory conditions. Misoprostol acts locally on the gastrointestinal mucosa to exert a cytoprotective effect by inhibiting gastric acid secretion and by increasing bicarbonate secretion from mucosal cells. Diarrhea, one of the most common adverse effects of misoprostol use, can be minimized by starting patients on a low dose of the drug and then gradually increasing the dose. In pregnant women, misoprostol is absolutely contraindicated because it may stimulate uterine contractions and cause premature labor.

Prostaglandin E₂ and F₂ₐ Derivatives

Dinoprostone and **carboprost tromethamine** are prostaglandin derivatives that have oxytocic activity and increase the uterine contractions of pregnant women. Dinoprostone is a formulation of PGE_2, whereas carboprost is an analogue of $PGF_{2\alpha}$.

Dinoprostone is available as a vaginal insert, gel, or suppository. In pregnant women, the vaginal insert or gel is applied to the vagina or cervix to produce **cervical ripening** prior to labor induction. The insert may provide more accurate dosing than the gel. The suppository is used for **evacuation of the uterine contents** in cases of intrauterine fetal death, benign hydatidiform mole, or second-trimester termination of pregnancy.

Carboprost is administered intramuscularly for the **control of postpartum bleeding** when other measures have failed and for the **termination of pregnancy.** It may cause flushing, diarrhea, vomiting, altered blood pressure, blurred vision, respiratory distress, and other adverse reactions.

Latanoprost is the first and only prostaglandin indicated for the treatment of **glaucoma.** It is administered topically as eye drops and is used to treat open-angle glaucoma that is resistant to other pharmacologic treatments. Latanoprost is a $PGF_{2\alpha}$ analogue that acts by increasing aqueous humor outflow via the uveoscleral pathway (see Box 6–1). It may alter the color of the iris and cause a permanent eye color change by increasing the amount of melanin in melanocytes.

Prostaglandin I₂ Derivatives

Epoprostenol is a PGI_2 (prostacyclin) derivative that is used to treat **pulmonary hypertension.** Epoprostenol dilates pulmonary blood vessels and increases pulmonary blood flow, thereby counteracting the pathophysiologic consequences of pulmonary hypertension. The drug is administered by continuous intravenous infusion, and the dosage is titrated on the basis of clinical improvement and adverse effects. The most common adverse reactions include flushing, tachycardia, hypotension, diarrhea, nausea, vomiting, and flu-like symptoms.

TABLE 26–4.   Effects and Clinical Uses of Prostaglandin (PG) Drugs

Drug	PG Class	Effect	Clinical Use
Alprostadil	PGE_1	Vasodilation.	Erectile dysfunction; patency of the ductus arteriosus.
Carboprost tromethamine	$PGF_{2\alpha}$ analogue	Contraction of uterine muscle.	Abortifacient; postpartum bleeding.
Dinoprostone	PGE_2	Contraction of uterine muscle.	Abortifacient; cervical ripening.
Epoprostenol	PGI_2	Vasodilation.	Pulmonary hypertension.
Latanoprost	$PGF_{2\alpha}$ analogue	Increase in aqueous humor outflow.	Glaucoma.
Misoprostol	PGE_1 analogue	Gastric cytoprotection.	Gastric and duodenal ulcers induced by use of nonsteroidal anti-inflammatory drugs (NSAIDs).

Eicosanoid Inhibitors

Among the groups of drugs that inhibit eicosanoid synthesis are **leukotriene inhibitors** (see Chapter 27), **NSAIDs** (see Chapter 30), and **corticosteroids** (see Chapter 33).

Leukotriene inhibitors act either by inhibiting 5-lipoxygenase or by blocking leukotriene receptors. They are currently used in the management of **asthma,** but other therapeutic applications are being explored.

NSAIDs act by inhibiting cyclooxygenase and are primarily used to alleviate **pain** and **inflammation.**

Corticosteroids block the formation of all eicosanoids, partly by inhibiting phospholipase A_2. They have **anti-inflammatory, antiallergic, and antineoplastic effects** and are used in the treatment of a wide variety of adrenal diseases and nonadrenal disorders.

Summary of Important Points

- Autacoids include histamine, serotonin, prostaglandins, and leukotrienes. These substances usually act on the same tissue in which they are produced.
- Histamine is the primary mediator of allergic reactions. Stimulation of H_1 receptors causes vasodilation, edema, congestion, and pruritus. Stimulation of H_2 receptors mediates gastric acid secretion.
- The first-generation H_1 receptor antagonists (chlorpheniramine, diphenhydramine, meclizine, promethazine, and others) produce varying degrees of sedation and also have anticholinergic side effects. The second-generation drugs (astemizole, cetirizine, loratadine, fexofenadine, and terfenadine) are largely devoid of central nervous system effects.
- The H_1 receptor antagonists are primarily used to treat allergies, but meclizine is used to prevent motion sickness and promethazine is used to treat nausea and vomiting.
- Fexofenadine is the active metabolite of terfenadine. Unlike terfenadine, fexofenadine does not prolong the QT interval and cause torsade de pointes. Cetirizine and loratadine also lack cardiac effects.
- Drugs that affect serotonin (5-hydroxytryptamine, or 5-HT) are classified as serotonin agonists, serotonin antagonists, and serotonin reuptake inhibitors.
- Some 5-HT_1 receptor agonists (such as sumatriptan) can be used to treat migraine headaches, whereas some 5-HT_2 receptor antagonists (such as methysergide) can be used to prevent migraine headaches.
- Cyproheptadine and methysergide, both of which are 5-HT_2 receptor antagonists, are used in the management of carcinoid syndrome, which is caused by excessive production of serotonin and other vasoactive substances in patients with carcinoid tumors.
- Cisapride is a 5-HT_4 receptor agonist that is used to increase gastrointestinal motility, and ondansetron is a 5-HT_3 receptor antagonist that is used in the treatment of nausea and vomiting.
- Eicosanoids are derived from arachidonic acid and other 20-carbon fatty acids. The two main groups of eicosanoids are prostaglandins and leukotrienes.
- Alprostadil and misoprostol are prostaglandin E_1 (PGE_1) derivatives. Alprostadil is used to maintain patency of the ductus arteriosus in neonates awaiting surgery for heart defects. It is also used to treat erectile dysfunction in men. Misoprostol is used to prevent gastric and duodenal ulcers in persons taking nonsteroidal anti-inflammatory drugs (NSAIDs).
- Dinoprostone is a prostaglandin E_2 (PGE_2) derivative used for cervical ripening prior to induction of labor and for evacuation of the uterine contents.
- Carboprost and latanoprost are prostaglandin $F_{2\alpha}$ ($PGF_{2\alpha}$) derivatives. Carboprost is used to control postpartum bleeding and to terminate pregnancy. Latanoprost increases the aqueous humor outflow and is used to treat glaucoma.
- Epoprostenol is a prostaglandin I_2 (PGI_2, or prostacyclin) derivative used to treat pulmonary hypertension.

Selected Readings

Graudins, A., et al. Treatment of the serotonin syndrome with cyproheptadine. J Emerg Med 16:615–619, 1998.

Jaanus, S. D. Oral and topical antihistamines: pharmacologic properties and therapeutic potential in ocular allergic disease. J Am Optom Assoc 69:77–87, 1998.

Lea, A. P., et al. Intracavernous alprostadil: a review of its pharmacodynamic and pharmacokinetic properties and therapeutic potential in erectile dysfunction. Drugs Aging 8:56–74, 1996.

Nicholson, A. N., and C. Turner. Central effects of an H_1 antihistamine, cetirizine. Aviat Space Environ Med 69:166–171, 1998.

Simons, F. E., and K. J. Simons. Peripheral H_1 blockade effect of fexofenadine. Ann Allergy Immunol 79:530–532, 1997.

Wood-Baker, R., et al. Histamine and the nasal vasculature: the influence of H_1 and H_2 histamine receptor antagonism. Clin Otolaryngol Appl Sci 21:348–352, 1996.

CHAPTER TWENTY-SEVEN

DRUGS FOR RESPIRATORY

TRACT DISORDERS

CLASSIFICATION OF DRUGS FOR RESPIRATORY TRACT DISORDERS

ANTI-INFLAMMATORY DRUGS
Glucocorticoids
- Beclomethasone
- Fluticasone
- Triamcinolone

Mast cell stabilizers
- Cromolyn sodium
- Lodoxamide
- Nedocromil

Leukotriene inhibitors
- Montelukast
- Zafirlukast
- Zileuton

BRONCHODILATORS
Selective β₂-adrenergic receptor agonists
- Albuterol
- Pirbuterol
- Salmeterol
- Terbutaline

Other bronchodilators
- Ipratropium
- Theophylline

ANTITUSSIVES
- Codeine
- Dextromethorphan
- Hydrocodone

EXPECTORANTS
- Guaifenesin

OVERVIEW

Disorders of the respiratory tract include asthma, chronic obstructive pulmonary disease (COPD), and other restrictive diseases of the airways; allergic rhinitis, viral rhinitis, and other upper or lower respiratory tract infections and diseases; and lung cancer. This chapter is primarily concerned with the drugs used in the treatment of asthma and rhinitis. The therapy of both of these conditions rests on a foundation of environmental control and preventive anti-inflammatory medication, with other drugs being used chiefly to treat acute exacerbations.

Asthma

Asthma is characterized by airway inflammation and hyperresponsiveness to stimuli that produce bronchoconstriction. These stimuli include **cold air, exercise,** a wide variety of **allergens,** and **emotional stress.**

Exposure to a stimulus triggers the release of various mediators from mast cells, eosinophils, basophils, neutrophils, macrophages, and other cells. Preformed mediators are stored in cell granules and include **histamine, adenosine, bradykinin,** and **major basic protein,** whereas lipid mediators are formed from arachidonic acid and include **leukotrienes** and **prostaglandins.** The release of these agents causes inflammation of the airway, edema and desquamation of the bronchial epithelium, and hypertrophy of smooth muscles in the respiratory tract. It also increases the responsiveness of smooth muscles and the permeability of bronchioles to allergens, infectious agents, mediators of inflammation, and other irritants. Increased mucus production then leads to mucus plugging and decreases the ability of the airways to remove these irritants. As a result, patients suffer from airway obstruction and must use accessory muscles to breathe.

Airway obstruction results from a combination of bronchial inflammation, smooth muscle constriction, and obstruction of the lumen with mucus, inflammatory cells, and epithelial debris. Symptoms of obstruction include dyspnea (difficulty in breathing), coughing, wheezing, headache, tachycardia, syncope, diaphoresis, pallor, and cyanosis. Patients experience a **biphasic reduction in pulmonary function,** with an **early phase** that occurs within 10–30 minutes of exposure to an allergen and lasts for 2–3 hours and with a **later phase** that occurs 2–8 hours after exposure. The late phase is believed to be responsible for inducing and maintaining bronchial hyperreactivity in asthmatic patients. Because of the circadian variation in bronchial responsiveness, some patients have up to an eightfold increase in airway hyperresponsiveness at night, and nearly 70% of asthma-related deaths occur at night.

The drugs used to treat asthma include anti-inflammatory drugs and bronchodilators. The pathophysiology of asthma and sites of anti-inflammatory drug action are shown in Fig. 27–1.

Rhinitis

Rhinitis is most frequently caused by allergic reactions to **pollens, mold spores, dust mites,** and **other environmental allergens** or by infections with **viruses,** such as rhinoviruses and other agents of the common cold.

Allergic rhinitis may be seasonal or nonseasonal (perennial), while **viral rhinitis** is an acute, self-limiting condition. Both types of rhinitis are characterized by sneezing, nasal congestion, and rhinorrhea. Nasal pruritus and conjunctivitis are more commonly associated with allergic rhinitis than with viral rhinitis. Malaise, pain, and general discomfort are generally associated with viral rhinitis.

Table 27–1 shows the relative efficacy of various types of respiratory tract drugs, including those used in the treatment of allergic rhinitis and viral rhinitis.

ANTI-INFLAMMATORY DRUGS
Glucocorticoids

Glucocorticoids are effective in the treatment of a wide variety of diseases and are available for oral, parenteral, topical, and inhalational administration. The discussion here focuses on the use of inhaled

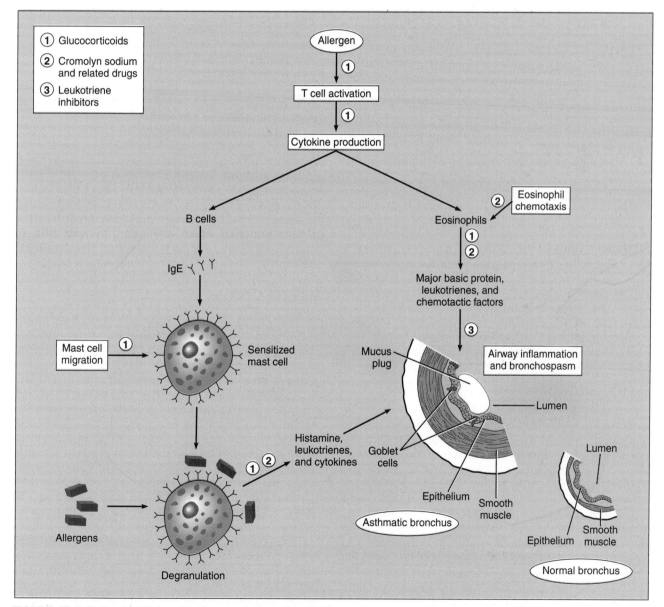

FIGURE 27–1. Pathophysiology of asthma and sites of anti-inflammatory drug action. When allergens activate T cells, cytokine production is stimulated. The cytokines in turn trigger the recruitment, activation, and release of a variety of cells and mediators. Glucocorticoids inhibit numerous steps in this process, including T cell activation, cytokine production, eosinophil recruitment and activation, and mast cell migration. Glucocorticoids, cromolyn sodium, and other cromolyn-related drugs all inhibit the release of mediators from mast cells and eosinophils. Cromolyn and related drugs also inhibit eosinophil chemotaxis induced by cytokines and other mediators. Leukotriene inhibitors either block leukotriene receptors or inhibit leukotriene synthesis. IgE = immunoglobulin E.

TABLE 27–1. Relative Efficacy of Anti-inflammatory Drugs, Bronchodilators, and Miscellaneous Agents in the Management of Respiratory Tract Disorders*

Drug	Asthma	COPD	Allergic Rhinitis	Viral Rhinitis
Anti-inflammatory drugs				
Glucocorticoids	++++	0 to ++	++++	0
Mast cell stabilizers	+++	0 to ++	+++	0
Leukotriene inhibitors	+++	0 to +	Unknown	0
Bronchodilators				
Selective β₂-adrenergic receptor agonists	++++	++	0	0
Other bronchodilators				
Ipratropium	+	+++	++	++
Theophylline	++ to +++	++ to +++	0	0
Miscellaneous agents				
Analgesics	0	0	0	+++
Antihistamines	0 to ++	0	++++	+
Decongestants	0 to ++	0 to ++	+++	+++

*COPD = chronic obstructive pulmonary disease, such as emphysema. Ratings range from 0 (not efficacious) to ++++ (highly efficacious).

glucocorticoids for **asthma** and **allergic rhinitis.** Chapter 33 provides a detailed description of drug properties and discusses other indications for glucocorticoid use.

The recognition that asthma is primarily an inflammatory disease has increased the role of glucocorticoids in asthma therapy over the past decade. For persons with moderate to severe asthma, glucocorticoids have become the cornerstone of therapy, and some patients with mild asthma may derive significant benefit as well. Although glucocorticoids are the most efficacious anti-inflammatory drugs available for the treatment of both asthma and allergic rhinitis (see Table 27–1), they have the potential to cause the greatest number of adverse effects. The incidence of adverse effects is markedly reduced when these drugs are given by inhalation, so this route of administration is employed under most circumstances. Other routes are reserved for the treatment of chronic severe asthma or acute exacerbations of asthma.

Among the glucocorticoids that are available as metered-dose inhalers are **beclomethasone, fluticasone,** and **triamcinolone.** Beclomethasone and triamcinolone are usually administered three or four times a day, whereas fluticasone needs to be administered only twice a day. The proper use of metered-dose inhalers requires considerable skill and the utilization of a spacer device between the mouth and the inhaler. The spacer decreases the amount of drug that is deposited in the mouth and upper airway and facilitates the delivery of the drug to the bronchioles.

Like other anti-inflammatory drugs, glucocorticoids are primarily used on a long-term basis for the prevention of asthmatic attacks, rather than for the treatment of acute bronchospasm. The maximal response to glucocorticoids usually requires up to 8 weeks to develop. Glucocorticoids can reduce the number and severity of symptoms and decrease the need for β₂-adrenergic receptor agonists and other bronchodilators.

Adverse effects associated with inhaled glucocorticoids are usually mild. Excessive deposition of the drugs in the mouth and upper airway may lead to oral candidiasis (thrush). There is also concern about the potential for glucocorticoids to suppress growth in children. This problem is difficult to evaluate because asthmatic children may have growth disturbances related to their disease. However, a meta-analysis of 21 studies concluded that inhaled beclomethasone does not cause growth impairment.

Mast Cell Stabilizers
Cromolyn Sodium

Chemistry and Mechanisms. Cromolyn sodium (Fig. 27–2A) and related drugs stabilize the plasma membranes of mast cells and eosinophils and thereby prevent degranulation and release of histamine, leukotrienes, and other mediators of allergic reactions that lead to airway inflammation (see Fig. 27–1). Some investigators postulate that cromolyn inhibits calcium influx into mast cells, but the exact mechanism of action remains uncertain. Cromolyn does not interfere with the binding of immunoglobulin E (IgE) to mast cells or with the binding of antigen to IgE. The drug is not a bronchodilator, and its beneficial effects in asthma and other conditions are largely prophylactic.

Pharmacokinetics. Cromolyn and other mast cell stabilizers are rather insoluble in body fluids, and minimal systemic absorption occurs following their oral administration or inhalation. The oral bioavailability of cromolyn is about 1%. When the drug is administered by inhalation, its major effect is exerted on the respiratory tract and very little is absorbed into the circulation. Most of the drug is swallowed following inhalation, and about 98% of it is excreted in the feces.

Indications. Cromolyn is administered by inhalation for the treatment of **asthma** or **allergic rhinitis** and is available in an ophthalmic solution for the treatment of **vernal (seasonal) conjunctivitis.** Cromolyn and related compounds are primarily used for the long-term prophylaxis of asthmatic bronchoconstriction and allergic reactions, and they have no role in the treatment of acute bronchospasm. For perennial asthma, the drug is usually given several times a day at regular intervals until symptoms resolve. Improvement may require several weeks, and then the dosage can be reduced to the lowest effective level. For exercise-induced asthma, cromolyn is inhaled not more than 1 hour before the anticipated exercise or other precipitating factor. For allergic rhinitis or vernal conjuncti-

vitis, cromolyn is administered several times a day at regular intervals.

Cromolyn is administered orally before meals and at bedtime for the treatment of **systemic masto-cytosis,** a rare condition characterized by infiltration of the liver, spleen, lymph nodes, and gastrointestinal tract with mast cells. A similar dosage schedule has been used for the treatment of **ulcerative colitis** and **food allergy.**

Adverse Effects and Interactions. Cromolyn and other mast cell stabilizers are remarkably non-toxic, partly because of their low solubility and systemic absorption. In some patients, however, inhalation of cromolyn may irritate the throat and cause cough and bronchospasm. Administration of a β_2-adrenergic receptor agonist can prevent or relieve

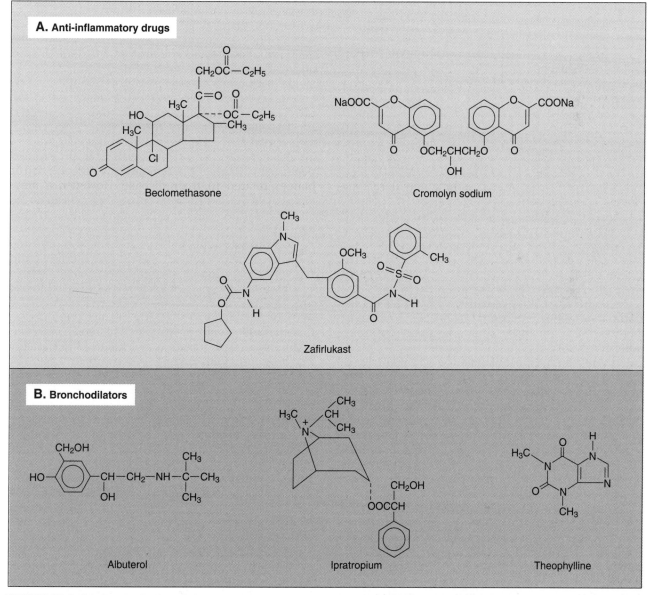

FIGURE 27–2. Structures of selected drugs used in the management of asthma. (A) Beclomethasone is a glucocorticoid. Cromolyn sodium is a mast cell stabilizer, and zafirlukast is a leukotriene receptor antagonist. **(B)** Albuterol is a selective β_2-adrenergic receptor agonist. Ipratropium is a muscarinic receptor antagonist, and theophylline is a phosphodiesterase inhibitor.

this reaction. Nasal and ocular preparations may cause localized pain and irritation, but these effects are usually mild and transient. Cromolyn does not interact significantly with other drugs.

Lodoxamide and Nedocromil

Lodoxamide is formulated as an ophthalmic solution for the treatment of ocular allergies, including **vernal keratitis** and **vernal conjunctivitis.** Like other mast cell stabilizers, lodoxamide appears to prevent calcium influx into mast cells and mast cell degranulation. It may cause ocular discomfort but is generally well tolerated.

Nedocromil has properties that are quite similar to those of cromolyn. However, nedocromil is only available as an aerosol for the prevention of bronchoconstriction in patients with **asthma.** It is initially administered as two inhalations four times a day at regular intervals, but the frequency of doses can be reduced to two or three times a day in persons whose asthma is well controlled.

Leukotriene Inhibitors

Leukotrienes are a group of arachidonic acid metabolites formed via the **5-lipoxygenase pathway** (see Chapter 26). These substances serve as mediators in the inflammatory events that contribute to bronchospasm in patients with asthma.

Pranlukast was the world's first **leukotriene receptor antagonist** and was marketed in Japan in 1995; it is still undergoing clinical trials in the USA. Two other leukotriene receptor antagonists, zafirlukast and montelukast, are now available in the USA. Zileuton, a **leukotriene synthesis inhibitor,** is also available.

Zafirlukast and Montelukast

Chemistry and Mechanisms. Zafirlukast (see Fig. 27–2A) and montelukast each have a complex structure that contains a sulfur moiety and resembles the structure of the **cysteinyl leukotrienes,** which are called **sulfidopeptide leukotrienes** or **leukotrienes C_4, D_4, and E_4** (LTC_4, LTD_4, and LTE_4). Because of their structural resemblance, the drugs are able to compete with the leukotrienes for their receptor, the **$CysLT_1$ receptor.** This receptor mediates airway inflammation, edema, bronchoconstriction, and the secretion of thick, viscous mucus. The leukotriene antagonists have been shown to inhibit both the early and the late phases of bronchoconstriction induced by antigen challenge.

Pharmacokinetics. Zafirlukast and montelukast are administered orally and are well absorbed from the gut. They are both highly bound to plasma proteins (>99%) and are extensively metabolized by hepatic cytochrome P450 enzymes. While the half-life of zafirlukast is about 10 hours, that of montelukast is only about 4 hours. Nevertheless, montelukast is administered as a single daily dose in the evening, whereas zafirlukast is usually given twice a day. It

would appear that the biologic activity of montelukast persists longer than the serum levels of the drug.

Pharmacologic Effects and Indications. The leukotriene receptor antagonists are considered alternatives to other anti-inflammatory drugs for the long-term control of mild to moderate **asthma.** The receptor antagonists improve pulmonary function, control symptoms, and may significantly reduce the incidence of asthmatic attacks. Their beneficial effects appear to be cumulative, and maximal effectiveness may require several weeks to months of therapy. While their main benefit seems to be a reduction in airway inflammation, they also produce significant bronchodilation within 1 hour of administration. Although they are not indicated for the treatment of acute bronchospasm, they do enhance the bronchodilating effect of therapy with β_2-adrenergic receptor agonists, and they reduce the requirement for this therapy in patients with asthma.

Leukotriene receptor antagonists offer the advantages of convenient oral administration and minimal side effects, but they are not as efficacious as glucocorticoids in the management of moderate to severe asthma. Furthermore, they are not recommended as monotherapy for the management of exercise-induced asthma.

Adverse Effects and Interactions. The leukotriene receptor antagonists are relatively free of serious adverse effects. However, allergic granulomatous angiitis (Churg-Strauss syndrome) developed in some patients who were being withdrawn from glucocorticoid therapy while receiving zafirlukast, so careful monitoring is necessary under these circumstances.

Zafirlukast inhibits the CYP2C9 and CYP3A4 isozymes of cytochrome P450 and may thereby interfere with the metabolism of phenytoin and warfarin (drugs metabolized by CYP2C9) and of astemizole, cisapride, felodipine, lovastatin, and triazolam (drugs metabolized by CYP3A4). Montelukast does not inhibit these isozymes or exhibit significant drug interactions. Hence, its use may be preferred in patients receiving concomitant drug therapy.

Zileuton

Mechanisms. Zileuton inhibits 5-lipoxygenase, the enzyme responsible for catalyzing the formation of leukotrienes from arachidonic acid. By blocking leukotriene synthesis, the drug protects the airways from the inflammatory and bronchoconstricting effects of leukotrienes.

Pharmacokinetics. Zileuton is administered orally four times a day (with meals and at bedtime). It is rapidly absorbed from the gut but undergoes some first-pass hepatic inactivation. Once in the systemic circulation, it is almost entirely metabolized by glucuronidation, with an elimination half-life of about 2 hours.

Pharmacologic Effects and Indications. Studies have shown that leukotriene synthesis increases during an asthmatic attack and that this increase can be prevented by the long-term use of zileuton in patients with mild to moderate **asthma.** Studies have also shown benefits of zileuton use in patients with **rheumatoid arthritis** and **ulcerative colitis,** but the drug is not officially approved for these indications in the USA.

Adverse Effects and Interactions. Because zileuton must be taken four times a day, patient noncompliance is sometimes a problem. Mild and transient adverse reactions to zileuton use include a flulike syndrome, headache, drowsiness, and dyspepsia. Zileuton elevates hepatic enzyme levels, so patients taking the drug should be closely monitored for signs of hepatitis. Patients with transaminase levels greater than three times the upper limit of normal should not take the drug. Zileuton should also be used cautiously in patients who consume substantial quantities of alcohol.

Zileuton inhibits isozymes CYP1A2 and CYP3A4, and it may elevate plasma concentrations of theophylline and warfarin. Patients who take these drugs concurrently with zileuton should be closely monitored. The potential of zileuton to interact with other drugs has not been fully evaluated.

BRONCHODILATORS

The bronchodilators include selective β_2-adrenergic receptor agonists, ipratropium, and theophylline. All of these drugs relax bronchial smooth muscle and prevent or relieve bronchospasm. The β_2 receptor agonists are the only type of bronchodilator used to counteract an acute asthmatic attack. Ipratropium is less useful in asthma and is primarily used to treat patients with a COPD such as emphysema. Theophylline can be administered on a long-term basis to prevent bronchoconstriction in patients with either asthma or emphysema.

Selective β_2-Adrenergic Receptor Agonists

The selective β_2-adrenergic receptor agonists are the primary bronchodilators used in the treatment of **asthma.** By activating β_2 receptors, these drugs increase cyclic adenosine monophosphate (cAMP) concentrations in smooth muscle and thereby cause the muscle to relax (Fig. 27–3). The selective β_2 receptor agonists relax bronchial smooth muscle without producing as much cardiac stimulation as do their nonselective counterparts, which also activate β_1 receptors in the heart (Fig. 27–4). However, the selectivity of β_2 receptor agonists is limited, and higher doses can activate cardiac β_1 receptors and thereby increase heart rate and contractility.

Chapter 8 describes the pharmacologic and other properties of various types of adrenergic receptor agonists, and Table 27–2 compares the properties of selective β_2-adrenergic receptor agonists that are administered by inhalation.

Rapid-acting β_2 receptor agonists, such as **albuterol, pirbuterol,** and **terbutaline,** are usually

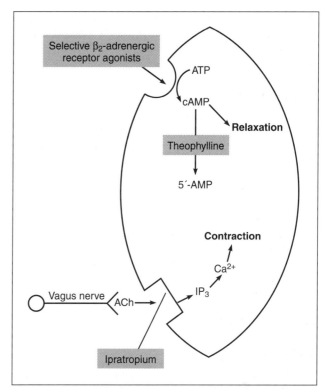

FIGURE 27–3. Mechanisms of action of bronchodilators. Selective β_2-adrenergic receptor agonists activate β_2 receptors. This increases cyclic adenosine monophosphate (cAMP) concentrations in smooth muscle and thereby causes the muscle to relax. Theophylline inhibits phosphodiesterase isozymes and thereby blocks the degradation of cAMP to 5′-AMP. Ipratropium blocks the stimulation of muscarinic receptors by acetylcholine (ACh) released from vagus nerves and thereby attenuates reflex bronchoconstriction. The effect of ACh is mediated by IP$_3$-induced calcium release and leads to smooth muscle contraction. ATP = adenosine triphosphate; and IP$_3$ = inositol triphosphate.

given by the inhalational route to prevent or treat **acute bronchospasm.** Although oral formulations of albuterol and terbutaline are available for children or adults who are unable to use a metered-dose inhaler, the oral formulations have a slower onset of action and may cause more systemic side effects. Pirbuterol is available only as an aerosol inhaler.

Salmeterol is a slower- and longer-acting β_2 receptor agonist that is given by inhalation. It is particularly useful in preventing **nocturnal asthmatic attacks,** which are sometimes life-threatening, and preventing **exercise-induced asthma.** It also appears to inhibit the late phase of **allergen-induced bronchoconstriction,** which usually occurs after the bronchodilating effects of shorter-acting drugs have dissipated.

Other Bronchodilators
Ipratropium

Ipratropium (see Fig. 27–2B) is the isopropyl derivative of atropine, a muscarinic receptor antagonist whose pharmacologic and other properties are described in Chapter 7. The addition of the isopropyl group results in a quaternary ammonium

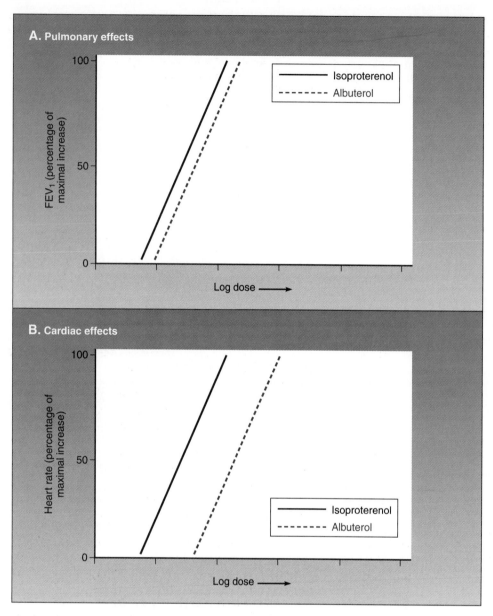

A. Pulmonary effects

B. Cardiac effects

FIGURE 27–4. **Pulmonary effects (A) and cardiac effects (B) of two types of β-adrenergic receptor agonists.** Albuterol, a selective β_2-adrenergic receptor agonist, produces bronchodilation and increases the forced expiratory volume in 1 second (FEV_1) at doses that produce relatively little cardiac stimulation. Isoproterenol, a nonselective β-adrenergic receptor agonist, produces equal effects on pulmonary function and heart rate.

compound that is not well absorbed into the circulation. Ipratropium is administered by oral inhalation or nasal spray and produces very few systemic side effects. It acts by blocking the

TABLE 27–2. Pharmacologic Properties of Selective β_2-Adrenergic Agonists Administered by Inhalation

Drug	Onset of Action (Minutes)	Duration of Action (Hours)	Dosage
Albuterol	5	3–8	2 puffs every 4–6 hours
Pirbuterol	5	5	2 puffs every 4–6 hours
Salmeterol	20	12	2 puffs every 12 hours
Terbutaline	5–15	3–6	2 puffs every 4–6 hours

bronchoconstricting effect of vagus nerve stimulation (see Fig. 27–3).

In patients with a **chronic obstructive pulmonary disease** (COPD) such as **emphysema,** the bronchodilating effect of ipratropium is slower to develop than that of albuterol (a β_2 receptor agonist described above), but it lasts longer. In one study, for example, investigators found that the effect of ipratropium was sustained after 12 weeks of treatment, whereas the effect of albuterol on the forced expiratory volume in 1 second (FEV_1) appeared to diminish over a 12-week period. Other studies have demonstrated that ipratropium improves the quality of life in patients with moderate to severe COPD, reduces rhinorrhea in patients with **allergic or viral rhinitis,** and benefits infants with **acute bronchitis.**

Ipratropium is less effective than a β_2 receptor agonist in the treatment of most patients with **asthma.** However, some studies indicate that combined therapy with ipratropium and a β_2 receptor agonist has a greater bronchodilating effect than does therapy with either drug alone in patients who have acute asthma.

Theophylline

Chemistry, Mechanisms, and Pharmacologic Effects. The structure of theophylline is shown in Fig. 27–2B. Like caffeine, theophylline is a **methylxanthine drug.** These drugs produce various degrees of central nervous system (CNS) stimulation, bronchodilation, diuresis, and other pharmacologic effects. In comparison with caffeine, for example, theophylline produces less CNS stimulation and more bronchodilation.

Theophylline has several actions at the cellular level, including inhibition of phosphodiesterase (PDE) isozymes, antagonism of adenosine receptors, inhibition of calcium influx, and enhancement of catecholamine secretion. All of these effects have been purported to contribute to the drug's beneficial bronchodilating effects in patients with asthma, yet each has also been subject to criticism. Recently, theophylline has also been found to elicit several anti-inflammatory and immunosuppressant effects that may contribute to its efficacy in asthma. It seems likely that theophylline exerts its beneficial effects through multiple actions and interactions involving numerous types of cells and receptors.

Theophylline is a nonspecific inhibitor of several PDE isozymes found in bronchial smooth muscle and inflammatory cells. As discussed above and shown in Fig. 27–3, cAMP mediates the bronchodilating effect of β_2 receptor agonists, and the traditional understanding has been that theophylline produces its bronchodilating effect by inhibiting PDE isozymes that catalyze the degradation of cAMP. Some studies have suggested that therapeutic levels of theophylline do not produce significant PDE inhibition. However, when asthmatic patients are compared with healthy individuals, it now appears that the asthmatic patients have higher PDE levels in their airways and that theophylline has a greater effect on their airways. Furthermore, studies show that investigational drugs that selectively inhibit type III and IV PDE can also relax human bronchial smooth muscle. Therefore, most authorities believe that inhibition of PDE remains a viable mechanism for the bronchodilating effect of theophylline and related drugs.

There is also evidence that theophylline exerts anti-inflammatory and immunomodulating effects that may be relevant to the treatment of asthma. Some of these actions are mediated by PDE inhibition, while others are caused by inhibition of T lymphocyte proliferation and cytokine production. In patients with asthma, theophylline reduces the number of eosinophils, lymphocytes, and monocytes that infiltrate the airway epithelium. It also impairs the release of cationic basic protein and eosinophil-derived neurotoxin, which are substances that contribute to the pathogenesis of asthma by damaging the epithelial lining of bronchioles.

Adenosine is a naturally occurring purine nucleoside formed from adenosine monophosphate. It has been shown to cause bronchospasm when inhaled by patients with asthma. While therapeutic levels of theophylline can block adenosine receptors, other xanthine drugs that have minimal adenosine antagonist activity are also able to act as potent bronchodilators. Hence, adenosine antagonism is probably not the major mechanism of the bronchodilating effect of theophylline. Adenosine antagonism may be responsible, however, for some of the CNS, cardiac, and diuretic effects of theophylline.

Pharmacokinetics. After oral administration, theophylline is well absorbed from the gut and has relatively little first-pass inactivation. The drug is widely distributed and crosses the blood-brain barrier to enter the CNS. Via the actions of a cytochrome P450 isozyme called CYP1A2, theophylline is extensively metabolized to inactive agents. These metabolites are primarily excreted in the urine, along with 10% of the parent drug. The half-life of theophylline is about 8 hours in adults who do not smoke. In contrast, it is about 4.5 hours in adults who smoke and in children from 1 to 9 years of age, because these populations metabolize the drug more rapidly.

The use of theophylline began to decline because of the drug's perceived narrow therapeutic index, its pronounced side effect profile, and its potential for interactions with other drugs (see below). However, the availability of sustained-release preparations of theophylline and the recognition that lower doses of the drug can provide significant benefits have renewed the interest of clinicians in prescribing theophylline. Nevertheless, because of the drug's narrow margin of safety, theophylline serum levels should be monitored carefully, especially when therapy is initiated. Therapeutic serum levels are considered to be in the range of 5–15 mg/L. Higher levels are associated with a greater risk of adverse reactions.

Indications. Theophylline is primarily used to treat obstructive lung disorders and asthma, but it is also used to treat apnea.

In patients with **chronic obstructive pulmonary disease** (COPD), theophylline is an effective bronchodilator whose long-term use is associated with a 20% increase in FEV_1 and with improvement in minute ventilation and gas exchange. Treatment with theophylline is reported to reduce dyspnea, increase diaphragmatic contractility, improve the exercise performance and sense of well-being of patients, and reduce fatigue. Theophylline may also increase the central respiratory drive and has favorable cardiovascular effects, including a reduction in pulmonary artery pressure and vascular resistance and an increase in right and left ventricular ejection fractions. The drug's other beneficial effects include increased mucociliary clearance and reduced airway inflammation. Hence, there is a good rationale for using theophylline to treat COPD in patients whose symptoms are not controlled with optimal doses of β_2 receptor agonists and ipratropium. Theophylline is most beneficial in patients with moderate to severe COPD.

Although the use of theophylline in the management of **asthma** is declining, recent studies support a continuing role for this drug in specific situations. It is useful in controlling nocturnal asthma, and it can improve pulmonary function in patients who require large doses of glucocorticoids. Patients who have moderate to severe asthma and are already being treated with glucocorticoids and β_2 receptor agonists may benefit from the addition of theophylline to their regimen, and the drug may be particularly useful in controlling refractory symptoms in patients with severe asthma.

Theophylline is an important treatment for **recurrent apnea in premature infants.** The drug appears to act via adenosine antagonism to increase the sensitivity of respiratory centers to carbon dioxide and to increase the contractility of respiratory muscles. Theophylline has also been used to treat **obstructive sleep apnea** and periodic breathing. However, the drug may reduce sleep quality via CNS stimulation.

Adverse Effects. Major adverse effects of theophylline include gastrointestinal distress, CNS stimulation, and cardiac stimulation.

Adverse gastrointestinal effects, such as abdominal pain, nausea, and vomiting, may be minimized by taking the drug with food or antacids or with a full glass of water or milk. After swallowing the drug, patients should remain upright for 30 minutes to prevent reflux esophagitis.

CNS effects include headache, anxiety, restlessness, insomnia, dizziness, and seizures. A reduction in dosage will often eliminate these problems.

Theophylline can affect the cardiovascular system, causing hypotension, bradycardia, extrasystoles, premature ventricular contractions, and tachycardia. These events are usually mild and transient, but serious reactions occasionally develop. Long-term overmedication is more likely than an incident of overdosage to cause severe toxicity. Seizures and serious arrhythmias may occur at concentrations over 25 mg/L.

Interactions. Cimetidine inhibits CYP1A2 and thereby prevents the metabolism of theophylline in the liver. Erythromycin and other macrolide antibiotics can reduce theophylline clearance and increase theophylline plasma concentrations, but the interaction only seems significant when theophylline concentrations are already in the high therapeutic range. Other drugs that can reduce the clearance and increase the plasma concentrations of theophylline include fluoroquinolone antimicrobial drugs, fluvoxamine, isoniazid, ticlopidine, and verapamil. Careful monitoring of patients is important, since it is difficult to predict which patients will require dosage adjustments when these drugs are given concomitantly.

ANTITUSSIVES

Coughing usually serves a beneficial purpose by expelling irritating substances such as dust, pollen, and accumulated fluids and inflammatory cells from the upper airways. However, an incessant nonproductive cough may lead to loss of sleep, rib fractures, pneumothorax, rupture of surgical wounds, or even syncope. Antitussive drugs are frequently used to **suppress coughing,** but the first-line therapy consists of determining and controlling the infection, allergy, or other condition responsible for the cough.

The **cough reflex** is initiated by stimulation of sensory receptors on afferent nerve endings located between mucosal cells of the pharynx, larynx, and larger airways. The impulses ascend via the vagus nerve to the dorsal medulla. The efferent limb of the reflex consists of somatic nerves innervating the larynx and thoracoabdominal muscles. Some antitussives act locally to anesthetize the afferent nerves that initiate the cough reflex, while other antitussives act by inhibiting the cough center in the medulla.

The locally acting antitussives include **menthol and related drugs** that are administered as throat sprays or lozenges. The centrally acting antitussives consist of **opioids,** and these are usually administered orally. Almost all of the opioid agonist drugs will exert an antitussive effect, but opioids that have a higher ratio of antitussive effects to analgesic and euphoric effects are usually employed for this purpose. These include **dextromethorphan, codeine,** and **hydrocodone.**

Dextromethorphan is the D-isomer of a potent opioid agonist. Although dextromethorphan has potent antitussive activity, it will not cause drowsiness, euphoria, analgesia, or other CNS effects except at extremely high doses. For these reasons, it is available in many nonprescription products for cough and other respiratory tract conditions, and it is the most widely used opioid antitussive drug.

Codeine and hydrocodone are moderate opioid agonists whose analgesic effects are described in Chapter 23. These drugs exhibit excellent antitussive activity at doses that produce relatively little CNS depression or euphoria. They are available in a number of liquid cough preparations that may also include guaifenesin, antihistamines, and decongestants. In the USA, preparations containing codeine and hydrocodone are classified as schedule V controlled substances, but pharmacies in some states are permitted to sell small quantities of these preparations without a prescription.

EXPECTORANTS

An expectorant is a drug that facilitates the coughing up of mucus and other material from the lungs. **Guaifenesin** is an oral nonprescription drug that has been used for this purpose for many years. It is purported to reduce the adhesiveness and surface tension of respiratory tract secretions and thereby facilitate their expectoration, but the exact mechanism by which the drug produces this effect is unknown. Through its expectorant effect, guaifenesin may also reduce the frequency of coughing. The drug may be useful in patients with **thick, tenacious respiratory tract secretions;** in patients with **dry, nonproductive coughing;** and in patients with **sinusitis.**

THE MANAGEMENT OF RHINITIS
Allergic Rhinitis

The effective management of allergic rhinitis usually requires environmental control of exposure to allergens and prophylactic use of anti-inflammatory medications. **Glucocorticoids** are the most efficacious anti-inflammatory drugs for this condition (see Table 27–1), and several inhalational formulations of **beclomethasone** and other glucocorticoids are now available. These products are convenient and effective, and they cause very few adverse reactions. **Cromolyn sodium** is slightly less effective but can be used in patients who do not tolerate glucocorticoids.

While anti-inflammatory drugs can significantly reduce symptoms in most cases, some patients will continue to experience symptoms during peak seasonal exposure to pollens such as ragweed pollen. At that time, antihistamines can be added to the treatment regimen. A long-acting nonsedating antihistamine such as **loratadine** or **fexofenadine** (see Chapter 26) is particularly suitable for most patients. If anti-inflammatory drugs and antihistamines are unable to control nasal congestion, a decongestant drug such as **pseudoephedrine** (see Chapter 8) can also be added to the regimen. However, decongestants are often not needed if patients begin taking anti-inflammatory drugs before the onset of seasonal allergies and if they add an antihistamine drug at the first sign of allergic symptoms.

Ipratropium, a bronchodilator, is now approved for the treatment of rhinorrhea associated with rhinitis. A nasal spray formulation is available for this purpose, but it does not relieve nasal itching or congestion.

Ocular inflammation, discomfort, and pruritus can be a particularly troublesome aspect of seasonal allergies. **Cromolyn** and **lodoxamide** are available in topical ocular formulations that are quite effective in preventing symptoms of allergic conjunctivitis. Mild ocular symptoms can be treated with topical decongestants and oral or topical antihistamines. More severe ocular symptoms may be controlled with a topical nonsteroidal anti-inflammatory drug such as **ketorolac** (see Chapter 30). Glucocorticoids are not usually employed for allergic conjunctivitis, because their long-term use is associated with adverse effects such as increased intraocular pressure and cataracts.

Viral Rhinitis

Viral rhinitis (the common cold) is a self-limiting condition that is best treated conservatively. Analgesics such as **acetaminophen, aspirin,** or **ibuprofen** (see Chapter 30) may be used to relieve the aches and discomfort associated with viral rhinitis. An increased intake of **zinc** has been advocated, but data supporting its effectiveness are limited. Decongestants such as **pseudoephedrine** (see Chapter 8) may be used to relieve nasal congestion, and **ipratropium** is approved for the treatment of rhinorrhea in persons with viral or allergic rhinitis.

Summary of Important Points

- Drugs used in the management of asthma are classified as anti-inflammatory agents or bronchodilators, but some drugs exhibit both anti-inflammatory and bronchodilating action.
- Glucocorticoids are the most efficacious anti-inflammatory drugs and are usually given by inhalation on a long-term basis to prevent asthmatic attacks. Orally or parenterally administered glucocorticoids are used for the management of chronic severe asthma or acute exacerbations of asthma.
- Cromolyn sodium and related drugs are used prophylactically in the management of mild to moderate asthma, allergic rhinitis, and related disorders. They have few adverse effects.
- Leukotriene inhibitors have anti-inflammatory and bronchodilating activity and offer convenient oral therapy for the prevention of asthmatic attacks. Montelukast and zafirlukast are leukotriene receptor antagonists, and zileuton is a leukotriene synthesis inhibitor.
- Selective β_2-adrenergic receptor agonists are the most efficacious bronchodilators for the treatment of acute bronchospasm. Examples are albuterol, pirbuterol, and terbutaline.
- Ipratropium is a muscarinic receptor antagonist that is useful for the treatment of chronic obstructive pulmonary disease (COPD) but has little efficacy in the treatment of asthma.
- Theophylline has anti-inflammatory and bronchodilating activity and is useful for the treatment of asthma and COPD. The metabolism of theophylline is affected by smoking and by the concurrent administration of drugs that inhibit cytochrome P450. Children metabolize theophylline more rapidly than do adults.
- Theophylline levels should be monitored to ensure efficacy and prevent toxicity. Adverse effects include central nervous system and cardiac toxicity.
- Antitussives are used to suppress dry, nonproductive coughing. Dextromethorphan is available without a prescription, whereas codeine and hydrocodone are contained in many prescription cough preparations.
- Guaifenesin is an expectorant that appears to facilitate removal of mucus and other material from the airways. It is also used in the treatment of sinusitis.

Selected Readings

Adkins, J. C., and R. N. Brogden. Zafirlukast: a review of its pharmacology and therapeutic potential in the management of asthma. Drugs 55:121–144, 1998.

Clark, D. J., and B. J. Lipworth. Dose response of inhaled drugs in asthma: an update. Clin Pharmacokinet 32:58–74, 1997.

Colice, G. L. Nebulized bronchodilators for outpatient management of stable chronic obstructive pulmonary disease. Am J Med 100:11S–18S, 1996.

D'Alonzo, G. E., and K. A. Tolep. Salmeterol in the treatment of chronic asthma. Am Fam Physician 56:558–562, 1997.

Drazen, J. M. New directions in asthma drug therapy. Hosp Pract (Off Ed) 33:25–38, 1998.

Hoekx, J. C., et al. Fluticasone propionate compared with budesonide: a double-blind trial in asthmatic children using powder devices at a dosage of 400 micrograms per day. Eur Respir J 9:2263–2272, 1996.

Kelly, H. W. Comparison of inhaled corticosteroids. Ann Pharmacother 32:220–232, 1998.

Schwartz, H. J., et al. A randomized controlled trial comparing zileuton with theophylline in moderate asthma. Arch Intern Med 158:141–148, 1998.

Simons, F. E. A comparison of beclomethasone, salmeterol, and placebo in children with asthma. N Engl J Med 337:1659–1665, 1997.

Vassallo, R., and J. J. Lipsky. Theophylline: recent advances in the understanding of its mode of action and uses in clinical practice. Mayo Clin Proc 73:346–354, 1998.

CHAPTER TWENTY-EIGHT

DRUGS FOR GASTROINTESTINAL

TRACT DISORDERS

CLASSIFICATION OF DRUGS FOR GASTROINTESTINAL TRACT DISORDERS*

DRUGS THAT REDUCE GASTRIC ACIDITY
Histamine H_2 receptor antagonists
- Cimetidine, famotidine, and ranitidine

Proton pump inhibitors
- Lansoprazole and omeprazole

Muscarinic receptor antagonists
- Atropine and pirenzepine

Gastric antacids
- Aluminum and magnesium hydroxides and calcium carbonate

CYTOPROTECTIVE DRUGS
- Misoprostol and sucralfate

DRUGS FOR *HELICOBACTER PYLORI* INFECTION
- Amoxicillin, bismuth, clarithromycin, metronidazole, and tetracycline

DRUGS FOR INFLAMMATORY BOWEL DISEASES
- Azathioprine, hydrocortisone, infliximab, mercaptopurine, mesalamine, metronidazole, prednisolone, and sulfasalazine

PROKINETIC DRUGS
- Cisapride and metoclopramide

LAXATIVES
- Bisacodyl, cascara, castor oil, docusate sodium, lactulose, magnesium oxide, magnesium sulfate, psyllium, senna, and sodium phosphate

ANTIDIARRHEAL AGENTS
- Bismuth subsalicylate, diphenoxylate, kaolin-pectin, loperamide, and polycarbophil

ANTIEMETICS
Serotonin 5-HT_3 receptor antagonists
- Granisetron and ondansetron

Dopamine D_2 receptor antagonists
- Metoclopramide and prochlorperazine

Other antiemetics
- Dimenhydrinate, dronabinol, meclizine, promethazine, and scopolamine

*Note that some drugs are listed more than once.

OVERVIEW

Gastrointestinal tract disorders are among the most common reasons that people seek assistance from health care providers. A vast array of drugs are available to treat the causes and relieve the many symptoms of gastrointestinal diseases. This chapter focuses on drugs used in the management of peptic ulcer disease, inflammatory bowel diseases, chronic gastrointestinal motility disorders, dyspepsia, constipation, diarrhea, nausea, and vomiting.

Peptic Ulcer Disease

Peptic ulcer disease is characterized by inflamed lesions or excavations (ulcers) of the mucosa and underlying tissue of the upper gastrointestinal tract. The ulcers are the result of damage to the mucous membrane that normally protects the esophagus, stomach, and duodenum from gastric acid and pepsin. This damage may be caused by several factors, including excessive acid and pepsin production, bile acid reflux, advancing age, ischemia, inhibition of prostaglandin synthesis, and infection with *Helicobacter pylori*.

In Western countries, the number of persons who harbor *H. pylori* increases from under 5% at birth to about 20% at the age of 45 years. However, only a small proportion of persons harboring this bacterial organism will develop peptic ulcer disease. Those at greatest risk include individuals who smoke, ingest excessive amounts of alcohol or nonsteroidal anti-inflammatory drugs (NSAIDs), are elderly, or have gastrointestinal ischemia. Prolonged use of glucocorticoids may also be a risk factor for peptic ulcer disease.

H. pylori–induced gastritis is believed to precede the development of peptic ulcers in most persons. *H. pylori* is found in the gastrointestinal tract of almost all patients with **duodenal ulcers** and about 80% of patients with **gastric ulcers.** There is evidence that the organism can penetrate the mucosa, attach to mucosal epithelial cells, release enzymes that damage the mucous membrane and mucosal cells, and cause inflammation and tissue destruction. There is also evidence that the eradication of *H. pylori* heals peptic ulcers and significantly reduces the recurrence rate for gastric and duodenal ulcers.

The agents that are used to treat peptic ulcer disease include drugs that reduce gastric acidity (primarily histamine H_2 receptor antagonists and proton pump inhibitors), drugs that eliminate *H. pylori,* and drugs that exert a cytoprotective effect on the gastrointestinal mucosa.

Inflammatory Bowel Diseases

The two most common inflammatory bowel diseases are **ulcerative colitis** and **Crohn's disease.** In ulcerative colitis, inflammation of the gastrointestinal mucosa is limited to the colon and rectum. In Crohn's disease, inflammation is transmural and may occur in any part of the gastrointestinal tract. Crohn's disease is sometimes incorrectly described as regional enteritis.

Abdominal cramping and diarrhea are among the most common complaints of patients with an inflammatory bowel disease. The clinical presentation of the disease can vary widely. Many patients experience acute exacerbations separated by periods of remission, but prolonged illness can occur in persons with severe disease. Because the symptoms and clinical course of ulcerative colitis and Crohn's disease are similar, a definitive diagnosis is often quite difficult and may require extensive laboratory, endoscopic, and radiologic testing.

Ulcerative colitis and Crohn's disease are generally treated with glucocorticoids, mesalamine, and sulfasalazine.

Gastrointestinal Motility Disorders

A number of gastrointestinal tract disorders are characterized by inadequate gastrointestinal motility. These include gastroesophageal reflux disease, gastroparesis, and irritable bowel syndrome.

Gastroesophageal reflux disease (GERD) is characterized by esophagitis and is due to the reflux of gastric acid into the esophagus. The disease is often associated with excessive secretion of gastric acid and decreased pressure in the lower esophageal sphincter. Pharmacologic agents used in the treatment of GERD include drugs that reduce gastric acidity (such as H_2 receptor antagonists and proton pump inhibitors) and drugs that increase esophageal sphincter pressure (such as cisapride). Nonpharmacologic measures are also useful and include avoid-

ance of certain foods (such as chocolate), avoidance of bedtime snacks, and elevation of the upper body during sleep. Because obesity contributes to GERD, weight reduction may help alleviate symptoms.

Acute gastroparesis is a delay in gastric emptying that is typically seen in patients recovering from surgery, trauma, or abdominal infections. **Chronic gastroparesis** is seen in patients with neuropathies that affect the stomach, such as patients with diabetes mellitus. Like other forms of gastroparesis, **diabetic gastroparesis** can be treated with prokinetic drugs.

Irritable bowel syndrome is a common, noninflammatory disorder characterized by abnormal bowel movements, which may consist of diarrhea, constipation, or both. The bowel is anatomically normal. Prokinetic drugs may be helpful in patients with irritable bowel syndrome.

Dyspepsia

Dyspepsia, or **heartburn,** is characterized by epigastric discomfort following meals. It is often associated with impaired digestion and excessive stomach acidity, but it is also caused by other factors. Several low-dose formulations of H_2 receptor antagonists are available as nonprescription drugs for the prevention and treatment of dyspepsia.

Constipation

Constipation may be an acute or chronic condition and is characterized by the difficult passage of hard, dry feces. The treatment of constipation rests on a foundation of increased dietary fiber ingestion, adequate fluid intake, and regular exercise. Patients should be encouraged to eat fruits, vegetables, and whole grain foods that add bulk to the diet. If dietary modifications are not sufficient to alleviate constipation, a laxative may be used to facilitate peristalsis. Bulk-forming laxatives can be used on a long-term basis without noticeable side effects, but the other types of laxatives described below should be used only to relieve acute constipation.

Diarrhea

The frequency of elimination and consistency of stools vary from person to person. Diarrhea is a condition characterized by an increase in the number and liquidity of a person's stools. Diarrhea has many causes, and it ranges in severity from mild to life-threatening. Most cases of diarrhea are self-limiting and subside within 1 or 2 days without treatment. Severe diarrhea due to bacterial infections and other causes may lead to significant loss of fluids and electrolytes and should be treated promptly.

If fever and systemic symptoms (such as anorexia and volume depletion) are absent, patients with acute diarrhea can usually be managed with dietary restrictions and with fluid and electrolyte replacement. An antidiarrheal agent may be given as adjunct treatment. Dietary guidelines usually consist of avoiding solid food and milk products for 24 hours. As bowel movements decrease, a bland diet can be started. Several preparations that contain the correct proportions of glucose and electrolytes are available for fluid and electrolyte replacement.

If fever or systemic symptoms are present, patients with diarrhea should be examined for microbial or parasitic infections. If cultures are positive, an appropriate antimicrobial or antiparasitic drug should be given. Chronic diarrhea is defined as diarrhea lasting for 14 days or longer. This condition requires a more thorough diagnostic work-up to determine the underlying cause and enable the selection of appropriate therapy.

A number of drugs can cause diarrhea, including antibiotics that eradicate the normal intestinal flora and predispose patients to superinfections. There is limited evidence that administration of *Lactobacillus* preparations may help restore the normal bowel flora and reduce diarrhea in these patients.

Nausea and Vomiting

Emesis, or vomiting, is a physiologic response to the presence of irritating and potentially harmful substances in the gut or blood stream. It sometimes occurs as a result of excessive vestibular stimulation (motion sickness) or psychologic stimuli such as fear,

dread, or obnoxious sights and odors. Vomiting is frequently preceded by nausea. A large number of antiemetic drugs are available to prevent vomiting.

DRUGS THAT REDUCE GASTRIC ACIDITY

The physiology of gastric acid secretion and sites of drug action are illustrated in Fig. 28–1.

The principal physiologic stimulants of gastric acid secretion are **gastrin, acetylcholine,** and **histamine.** Gastrin is a hormone secreted by G cells in the gastric antrum, while acetylcholine is released from vagus nerve terminals. Gastrin and acetylcholine directly stimulate acid secretion by parietal cells, and they also stimulate the release of histamine from paracrine (enterochromaffinlike) cells. Histamine stimulates H_2 receptors located on parietal cells and provokes acid secretion via cyclic adenosine monophosphate (cAMP) stimulation of the proton pump (H^+,K^+-ATPase).

The vagus nerve mediates the cephalic phase of gastric acid secretion evoked by the smell, taste, and thought of food. Gastrin mediates the gastric phase of acid secretion evoked by the presence of food in the stomach. Histamine contributes to the cephalic and gastric phases of acid secretion, and it also mediates basal acid secretion in the fasting state.

The level of gastric acidity can be reduced either by neutralizing gastric acid (as occurs with antacids) or by inhibiting gastric acid secretion (as occurs with

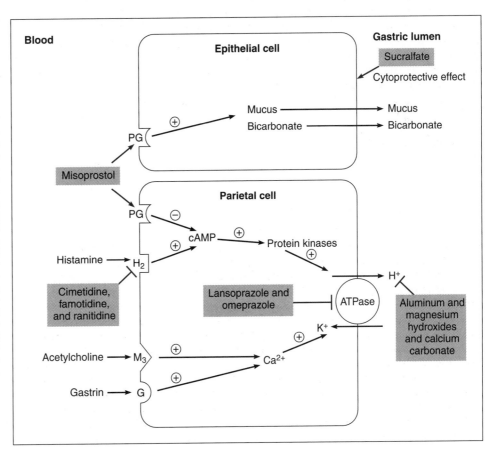

FIGURE 28–1. Physiology of gastric acid secretion and sites of drug action. Gastric acid is secreted by the proton pump (H^+,K^+-ATPase) located in the luminal membrane of parietal cells. H^+,K^+-ATPase is stimulated by histamine, acetylcholine, and gastrin, and it is irreversibly blocked by the proton pump inhibitors (lansoprazole and omeprazole). The effect of histamine is blocked by H_2 receptor antagonists (cimetidine, famotidine, and ranitidine). Prostaglandins such as misoprostol inhibit gastric acid secretion and stimulate secretion of mucus and bicarbonate by epithelial cells. Sucralfate binds to proteins of the ulcer crater and exerts a cytoprotective effect, while antacids (aluminum and magnesium hydroxides and calcium carbonate) neutralize acid in the gastric lumen. PG = prostaglandin receptor; H_2 = histamine H_2 receptor; M_3 = muscarinic M_3 receptor; G = gastrin receptor; and cAMP = cyclic adenosine monophosphate.

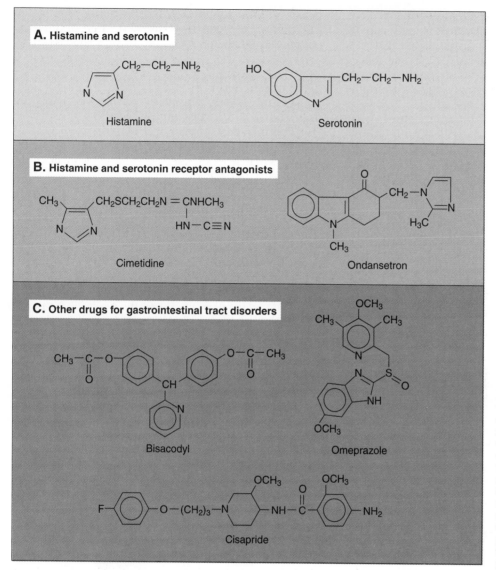

FIGURE 28–2. Structures of histamine and serotonin (A) and selected drugs for gastrointestinal tract disorders (B and C). Cimetidine is a histamine H_2 receptor antagonist whose structure is similar to that of histamine. Ondansetron is a serotonin 5-HT_3 receptor antagonist whose structure is similar to that of serotonin. Bisacodyl is a stimulant (secretory) laxative. Cisapride is a serotonin 5-HT_4 receptor agonist. Omeprazole is a proton pump inhibitor.

histamine H_2 receptor antagonists, proton pump inhibitors, or muscarinic receptor antagonists). Today, the most widely used drugs to inhibit gastric acid secretion are the H_2 receptor antagonists and the proton pump inhibitors.

Histamine H_2 Receptor Antagonists

The H_2 receptor antagonists, or **H_2-blockers,** include **cimetidine, famotidine,** and **ranitidine.**

Chemistry, Mechanisms, and Pharmacologic Effects. The H_2-blockers each contain a 5-membered imidazole, thiazole, or furan ring with an attached side chain. The structure of H_2-blockers is similar to that of histamine (Fig. 28–2A and 28–2B), and this enables the drugs to compete with histamine for binding to H_2 receptors on gastric parietal cells (see Fig. 28–1). The H_2-blockers have been shown to be potent inhibitors of both meal-stimulated secretion and basal secretion of **gastric acid.** When they reduce the volume and concentration of gastric acid, they produce a proportionate decrease in the produc-

tion of **pepsin** because gastric acid catalyzes the conversion of inactive pepsinogen to pepsin. The H_2-blockers also reduce the secretion of **intrinsic factor,** but not enough to significantly reduce vitamin B_{12} absorption. They have no effect on gastric emptying time, esophageal sphincter pressure, or pancreatic enzyme secretion.

Pharmacokinetics. The H_2-blockers are well absorbed from the gut and undergo varying degrees of hepatic inactivation before being excreted in the urine. While the half-life of most H_2-blockers is only 2–3 hours, their duration of action is considerably longer (Table 28–1). Therefore, these drugs can be administered only once or twice daily.

Indications. The H_2-blockers are used to treat several conditions associated with excessive acid production. These include **dyspepsia, peptic ulcer disease,** and **gastroesophageal reflux disease** (GERD). An H_2-blocker is also occasionally used in combination with an H_1-blocker for the treatment of **allergic reactions** that do not respond when an H_1-blocker is used alone.

TABLE 28–1. Properties of Selected Drugs for Peptic Ulcer Disease

Drug Class	Duration of Action (Hours)	Duration of Therapy (Weeks)	Recurrence Rate*
Antimicrobial agents	Varies	2	<5%
Cytoprotective drugs (sucralfate)	6–12	6–8	80–90%
Gastric antacids	3–4	6–8	80–90%
Histamine H_2 receptor antagonists	12	6–8	80–90%
Proton pump inhibitors	24–48	6–8	80–90%

*Recurrence rates are high when patients with peptic ulcer disease are not treated for *Helicobacter pylori* infection. To reduce the recurrence rate, patients should be treated concomitantly with two or three appropriate antimicrobial agents (such as amoxicillin, bismuth, clarithromycin, metronidazole, and tetracycline) for 2 weeks plus an inhibitor of gastric acid secretion (either a histamine H_2 receptor antagonist or a proton pump inhibitor) for 6–8 weeks.

For the prevention or treatment of dyspepsia, several low-dose formulations of H_2-blockers are available as nonprescription drugs. These formulations are most effective when taken 30 minutes prior to ingestion of a dyspepsia-provoking meal.

For the treatment of peptic ulcer disease, H_2-blockers are administered once or twice daily at doses that raise the gastric pH above 4 for about 13 hours a day. Most authorities currently recommend giving a single daily dose at bedtime on an empty stomach and continuing the treatment for 6–8 weeks. The bedtime dose ensures that acid secretion is suppressed all night.

When cimetidine was introduced as the first H_2-blocker, it quickly revolutionized the treatment of peptic ulcers and became the most profitable drug marketed at the time. Studies have shown that cimetidine and other H_2-blockers rapidly suppress acid secretion and relieve pain in persons with peptic ulcers, and they heal about 70% of ulcers in 4 weeks and about 85% in 8 weeks. According to controlled trials, all of the available H_2-blockers produce comparable healing rates. Unfortunately, 80–90% of patients who undergo monotherapy with an H_2-blocker have an ulcer recurrence within 1 year after discontinuing this therapy. In contrast, fewer than 5% of patients who undergo therapy with both an H_2-blocker and an agent to eliminate *H. pylori* infection have an ulcer recurrence. For this reason, combination therapy is recommended.

Adverse Effects. Cimetidine has weak antiandrogenic activity and may cause gynecomastia in elderly men, but this reaction is less common with other H_2-blockers. The fact that the H_2-blockers have proved remarkably nontoxic has led to their approval as nonprescription drugs.

Interactions. Cimetidine is a well-known inhibitor of cytochrome P450 isozymes CYP2C9, CYP2D6,

and CYP3A4. These isozymes are involved in the metabolism of numerous drugs, including alprazolam, carbamazepine, cisapride, disopyramide, felodipine, lovastatin, phenytoin, saquinavir, triazolam, and warfarin. The dosage of these drugs may need to be reduced in patients taking cimetidine concurrently, and patients should be monitored closely for signs of toxicity. Another H_2-blocker, such as ranitidine or famotidine, is often used instead of cimetidine in patients receiving concomitant drug therapy, because these H_2-blockers are much less likely to cause drug interactions.

Proton Pump Inhibitors

The proton pump inhibitors include **lansoprazole** and **omeprazole**.

Chemistry and Pharmacokinetics. The proton pump inhibitors are benzimidazole compounds. The chemical structure of omeprazole is shown in Fig. 28–2C.

Lansoprazole and omeprazole are acid-labile prodrugs that are administered orally as sustained-release enteric-coated preparations. After they are absorbed from the gut, the prodrugs are distributed to the secretory canaliculi in the gastric mucosa and converted to active metabolites that bind to the proton pump. Lansoprazole and omeprazole are eventually metabolized to inactive compounds in the liver, and these compounds are excreted in the urine and feces.

Mechanisms and Pharmacologic Effects. The active metabolites of lansoprazole and omeprazole form a covalent disulfide link with a cysteinyl residue in the proton pump (H^+,K^+-ATPase) located in the luminal membrane of gastric parietal cells (see Fig. 28–1). This enables the drugs to irreversibly inhibit the proton pump and to prevent the secretion of gastric acid for an extended period of time. The drugs can produce a dose-dependent inhibition of up to 95% of gastric acid secretion, and a single dose can inhibit acid secretion for 1–2 days. This makes the proton pump inhibitors more efficacious and longer-acting than the H_2-blockers (see Table 28–1).

Indications. Proton pump inhibitors are useful in the treatment of **peptic ulcer disease.** They typically heal 75–80% of peptic ulcers in 4 weeks, whereas H_2-blockers heal about 70% in 4 weeks. Patients who have been treated with proton pump inhibitors appear to relapse at the same rate as those who have been treated with H_2-blockers. Because the recurrence of ulcers is usually due to persistent *H. pylori* infection, experts recommend that proton pump inhibitors be given in combination with drugs that eliminate *H. pylori* infection.

Proton pump inhibitors are the drugs of choice for patients with **Zollinger-Ellison syndrome,** a condition characterized by severe ulcers resulting from **gastrin-secreting tumors (gastrinomas).** Higher doses are required for treating patients with this condition than for treating patients with typical peptic ulcer disease.

Omeprazole and lansoprazole appear to be the most effective drugs for treating **gastroesophageal reflux disease** (GERD).

Adverse Effects. Proton pump inhibitors are usually well tolerated. Minor gastrointestinal and central nervous system side effects have occurred in some patients, and skin rash and elevated hepatic enzyme levels have also been reported. However, patients with GERD have been treated for several years without significant side effects.

Muscarinic Receptor Antagonists

Before H_2-blockers and proton pump inhibitors were developed, **atropine** and other nonselective muscarinic receptor antagonists (see Chapter 7) were used to treat **peptic ulcer disease.** Although administering high doses of atropine can effectively reduce gastric acid secretion, it often causes blurred vision, urinary retention, and other intolerable side effects. Hence, the role of atropine in treating peptic ulcers is currently quite limited.

Unlike atropine, **pirenzepine** is a selective muscarinic M_1 antagonist. Pirenzepine and other selective antagonists are being investigated for ulcer treatment, because they may be able to reduce gastric acid secretion at doses that produce fewer adverse effects than atropine produces. The M_1 receptor appears to mediate the release of histamine from gastric paracrine cells.

Gastric Antacids

Mechanisms and Pharmacologic Effects. Gastric antacids chemically neutralize stomach acid. This raises the gastrointestinal pH sufficiently to relieve the pain of dyspepsia and acid indigestion and to enable peptic ulcers to heal.

Pharmacokinetics and Adverse Effects. The most commonly used antacids are **aluminum and magnesium hydroxides** and **calcium carbonate.** These substances are available in chewable tablets and in liquid suspensions. When used alone, aluminum hydroxide may cause constipation, while magnesium hydroxide often causes diarrhea. For this reason, the combination of aluminum and magnesium hydroxides usually has a relatively neutral effect on gastrointestinal motility. Calcium carbonate may also cause constipation, and large doses of calcium carbonate may lead to a rebound in acid secretion.

Indications. Antacids are available without a prescription and are commonly used to treat **acid indigestion** and **dyspepsia.**

While some studies have shown that antacids can be as effective as acid secretion inhibitors for treating **peptic ulcer disease,** antacids are more difficult for patients to use correctly. For antacids to be effective, they must be taken in large quantities at frequent intervals. For example, 30 mL (1 ounce) of the aluminum and magnesium hydroxide suspension must be taken several times a day (1–3 hours after each meal and at bedtime) for 6–8 weeks. Nocturnal acid secretion is particularly difficult to control with antacids and may require multiple nighttime doses. For these reasons, antacids are not widely employed as the primary treatment for peptic ulcer disease today.

In addition to its utility as a gastric antacid, calcium carbonate is also used as a **calcium supplement.**

CYTOPROTECTIVE DRUGS

Sucralfate and misoprostol both protect the gastrointestinal mucosa, but they do so by different means (see Fig. 28–1).

Sucralfate

Chemistry, Mechanisms, and Pharmacologic Effects. Sucralfate is a viscous polymer of sucrose octasulfate and aluminum hydroxide. This sulfated polysaccharide adheres to ulcer craters and epithelial cells, and it inhibits pepsin-catalyzed hydrolysis of mucosal proteins. Sucralfate also stimulates prostaglandin synthesis in mucosal cells. These actions contribute to the formation of a protective barrier to acid and pepsin and thereby facilitate the healing of ulcers.

Pharmacokinetics. Sucralfate is administered orally as a tablet or suspension. The drug is not absorbed significantly from the gut, and it is primarily excreted in the feces. Patients absorb a small amount of aluminum from the drug, so sucralfate should be used cautiously in patients with renal impairment.

Indications. In the management of **peptic ulcer disease,** sucralfate can be used to treat active ulcers or to suppress the recurrence of ulcers. Because it is somewhat less effective than drugs that inhibit gastric acid secretion, it is primarily used in patients who cannot tolerate H_2-blockers or proton pump inhibitors.

Adverse Effects and Interactions. Although sucralfate causes very few systemic adverse effects, there have been occasional reports of constipation, other gastrointestinal disturbances, and laryngospasm. The use of sucralfate may impair the absorption of other drugs, such as digoxin, fluoroquinolones, ketoconazole, and phenytoin. To prevent this problem, sucralfate should be ingested 2 hours before or after these other drugs are taken.

Misoprostol

As discussed in Chapter 26, misoprostol is a prostaglandin E_1 analogue. The drug exerts a cytoprotective effect by inhibiting gastric acid secretion and promoting the secretion of mucus and bicarbonate. It is primarily indicated for the prevention of **gastric and duodenal ulcers** in patients who are taking NSAIDs on a long-term basis for the treatment of arthritis and other conditions. Because misoprostol is expensive, it is usually reserved for patients at high risk of NSAID-induced ulcers, including the elderly and those with a history of peptic ulcer disease.

Misoprostol is administered orally four times daily with food for the duration of NSAID therapy. Diarrhea and intestinal cramping are the most common adverse effects, but other gastrointestinal reactions may also occur.

Misoprostol can stimulate uterine contractions and induce labor in pregnant women, so its use is contraindicated during pregnancy.

DRUGS FOR *HELICOBACTER PYLORI* INFECTION

The discovery that *H. pylori* plays a role in peptic ulcer disease has led to the development of effective methods to treat infections caused by this bacterium. Single-drug therapy is rarely effective in eradicating *H. pylori* organisms. Therefore, multiple-drug therapy must be used, despite the fact that it is complicated and costly and is sometimes associated with compliance problems and significant side effects.

For the treatment of **peptic ulcer disease,** most regimens include a gastric acid secretion inhibitor (either a proton pump inhibitor or H_2-blocker, as described above) and two or more of the following agents: **amoxicillin, bismuth, clarithromycin, metronidazole,** and **tetracycline.** At the present time, experts recommend that gastric acid secretion inhibitors be given for 6–8 weeks and that antimicrobial agents be given for 2 weeks. Studies indicate that three-drug regimens consisting of one proton pump inhibitor and two antimicrobial agents achieve eradication rates of about 90%. Based on some reports, regimens that include clarithromycin may provide higher eradication rates in a shorter period of time (7–10 days) than do regimens that include antimicrobial agents other than clarithromycin.

The properties of antimicrobial agents are discussed in the chapters of Section VII.

DRUGS FOR INFLAMMATORY BOWEL DISEASES
Glucocorticoids

Hydrocortisone, prednisolone, and other glucocorticoids (see Chapter 33) have been extensively used for the treatment of both **ulcerative colitis** and **Crohn's disease.** In cases of mild ulcerative colitis, they may be effectively administered as rectal enemas. In cases of Crohn's disease or more severe ulcerative colitis, they are usually administered orally or parenterally.

Glucocorticoids are often able to induce the remission of ulcerative colitis or Crohn's disease, but they have proven less valuable in maintaining remission, particularly without causing significant toxicity. The long-term maintenance of remission usually requires treatment with an aminosalicylate.

Aminosalicylates

Sulfasalazine and its active metabolite, **mesalamine,** are used to induce and maintain the remission of inflammatory bowel diseases.

Sulfasalazine has been the foundation of therapy for **ulcerative colitis** for many years, and it is also helpful in the treatment of **Crohn's disease.** The drug is a modified sulfonamide compound (see Chapter 41) and is not well absorbed from the gut. In the gastrointestinal tract, bacteria convert sulfasalazine to 5-aminosalicylic acid (5-ASA, or mesalamine) and sulfapyridine. Although 5-ASA is believed to mediate the inflammatory effects of sulfasalazine, the exact mechanism is uncertain. Some investigators hypothesize that 5-ASA acts by inhibiting prostaglandin synthesis or by inhibiting the migration of inflammatory cells into the bowel wall. Others hypothesize that 5-ASA is a superoxide free radical scavenger.

Mesalamine can be administered as a rectal suppository, rectal suspension, or delayed-release oral tablet. It acts primarily in the gut, but about 15% of the drug is absorbed into the circulation.

Other Agents

Although the primary therapy for inflammatory bowel disease consists of glucocorticoids and aminosalicylates, a few other agents have also been used. **Azathioprine** and **mercaptopurine** are immunosuppressive agents whose use is reserved for the treatment of patients who fail to respond to glucocorticoid therapy. **Metronidazole** is an antimicrobial agent that has demonstrated value in some cases of Crohn's disease and may work by eradicating bacteria that contribute to mucosal inflammation in this disease. **Infliximab** is a monoclonal antibody to tumor necrosis factor alpha (TNF-α), a substance believed to play a role in the pathogenesis of Crohn's disease. According to one study, a single 2-hour intravenous infusion of infliximab resulted in improvement in 82% of patients with moderate to severe Crohn's disease.

PROKINETIC DRUGS

Prokinetic drugs are used in the management of a number of disorders that are characterized by gastrointestinal hypomotility. Prokinetic drugs and laxatives both increase gastrointestinal motility, but they do so by different means. Prokinetic drugs increase the activity of gastrointestinal smooth muscle, particularly in the esophagus, stomach, and small intestine, whereas laxatives stimulate intestinal peristalsis primarily by increasing the amount of water in the intestinal lumen.

The most widely used prokinetic drugs are cisapride, which acts by stimulating **serotonin 5-HT$_4$ receptors,** and metoclopramide, which acts by blocking **dopamine D$_2$ receptors.** Investigators have recently discovered that the antibiotic erythromycin has a prokinetic effect caused by stimulation of **motilin receptors.** While erythromycin is usually not employed as a prokinetic drug, this discovery about its association with motilin, a polypeptide hormone that mediates intestinal smooth muscle contraction, may lead to the development of selective motilin receptor agonists for this purpose.

Cisapride

Chemistry, Mechanisms, and Pharmacologic Effects. Cisapride is a substituted methoxybenzamide drug (see Fig. 28–2C). By stimulating serotonin 5-HT_4 receptors in the enteric nervous system, the drug enhances the release of acetylcholine and increases the activity of esophageal, gastric, and intestinal smooth muscles.

Pharmacokinetics. Cisapride is usually administered orally four times a day (before each meal and at bedtime). After it is absorbed, the drug is metabolized extensively by CYP3A4, a hepatic cytochrome P450 isozyme. The half-life of cisapride is about 9 hours.

Indications. In patients with **gastroesophageal reflux disease** (GERD), cisapride increases pressure in the lower esophageal sphincter and inhibits the reflux of gastric acid into the esophagus. In patients with **diabetic gastroparesis,** the drug increases gastric motility and thereby facilitates gastric emptying and relieves symptoms of nausea, vomiting, and indigestion. It acts similarly in patients with other forms of gastroparesis, including forms resulting from gastric surgery. Cisapride has been used to treat **colonic hypomotility** and **chronic constipation,** but further studies are needed to determine its ultimate role in these disorders.

Adverse Effects and Interactions. Cisapride treatment is associated with a significant incidence of headache, diarrhea, and abdominal pain. Cisapride metabolism can be inhibited by concurrent ingestion of grapefruit or by concurrent administration of drugs such as clarithromycin, erythromycin, itraconazole, ketoconazole, verapamil, zafirlukast, and human immunodeficiency virus (HIV) protease inhibitors. Inhibition of cisapride metabolism may elevate plasma levels of the drug, prolong the QT interval on the electrocardiogram, and precipitate polymorphic ventricular tachycardia (torsade de pointes). For this reason, cisapride should not be used concurrently with drugs that inhibit its metabolism.

Metoclopramide

Mechanisms and Pharmacologic Effects. Metoclopramide is an older prokinetic drug that acts primarily by blocking dopamine D_2 receptors. It is also a weak antagonist at serotonin 5-HT_3 receptors. Metoclopramide blocks presynaptic dopamine receptors that inhibit the release of acetylcholine from cholinergic motor neurons in the enteric nervous system. It thereby promotes the release of acetylcholine and increases stimulation of muscarinic receptors in gastrointestinal smooth muscle. By facilitating normal cholinergic neurotransmission, metoclopramide enhances propulsive activity in a coordinated manner, leading to increased tone and motility in the esophagus and stomach. At the same time, it relaxes the proximal duodenum so that it can accept gastric material as antral contractions arrive at the pyloric sphincter. These actions facilitate gastric emptying.

Pharmacokinetics. Metoclopramide can be administered orally or parenterally. It is rapidly absorbed from the gut and has an average bioavailability of 85%. The drug is conjugated with sulfate and glucuronate, and these metabolites are excreted in the urine, along with 20% of the parent compound. The terminal half-life is about 4 hours.

Indications. Metoclopramide is used to treat **gastroesophageal reflux disease** (GERD), **diabetic gastroparesis,** and **intractable hiccup.** It is sometimes used to facilitate **intubation of the small bowel** during radiologic examination. Metoclopramide serves as a **radiation sensitizer** when it is used in combination with radiation therapy for the treatment of **non–small cell lung cancer.** In addition, metoclopramide exerts **antiemetic effects** by blocking dopamine receptors in the chemoreceptor trigger zone (see the discussion of antiemetics, below).

Adverse Effects. The major adverse effects of metoclopramide are central nervous system reactions such as drowsiness, extrapyramidal effects, and seizures. Hyperprolactinemia, diarrhea, and hematologic toxicity have also been reported. Metoclopramide is contraindicated in persons with seizure disorders, mechanical obstruction of the gastrointestinal tract, gastrointestinal hemorrhage, or pheochromocytoma.

LAXATIVES

Laxatives are drugs that stimulate intestinal peristalsis and increase the movement of material through the bowel. By these actions, laxatives decrease the intestinal transit time and facilitate defecation. Laxatives are used to **treat constipation** and to **evacuate the bowel prior to surgery or diagnostic examination.** They are also used to **eliminate drugs or poisons from the intestinal tract** in cases of drug overdose or poisoning.

Laxatives are classified according to their mechanism of action as bulk-forming, surfactant, osmotic, and stimulant. Lubricant laxatives, such as mineral oil, are essentially obsolete.

Of the various types of laxatives, only the bulk-forming ones can be used on a long-term basis without noticeable side effects. Long-term use of osmotic or stimulant laxatives may lead to electrolyte depletion, serum electrolyte abnormalities, and dependence on laxative use. Patients with renal impairment are particularly susceptible to these adverse effects, because they may not be able to properly excrete osmotic substances that are absorbed into the circulation.

Bulk-Forming Laxatives

Bulk-forming laxatives are undigestible hydrophilic substances, such as **psyllium,** that resemble natural dietary fiber. They induce retention of water in the intestinal lumen and thereby increase the mass of intestinal material. These actions cause mechanical distention of the intestinal wall and stimulate

Agonists

M1 (neura) — modulate neuro tx
M2 (cardia? — ↓ ⊗ rate ↓ cont
M3 (gla) — ↑ smoth musc contr
— ↑ gland secr'ns.

Nm : contraction of muscles
Nn = excite post ganglionic neurons

Antagonists

block above ↗

Mblockers → Belladonna
+ Synthetr

Nblocks → ganglion blocking (Nn)
— neuromuscular block (Nm)

Adre Antagonists Agonists

$\alpha_1 \rightarrow$ smooth musc contrac'!, vasoconstrict

$\alpha_2 \rightarrow$ ↓NE release
↓aqueous humour & cns
↓insulin
↑platelet aggregation

↑cAMP

$B_1 =$ ↑renin , ↑ ♡rate, ♡contra

$B_2 =$ glycogenolysis
= smooth muscle relaxed → vasodilation
bronchodil
= ↑ICF into skeletal muscle

$B_3 =$ lipolysis

$D_1 =$ vasodilation

$D_2 =$ moedul at'r of neurotrans. to sym SNS + CNS

Antag

peristalsis. Bulk-forming laxatives are available in several preparations, including fiber tablets and packets of psyllium granules. They must be taken with a full glass of water to ensure adequate hydration of the preparation and avoid intestinal obstruction. Bulk-forming laxatives are the safest and most physiologic type of laxative, and they rarely cause adverse effects.

Surfactant Laxatives

The surfactant laxatives include **docusate sodium** (dioctyl sodium sulfosuccinate) and other docusate salts. These laxatives are also called **stool softeners** because they facilitate the incorporation of water into fatty intestinal material and thereby soften the feces. Stool softeners are primarily beneficial when fecal materials are hard or dry and when their passage is irritating and painful (as occurs, for example, with anorectal conditions such as hemorrhoids). They are also useful when patients must avoid straining during defecation (for example, after undergoing abdominal or other surgery). Surfactants produce few adverse effects but occasionally cause mild gastrointestinal reactions.

Osmotic (Saline) Laxatives

Osmotic laxatives consist of poorly absorbed inorganic salts, such as **magnesium oxide** (milk of magnesia), **magnesium sulfate** (Epsom salt), and **sodium phosphate.** These substances attract and retain water in the intestinal lumen and increase intraluminal pressure, thereby stimulating peristalsis. They may be taken orally as a liquid or chewable tablet, or they may be administered as an enema. Sufficient doses of osmotic laxatives act rapidly to stimulate defecation. They are often employed to evacuate the bowel in patients scheduled for surgery or diagnostic examination or in patients suffering from drug overdose or poisoning. Lower doses of magnesium oxide can be used to prevent constipation in some patients, such as those receiving opioid analgesics. However, use of osmotic laxatives may lead to excessive loss of fluids and electrolytes, so these laxatives are generally not well suited for the treatment of chronic constipation.

Stimulant (Secretory) Laxatives

The stimulant laxatives include a large group of natural and synthetic compounds that act directly on the intestinal mucosa to alter fluid secretion and stimulate peristalsis. These compounds include **castor oil,** plant extracts of **senna** or **cascara,** and synthetic compounds such as **bisacodyl** (see Fig. 28–2C). Some of these laxatives are frequently used and abused in the treatment of constipation. Bisacodyl is available in oral and rectal suppository formulations that are used in evacuating the bowel prior to surgery or examination. The stimulant laxatives can cause a number of adverse effects, including abdominal cramping and significant electrolyte and fluid depletion.

ANTIDIARRHEAL AGENTS

Diarrhea may be acute or chronic, can range in severity from mild to life-threatening, and has many causes and pathophysiologic mechanisms. For example, **secretory diarrhea** may be caused by microbial toxins, laxatives, vasoactive intestinal polypeptide (VIP) secreted by a pancreatic tumor, excessive bile acids, or unabsorbed fat in malabsorption syndromes (steatorrhea). Most of the mediators of secretory diarrhea act by stimulating cAMP formation or inhibiting membrane Na^+,K^+-ATPase, and this leads to an increase in the secretion of water and electrolytes by the intestinal mucosa. Cholera toxin, for instance, stimulates adenylyl cyclase activity and increases cAMP levels in intestinal cells. This in turn causes active secretion of electrolytes and water into the intestinal lumen. Some mediators of diarrhea also inhibit ion absorption by intestinal cells.

General guidelines for the treatment of diarrhea are outlined at the beginning of this chapter. In cases of severe or chronic diarrhea, efforts should focus on eliminating or controlling the underlying cause and giving appropriate fluid and electrolyte replacement. Antidiarrheal agents may be used as adjuncts to provide symptomatic relief. These agents include systemically acting opioid drugs and locally acting drugs.

Opioid Drugs

The opioids are the most efficacious antidiarrheal drugs. They exert a nonspecific effect that can control diarrhea due to almost any cause. Opioids act by inducing a sustained segmental contraction of intestinal smooth muscle, which prevents the rhythmic waves of contraction and relaxation of smooth muscle that occur with normal peristalsis.

The effects of opioids are mediated by activation of **opioid receptors** in smooth muscle. All of the more potent opioid receptor agonists are effective antidiarrheal compounds. In most cases, the opioid chosen for treatment is one that selectively activates intestinal opioid receptors while having relatively little effect on the central nervous system. **Diphenoxylate** and **loperamide** are the opioid agonists with the greatest ratio of intestinal smooth muscle activity to central nervous system activity, so they are the most widely used opioids for treating diarrhea. Loperamide is available without a prescription and can effectively control mild diarrhea.

Locally Acting Drugs

Several drugs purportedly reduce diarrhea by acting locally within the intestinal tract either to adsorb water and toxins or to inhibit intestinal secretions.

Kaolin-pectin and **polycarbophil** are examples of drugs that adsorb water and toxins. Of the two, polycarbophil appears to be more effective and is the only adsorbent recommended by the Food and Drug Administration panel appointed to review over-the-counter (OTC) drugs.

Bismuth subsalicylate is an example of a drug that inhibits intestinal secretions. It appears to be particularly effective in infectious diarrhea, which often has a strong secretory component. In patients with traveler's diarrhea and other forms of infectious diarrhea, clinical studies demonstrated that bismuth subsalicylate caused a greater reduction in the number of diarrheal episodes than did a placebo. However, bismuth subsalicylate suspension must be given frequently and repeatedly for maximum efficacy (30 mL every 30 minutes for up to eight doses per day). This preparation causes few side effects, but excessively large doses may expose the patient to bismuth or salicylate toxicity.

ANTIEMETICS

Emesis, or **vomiting,** is initiated by a nucleus of cells that is located in the medulla and called the **vomiting center (emesis center).** This center coordinates a complex series of events involving pharyngeal, gastrointestinal, and abdominal wall contractions that lead to expulsion of the gastric contents. These include orally migrating intestinal contractions (reverse peristalsis), gastric contractions, contractions of the diaphragm and abdominal wall, and relaxation of the esophageal sphincter and wall. The reverse intestinal contractions are associated with **nausea,** which is an intensely unpleasant feeling of the imminent need to vomit. Nausea may also occur in the absence of vomiting.

The neural pathways involved in emesis and the sites of antiemetic drug action are shown in Fig. 28–3. The vomiting center may be activated by afferent fibers arising from the gut, **chemoreceptor trigger zone** (CTZ), cerebral cortex, or vestibular apparatus. The CTZ is located in the area postrema and responds to blood-borne substances, including cytotoxic cancer chemotherapy drugs. These substances activate the CTZ via stimulation of **serotonin 5-HT$_3$, dopamine D$_2$, or muscarinic M$_1$ receptors.** The vestibular apparatus activates the vomiting center via fibers that project to the cerebellum and release acetylcholine or histamine. Noxious substances in the gut can activate afferent pathways to the solitary tract nucleus, which projects to the vomiting center, as well as pathways to the nerve tracts that stimulate the CTZ. The D$_2$ and 5-HT$_3$ receptors also have a major role in these pathways.

Most antiemetic drugs act by blocking **dopamine, serotonin, muscarinic, or histamine receptors.** Some drugs appear to inhibit several pathways that lead to vomiting center activation. The D$_2$ and 5-HT$_3$ receptor antagonists inhibit activation of both the CTZ and the solitary tract nucleus. Muscarinic

receptor antagonists may block the CTZ, solitary tract, and vestibular pathways involved in emesis.

Serotonin 5-HT$_3$ Receptor Antagonists

Ondansetron was the first selective 5-HT$_3$ receptor antagonist to be developed for the treatment of cancer chemotherapy–induced nausea and vomiting. It was found to significantly reduce the number of episodes of emesis in patients treated with cisplatin, which is one of the most highly emetogenic chemotherapy agents. **Granisetron** is a newer drug whose clinical efficacy and adverse effect profile appear to be essentially identical to those of ondansetron.

Chemistry, Mechanisms, and Pharmacologic Effects. Granisetron and ondansetron are carbazole derivatives whose structures are similar to the structure of serotonin (see Fig. 28–2A and 28–2B). Each drug competitively blocks 5-HT$_3$ receptors located on visceral afferent nerves in the gastrointestinal tract, in the solitary tract nucleus, and in the CTZ. This enables the drug to prevent both peripheral and central stimulation of the vomiting center.

Pharmacokinetics and Indications. The 5-HT$_3$ receptor antagonists can be administered orally or intravenously. They are extensively metabolized by cytochrome P450, and the metabolites are primarily eliminated in the urine. The half-lives of granisetron and ondansetron are 4 hours and 6 hours, respectively.

Both drugs are primarily used for the prevention and treatment of **cancer chemotherapy–induced emesis.** Ondansetron is also approved for the treatment of **postoperative emesis.** Neither drug is indicated for the treatment of less serious nausea and vomiting, partly because granisetron and ondansetron cost more than other antiemetic drugs.

Oral ondansetron is usually administered just prior to chemotherapy and is continued for 3–5 days after the course of chemotherapy is completed. Other antiemetic drugs appear to exert an additive or synergistic effect in combination with ondansetron. Studies have shown that a combination of ondansetron and dexamethasone, for example, was able to control emesis in persons who had failed to respond to ondansetron alone. Studies have also confirmed the usefulness of ondansetron in controlling postoperative nausea and vomiting. In patients who underwent laparoscopic cholecystectomy, for example, ondansetron was found to be more effective than metoclopramide or a placebo in controlling emesis.

Adverse Effects and Interactions. Granisetron and ondansetron are well tolerated and usually produce few adverse effects. The most common side effects are headache, constipation, and diarrhea. Less common reactions include hypertension and elevated hepatic enzyme levels. In several cases, use of ondansetron resulted in an anaphylactoid reaction consisting of bronchospasm, angioedema, hypotension, and urticaria. Clinically significant drug interactions with 5-HT$_3$ receptor antagonists have not

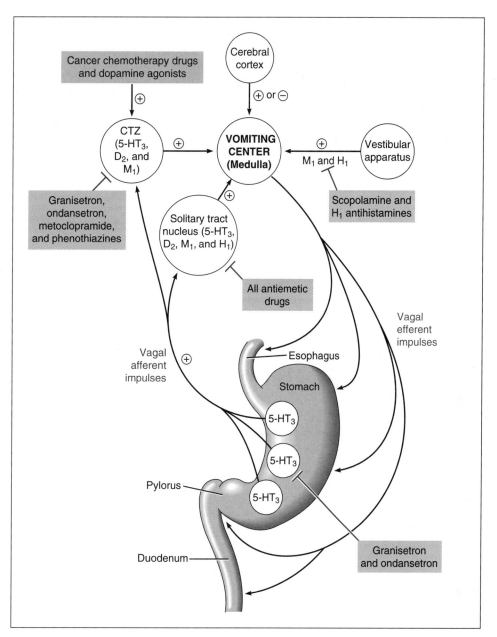

FIGURE 28–3. Physiology of emesis and sites of drug action. Emetic stimuli travel from the gastrointestinal tract via the solitary tract nucleus to arrive at the vomiting center in the medulla. Emetic stimuli also reach the vomiting center via afferent fibers from the chemoreceptor trigger zone (CTZ), cerebral cortex, and vestibular apparatus. Granisetron and ondansetron prevent emesis by blocking serotonin 5-HT$_3$ receptors in the gastrointestinal tract, solitary tract nucleus, and CTZ. Metoclopramide and phenothiazines prevent emesis by blocking dopamine D$_2$ receptors in the solitary tract nucleus and CTZ. Scopolamine and the H$_1$ antihistamines prevent emesis by blocking muscarinic M$_1$ receptors, histamine H$_1$ receptors, or both types of receptors in the vestibular tracts that project to the vomiting center and in the solitary tract nucleus and CTZ. Note that cancer chemotherapy drugs and dopamine agonists cause emesis by stimulating the CTZ.

been identified, although ketoconazole appears to inhibit the metabolism of granisetron.

Dopamine D$_2$ Receptor Antagonists

The D$_2$ receptor antagonists include **prochlorperazine** and a large number of other **phenothiazine drugs.** They also include **metoclopramide.** All of the D$_2$ receptor antagonists appear to act primarily on the CTZ to inhibit stimulation of the vomiting center, but they may also inhibit afferent impulses from the gut by antagonizing receptors in the solitary tract nucleus. In addition to blocking D$_2$ receptors, metoclopramide appears to inhibit vomiting by blocking 5-HT$_3$ receptors in the gut and central nervous system.

The phenothiazines, as a class, have antiemetic, antipsychotic, anticholinergic, antihistamine, and sedative properties (see Chapter 22). Prochlorperazine has been one of the most widely used phenothiazines for the management of **nausea and vomiting in a wide range of clinical applications.** It can be administered parenterally or as a rectal suppository in patients who are unable to take oral medication. In patients with **cancer chemotherapy–induced emesis,** the efficacy of prochlorperazine and other phenothiazines appears to be less than that of ondansetron, dexamethasone, or metoclopramide. Higher doses of phenothiazines are more effective than lower doses but often cause considerable hypotension and extrapyramidal side effects.

Metoclopramide is a D_2 receptor antagonist that also has prokinetic activity (see above). Metoclopramide has been found to be somewhat less effective than ondansetron for the prevention of **cisplatin-induced emesis.**

With the advent of selective 5-HT$_3$ receptor antagonists such as ondansetron, the use of D_2 receptor antagonists for cancer chemotherapy–induced emesis appears to be declining. However, phenothiazine compounds and metoclopramide remain viable options for treating nausea and vomiting due to other causes.

Other Antiemetics

Dronabinol is an oral formulation of Δ^9-tetrahydrocannabinol (THC) and is approved for the treatment of **cancer chemotherapy–induced emesis** when conventional antiemetic drugs have failed. Dronabinol is usually administered several hours before chemotherapy and is then administered every 4–6 hours during a 12-hour period after chemotherapy. The drug probably acts on the vomiting center in the medulla, but its exact site and mechanism of action are uncertain. It has about the same antiemetic efficacy as the phenothiazines, but it is usually less effective than ondansetron or metoclopramide. Dronabinol is also approved as an **appetite stimulant** in acquired immunodeficiency syndrome (AIDS) patients with anorexia.

Several histamine H$_1$ receptor antagonists (H$_1$ antihistamines) have antiemetic actions and are discussed in Chapter 26. Two of these agents, **dimenhydrinate** and **meclizine,** are used in the management of **motion sickness.** Another of these agents, **promethazine,** is an H$_1$ antihistamine that also has significant antimuscarinic activity and is used for the prevention and treatment of **nausea and vomiting** induced by medications and a wide variety of neurologic, psychogenic, and gastrointestinal stimuli. Promethazine is usually administered as a rectal suppository or by injection.

Scopolamine is a muscarinic receptor antagonist that is similar to atropine and is primarily used for the prevention of **motion sickness.** In addition to being used by persons traveling in cars, planes, or boats for extended times, it has been used by astronauts in space. Scopolamine is available as a skin patch that slowly releases the drug over 72 hours.

Summary of Important Points

- Peptic ulcer disease may result from gastrointestinal mucosal damage caused by *H. pylori* infection, decreased prostaglandin synthesis, excessive acid and pepsin production, bile acid reflux, and life-style factors such as smoking and excessive alcohol ingestion.
- Drugs used to treat peptic ulcers include inhibitors of gastric acid secretion, cytoprotective agents, and drugs for *H. pylori* infection. The histamine H$_2$ receptor antagonists (cimetidine, famotidine, ranitidine, and others) and the proton pump inhibitors (lansoprazole and omeprazole) are the primary gastric acid inhibitors. Gastric antacids (aluminum and magnesium hydroxides and calcium carbonate) are also used.
- The H$_2$ receptor antagonists inhibit basal and meal-stimulated acid secretion and can be used to treat gastroesophageal reflux disease (GERD) and dyspepsia as well as peptic ulcer disease. Cimetidine inhibits cytochrome P450 isozymes and may increase the plasma concentrations of many other drugs, leading to potential toxicity. Other H$_2$ receptor antagonists usually do not cause such interactions.
- Lansoprazole and omeprazole irreversibly inhibit the proton pump (H$^+$,K$^+$-ATPase) and acid secretion. They are the most efficacious drugs for treating GERD, and they are the drugs of choice for use in patients with gastrin-secreting tumors (gastrinomas) and Zollinger-Ellison syndrome.
- Sucralfate is a cytoprotective drug that binds to the ulcer crater and forms a barrier to acid and pepsin. Misoprostol is a prostaglandin E$_1$ analogue that increases the production of mucus and bicarbonate while reducing the secretion of gastric acid. Misoprostol is used to prevent ulcers caused by long-term therapy with nonsteroidal anti-inflammatory drugs (NSAIDs).
- Amoxicillin, bismuth, clarithromycin, metronidazole, and tetracycline are the most commonly used drugs for *H. pylori* infection. They are usually given in combination with a gastric acid secretion inhibitor for the treatment of peptic ulcer disease.
- Inflammatory bowel diseases (ulcerative colitis and Crohn's disease) are primarily treated with glucocorticoids and aminosalicylates (sulfasalazine and mesalamine).
- Prokinetic drugs increase gastrointestinal motility and are used to treat GERD, diabetic gastroparesis, and other disorders. Cisapride activates serotonin 5-HT$_4$ receptors, while metoclopramide inhibits dopamine D$_2$ receptors. Both drugs facilitate the release of acetylcholine from enteric system neurons and thereby increase coordinated smooth muscle contractions.
- Laxatives are drugs used to facilitate defecation and evacuate the bowels. They include bulk-forming laxatives (psyllium), surfactant laxatives (docusate sodium), osmotic laxatives (magnesium oxide, magnesium sulfate, and sodium phosphate), and stimulant laxatives (bisacodyl and many others). Bulk-forming laxatives are preferred for the treatment of chronic constipation. Osmotic and stimulant laxatives are used to clear the bowels of patients preparing for intestinal surgery or diagnostic examination and patients being treated for a drug overdose or poisoning.
- Opioids are the most efficacious antidiarrheal drugs. Loperamide and diphenoxylate cause lit-

tle or no central nervous system effects at doses that control diarrhea.

- Serotonin 5-HT$_3$ receptor antagonists (granisetron and ondansetron) are the most efficacious antiemetics for the management of cancer chemotherapy–induced nausea and vomiting. Metoclopramide and other D$_2$ receptor antagonists, such as prochlorperazine, are also effective antiemetics. Promethazine, a highly sedating histamine H$_1$ receptor antagonist, is often used for mild nausea and vomiting. Motion sickness can be prevented by meclizine, a less-sedating H$_1$ receptor antagonist, or by scopolamine, a muscarinic receptor antagonist.

Selected Readings

Brynskov, J., and S. N. Rasmussen. Clinical pharmacology in gastroenterology: development of new forms of treatment for inflammatory bowel disease. Scand J Gastroenterol 216(supplement):175–180, 1996.

Campieri, M., et al. Oral budesonide is as effective as oral prednisolone in active Crohn's disease. Gut 41:209–214, 1997.

Fass, R., et al. Contemporary medical therapy for gastroesophageal reflux disease. Am Fam Physician 55:205–218, 1997.

Galmiche, J. P., et al. Treating the symptoms of gastroesophageal reflux disease: a double-blind comparison of omeprazole and cisapride. Aliment Pharmacol Ther 11:765–773, 1997.

Hoffman, J. S. Pharmacologic therapy of *Helicobacter pylori* infection. Semin Gastrointest Dis 8:156–163, 1997.

Langtry, H. D., and M. I. Wilde. Lansoprazole: an update of its pharmacologic properties and clinical efficacy in the management of acid-related disorders. Drugs 54:473–500, 1997.

Marcon, M. A. Advances in the diagnosis and treatment of gastroesophageal reflux disease. Curr Opin Pediatr 9:490–493, 1997.

Perez, E. A. A risk-benefit assessment of serotonin 5-HT$_3$ receptor antagonists in antineoplastic therapy–induced emesis. Drug Saf 18:43–56, 1998.

Pipkin, G. A., et al. Clarithromycin dual-therapy regimens for eradication of *Helicobacter pylori:* a review. Helicobacter 2:159–171, 1997.

Schepp, W. Proton pump inhibitory therapy: then and now. Yale J Biol Med 69:175–186, 1996.

Veyrat-Follet, C., et al. Physiology of chemotherapy-induced emesis and antiemetic therapy. Drugs 53:206–234, 1997.

Walker, A. M., et al. 5-Aminosalicylates, sulfasalazine, steroid use, and complications in patients with ulcerative colitis. Am J Gastroenterol 92:816–820, 1997.

CHAPTER TWENTY-NINE

DRUGS FOR HEADACHE DISORDERS

CLASSIFICATION OF DRUGS FOR HEADACHE DISORDERS*

DRUGS FOR MIGRAINE HEADACHES
Drugs for preventing headaches
  Anticonvulsants and antidepressants
- Amitriptyline
- Fluoxetine
- Phenelzine
- Valproate

  Nonsteroidal anti-inflammatory drugs
- Naproxen

  β-Adrenergic receptor antagonists
- Timolol

  Calcium channel blockers
- Verapamil

  Serotonin 5-HT₂ receptor antagonists
- Methysergide

Drugs for aborting headaches
  Serotonin 5-HT$_{1D/1B}$ receptor agonists
- Dihydroergotamine
- Ergotamine
- Naratriptan
- Rizatriptan
- Sumatriptan
- Zolmitriptan

  Other drugs
- Isometheptene
- Naproxen
- Tramadol

DRUGS FOR OTHER HEADACHES
See Table 29–1

*Note that some drugs are listed more than once.

OVERVIEW

The International Headache Society divides headache disorders into two large groups. The first consists of **primary headache disorders** and includes **cluster, migraine, and tension headaches.** The characteristics and management of these three types of headaches, which together account for 97–98% of all headaches, are compared in Table 29–1. The second group consists of **secondary headache disorders,** which arise from organic disorders (such as hemorrhage, infection, neuropathy, stroke, and tumor) and are responsible for the remaining 2–3% of headaches. In patients with secondary headaches, management focuses on treating the underlying disorder.

Because migraine is the most common headache disorder, it is the focus of this chapter.

CHARACTERISTICS AND PATHOGENESIS OF MIGRAINE HEADACHES

In the USA, approximately 24 million people suffer from migraine headache disorder. The pathophysiologic mechanisms of the disorder are not completely understood, but the headaches appear to result from neurovascular dysfunction caused by an imbalance between excitatory and inhibitory neuronal activity at various levels in the central nervous system (CNS). This imbalance may be triggered by hormones, stress, fatigue, hunger, and circulating food- or drug-derived substances.

About 15% of patients who have migraine headache disorder report that they experience an **aura** that precedes each headache attack and lasts for about 15–20 minutes. A **visual aura** may take the form of brightly flashing lights or rippling images that spread from the corner of the visual field (teichopsia). A **sensory aura** may take the form of a paresthesia that involves the arm and face and tends to "march" sequentially from the fingers to the hand and then to the body. Auras are believed to result from the cerebral vasoconstriction and ischemia that precipitate migraine attacks. A migraine without an aura (previously known as a common migraine) is often accompanied by an attack of photophobia, phonophobia, nausea, or vomiting.

Each migraine attack has two phases. The **first phase** is characterized by **cerebral vasoconstriction** and **ischemia.** The release of **serotonin,** or 5-hydroxytryptamine (5-HT), from CNS neurons and circulating platelets contributes to this phase. Hence, antiplatelet drugs and serotonin receptor antagonists have demonstrated efficacy in the prevention of migraine headaches. The **second phase** is longer than the first one and is characterized by **cerebral vasodilation** and **pain.** The trigeminal neurovascular system appears to play a central role in the second phase. Neurons in the trigeminal complex release various peptides, including **substance P** and **calcitonin gene–related peptide** (CGRP). The peptides trigger vasodilation and inflammation of pial and dural vessels, and this in turn stimulates nociceptive fibers of the trigeminal nerve and causes pain.

TABLE 29–1. Classification and Pharmacologic Management of Headache Disorders*

Classification	Characteristics	Drugs for Preventing Headaches	Drugs for Aborting Headaches
Primary headaches			
Cluster headaches	Severe, unilateral, retro-orbital; clustered over time.	Lithium, methysergide, and verapamil.	DHE, ergotamine, glucocorticoids, lidocaine, oxygen, and sumatriptan.
Migraine headaches	Moderate or severe, often unilateral, usually pulsatile; occur with or without aura.	β-Adrenergic receptor antagonists, anticonvulsants, antidepressants, calcium channel blockers, NSAIDs, and serotonin 5-HT₂ receptor antagonists.	DHE, ergotamine, isometheptene, NSAIDs, tramadol, and triptans.†
Tension headaches	Mild or moderate, bilateral, nonpulsatile; exert bandlike pressure.	Amitriptyline.	Muscle relaxants and NSAIDs.
Secondary headaches	Characteristics vary, depending on the underlying cause.‡	None.	None (treat underlying disorder).

*DHE = dihydroergotamine; and NSAIDs = nonsteroidal anti-inflammatory drugs.
†Triptans include naratriptan, rizatriptan, sumatriptan, and zolmitriptan.
‡Examples of causes are hemorrhage, infection, neuropathy, stroke, and tumor.

Fig. 29–1 depicts these events and the mechanisms of drugs that are used to terminate migraine headaches.

DRUGS FOR MIGRAINE HEADACHES

The drugs used to manage patients with migraine headaches can be classified as **prophylactic drugs** and **abortive (symptomatic) drugs.** Many prophylactic drugs act by preventing the vasoconstrictive phase of the disorder, whereas abortive drugs reverse the vasodilative phase of migraine or relieve pain and inflammation.

Several drugs for migraine are antagonists or agonists at specific types of **serotonin receptors.** These receptors have been classified into four main types, 5-HT₁ through 5-HT₄.

The **5-HT₂ receptors** are widely distributed in the CNS, smooth muscle, and platelets, where they mediate vasoconstriction and platelet aggregation. Drugs that block 5-HT₂ receptors, such as methysergide, can prevent the vasoconstrictive phase of migraine and are used as migraine prophylactics.

The **5-HT₁ receptors** are the predominant serotonin receptors in the CNS, and many of them function as presynaptic autoreceptors whose activation inhibits the release of serotonin and other neurotransmitters. The 5-HT₁ receptors also mediate cerebral vasoconstriction. Drugs that activate these receptors, such as sumatriptan, are used to terminate a migraine attack.

Drugs for Preventing Headaches

Numerous classes of drugs are used to prevent migraine headaches in persons who experience frequent attacks. These include anticonvulsants, antidepressants, anti-inflammatory drugs, β-adrenergic receptor antagonists, calcium channel blockers, and

serotonin receptor antagonists. A trial of several different types of drugs may be useful to determine the most effective drug for a particular patient. Each drug requires several weeks of therapy before its effectiveness can be observed.

Anticonvulsants and Antidepressants

The properties of anticonvulsants and antidepressants are described in Chapters 20 and 22, respectively. Studies have shown that these two classes of drugs are able to prevent migraine in some persons, but the mechanisms underlying their effect are poorly understood.

Valproate (divalproex) is the most widely used anticonvulsant for migraine prophylaxis. Its onset of efficacy (2–3 weeks) is somewhat shorter than that of other prophylactic drugs. Its common adverse effects include sedation, tremor, and weight gain.

Three types of antidepressants can be used to prevent migraine. The first consists of selective serotonin reuptake inhibitors (SSRIs), such as **fluoxetine.** The second consists of tricyclic antidepressants. In this second group, tertiary amines such as **amitriptyline** are more potent inhibitors of serotonin reuptake and may be more effective in preventing migraine than are secondary amines such as desipramine. The third group consists of monoamine oxidase (MAO) inhibitors, such as **phenelzine.** MAO inhibitors are able to block serotonin degradation and are occasionally used in persons who fail to respond to other antidepressants.

Patients must take antidepressants for 3–4 weeks before the drugs become effective in preventing headaches or in alleviating the symptoms of depression. The inhibition of serotonin reuptake by the antidepressants leads to down-regulation of postsynaptic serotonin receptors and a compensatory in-

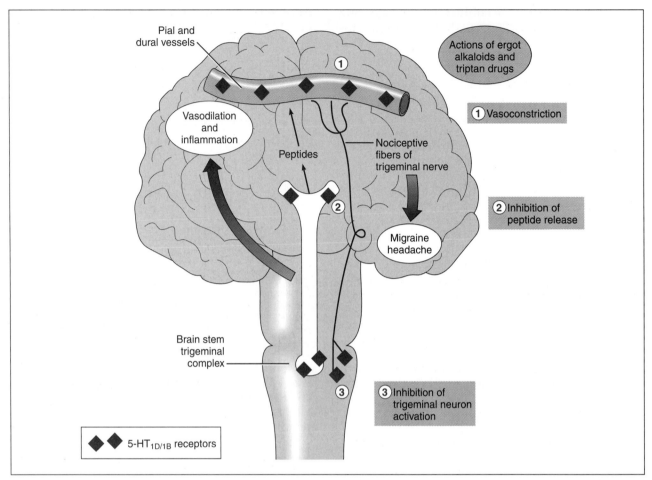

FIGURE 29–1. Mechanisms of ergot alkaloids and triptan drugs used in the treatment of migraine headache disorder. Migraine attacks are thought to result from trigeminal neurovascular dysfunction. When neurons in the trigeminal complex release peptides such as substance P and calcitonin gene–related peptide (CGRP), this causes vasodilation and inflammation of pial and dural vessels. These events activate nociceptive trigeminal fibers and cause the moderate to severe pain that is characteristic of migraine headaches. Ergot alkaloids and triptan drugs terminate the pain by activating serotonin 5-HT$_{1D/1B}$ receptors at several sites: (1) They activate receptors on pial and dural vessels and thereby cause vasoconstriction. (2) They activate presynaptic receptors so as to inhibit the release of peptides and other mediators from trigeminal neurons. (3) They activate receptors in the brain stem, and this is believed to inhibit activation of trigeminal neurons responsible for migraine attacks.

crease in the firing rate of serotonin neurons. However, the relationship between these actions and migraine prophylaxis has not been clearly established.

SSRIs sometimes cause anxiety, insomnia, tremor, anorexia, and sexual dysfunction. Tricyclic antidepressants may cause drowsiness, tremor, and anticholinergic effects such as dry mouth, blurred vision, and urinary retention. MAO inhibitors may cause a hypertensive crisis if they are taken with tyramine-containing foods or with sympathomimetic amine drugs.

Nonsteroidal Anti-inflammatory Drugs

Nonsteroidal anti-inflammatory drugs (NSAIDs), including **naproxen,** can be used for the prevention and treatment of migraine. As discussed in Chapter 30, these drugs act by blocking thromboxane synthesis and platelet aggregation and thereby reducing the

release of serotonin. NSAIDs may be used continuously or on an intermittent basis for the prevention of predictable headaches. For example, administration beginning 1 week before menses and continuing through menstruation may prevent associated migraine headaches.

β-Adrenergic Receptor Antagonists

Of the various types of β-adrenergic receptor antagonists that are available (see Chapter 9), only the β-blockers that lack intrinsic sympathomimetic activity are effective for the prevention of migraine headaches. One example of these β-blockers is **timolol.** Another example, propranolol, has been widely used for migraine prophylaxis but may cause more CNS side effects than timolol.

The mechanism of action of β-blockers in migraine prophylaxis is uncertain. The drugs may attenuate the vasodilative phase of migraine by blocking β_2-mediated vasodilation. They may also reduce platelet aggregation and thereby decrease the release of serotonin from platelets.

Calcium Channel Blockers

Although **verapamil** and other calcium channel blockers have been used for migraine prophylaxis, some authorities believe that the calcium channel blockers are less effective in preventing migraine attacks than are other classes of drugs.

Calcium channel blockers probably act by preventing the vasoconstrictive phase of migraine headaches. The properties of these drugs are described in Chapter 10.

Serotonin 5-HT$_2$ Receptor Antagonists

Methysergide is a drug that blocks 5-HT$_2$ receptors and thereby prevents the vasoconstrictive phase of migraine from occurring. However, because of the drug's potential toxicity, other prophylactic drugs are usually chosen initially for migraine prophylaxis.

The properties of methysergide are discussed in Chapter 26. The drug is associated with a number of relatively mild adverse effects, including abdominal pain, weight gain, and hallucinations. It is also associated with a risk of life-threatening retroperitoneal, pleural, and cardiac valve fibrosis. For this reason, it should not be used longer than 6 months without a 1-month drug-free period initiated by a 2-week taper of the drug dosage. Serum creatinine measurements should be monitored and chest x-rays should be taken to detect early signs of fibrosis in patients treated with methysergide.

Drugs for Aborting Headaches

Numerous drugs can be used to terminate a migraine headache after it has begun. Most of these drugs are serotonin 5-HT$_{1D/1B}$ receptor agonists, and their sites of action are shown in Fig. 29–1. The structures of serotonin and two of the receptor agonists are illustrated in Fig. 29–2A and 29–2B.

Serotonin 5-HT$_{1D/1B}$ Receptor Agonists
Ergotamine and Dihydroergotamine

Ergotamine and dihydroergotamine (DHE) are **ergot alkaloids** that are effective in the treatment of migraine headaches and cluster headaches. A number of other ergot alkaloids are available and are used in the treatment of Parkinson's disease, hyperprolactinemia, and other disorders.

Chemistry and Mechanisms. Like other ergot alkaloids, ergotamine and DHE are isolated from *Claviceps purpurea,* a fungus that grows primarily on rye. Ergotamine and DHE relieve migraine primarily by activating serotonin 5-HT$_{1D/1B}$ receptors at several levels in the trigeminal neurovascular system. Activa-

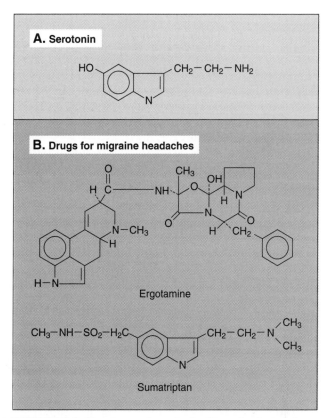

FIGURE 29–2. Structures of serotonin (A) and selected drugs for migraine headaches (B). Serotonin is also called 5-hydroxytryptamine (5-HT). Ergotamine is an ergot alkaloid, and sumatriptan is a structural analogue of serotonin. Both drugs are serotonin 5-HT$_{1D/1B}$ receptor agonists.

tion of 5-HT$_{1D/1B}$ receptors in cerebral blood vessels produces vasoconstriction, thereby reversing the vasodilation that contributes to the throbbing migraine headache. Stimulation of presynaptic 5-HT$_{1D/1B}$ receptors on trigeminal nerve endings inhibits the release of peptides that cause vasodilation, neurogenic inflammation, and pain. Finally, stimulation of 5-HT$_{1D/1B}$ receptors in the brain stem prevents activation of trigeminal nerves involved in migraine headache.

Pharmacokinetic and Pharmacologic Effects. The ergot alkaloids are most effective when they are given early in a migraine attack.

Ergotamine is marketed in parenteral, oral, and rectal formulations. When it is given orally, it has a relatively slow onset of action because of its poor oral bioavailability. Although it is available as a rectal suppository for use by persons with nausea and vomiting, it may actually worsen these symptoms by stimulating the vomiting center. Some oral and rectal ergotamine preparations contain caffeine, which appears to increase the absorption of ergotamine and may exert a mild vasoconstrictive effect that helps relieve migraine.

DHE is available in intranasal and injectable preparations. The intranasal preparation, which was recently approved, offers patients a convenient method of administering DHE and has a moderately rapid onset of action. The injectable DHE preparation is usually more rapid-acting and reliable than the various ergotamine preparations and can be administered subcutaneously, intramuscularly, or intravenously. When administered parenterally, DHE is often given with an antiemetic drug, such as metoclopramide, to prevent drug-induced nausea and vomiting.

Adverse Effects. The relatively mild adverse effects of ergot alkaloids include nausea and vomiting, diarrhea, muscle cramps, cold skin, paresthesias, and vertigo.

Ergotamine and DHE may cause peripheral vasoconstriction by stimulating α-adrenergic receptors and by directly stimulating vascular smooth muscle. These drugs are therefore contraindicated in persons with coronary artery disease or peripheral vascular disease. Excessive doses of ergotamine or DHE may cause severe cerebral vasoconstriction, ischemia, and rebound vasodilation and headache. A rebound headache may last several days, and hospitalization may be required to wean the patient from ergotamine and alleviate the pain. Strict dosage guidelines must be followed to prevent rebound headache and other forms of toxicity. To prevent cumulative toxicity, daily use of ergotamine should be avoided.

Interactions. Concomitant use of ergot alkaloids and β-adrenergic receptor antagonists may cause severe peripheral ischemia resulting from α-mediated vasoconstriction that is unopposed by β_2-mediated vasodilation. Hence, this drug combination should be used with caution.

Sumatriptan, Naratriptan, Rizatriptan, and Zolmitriptan

Sumatriptan was the first of a new group of selective serotonin 5-HT$_{1D/1B}$ agonists to be developed. These so-called **triptan drugs** include naratriptan, rizatriptan, and zolmitriptan. The newer triptans are quite similar to sumatriptan, but their improved pharmacokinetic properties may be advantageous in some cases.

Chemistry and Mechanisms. Sumatriptan and other 5-HT$_{1D/1B}$ agonists are structural analogues of serotonin (see Fig. 29–2). Their mechanisms for terminating migraine headaches appear to be similar to those of ergotamine and DHE (see above).

Pharmacokinetic and Pharmacologic Effects. A sumatriptan preparation for subcutaneous administration was introduced in 1992, and oral and intranasal preparations were introduced several years later. Peak plasma levels of sumatriptan are achieved most rapidly with subcutaneous administration and least rapidly with oral administration. Relief of migraine usually takes an hour when the drug is given subcutaneously but takes up to 3 hours when it is given orally.

Naratriptan, rizatriptan, and zolmitriptan are currently limited to oral administration. In comparison with sumatriptan, these newer triptan drugs are more lipophilic, have higher oral bioavailabilities,

and achieve higher concentrations in the CNS. The fact that they penetrate the CNS more readily may enable them to inhibit the brain stem mechanisms involved in migraine more effectively than does sumatriptan.

In a clinical trial comparing the effects of sumatriptan treatment with those of DHE treatment in patients who suffer from migraine headache disorder, subcutaneously administered sumatriptan was found to relieve 85% of migraine attacks and to be slightly superior to DHE in this regard. Nevertheless, studies show that sumatriptan is not efficacious in 10–20% of patients who have migraine headache disorder, and about 40% of patients who initially obtain relief with sumatriptan have a recurrence of their headache on the same day. Recurrences are more prevalent in patients who have more severe and longer attacks. If a headache recurs, treatment can be repeated at specified intervals until a maximum daily dose has been administered. Because sumatriptan and other triptan drugs cost more than ergotamine alkaloids, the need to repeat doses is an important consideration in drug selection.

According to some clinical trials, the newer triptans have a 10–20% greater efficacy than sumatriptan, and their rates of headache recurrence are smaller (30% for newer triptans versus 40% for sumatriptan). Naratriptan has a longer half-life than sumatriptan, and this may explain its lower rate of headache recurrence. Further clinical studies are needed to confirm these differences.

Adverse Effects and Interactions. In clinical trials, the incidence of chest tightness, weakness, somnolence, and dizziness in subjects treated with a triptan was 50%, while the incidence in subjects treated with a placebo was 30%. The incidence of adverse effects appears to be similar for all triptan drugs.

The triptans have been reported to cause abnormal tingling or burning sensations in the skin covering various parts of the body. These sensations are benign, but they may be mistaken for a serious adverse effect by the patient.

Triptan drugs may cause coronary vasospasm and should not be used in patients with a history of angina pectoris, myocardial infarction, or other coronary artery disease. The triptans should not be used concurrently with MAO inhibitors, nor should they be used within 24 hours of administering an ergot alkaloid or methysergide.

Other Drugs for Aborting Headaches

An NSAID such as **naproxen** can be used either to prevent or abort a migraine attack.

Isometheptene is an agent that acts as a sympathomimetic and is able to terminate migraine headaches. It is available in a preparation that also contains acetaminophen and a mild sedative drug.

Opioid analgesics are able to relieve the pain of migraine headaches, but their use should be reserved for patients in whom other agents are contraindicated or ineffective. **Tramadol** has been particularly useful in chronic pain syndromes (see Chapter 23) and is one of the most widely used opioid drugs for the treatment of migraine. Tramadol acts as an agonist at opioid receptors, and it also inhibits norepinephrine and serotonin reuptake in the CNS. The latter action may contribute to the drug's analgesic effect.

GUIDELINES FOR MANAGING MIGRAINE HEADACHES
Prophylactic Therapy

Nonpharmacologic measures can play a significant role in the prevention of migraine attacks. These measures include appropriate patient education; the identification and avoidance of factors that contribute to migraine attacks, including particular foods, beverages, and environmental factors; biofeedback and relaxation therapy; and psychotherapy. Acupuncture and physiotherapy may be beneficial, but their efficacy has not been established in controlled trials.

Many pharmacologic agents are known to prevent migraine attacks. However, the efficacy of these agents varies from patient to patient, so finding a drug that works well is largely a matter of trial and error. The characteristics of individual patients should help guide drug selection. For example, β-blockers have negative effects on cardiac output, so they are usually less suitable than other drugs for competitive athletes. The goal of prophylactic drug use is to reduce the frequency of migraine attacks by at least 50%, and the criteria for evaluating the efficacy of particular drugs should be clearly established and understood by the physician and patient. It usually takes 3–4 weeks of therapy before the benefit of a given drug is observed, so authorities recommend a trial of 4–6 weeks before switching to another drug.

Abortive Therapy

The ideal drug to terminate migraine headaches would act rapidly, be highly efficacious, and have a low potential to cause serious adverse effects. No available drug meets all of these criteria. The newer serotonin agonists (triptans) appear to be less toxic and slightly more effective than the ergot preparations. However, DHE has the advantage of a longer duration of action than the triptan drugs. Intranasal preparations of sumatriptan and DHE offer a more rapid onset of action than do oral preparations, and they are more convenient than parenteral therapy.

The optimal use of abortive treatment requires prudent drug selection and reasonable restrictions on drug use to avoid toxicity or habituation. The effectiveness of a given drug varies widely from patient to patient, so a judicious trial of several drugs is usually required to determine the most effective drug for a particular patient. Some authorities recommend starting abortive therapy with an NSAID such as naproxen. If use of an NSAID consistently fails

to relieve pain within an hour, then the patient should be encouraged to switch to a different agent, such as tramadol, a triptan drug, or DHE. While this approach may work well for some patients, others may derive more benefit from the initial use of a triptan or DHE. To evaluate the effects of drug therapy, the patient should be instructed to keep an accurate log of drug dosage and symptom severity, especially during a trial period.

The overuse of abortive drugs can lead to serious toxicity, so patients must be properly instructed about limiting their use of these drugs. According to the guidelines of the National Headache Foundation, patients should limit their use of ergotamine to 8 treatment days per month, with an ample interval between treatment days. They should limit their use of sumatriptan and other triptan drugs to 6 treatment days per month and 2 treatment days per week, and they should limit their use of opioid drugs to 2 treatment days per week.

CHARACTERISTICS AND MANAGEMENT OF CLUSTER HEADACHES

Cluster headaches are severe, unilateral, retro-orbital headaches that tend to group or cluster over time. Patients often describe a searing or burning pain that arises behind one eye, occurs without warning, and can be excruciating. Pain often lasts from 15 minutes to 3 hours and usually occurs at the same time each day. Unlike patients with migraine headaches, who are highly sensitive to movement and external stimuli, those with cluster headaches often pace in an agitated fashion, apply pressure to the orbit, or even strike the face to provide distraction from the pain. Fortunately, the incidence of cluster headache disorder is quite low, affecting less than 0.5% of the population.

Drugs to prevent cluster headaches include lithium (see Chapter 22), methysergide, and verapamil. Like migraine headaches, cluster headaches can be aborted by administering DHE, ergotamine, or sumatriptan. Other agents that are effective in aborting cluster headaches include inhaled oxygen, intranasal lidocaine, and glucocorticoids. Guidelines for selecting drugs to manage cluster headaches are similar to those outlined above for migraine headaches.

CHARACTERISTICS AND MANAGEMENT OF TENSION HEADACHES

Tension headaches are characterized by bilateral, nonpulsatile, bandlike pressure that is mild or moderate in intensity. This common type of headache often responds to physiologic approaches that correct cervical or dental alignment or visual refractive error. Nonpharmacologic therapies such as biofeedback, acupuncture, and physiotherapy are also useful in controlling both episodic and chronic tension headaches. Pharmacologic therapy usually consists of NSAIDs and muscle relaxants, but patients with chronic tension headaches may also respond to prophylactic use of amitriptyline. This drug is usually tolerated better when therapy is initiated with a low dose at bedtime and the dosage is gradually increased over a period of several weeks.

Summary of Important Points

- Migraine, the most common headache disorder, is believed to result from neurovascular dysfunction at several levels in the central nervous system. Cerebral vasoconstriction and ischemia are followed by vasodilation, inflammation, and a unilateral, pulsatile headache.
- Drugs for migraine prophylaxis should aim to reduce the frequency of migraine attacks by 50%. These include anticonvulsants (valproate), antidepressants (amitriptyline and fluoxetine), nonsteroidal anti-inflammatory drugs (NSAIDs, such as naproxen), β-adrenergic receptor antagonists (timolol), calcium channel blockers (verapamil), and serotonin 5-HT$_2$ receptor antagonists (methysergide). Prophylactic drugs often must be taken for 3–4 weeks before benefits are observed.
- Drugs for aborting migraine headaches include ergot alkaloids (ergotamine and dihydroergotamine) and so-called triptan drugs (sumatriptan and others). These drugs act primarily by stimulating serotonin 5-HT$_{1D/1B}$ receptors. This stimulation causes cerebral vasoconstriction, inhibits the release of peptides and other mediators of inflammation and vasodilation from trigeminal neurons, and inhibits activation of the trigeminal nucleus in the brain stem.
- Ergot alkaloids and triptan drugs can cause marked vasoconstriction, so their dosage and frequency of use must be restricted to avoid rebound headache and adverse effects. Common adverse effects of ergots include nausea, vomiting, and muscle cramps; those of triptans include chest tightness and drowsiness. Use of ergots or triptans is contraindicated in patients with coronary artery disease.
- Other agents for aborting migraine headaches include NSAIDs, such as naproxen; opioid analgesics, such as tramadol; and a sympathomimetic drug called isometheptene.
- Cluster headaches can be prevented with lithium, methysergide, or verapamil. They can be terminated with ergot alkaloids, sumatriptan, inhaled oxygen, intranasal lidocaine, or glucocorticoids.
- Tension headaches often respond to NSAIDs and muscle relaxants. Nonpharmacologic therapies, such as biofeedback and physiotherapy, are also useful.

Selected Readings

Deleu, D., et al. Symptomatic and prophylactic treatment of migraine: a critical reappraisal. Clin Neuropharmacol 21:267–279, 1998.

Jackson, C. M. Effective headache management: strategies to help patients gain control over pain. Postgrad Med 104:133–136, 1998.

Mathew, N. T. Serotonin 1D (5-HT$_{1D}$) agonists and other agents in acute migraine. Neurol Clin 15:61–83, 1997.

Saper, J. R. Diagnosis and symptomatic treatment of migraine. Headache 37(supplement 1):S1–S14, 1997.

Schoenen, J. Acute migraine therapy: the newer drugs. Curr Opin Neurol 10:237–243, 1997.

Solomon, G. D., et al. National Headache Foundation: Standards of care for treating headache in primary care practice. Cleve Clin J Med 64:373–383, 1997.

Solomon, S., et al. The site of common side effects of sumatriptan. Headache 37:289–290, 1997.

CHAPTER THIRTY

DRUGS FOR PAIN, INFLAMMATION,

AND ARTHRITIC DISORDERS

CLASSIFICATION OF DRUGS FOR PAIN, INFLAMMATION, AND ARTHRITIC DISORDERS*

NONSTEROIDAL ANTI-INFLAMMATORY DRUGS
Nonselective cyclooxygenase inhibitors
- Acetaminophen
- Aspirin and other salicylates
- Ibuprofen
- Indomethacin
- Ketoprofen
- Ketorolac
- Naproxen

Selective cyclooxygenase-2 inhibitors
- Celecoxib

DISEASE-MODIFYING ANTIRHEUMATIC DRUGS
Gold salts
- Auranofin
- Gold sodium thiomalate

Glucocorticoids
- Prednisone

Other disease-modifying antirheumatic drugs
- Etanercept
- Hydroxychloroquine
- Infliximab
- Leflunomide
- Methotrexate

DRUGS FOR GOUT
Drugs for preventing gout attacks
- Allopurinol
- Probenecid

Drugs for treating gout attacks
- Colchicine
- Indomethacin and other nonsteroidal anti-inflammatory drugs

*Note that some drugs are listed more than once.

OVERVIEW

A variety of medical disorders and injuries are characterized by pain and inflammation. This chapter describes the pharmacologic properties of nonsteroidal anti-inflammatory drugs (NSAIDs), which are widely used to alleviate the symptoms of rheumatoid arthritis, osteoarthritis, and gout, as well as to relieve the pain and fever that accompany many nonarthritic disorders. The chapter also discusses disease-modifying antirheumatic drugs (DMARDs) and drugs for the prevention and treatment of gout.

Rheumatoid Arthritis

Rheumatoid arthritis affects 2–3% of the population in the USA, making it the most common systemic inflammatory disease. It is three times more common in women than in men and is characterized by symmetric joint inflammation. The joints that are most frequently affected are the small joints of the hands, wrists, and feet, but the joints of the ankles, elbows, hips, knees, and shoulders may also be involved. Cardiopulmonary, neurologic, and ocular inflammation are commonly found in patients with rheumatoid arthritis, and many patients develop rheumatoid nodules on the extensor surfaces of the elbows, forearms, and hands. In addition, many patients have extraarticular manifestations, such as vasculitis, lymphadenopathy, and splenomegaly.

The etiology of rheumatoid arthritis is unknown. Although infectious agents have been postulated to cause the disease, none of them have been isolated from tissues of affected patients. Studies have demonstrated, however, that most patients express specific human lymphocyte antigens in the major histocompatibility complex located on T lymphocytes. As shown in Fig. 30–1, rheumatoid arthritis is believed to involve autoimmune mechanisms that lead to the destruction of synovial tissue and other connective tissue. Both humoral and cellular immunologic mechanisms are involved in the pathogenesis of the disease. These mechanisms include the cytokine-mediated activation of T and B lymphocytes and the recruitment and activation of polymorphonuclear leukocytes. The inflammatory leukocytes then release a variety of prostaglandins, cytotoxic compounds, and free radicals that cause joint inflammation and destruction.

In patients with rheumatoid arthritis, NSAIDs are used to relieve pain and inflammation, and DMARDs

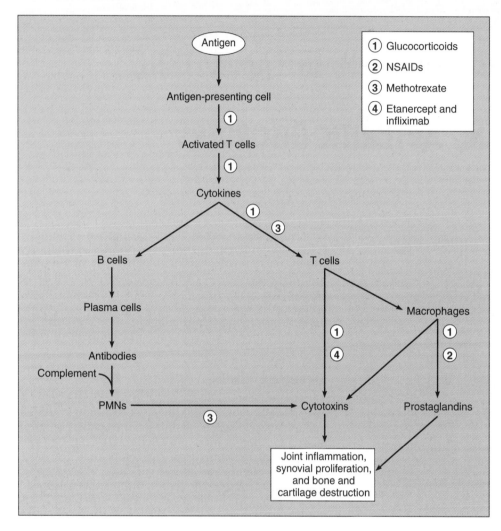

FIGURE 30–1. Pathogenesis of rheumatoid arthritis and sites of action of selected antirheumatic drugs. Antigen-presenting cells phagocytose antigens and present them to T cells, thereby activating the T cells. Activated T cells produce cytokines that stimulate the production of B and T cells. B cells produce plasma cells that form antibodies, and these combine with complement to stimulate accumulation of polymorphonuclear leukocytes (PMNs). T helper cells activate macrophages. Together, T cells, PMNs, and macrophages produce cytotoxic substances and prostaglandins that cause joint inflammation, synovial proliferation, and bone and cartilage destruction. Glucocorticoids inhibit T cell activation and cytokine production. Glucocorticoids and nonsteroidal anti-inflammatory drugs (NSAIDs) inhibit the formation of prostaglandins. Methotrexate inhibits the proliferation and activity of T cells and PMNs. Etanercept and infliximab inactivate a cytokine called tumor necrosis factor.

are used to suppress the underlying disease process and slow the progression of joint destruction. The sites of action and the structures of selected antirheumatic drugs are depicted in Figs. 30–1 and 30–2.

Osteoarthritis

Osteoarthritis, also called **degenerative joint disease,** is the most common joint disease in the world. It affects about 10% of persons over 60 years of age, and radiographic evidence of osteoarthritis can be found in most persons over 65. However, the disease is not simply associated with aging. Other factors that increase the risk for osteoarthritis include obesity, osteoporosis, smoking, heredity, repetitive use of joints through work or leisure activities, and joint trauma.

Osteoarthritis primarily affects weight-bearing joints and causes deformity, limitation of motion, and progressive disability. The cartilage undergoes thickening, inflammation, splitting, and thinning. Eventually, the cartilaginous layer is completely destroyed, leading to erosion and microfractures in the underlying bone. The major symptoms of osteoarthritis are pain, stiffness, and muscle weakness around affected joints.

Nonpharmacologic measures for treating osteoarthritis include joint protection and splinting, physiotherapy, orthotic prostheses to support the feet, and joint replacement surgery. Pharmacologic measures includes NSAIDs, local glucocorticoid injections, and experimental chondroprotective drugs, such as chondroitin sulfate and glucosamine.

Gout

Gout is an arthritic syndrome caused by an inflammatory response to crystals of **monosodium urate monohydrate** in joints, renal tubules, and other tissues. The deposition of these crystals occurs as a consequence of **hyperuricemia,** which may be caused by overproduction or underexcretion of uric acid. Other risk factors for gout include obesity, alcohol consumption, and hypertension.

Acute gout is treated with an NSAID or colchicine to relieve joint inflammation. Subsequent attacks of gout can be prevented by long-term therapy with a drug that either increases uric acid excretion or inhibits uric acid formation and thereby reduces the serum level of uric acid.

NONSTEROIDAL ANTI-INFLAMMATORY DRUGS
Mechanisms of Action

The nonsteroidal anti-inflammatory drugs, or NSAIDs, comprise a large family of weakly acidic drugs whose pharmacologic effects result primarily from the inhibition of **cyclooxygenase** (COX), an enzyme that catalyzes the first step in the synthesis of **prostaglandins** from arachidonic acid and other 20-carbon fatty acids (see Chapter 26). Arachidonic acid is released from cell membranes by the action of phospholipase A_2, an enzyme that is activated by physical trauma and various chemical stimuli.

NSAIDs also appear to inhibit B and T cell proliferation by mechanisms that do not involve inhibition of COX and prostaglandin formation. For example, the drugs may exert their anti-inflammatory effects by inhibiting G protein signal transduction and phospholipase C activation in leukocytes and thereby decreasing the adhesiveness of cells in inflamed tissue.

Prostaglandins

Prostaglandins play an important role in the development of pain, inflammation, and fever.

Prostaglandins are released from cells in response to chemical stimuli or physical trauma. They sensitize sensory nerves to nociceptive stimuli and thereby amplify the formation of pain impulses. They also promote tissue inflammation by stimulating inflammatory cell chemotaxis, causing vasodilation, and increasing capillary permeability and edema.

Fever, defined as the elevation of body temperature to a level above 37°C (98.6°F), often results from an alteration of hypothalamic thermoregulatory mechanisms. Bacterial toxins and other pyrogens stimulate the production of cytokines by leukocytes, and these cytokines increase prostaglandin synthesis in the preoptic area of the hypothalamus. The prostaglandins then act to reset the body's thermostat to a new point above 37°C. This in turn activates temperature-raising mechanisms, such as a reduction in heat loss via cutaneous vasodilation, and causes the temperature to rise. All NSAIDs relieve fever by inhibiting prostaglandin synthesis in the hypothalamus, but these drugs are not capable of reducing body temperature below normal.

Cyclooxygenase Isozymes

COX is now known to occur in two major isoforms, **cyclooxygenase-1** (COX-1) and **cyclooxygenase-2** (COX-2). COX-1 is a constitutive or "housekeeping" enzyme that is found in relatively constant

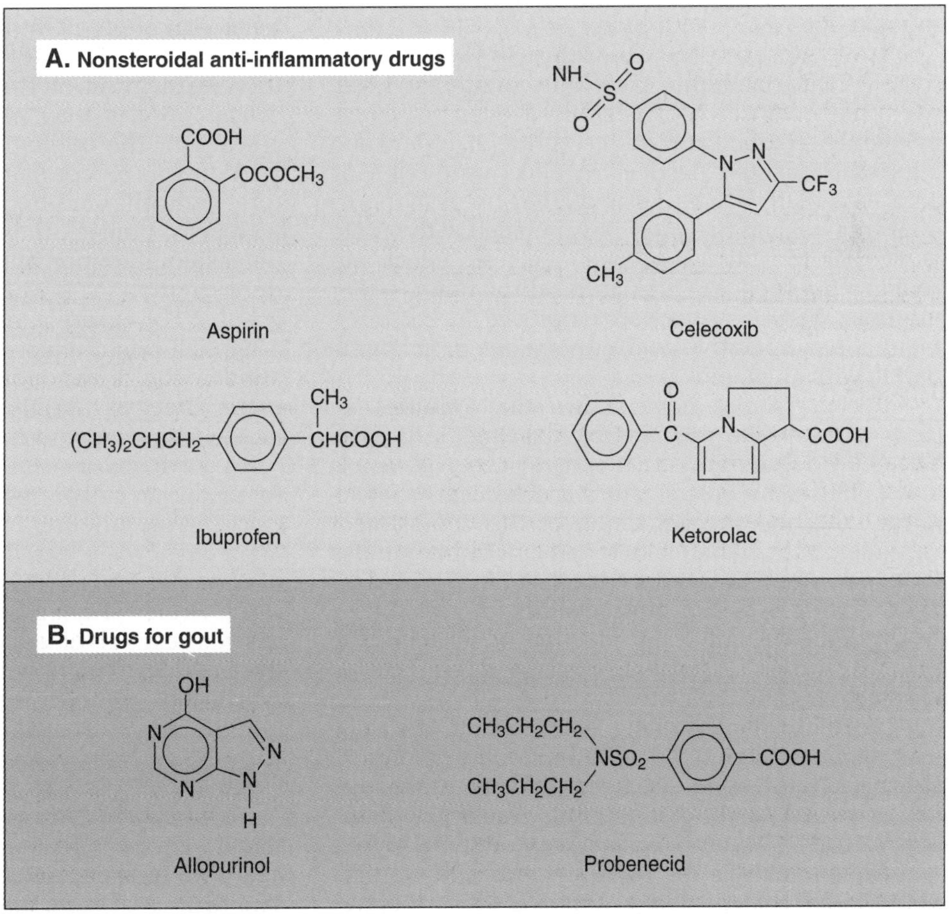

FIGURE 30–2. Structures of selected drugs for pain, inflammation, and arthritic disorders. (A) Aspirin (acetylsalicylic acid), ibuprofen, and ketorolac are nonselective cyclooxygenase inhibitors. Celecoxib is a selective cyclooxygenase-2 inhibitor. (B) Allopurinol is a xanthine oxidase inhibitor. Probenecid is a uricosuric drug.

levels in various tissues. COX-1 participates in the synthesis of prostaglandins that have a cytoprotective effect on the gastrointestinal tract. It also catalyzes the formation of thromboxane A_2 in platelets, leading to platelet aggregation and hemostasis. In contrast, COX-2 is an inducible enzyme. Its levels are normally quite low in most tissues but are rapidly up-regulated during the inflammatory process by proinflammatory substances, such as cytokines, endotoxins, and tumor promoters. Both COX-1 and COX-2 appear to participate in renal homeostasis.

Most of the NSAIDs available today are nonselective inhibitors of COX-1 and COX-2. The discovery of COX isozymes recently led to the development of selective COX-2 inhibitors, such as celecoxib. These selective inhibitors are effective anti-inflammatory drugs, and they have a lower tendency to cause gastrointestinal bleeding and peptic ulcer disease than do the nonselective COX inhibitors.

Nonselective Cyclooxygenase Inhibitors

Among the nonselective COX inhibitors are many well-known NSAIDs that are available without a prescription, including aspirin, ibuprofen, ketoprofen, and naproxen. Acetaminophen is only a weak anti-inflammatory agent, but it is also included in this class of drugs because it exerts analgesic and antipyretic effects via inhibition of COX. As shown in Table 30–1, the NSAIDs vary greatly in potency and half-life, but most of them are administered from two to four times a day with food.

Lower doses of NSAIDs are usually sufficient to treat mild to moderate pain and counteract fever, while higher doses are generally needed to relieve inflammation associated with arthritic disorders and injuries. NSAIDs are particularly effective in relieving pain caused by tissue inflammation or by bone or joint trauma, and they may be combined with opioid analgesics to obtain a greater analgesic effect and reduce the need for higher doses of opioids. For example, NSAIDs are widely employed in the treatment of postoperative pain, either alone or in combination with an opioid.

Recent studies have shown that NSAIDs can delay or slow the progress of Alzheimer's disease. The neurodegeneration that occurs in this disease is accompanied by inflammatory mechanisms that involve COX and the activation of the complement cascade. Other epidemiologic and laboratory studies indicate that NSAIDs reduce the risk of colon cancer by inhibiting COX and prostaglandin formation.

Although NSAIDs are effective in relieving the pain of chronic disorders, their long-term use is associated with a number of adverse effects, including gastrointestinal bleeding, peptic ulcers, and renal and hepatic dysfunction. Acetaminophen produces fewer gastrointestinal problems than do other nonselective COX inhibitors, but it also lacks significant antiplatelet and anti-inflammatory activity. While acetaminophen may be used concurrently with another NSAID for supplemental analgesia, alternative

TABLE 30–1. Properties of Nonsteroidal Anti-inflammatory Drugs

Drug	Relative Potency	Half-Life (Hours)	Daily Doses
Nonselective cyclooxygenase inhibitors			
Acetaminophen	1	3	4
Aspirin	1	2*	4
Ibuprofen	4	2	2–4
Indomethacin	40	4	1–3
Ketoprofen	20	2	2–4
Ketorolac	100	7	4
Naproxen	4	14	2
Selective cyclooxygenase-2 inhibitors			
Celecoxib	20	11	2

*For aspirin, the value shown is the half-life of the active metabolite, salicylic acid.

combinations of two NSAIDs should generally be avoided, not only because they increase the risk of gastrointestinal and other side effects but also because they sometimes have adverse interactions. For example, aspirin and other salicylates displace some NSAIDs, such as ketorolac, from plasma proteins and thereby increase their serum levels significantly.

NSAIDs may interact with a large number of other drugs through pharmacokinetic and pharmacodynamic mechanisms. Most NSAIDs inhibit the renal excretion of lithium and may increase lithium serum levels and toxicity. NSAIDs may reduce the clearance of methotrexate and aminoglycoside drugs. NSAIDs may also interfere to varying degrees with the antihypertensive effect of diuretics, β-adrenergic receptor antagonists, angiotensin inhibitors, and other antihypertensive drugs. When given with potassium-sparing diuretics, NSAIDs may cause potassium retention and lead to hyperkalemia. Some drug interactions are only associated with particular NSAIDs. For example, high doses of salicylates exert a hypoglycemic effect that may alter the effects of antidiabetic drugs. Indomethacin reduces the natriuretic effect of diuretics and may cause nephrotoxicity when given with triamterene.

Low doses of acetaminophen may be safely used for analgesia and antipyresis during pregnancy. However, the use of other NSAIDs during the second half of pregnancy is generally not recommended, because of potential adverse effects to the fetus. These effects result from prostaglandin inhibition and include gastrointestinal bleeding, platelet inhibition, renal dysfunction, and premature closure of the ductus arteriosus.

Acetaminophen

Chemistry, Pharmacologic Effects, and Indications. For over 100 years, acetaminophen has been available for the treatment of **mild pain and fever.** The drug is a *p*-aminophenol derivative that exerts analgesic and antipyretic effects at doses that are well tolerated and produce remarkably few adverse effects during short-term administration. Unlike aspirin use, acetaminophen use has not been associated with Reye's syndrome, so acetaminophen can be safely given to patients with fever due to viral illnesses.

Acetaminophen has only weak anti-inflammatory activity because it is inactivated by peroxides produced in the cells of inflamed tissue. Although acetaminophen is not considered a first-line drug for patients with arthritic disorders, it is sometimes used as an analgesic in those with **mild arthritis.** Because

acetaminophen lacks the ability to inhibit thromboxane synthesis and platelet aggregation, it is not used for the prophylaxis of myocardial infarction, stroke, or other thromboembolic disorders.

Pharmacokinetics. Acetaminophen is rapidly absorbed from the gut, exhibits minimal binding to plasma proteins, and is widely distributed to peripheral tissues and the central nervous system.

As shown in Fig. 30–3A, acetaminophen is extensively metabolized by several pathways in the liver. Most of the drug is conjugated with sulfate and glucuronide, and these metabolites are excreted in

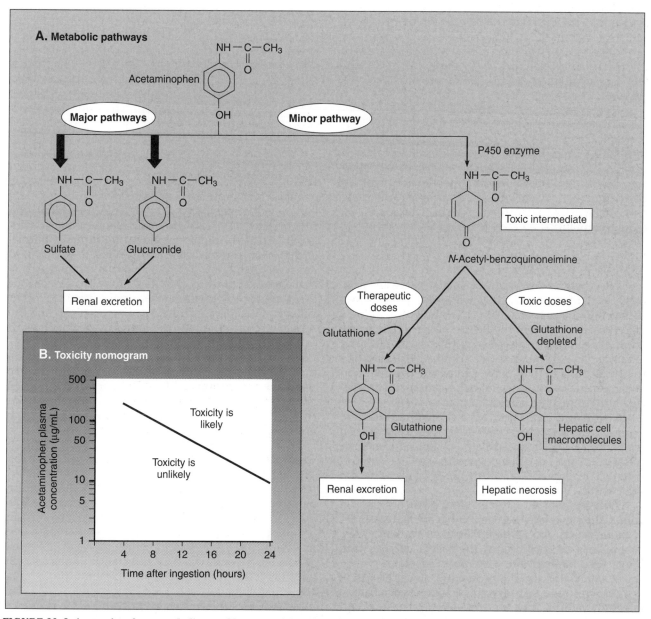

FIGURE 30–3. Acetaminophen metabolism and hepatotoxicity. (A) Acetaminophen is primarily metabolized by conjugation with sulfate and glucuronate. A minor pathway involves oxidation of acetaminophen by cytochrome P450 enzymes to form a potentially toxic intermediate, *N*-acetyl-benzoquinoneimine. When a therapeutic dose of acetaminophen is taken, this quinone intermediate is conjugated with glutathione and excreted in the urine. When a toxic dose of acetaminophen is taken, glutathione stores are depleted, and the quinone intermediate attacks hepatic cell macromolecules. This process results in hepatic necrosis. **(B)** The nomogram shows the plasma concentrations of acetaminophen at various times after a drug overdose is ingested. If the patient's drug concentration is above the curve, acetylcysteine should be administered as an antidote. If the drug concentration is below the curve, hepatotoxicity is unlikely and acetylcysteine administration is not necessary.

the urine. A small amount of acetaminophen is converted by cytochrome P450 to a potentially hepatotoxic quinone intermediate. When a therapeutic dose of acetaminophen is taken, the quinone intermediate is rapidly inactivated by conjugation with glutathione. However, toxic doses of acetaminophen deplete hepatic glutathione, cause accumulation of the quinone intermediate, and lead to hepatic necrosis. To prevent liver damage, patients who ingest an overdose and are determined to be at risk for hepatotoxicity can be given acetylcysteine, a sulfhydryl compound that conjugates the quinone intermediate and renders it harmless.

Adverse Effects. There is some epidemiologic evidence that long-term use of acetaminophen is associated with an increased risk of renal dysfunction.

Although therapeutic doses of acetaminophen are remarkably nontoxic, the ingestion of 20–30 tablets is sufficient to cause life-threatening hepatotoxicity.

Treatment of Acetaminophen Overdose. Because hepatotoxicity gradually progresses over several days following an acetaminophen overdose, prompt treatment with **acetylcysteine** can prevent or significantly reduce hepatotoxicity. The nomogram in Fig. 30–3B shows the plasma concentrations of acetaminophen at various times after an overdose and can be used to determine the need for acetylcysteine treatment.

Aspirin and Other Salicylates

The therapeutic value of salicylates was originally recognized when they were identified as the active ingredients of willow bark and other plant materials used in folk medicine to relieve pain and fever. Aspirin was synthesized in 1899 during a search for a salicylate derivative that would be less irritating to the stomach than salicylic acid. Aspirin soon became widely used around the world as an analgesic, antipyretic, and anti-inflammatory drug.

Chemistry. Salicylic acid derivatives include aspirin (acetylsalicylic acid) and several nonacetylated drugs, such as salsalate, choline magnesium salicylate, and methyl salicylate (oil of wintergreen). The chemical structure of aspirin is shown in Fig. 30–2A.

Pharmacologic Effects and Indications. In adults, the salicylates can be used in the management of **pain, fever,** and **inflammation,** as well as in the prophylaxis of **myocardial infarction, stroke, and other thromboembolic disorders.** In children, the use of salicylates should be avoided, since the risk of Reye's syndrome appears to be increased in virus-infected children who are treated with these drugs.

The analgesic, antipyretic, and anti-inflammatory effects of aspirin and other salicylates result from nonspecific inhibition of COX in peripheral tissues and the central nervous system. Aspirin irreversibly acetylates platelet COX and has a longer-lasting effect on thromboxane synthesis than do other salicylates. The antiplatelet effect of aspirin persists for about

14 days, while that of most other NSAIDs is much shorter.

The salicylates are usually administered orally, but formulations are also available for topical and rectal administration. The oral dosage of aspirin that is needed to inhibit platelet aggregation is somewhat lower than the oral dosage needed to obtain analgesic and antipyretic effects, and it is much lower than the oral dosage needed to relieve inflammation caused by arthritic and other inflammatory disorders. Fig. 30–4 shows the relationship between the dosage of aspirin and the pharmacologic and toxic effects of the drug.

Pharmacokinetics. Aspirin is well absorbed from the gut. Although its concurrent administration with antacids may slow its absorption rate, it will not significantly reduce its bioavailability. Aspirin is rapidly hydrolyzed to salicylic acid by plasma esterases, and this accounts for its short plasma half-life (about 15 minutes). Most of the pharmacologic effects of aspirin are attributed to its salicylic acid metabolite, which has a half-life of about 2 hours. However, aspirin itself is responsible for irreversible inhibition of platelet COX and platelet aggregation.

Most of the salicylic acid formed from aspirin and other salicylate drugs is conjugated with glycine to form salicyluric acid. This substance is then excreted in the urine, along with about 10% of free salicylate and a similar amount of glucuronide conjugates. The rate of excretion of salicylate is affected by urine pH. For this reason, alkalinization of the urine by administration of sodium bicarbonate has been used to increase the ionization and elimination of salicylic acid in cases of drug overdose (see Chapter 2).

When a therapeutic dose of aspirin or other salicylate is ingested, the rate of metabolism and the rate of excretion of salicylic acid are proportional to the drug's plasma concentration (first-order elimination). When an excessive dose is taken, the elimination pathways become saturated, giving rise to zero-order elimination. For this reason, larger doses can rapidly elevate plasma salicylate concentrations to toxic levels, especially in the elderly, who are at greatest risk of aspirin toxicity.

Adverse Effects. The use of aspirin in children with chickenpox and other viral infections has been associated with Reye's syndrome. As mentioned above, treatment with salicylates should therefore be avoided in children.

Therapeutic doses of aspirin can cause gastric irritation and contribute to gastrointestinal bleeding and peptic ulcers. Moderately high therapeutic doses can cause tinnitus, which is described as an abnormal auditory sensation or noise.

Excessive doses of aspirin produce the toxic effects shown in Fig. 30–4. Hyperventilation is due to direct and indirect stimulation of the respiratory center in the medulla, and it often leads to increased exhalation of carbon dioxide and respiratory alkalosis. Higher plasma salicylate concentrations may cause fever, dehydration, and severe metabolic acidosis. If not treated promptly, these events may culminate in shock, coma, organ system failure, and

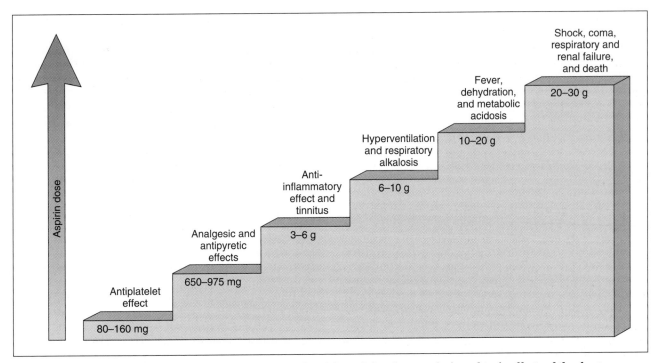

FIGURE 30–4. Relationship between the dosage of aspirin and the pharmacologic and toxic effects of the drug.

death. Excessive doses of aspirin may also cause a hypoprothrombinemic effect that impairs hemostasis and causes bleeding.

Aspirin hypersensitivity is an uncommon but serious condition that may result in severe and potentially fatal anaphylactic reactions. Symptoms of aspirin intolerance include vasomotor rhinitis, angioedema, and urticaria (hives). Aspirin sensitivity occurs most frequently in persons with asthma, nasal polyps, or chronic urticaria. Persons who have had a severe hypersensitivity reaction to aspirin or another salicylate should not be treated with another type of NSAID, because there is a 5% risk of cross-sensitivity between salicylates and other NSAIDs.

Treatment of Salicylate Overdose. The treatment of salicylate poisoning may include the following: (1) induction of vomiting and gastric lavage to remove unabsorbed drug; (2) intravenous administration of **sodium bicarbonate** to counteract metabolic acidosis, increase the ionization of salicylate in the kidneys, and thereby enhance the rate of excretion of salicylate; and (3) administration of fluids, electrolytes, and other supportive care as needed.

Ibuprofen, Ketoprofen, and Naproxen

Chemistry, Pharmacologic Effects, and Indications. Ibuprofen, ketoprofen, and naproxen are propionic acid derivatives that are among the most widely used NSAIDs for **pain and inflammation due to trauma, infection, autoimmune disorders, neoplasms, joint degeneration, and other causes.** By reversibly and nonselectively inhibiting COX isozymes, these drugs are able to exert their analgesic, antipyretic, and anti-inflammatory effects. Low-

dose formulations of the drugs are now available without prescription for the treatment of mild pain and inflammation. The higher-dose formulations used to treat most arthritic disorders still require a prescription.

Pharmacokinetics. Ibuprofen, ketoprofen, and naproxen are administered orally, are widely distributed, and are extensively metabolized to inactive metabolites in the liver before undergoing renal excretion. Naproxen has a longer half-life (14 hours) than does ibuprofen or ketoprofen (2 hours each). For this reason, naproxen is given twice daily, while ibuprofen or ketoprofen is usually administered from two to four times a day.

Adverse Effects. Ibuprofen and related drugs produce dose-dependent gastric irritation, nausea, dyspepsia, and bleeding. Long-term administration of high doses has been associated with peptic ulcer disease, but short-term use of low doses causes very few serious adverse effects. Among the serious effects that have been reported are hepatic toxicity and renal toxicity. In some cases, acute renal failure occurred following short-term use of therapeutic doses by patients who failed to ingest adequate fluids and became dehydrated.

Indomethacin

Indomethacin is an indoleacetic acid derivative that is often regarded as one of the most potent inhibitors of COX isozymes. Because of its greater tendency to cause adverse effects, this drug is usually reserved for the management of **moderate to severe acute inflammatory conditions.** It is also used to treat infants with a **patent ductus arteriosus.** In these infants, indomethacin inhibits the synthesis of prostaglandins and thereby causes closure of the ductus.

The incidence of gastrointestinal and central nervous system side effects is higher with the use of indomethacin than with the use of many other NSAIDs. Indomethacin therapy is also associated with a risk of serious hematologic toxicity. Hence, therapy should be limited to short-term use whenever possible, and patients should be closely monitored.

Ketorolac

Ketorolac is an arylacetic acid derivative (see Fig. 30–2A). It has potent analgesic activity and is one of the few NSAIDs that is available for parenteral use as well as oral and topical ophthalmic use.

In studies of postoperative pain, ketorolac produced a level of analgesia comparable to that produced by morphine but caused less nausea, vomiting, and drowsiness. Ketorolac has therefore been widely used for the short-term management of **moderate to severe pain,** such as **postoperative pain associated with dental surgery.** Although the drug has also been used to treat **migraine headaches,** it does not appear to be superior to ibuprofen for treatment of musculoskeletal pain. The ophthalmic solution of ketorolac is used to treat **allergic conjunctivitis** and **postoperative ocular inflammation.**

Ketorolac may cause fewer adverse gastrointestinal and central nervous system effects than do opioid analgesics, but it poses a significant risk of hematologic toxicity and other adverse effects. For this reason, oral or parenteral therapy with the drug must be limited to 5 or fewer days. In patients with renal or hepatic disease, ketorolac should be used with caution because it is associated with an increased risk of severe renal or hepatic impairment. A similar drug, **bromfenac,** was withdrawn from the market in 1998, following postmarketing reports of hepatic failure and death.

Selective Cyclooxygenase-2 Inhibitors

The selective cyclooxygenase-2 (COX-2) inhibitors are a new group of drugs that appear to provide potent anti-inflammatory activity without causing significant gastrointestinal toxicity. **Celecoxib** is the first selective COX-2 inhibitor to be marketed, and several other compounds with similar activity are being developed.

Chemistry, Pharmacologic Effects, and Indications. Celecoxib is a diaryl-substituted pyrazole compound (see Fig. 30–2A) that acts as a potent analgesic, antipyretic, and anti-inflammatory agent. The drug does not inhibit platelet aggregation, because platelets contain the COX-1 isozyme.

In clinical studies of **osteoarthritis** and **rheumatoid arthritis,** celecoxib was shown to be as efficacious as naproxen without causing significant side effects. In a study of postoperative pain management, however, celecoxib was reported to provide insufficient analgesia to control pain after general surgery.

In laboratory studies, investigators found that celecoxib was more effective than nonselective COX inhibitors in protecting against **colon carcinogenesis.** This finding suggests a role for prophylactic celecoxib use in persons with a high risk of colon cancer.

Pharmacokinetics. Celecoxib is available for oral administration and is usually taken twice daily. The drug is rapidly absorbed from the gut, is metabolized by cytochrome P450 isozyme CYP2C9, and is excreted in the feces and urine. The half-life is about 11 hours.

Adverse Effects and Interactions. Celecoxib appears to cause a low incidence of adverse reactions, the most common of which are diarrhea, dyspepsia, and abdominal pain. The drug is associated with a much lower incidence of gastroduodenal ulcers than are nonselective NSAIDs such as ibuprofen and naproxen.

Because celecoxib is metabolized by CYP2C9, drugs such as fluconazole, fluvastatin, and zafirlukast may inhibit its metabolism and increase its serum concentration. Lower doses of celecoxib should probably be used in patients treated concurrently with these interacting drugs.

DISEASE-MODIFYING ANTIRHEUMATIC DRUGS

The disease-modifying antirheumatic drugs (DMARDs) are agents capable of slowing the progression of joint erosions in patients with rheumatoid arthritis. Examples of DMARDs are gold salts, glucocorticoids, hydroxychloroquine, methotrexate (MTX), and a number of newer immunologic agents, including leflunomide, etanercept, and infliximab. These drugs have a delayed onset of action and require several weeks to months before their antirheumatic benefits are observed. Several studies suggest that using a combination of DMARDs is more effective than using a single DMARD in many patients with rheumatoid arthritis.

DMARDs act by various mechanisms to suppress the proliferation and activity of lymphocytes and polymorphonuclear leukocytes and thereby counteract their ability to cause joint inflammation and destruction. Because joint erosion is usually found within the first 2 years of rheumatoid arthritis, many rheumatologists prescribe DMARDs at the time of diagnosis. Unfortunately, the utility of DMARDs is often limited by their toxicity or by their loss of efficacy over time, and many patients must cease taking them within 5 years of commencing therapy.

Gold Salts

Gold salts were first used to treat rheumatoid arthritis in the late 1920s. They were once used extensively in the management of this disease, but their popularity has declined with the introduction of newer DMARDs, which tend to be more efficacious and less toxic. Both oral and parenteral gold preparations are available. However, the oral compound,

auranofin, is poorly absorbed from the gut and may be less efficacious than parenteral preparations, such as **gold sodium thiomalate.** The antirheumatic effects of gold salts are usually not observed until 3–6 months after starting therapy.

Gold salts can cause a variety of adverse hematologic, dermatologic, gastrointestinal, and renal effects. Flushing, hypotension, and tachycardia are sometimes observed. Skin rash and stomatitis are commonly observed and require discontinuation of treatment until they resolve.

Glucocorticoids

For many years, **prednisone** and other glucocorticoids have played an important role in the treatment of rheumatoid arthritis. These drugs induce the formation of lipocortin, a protein that inhibits phospholipase A_2 activity. By this mechanism, they inhibit the release of arachidonic acid from cell membranes and the formation of prostaglandins. Glucocorticoids also inhibit the production of numerous cytokines, including interleukins and tumor necrosis factor (TNF).

Glucocorticoids act more rapidly than other DMARDs, but their long-term use is limited by the development of serious adverse effects. In light of these facts, glucocorticoids have been used in various ways to manage patients with rheumatoid arthritis or other inflammatory joint diseases. For example, they have been used to induce a remission in the disease at the time that therapy with another (slower-acting) DMARD is started; to provide short courses of therapy during disease flare-ups; and to provide continuous low-dose background therapy in patients undergoing treatment with other DMARDs and NSAIDs.

Other Disease-Modifying Antirheumatic Drugs
Methotrexate

Methotrexate (MTX) is an antineoplastic and immunomodulating drug whose properties are discussed in detail in Chapter 45. The drug was first used to treat rheumatoid arthritis in the 1980s, and it remains the single most effective DMARD available today.

MTX has several mechanisms of action. It inhibits human folate reductase and thereby reduces the availability of active forms of folate that are required for thymidylate and DNA synthesis. It also inhibits lymphocyte proliferation and the production of cytokines and rheumatoid factor. In addition, it interferes with polymorphonuclear leukocyte chemotaxis and reduces the production of cytotoxins and free radicals that damage the synovial membrane and bone.

MTX is considered the DMARD of choice for most patients with rheumatoid arthritis. The drug can be given orally or intramuscularly and has a fairly rapid onset of action, with benefits observed as early as 2–3 weeks after therapy is started. From 45% to 55% of patients continue therapy for at least 5–7 years, and sustained efficacy for up to 15 years has been demonstrated in some patients. The combined use of MTX and other DMARDs is often more effective than single-drug therapy.

MTX treatment is generally well tolerated by patients with rheumatoid arthritis, but it may cause adverse gastrointestinal, hematologic, hepatic, and pulmonary reactions. Elevated liver enzyme levels are found in up to 15% of patients treated with MTX, but serious hepatotoxicity is rare. The administration of folic acid supplements does not reduce the drug efficacy and may prevent some of these adverse effects.

The use of MTX is contraindicated in pregnancy.

Leflunomide

Leflunomide is a new immunosuppressive drug that acts as a powerful inhibitor of mononuclear and T cell proliferation. The active metabolite of leflunomide inhibits a key enzyme in pyrimidine synthesis, dihydroorotate dehydrogenase, and thereby prevents replication of DNA and synthesis of RNA and protein in immune cells. Leflunomide is converted to its active metabolite in the intestinal wall and liver. The active metabolite is further metabolized and excreted in the urine and feces, with an elimination half-life of about 2 weeks.

Leflunomide is marketed as an alternative to MTX for the first-line management of rheumatoid arthritis. In a controlled trial, 41% of patients treated with leflunomide showed significant improvement in tender and swollen joints, compared with 35% of those treated with MTX and 19% given a placebo.

The adverse effects of leflunomide include diarrhea and reversible alopecia. The drug may increase serum levels of hepatic enzymes and increase the risk of hepatotoxicity when it is used in combination with MTX. The active metabolite of leflunomide inhibits CYP2C9 and may thereby increase the serum level of many drugs, including ibuprofen and some of the other NSAIDs.

Leflunomide is teratogenic, so its use is contraindicated in pregnancy.

Etanercept and Infliximab

Etanercept and infliximab are immunologic agents that both exert their antirheumatic effects by binding to and inactivating **tumor necrosis factor** (TNF). TNF is one of the proinflammatory cytokines produced by macrophages and activated T cells. In patients with rheumatoid arthritis, TNF triggers and enhances the function of various leukocytes and also mediates the cytokine cascade that causes joint inflammation and destruction (see Fig. 30–1).

Etanercept is a protein formed by recombining human p75 (75-kilodalton) TNF receptors with Fc fragments of human immunoglobulin G1 (IgG1). In comparison with the original protein, the recombined protein is able to antagonize TNF to a greater extent and has a much longer half-life. Experimental studies in several animal models of rheumatoid arthritis have found etanercept treatment to be effective, as have subsequent clinical trials in patients with this disease. According to a 3-month clinical study, 75% of patients with rheumatoid arthritis had a significant improvement in the signs and symptoms of their disease. The drug was generally well tolerated, although injection site reactions were common.

Etanercept must be administered subcutaneously twice a week and is quite expensive (a 6-month supply costs about $6300). The drug is currently intended for use in patients whose rheumatoid arthritis is refractory to treatment with MTX or other DMARDs. Etanercept may be used alone or in combination with MTX in these patients.

Infliximab is a chimeric human-murine monoclonal antibody that inactivates TNF. It has been used in the treatment of Crohn's disease and rheumatoid arthritis. In one clinical trial, infliximab treatment resulted in an improvement of rheumatoid arthritis manifestations in 80% of patients whose disease was refractory to other drugs. In another study, infliximab was found to be more effective when combined with MTX than when used alone. Infliximab is administered intravenously at 4- to 12-week intervals.

Hydroxychloroquine

Hydroxychloroquine, an antimalarial drug related to chloroquine, has been extensively used as a DMARD. It inhibits the function of lymphocytes, reduces the chemotaxis and phagocytosis of polymorphonuclear leukocytes, and decreases the production of superoxide radicals by these cells. The drug has a slow onset of action and may require 6 months of therapy before benefits are observed. However, it does not produce the myelosuppressive, hepatic, and renal toxicities that many other DMARDs produce. Hydroxychloroquine occasionally causes gastrointestinal disturbances, and patients undergoing hydroxychloroquine treatment must be monitored for adverse ocular effects, including blurred vision, scotomas, and night blindness.

DRUGS FOR GOUT

The effective management of gout often requires the use of various agents to prevent and treat acute attacks.

Drugs for Preventing Gout Attacks

Gout attacks can be prevented by lowering the serum concentration of uric acid. Probenecid accomplishes this goal by increasing the excretion of uric acid, whereas allopurinol does so by inhibiting the synthesis of uric acid. Uric acid metabolism and sites of drug action are depicted in Fig. 30–5.

Probenecid

A **uricosuric drug** such as probenecid (see Fig. 30–2B) is used to prevent gout attacks in persons who

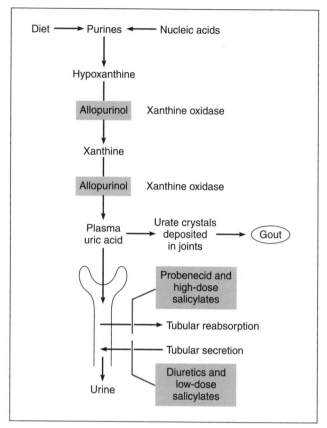

FIGURE 30–5. Uric acid metabolism and sites of drug action. Purines obtained from the diet or from catabolism of nucleic acids are converted to hypoxanthine. Under normal conditions, xanthine oxidase converts hypoxanthine to xanthine and then to uric acid. Allopurinol acts by inhibiting xanthine oxidase. Probenecid and high-dose salicylates inhibit the renal tubular reabsorption of uric acid, whereas diuretics and low-dose salicylates inhibit the renal tubular secretion of uric acid.

underexcrete uric acid, as indicated by a 24-hour uric acid excretion that is less than 800 mg.

Probenecid is a weak acid that competitively inhibits the reabsorption of uric acid by renal tubules and thereby increases the excretion of uric acid. The drug is taken orally and should be swallowed with a full glass of water to ensure adequate fluid intake. Treatment should begin with a low dose, and the dosage should be gradually increased until an adequate uricosuric effect is obtained or the maximal dosage is reached. Probenecid treatment is usually well tolerated.

The use of aspirin and other salicylates may alter or interfere with the uricosuric effect of probenecid, so patients should avoid using these agents. High doses of salicylates inhibit uric acid reabsorption and exert a uricosuric effect. However, low doses of salicylates inhibit uric acid secretion by renal tubules and thereby increase serum concentrations of uric acid.

Allopurinol

Allopurinol (see Fig. 30–2B) is used to prevent gout attacks in persons who overproduce uric acid, as indicated by a 24-hour uric acid excretion that is greater than 800 mg. It is also sometimes used to prevent hyperuricemia and gout in persons who are undergoing cancer chemotherapy and whose rate of purine catabolism is high because of the death of neoplastic cells.

Allopurinol is a competitive inhibitor of **xanthine oxidase,** an enzyme that converts the purine metabolite hypoxanthine to xanthine and then converts xanthine to uric acid. In contrast to uricosuric drugs, allopurinol causes a decrease in uric acid excretion and a corresponding increase in the urinary excretion of hypoxanthine. In addition to its effect on xanthine oxidase, allopurinol also decreases the de novo synthesis of purines.

Allopurinol is administered orally. Most of the drug is rapidly converted to its active metabolite, oxypurinol, in the liver. Oxypurinol has a half-life of about 20 hours, and the majority of this metabolite is excreted unchanged in the urine.

About 25% of patients are unable to tolerate allopurinol because of its adverse effects, which include nausea, vomiting, hepatitis, skin rashes, and other forms of hypersensitivity. Because allopurinol inhibits the catabolism of azathioprine and mercaptopurine, doses of these drugs may need to be reduced if allopurinol is given concurrently with either of them.

Drugs for Treating Gout Attacks

In patients with acute gout, a potent anti-inflammatory drug is given for the rapid relief of pain. Although **indomethacin** (see above) is widely used for this purpose, other NSAIDs are often effective when used in an adequate dosage. If these drugs do not provide relief or cannot be tolerated by the patient, **colchicine** can be given orally or parenterally.

Colchicine was traditionally used for the treatment of acute gout, but it is less frequently used today because of its unpleasant side effects, which include nausea, vomiting, diarrhea, and abdominal cramps. The drug is believed to act by inhibiting the motility of inflammatory leukocytes and thereby blocking their ability to cause crystal-induced joint inflammation. Colchicine is rapidly absorbed after oral administration. It is partly metabolized in the liver, and the drug and its metabolites are excreted by the biliary and fecal route. If colchicine treatment causes the adverse effects noted above, treatment should be stopped to avoid more serious toxicity.

Summary of Important Points

- Nonsteroidal anti-inflammatory drugs (NSAIDs) act primarily by inhibiting cyclooxygenase (COX) and the synthesis of prostaglandins. The drugs exhibit varying degrees of analgesic, anti-inflammatory, and antipyretic activity. Most of them also inhibit platelet aggregation. Long-term use of NSAIDs may lead to renal or hepatic toxicity.
- Nonselective COX inhibitors include acetaminophen, aspirin, ibuprofen, indomethacin, ketoprofen, ketorolac, and naproxen. Except for acetaminophen, the agents in this group can cause gastric irritation and bleeding, and their long-term use may lead to peptic ulcers.
- Acetaminophen is an effective analgesic and antipyretic agent, but it lacks significant anti-inflammatory and antiplatelet activity. A minor metabolite of acetaminophen is a potentially hepatotoxic quinone. This quinone metabolite is normally inactivated by conjugation with glutathione, but toxic doses of acetaminophen may deplete glutathione and cause fatal liver failure.
- Acetylcysteine is a sulfhydryl compound that conjugates and inactivates the quinone metabolite of acetaminophen and is used as an antidote for acetaminophen hepatotoxicity.
- Low doses of aspirin have potent antiplatelet effects because they acetylate and irreversibly inhibit platelet COX. Low doses of aspirin also produce analgesic and antipyretic effects, but higher doses are needed to counteract inflammation.
- High therapeutic doses of aspirin can cause tinnitus. Toxic doses cause hyperventilation and respiratory alkalosis, followed by metabolic acidosis. In cases of severe aspirin toxicity, sodium bicarbonate can be given to counteract acidosis and increase urinary excretion of salicylic acid.
- Ibuprofen, ketoprofen, and naproxen are potent NSAIDs that are widely used as analgesic, antipyretic, and anti-inflammatory agents. Ketorolac is a potent analgesic that may be given orally or parenterally. To avoid hematologic toxicity, ketorolac use should be limited to a few days.
- Indomethacin is a potent COX inhibitor that can be used to treat moderate to severe acute inflammatory conditions. It is also used to cause closure of the ductus arteriosus in infants.
- Celecoxib is the first selective COX-2 inhibitor and is a potent analgesic, antipyretic, and anti-inflammatory drug. Its associated incidence of gastrointestinal bleeding and peptic ulcers is lower than that of nonselective COX inhibitors.
- The disease-modifying antirheumatic drugs (DMARDs) are agents capable of slowing the progression of joint erosion in patients with rheumatoid arthritis. These drugs have a slow onset of action and may cause considerable toxicity. DMARDs act by inhibiting the proliferation and activity of lymphocytes and polymorphonuclear leukocytes.
- Methotrexate (MTX) is the most widely used and effective DMARD and can be combined with other drugs in this class for enhanced activity. It is generally well tolerated and may be used effectively for many years.
- Etanercept and infliximab are DMARDs that bind to and inactivate tumor necrosis factor (TNF). Etanercept is a recombinant form of the human TNF receptor fused to an Fc fragment of an immunoglobulin. Infliximab is a monoclonal antibody to TNF. These drugs are administered

intermittently by injection and appear to benefit many patients with rheumatoid arthritis.

- Other DMARDs include gold salts, glucocorticoids, leflunomide, and hydroxychloroquine.
- Gout is caused by hyperuricemia and the deposition of urate crystals in joints. Uricosuric drugs such as probenecid increase uric acid excretion, while allopurinol inhibits uric acid formation. These drugs are used for the prevention of gout attacks.
- Acute gout is treated with an anti-inflammatory drug, such as indomethacin, another NSAID, or colchicine. Colchicine inhibits the motility of leukocytes and thereby prevents their migration into joints and their ability to cause urate crystal–induced joint inflammation.

Selected Readings

Jouzeau, J. Y., et al. Cyclooxygenase isoenzymes: how recent findings affect thinking about nonsteroidal anti-inflammatory drugs. Drugs 53:563–582, 1997.

Kawamori, T., et al. Chemopreventive activity of celecoxib, a specific cyclooxygenase-2 inhibitor, against colon carcinogenesis. Cancer Res 58:409–412, 1998.

Lane, N. E. Pain management in osteoarthritis: the role of cyclooxygenase-2 inhibitors. J Rheumatol 24(supplement 49):20–24, 1997.

Moreland, L. W. Soluble tumor necrosis factor receptor (p75) fusion protein (ENBREL) as a therapy for rheumatoid arthritis. Rheum Dis Clin North Am 24:579–591, 1998.

Needleman, P., and P. C. Isakson. Selective inhibition of cyclooxygenase-2. Sci Med 5:26–35, 1998.

Pasero, G. The treatment of rheumatoid arthritis in this century: from spas to monoclonal antibodies. Clin Exp Rheumatol 15(supplement 17):S67–S70, 1997.

Pasinetti, G. M. Cyclooxygenase and inflammation in Alzheimer's disease: experimental approaches and clinical interventions. J Neurosci Res 54:1–6, 1998.

Schiff, M. Emerging treatments for rheumatoid arthritis. Am J Med 102(supplement 1):11S–15S, 1997.

Silva-Junior, H. T., and R. E. Morris. Leflunomide and malononitrilamides. Am J Med Sci 313:289–301, 1997.

SECTION VI

ENDOCRINE

PHARMACOLOGY

HYPOTHALAMIC AND PITUITARY DRUGS

CLASSIFICATION OF HYPOTHALAMIC AND PITUITARY DRUGS

ANTERIOR PITUITARY HORMONES
Adrenocorticotropic hormone and related drugs
- Corticotropin
- Cosyntropin

Growth hormone and related drugs
- Octreotide
- Sermorelin
- Somatostatin
- Somatotropin
- Somatrem

Gonadotropins and related drugs
- Chorionic gonadotropin
- Gonadorelin
- Goserelin
- Leuprolide
- Menotropins
- Nafarelin

Other hormones and related drugs
- Bromocriptine
- Cabergoline
- Prolactin
- Protirelin
- Thyrotropin

POSTERIOR PITUITARY HORMONES AND RELATED DRUGS
- Desmopressin
- Oxytocin
- Vasopressin

OVERVIEW

The hypothalamus and pituitary gland constitute an important neuroendocrine system that regulates growth, reproduction, metabolic rates, and other important body functions. The pituitary gland is divided into two major lobes, the adenohypophysis (anterior lobe) and the neurohypophysis (posterior lobe). Various hormones are secreted by each of these lobes and by the hypothalamus.

Adenohypophysis and Hypothalamus

The adenohypophysis secretes six hormones: (1) **corticotropin,** or **adrenocorticotropic hormone** (ACTH); (2) **somatotropin,** or **growth hormone** (GH);

(3) **follicle-stimulating hormone** (FSH); (4) **luteinizing hormone** (LH); (5) **thyrotropin,** or **thyroid-stimulating hormone** (TSH); and (6) **prolactin.** The actions of these **anterior pituitary hormones** are summarized in Fig. 31–1.

The secretion of anterior pituitary hormones is controlled by several hormone-releasing and hormone-inhibiting factors that are formed in the hypothalamus. These factors, or **hypothalamic hormones,** include the following: (1) **corticotropin-releasing hormone** (CRH); (2) **growth hormone–releasing hormone** (GHRH); (3) **somatostatin,** or **growth hormone–inhibiting hormone** (GIH); (4) **gonadotropin-releasing hormone** (GnRH), or **luteinizing hormone–releasing hormone** (LHRH); (5) **protirelin,** or **thyrotropin-releasing hormone** (TRH); and (6) **prolactin-inhibiting hormone** (PIH). There is also evidence suggesting the presence of one or more prolactin-releasing factors. The various hypothalamic hormones are secreted by the arcuate and other hypothalamic nuclei, and they are transported to the anterior pituitary via the hypophysioportal circulation.

The anterior pituitary hormones are transported to their target organs via the systemic circulation. In the target organs, they stimulate growth, development, and the secretion of other hormones, which not only activate specific functions in various organs but also exert negative feedback inhibition of the corresponding hypothalamic and pituitary hormones.

Neurohypophysis

The neurohypophysis secretes **oxytocin** and **vasopressin.** These **posterior pituitary hormones** are synthesized in the cell bodies of neurons in the supraoptic and paraventricular nuclei of the hypothalamus. The hormones are transported down the nerve axons to their endings in the posterior pituitary, where they are released in response to electrical activity in the nerve terminals.

Uses of Hypothalamic and Pituitary Hormones

Hypothalamic and pituitary hormones are used for both diagnostic and therapeutic purposes. Hypothalamic hormone-releasing factors are helpful in assessing the functional capacity of the anterior pituitary to secrete particular pituitary hormones. Anterior pituitary hormones are used to evaluate the functional capacity of their target organs, to stimulate

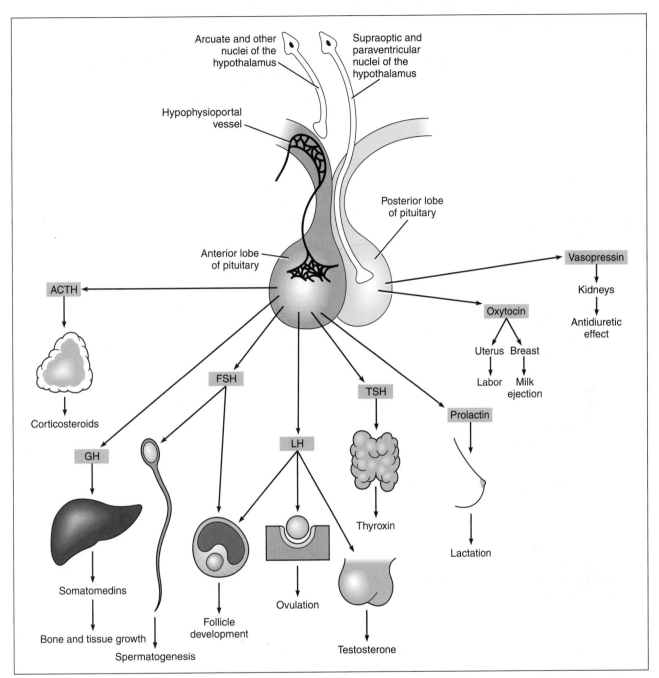

FIGURE 31–1. Relationships between hypothalamic hormones, pituitary hormones, and target organs. Numerous hormone-releasing and hormone-inhibiting factors are formed in the arcuate and other hypothalamic nuclei and are transported to the anterior pituitary by hypophysioportal vessels. In response to hypothalamic hormones, the anterior pituitary secretes the following: adrenocorticotropic hormone (ACTH), which evokes corticosteroid secretion by the adrenal cortex; growth hormone (GH), which elicits somatomedin production by the liver; follicle-stimulating hormone (FSH), which stimulates spermatogenesis and facilitates ovarian follicle development; luteinizing hormone (LH), which elicits testosterone secretion by the testes, facilitates ovarian follicle development, and induces ovulation; thyroid-stimulating hormone (TSH), which stimulates thyroxin secretion by the thyroid gland; and prolactin, which induces breast tissue growth and lactation. The posterior pituitary hormones are formed in the supraoptic and paraventricular nuclei and are transported by nerve axons to the posterior lobe, where they are released by physiologic stimuli. Oxytocin induces milk ejection by the breast and stimulates uterine contractions during labor. Vasopressin increases water and sodium reabsorption by the kidneys.

hypofunctional target organs, and to provide replacement therapy in hormone deficiency states. Posterior pituitary hormones are used therapeutically to activate specific physiologic functions.

All of the hypothalamic and pituitary hormones are peptides or small proteins that are extensively degraded in the gut following oral administration. For this reason, most of these hormones are administered parenterally. A few of them are available as a spray for intranasal administration.

ANTERIOR PITUITARY HORMONES

Adrenocorticotrophic Hormone and Related Drugs

ACTH (corticotropin) is a 39-amino-acid peptide that is released from the anterior pituitary in response to CRH stimulation. ACTH in turn stimulates the adrenal cortex to produce cortisol, aldosterone, and adrenal androgens by increasing the activity of the enzyme that converts cholesterol to pregnenolone and is the rate-limiting enzyme in corticosteroid production.

Adrenocorticotrophic Hormone Preparations

Two ACTH preparations are available for clinical use. One is derived from porcine ACTH and is simply referred to as **corticotropin,** while the other is a synthetic form of human ACTH and is called **cosyntropin.** Cosyntropin contains the first 24 amino acids of ACTH, which are the ones necessary for its biologic activity. Cosyntropin is preferable for clinical use because it produces fewer allergic reactions.

Cosyntropin is employed in two diagnostic tests. First, it is used to distinguish **congenital adrenal hyperplasia** from **ovarian hyperandrogenism.** Second and more commonly, it is used to diagnose **adrenal insufficiency** in a test that measures plasma cortisol levels before and after a cosyntropin injection. Cosyntropin increases cortisol levels in healthy individuals but fails to increase cortisol levels in persons with adrenal insufficiency. Then to distinguish primary adrenal insufficiency from secondary adrenal insufficiency, endogenous plasma ACTH concentrations are measured. In patients with primary adrenal insufficiency, ACTH concentrations are high because of the lack of negative feedback inhibition of the hypothalamus and pituitary gland by the adrenal corticosteroids. In patients with secondary adrenal insufficiency, ACTH concentrations are low because of inadequate production of ACTH by the pituitary gland.

Corticotropin-Releasing Hormone Preparations

A synthetic CRH preparation is being investigated for use in the differential diagnosis of **Cushing's syndrome.**

Growth Hormone and Related Drugs

GH (somatotropin) is a large peptide that contains 191 amino acids, is produced by the anterior pituitary, and has both direct and indirect actions on target organs. GH acts directly to stimulate lipolysis and antagonize insulin so as to elevate blood glucose levels. However, most of the effects of GH are mediated by **somatomedins** (insulinlike growth factors), which are peptides produced in the liver and cartilage. The somatomedins stimulate skeletal growth, amino acid transport, protein synthesis, nucleic acid synthesis, and cell proliferation.

The secretion of GH is stimulated by GHRH and is inhibited by GIH. Several preparations of GH, GHRH, and GIH are available for use in the diagnosis and treatment of **growth disorders** associated with excessive or inadequate secretion of GH.

Growth Hormone Preparations

GH preparations obtained from animal sources are not active in humans. In the past, GH obtained from human cadavers was used to treat patients with **growth hormone deficiency and short stature,** but some of the patients subsequently developed Creutzfeldt-Jakob disease. This fatal disease, like mad cow disease and kuru, is characterized by spongiform encephalopathy and is thought to be transmitted by unconventional neurotropic agents called prions.

Today, two biosynthetic GH preparations are available for treatment of GH deficiency. One is a recombinant human GH and is simply referred to as **somatotropin.** The other is a human GH analogue that contains one additional amino acid and is called **somatrem.** If a child has GH deficiency and a growth rate under 4 cm per year, either preparation can be used. The hormone is usually administered subcutaneously or intramuscularly three times a week, and treatment is extremely expensive (from $10,000 to $30,000 per year). GH deficiency is often accompanied by other pituitary hormone deficiencies, which should also be treated with appropriate hormones.

Growth Hormone–Releasing Hormone Preparations

Sermorelin, a synthetic analogue of GHRH, is available for use in a test to determine whether **growth hormone deficiency** is secondary to **hypothalamic insufficiency** or to **pituitary insufficiency.** In this test, plasma levels of GH are measured before and after a single injection of sermorelin is given. A normal response indicates that the pituitary is capable of secreting GH and that the patient's GH deficiency is due to hypothalamic insufficiency.

Sermorelin has orphan drug status for the treatment of GH deficiency and the treatment of weight loss associated with acquired immunodeficiency syndrome (AIDS).

Growth Hormone–Inhibiting Hormone Preparations

Somatostatin is an agent that inhibits GH secretion, but it also exerts effects on several endocrine glands, including the pancreas, and this limits its therapeutic usefulness. Scientists searching for GIH preparations that were more selective for GH inhibition discovered **octreotide,** a somatostatin analogue that consists of 8 amino acids. In comparison with somatostatin, octreotide is 45 times more potent in inhibiting GH secretion but only 2 times as potent in inhibiting insulin secretion by the pancreas.

Octreotide is used to treat patients with **acromegaly.** This endocrine disorder is caused by excessive GH secretion and is characterized by acral enlargement and soft tissue overgrowth of the hands and feet, coarsening of facial features, thickening and oiliness of the skin, and increased sweating. It is often accompanied by numerous other metabolic and endocrine abnormalities. In addition, octreotide has been used successfully in the treatment of several **neoplastic diseases,** including **carcinoid syndrome, pituitary adenomas that secrete thyrotropin,** and **tumors that produce vasoactive intestinal polypeptide** (VIP).

Octreotide is usually administered subcutaneously every 8 hours. A sustained-release preparation for intramuscular administration has also been developed. Adverse effects of octreotide treatment include nausea, vomiting, abdominal cramps, steatorrhea (excessive fat in the feces), and gallstones.

In patients with acromegaly, the use of cabergoline (see below) and other new dopamine agonists can reduce the circulating levels of GH, insulinlike growth factor, and prolactin. These drugs therefore appear to be a valuable addition to the medical management of acromegaly.

Gonadotropins and Related Drugs

The pituitary secretes two gonadotropins—namely, FSH and LH—in response to pulsatile stimulation by GnRH. The frequency and amplitude of the GnRH pulses at a particular time determine which gonadotropin is secreted. In females, FSH stimulates ovarian follicle maturation, whereas LH assists FSH in follicle development, induces ovulation, and stimulates the corpus luteum to produce progesterone and androgens. In males, FSH stimulates spermatogenesis, whereas LH stimulates Leydig cells in the testes to produce testosterone.

Gonadotropin Preparations

Several gonadotropin preparations are available for the treatment of infertility and hypogonadism. One of them contains both FSH and LH, is called **menotropins** (human menopausal gonadotropin, or hMG), and is obtained from the urine of menopausal women. Another primarily contains LH, is called **chorionic gonadotropin** (human chorionic gonadotropin, or hCG), and is produced by the placenta and isolated from the urine of pregnant women.

In women with **infertility** caused by failure to ovulate, menotropins and chorionic gonadotropin are used sequentially. A dose of menotropins is administered each day for 9–12 days to stimulate maturation of the ovarian follicle. On the day after the last dose is given, a single dose of chorionic gonadotropin is administered to induce ovulation. In men with **hypogonadotropic hypogonadism,** menotropins therapy is used to stimulate spermatogenesis. In prepubertal boys with **cryptorchidism** (undescended testes) and hypogonadism, chorionic gonadotropin is administered to stimulate testosterone production and descent of the testes.

Gonadotropin-Releasing Hormone Preparations

GnRH preparations that are currently available include **gonadorelin, goserelin, leuprolide,** and **naf-**

arelin. Gonadorelin is synthetic GnRH, and the other preparations are synthetic GnRH analogues. Like natural GnRH, these synthetic drugs affect the release of gonadotropins. The way in which they are administered determines their effects on the body. Pulsatile administration mimics the natural secretion of GnRH and is used therapeutically to stimulate the release of FSH and LH from the anterior pituitary. In contrast, continuous administration leads to down-regulation of FSH and LH secretion and is used therapeutically to suppress gonadotropin stimulation of target organs.

Gonadorelin has a half-life of about 5 minutes. Unlike the other GnRH preparations, gonadorelin can be administered in a pulsatile manner via a portable infusion pump that injects a small bolus of the drug subcutaneously every 60–120 minutes. In women with infertility caused by **hypothalamic amenorrhea,** pulsatile treatment for 10–20 days is given to induce ovulation. Ovulation rates exceeding 90% are achieved by this method, and most women become pregnant within 6 months of therapy. Gonadorelin is also used diagnostically to evaluate the functional capacity of the gonadotropin-secreting cells of the pituitary. For this purpose, plasma gonadotropin concentrations are measured before and after a single dose of gonadorelin is injected.

Goserelin, leuprolide, and nafarelin have half-lives of about 3 hours. Goserelin and leuprolide are administered as pellets that slowly release the drug following subcutaneous implantation, and nafarelin is available as a nasal spray. By suppressing gonadotropin secretion, these GnRH analogues reduce testosterone levels in males and estrogen levels in females. This in turn decreases testosterone stimulation of the prostate gland and estrogen stimulation of the breast and uterus. For this reason, the GnRH analogues are effective in the treatment of **precocious puberty** in boys or girls and in the treatment of **prostate cancer, breast cancer,** and **endometriosis** in adults.

Thyroid-Stimulating Hormone and Related Drugs

TSH is secreted in response to stimulation of the anterior pituitary by TRH. Both **thyrotropin** (TSH) and **protirelin** (TRH) have been employed as diagnostic agents, but their use has been largely supplanted by other methods.

Prolactin and Related Drugs

Prolactin contains 198 amino acids and acts on the mammary gland to stimulate tissue growth and promote lactation (milk production) in the presence of adequate levels of estrogens, progestins, and other hormones. Prolactin does not have any current clinical use.

The secretion of prolactin is inhibited by PIH (dopamine) and is stimulated by hypothalamic prolactin-releasing factors. Excessive prolactin secretion causes **hyperprolactinemia** and often leads to **galactorrhea** (excessive milk production), **hypogo-**

nadism, and **infertility.** In some cases, hyperprolactinemia occurs secondary to **prolactin-secreting pituitary adenomas.**

Both the idiopathic and secondary forms of hyperprolactinemia can be treated with a dopamine agonist such as **bromocriptine** or **cabergoline.** Each drug mimics the action of PIH and thereby reduces prolactin secretion. In patients with prolactin-secreting adenomas, treatment with either drug also produces a significant reduction in tumor size.

Bromocriptine and cabergoline are both ergot alkaloid derivatives. The pharmacologic properties of bromocriptine, a drug that is also used to treat Parkinson's disease, are described in Chapter 21. In comparison with bromocriptine, cabergoline appears to be more effective and better tolerated in patients with hyperprolactinemia. Cabergoline selectively activates dopamine D_2 receptors in the pituitary gland and thereby suppresses the secretion of prolactin. The drug has an elimination half-life of about 65 hours, which provides a long duration of action. The most common adverse effects of cabergoline are nausea, headache, and dizziness.

POSTERIOR PITUITARY HORMONES

Oxytocin and vasopressin are nonapeptides that are released from the posterior pituitary in response to specific physiologic stimuli (see Fig. 31–1).

Oxytocin and Related Drugs

Oxytocin is a hormone that increases the strength of uterine contractions and causes milk ejection (milk let-down) by contracting myoepithelial cells that line the ducts of the breast. The hormone is released via a reflex that is triggered by dilation of the uterine cervix, uterine contractions, or breast suckling. During late pregnancy, the uterus becomes highly sensitive to the actions of oxytocin owing to an increased number of oxytocin receptors. The sensitivity of the uterus is enhanced by estrogen and is inhibited by progesterone.

Synthetic oxytocin has several uses in obstetrics. The drug is given intravenously to **induce or enhance uterine contractions during labor,** and it is injected intramuscularly to **prevent postpartum uterine hemorrhage** by causing the uterine muscle to contract. In addition, a nasal spray preparation of oxytocin is available to **stimulate milk let-down in nursing mothers.** The spray is inhaled 2–3 minutes before breast-feeding. Adverse reactions to oxytocin are uncommon. They include cardiac arrhythmias, central nervous system stimulation, excessive uterine contraction, and hyponatremia.

Use of synthetic oxytocin is contraindicated in instances of fetal distress, abnormal fetal presentation, prematurity, or cephalopelvic disproportion.

Vasopressin and Related Drugs

Vasopressin (arginine vasopressin) is secreted by the posterior pituitary in response to a decrease in extracellular fluid volume or an increase in plasma osmotic pressure. The hormone interacts with two types of **vasopressin receptors** to exert its antidiuretic and vasoconstrictive effects.

To increase water reabsorption by the kidney, vasopressin stimulates the insertion of water channels (aquaporins) in the luminal membranes of renal tubule cells in the collecting ducts. This action concentrates the urine and reduces the urine volume. For this reason, vasopressin is also called **antidiuretic hormone** (ADH). The renal actions of vasopressin are mediated by V_2 **receptors** via production of cyclic adenosine monophosphate (cAMP).

Vasopressin causes vasoconstriction in several vascular beds by stimulating V_1 **receptors** in vascular smooth muscle.

A deficiency of pituitary vasopressin secretion leads to **diabetes insipidus,** a condition characterized by excessive water excretion (polyuria) and subsequent increased water intake (polydipsia). Diabetes insipidus is usually treated with **desmopressin,** a long-acting synthetic analogue of vasopressin. This agent has potent antidiuretic activity but causes much less vasoconstriction than natural vasopressin causes. Desmopressin solutions are available for subcutaneous, intramuscular, or intravenous administration. Desmopressin nasal spray is also available and is used to prevent nocturnal urine production and enuresis in patients with diabetes insipidus. Desmopressin overdosage may result in dilutional hyponatremia.

Synthetic vasopressin is available as an injectable preparation for the treatment of **bleeding due to esophageal varices or colonic diverticula.** In these conditions, the drug acts by producing vasoconstriction. Vasopressin should be used cautiously in persons with coronary artery disease.

Summary of Important Points

- Cosyntropin is a synthetic corticotropin analogue that is used to diagnose adrenal insufficiency.
- Recombinant human growth hormone and somatrem are growth hormone preparations used to treat growth hormone deficiency in children with a low growth rate.
- Sermorelin is a synthetic analogue of growth hormone–releasing hormone (GHRH). It is used diagnostically to differentiate hypothalamic from pituitary growth hormone deficiency.
- Octreotide is a synthetic somatostatin preparation that inhibits growth hormone secretion and is used in the treatment of acromegaly, carcinoid syndrome, pituitary adenomas that secrete thyrotropin, and tumors that secrete vasoactive intestinal polypeptide.
- Menotropins and chorionic gonadotropin are human gonadotropin preparations that are used to induce ovulation in infertile women. Chorionic gonadotropin is also used to stimulate spermatogenesis in men with hypogonadotropic hypogo-

nadism and to treat cryptorchidism in prepubertal boys.

- Gonadorelin is a gonadotropin-releasing hormone (GnRH) preparation administered in pulsatile fashion to induce ovulation in women with hypothalamic amenorrhea.
- Goserelin and leuprolide are synthetic GnRH preparations administered continuously to suppress gonadotropin secretion in children with precocious puberty and in adults with prostate cancer, breast cancer, and endometriosis.
- Nafarelin is a GnRH preparation administered as a nasal spray to treat precocious puberty in children and endometriosis in women.
- Dopamine agonists, such as bromocriptine and cabergoline, are used to suppress prolactin secretion in women with hyperprolactinemia. This condition is often associated with galactorrhea, hypogonadism, and infertility.
- Oxytocin stimulates uterine contractions at term and is used to induce or augment labor, to prevent postpartum uterine hemorrhage, and to stimulate milk let-down in nursing women.
- Desmopressin is a synthetic vasopressin analogue that retains the antidiuretic activity of the natural hormone but lacks the vasoconstrictive effect. It is administered parenterally and intranasally to treat diabetes insipidus resulting from deficient pituitary vasopressin secretion. Synthetic vasopressin is used to control gastrointestinal bleeding by causing vasoconstriction.

Selected Readings

Abs, R., et al. Cabergoline in the treatment of acromegaly: a study in 64 patients. J Clin Endocrinol Metab 83:374–378, 1998.

Bergqvist, A., et al. A double-blind randomized study of the treatment of endometriosis with nafarelin or nafarelin plus norethisterone. Gynecol Endocrinol 11:194–197, 1997.

Blethen, S. L., et al. Adult height in growth hormone–deficient children treated with biosynthetic growth hormone. J Clin Endocrinol Metab 82:418–420, 1997.

Ferreira, E., and S. R. Letwin. Desmopressin for nocturia and enuresis associated with multiple sclerosis. Ann Pharmacother 32:114–116, 1998.

Kuhn, J. M., et al. A randomized comparison of the clinical and hormonal effects of two GnRH agonists in patients with prostate cancer. Eur Urol 32:397–403, 1997.

Mannucci, P. M. Desmopressin (DDAVP) in the treatment of bleeding disorders: the first 20 years. Blood 90:2515–2521, 1997.

Muratori, M., et al. Use of cabergoline in the long-term treatment of hyperprolactinemic and acromegalic patients. J Endocrinol Invest 20:537–546, 1997.

Van der Lely, A. J., et al. A risk-benefit assessment of octreotide in the treatment of acromegaly. Drug Saf 17:317–324, 1997.

CHAPTER THIRTY-TWO

THYROID DRUGS

OVERVIEW

The thyroid gland synthesizes and secretes **triiodothyronine** (T_3) and **tetraiodothyronine** (T_4, or thyroxine). These **thyroid hormones** are necessary for normal growth and development, and they play a role in a number of metabolic processes, including those involved in the synthesis and degradation of essentially all other hormones. Thyroid hormones also augment sympathetic nervous system function, primarily by increasing the number of adrenergic receptors in target tissues.

Synthesis of Thyroid Hormones

Thyroid hormones are synthesized in a process that involves the uptake and organification of **iodide** and the subsequent coupling of iodotyrosine residues of **thyroglobulin**. These steps are illustrated in Fig. 32–1.

Iodide is actively transported into thyroid follicle cells. It diffuses across the cells to the apical membrane, where it is oxidized and attached to tyrosine residues of thyroglobulin. This process is called iodide organification. The iodinated tyrosine residues, monoiodotyrosine (MIT) and diiodotyrosine (DIT), are then coupled to form T_3 and T_4. Iodide organification and the coupling reactions are catalyzed by peroxidase.

T_4 accounts for about 80% of the hormones secreted by the thyroid, and T_3 accounts for the remainder. These hormones are transported to target organs by thyroid-binding globulin, thyroid-binding prealbumin, and albumin. In peripheral tissues, some of the T_4 is converted to T_3 and reverse T_3 (rT_3) by 5′-deiodinase and 5-deiodinase, respectively. T_3 is about five times more active than T_4, whereas rT_3 is completely inactive. For this reason, the deiodinase enzymes have an important role in controlling the level of thyroid activity. T_3 and rT_3 are eventually metabolized by deiodinase and sulfotransferase reactions to diiodothyronine sulfate.

When T_3 enters the cell nucleus, it binds to specific receptors that activate gene transcription, leading to increased synthesis of proteins necessary for growth, development, and calorigenesis (heat production).

Release of Thyroid Hormones

As discussed in Chapter 31, the secretion of thyroid hormones is modulated by an anterior pituitary hormone called **thyroid-stimulating hormone** (TSH, or thyrotropin) and by a hypothalamic hormone called **thyrotropin-releasing hormone** (TRH).

Thyroglobulin is stored as colloid in the follicular lumen. It reenters the follicular cell by endocytosis, and it undergoes proteolysis during release of the thyroid hormones. This release is stimulated by TSH via the formation of cyclic adenosine monophosphate (cAMP) in thyroid follicular cells.

The production of thyroid hormones is controlled in two ways. First, it is controlled by T_3, which inhibits TRH and TSH secretion by the hypothalamus and pituitary. Second, it is controlled by the rate of conversion of T_4 to T_3 and rT_3 in peripheral tissues. This rate is in turn affected by a variety of hormones, nutrients, and disease states.

Normal and Abnormal Thyroid Function

Normal thyroid function, or **euthyroidism,** is maintained via feedback inhibition of TSH secretion. This inhibition keeps the plasma concentration of free (circulating or unbound) T_4 within a narrow range.

Thyroid disorders are diagnosed primarily on the basis of clinical manifestations and plasma T_4 and TSH levels. **Hypothyroidism** is characterized by low T_4 and high TSH levels, which impair growth and development and cause a decrease in metabolic activity. In contrast, **hyperthyroidism** is associated with high T_4 and low TSH levels, which cause hyperactivity of organ systems (particularly the nervous and cardiovascular systems) and speed up the metabolism.

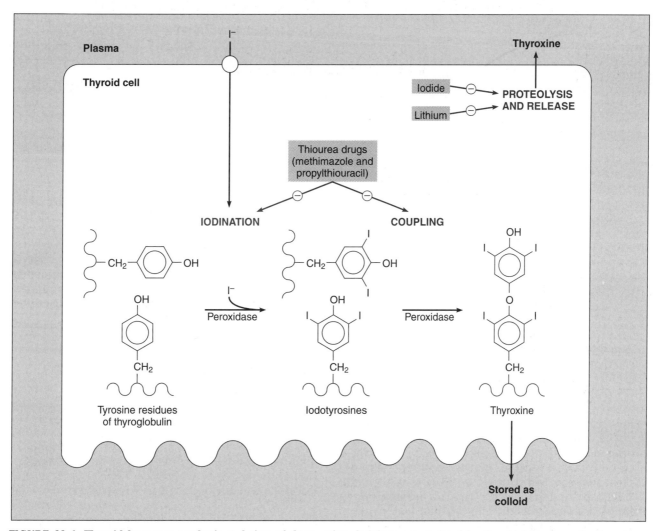

FIGURE 32–1. Thyroid hormone synthesis and sites of drug action. Iodide is accumulated by thyroid follicular cells. Peroxidase catalyzes the iodination of tyrosine residues of thyroglobulin and the coupling of iodotyrosines to form triiodothyronine (T_3) and tetraiodothyronine (T_4, or thyroxine). Thyroglobulin is stored as colloid in thyroid follicles and undergoes proteolysis to release T_4 when stimulated by thyroid-stimulating hormone (TSH, or thyrotropin). Thiourea drugs inhibit the synthesis of thyroid hormones by inhibiting iodination and coupling of tyrosine residues. Elevated iodide concentrations and lithium inhibit the release of thyroid hormones.

THYROID DISORDERS

Thyroid disorders are relatively common. In many cases, patients seek medical attention because they notice a diffuse or nodular thyroid gland enlargement **(goiter)** or suffer from other manifestations of abnormal thyroid function.

Hypothyroidism

In infants and children, hypothyroidism causes irreversible mental retardation and impairs growth and development. In adults, hypothyroidism is associated with impairment of physical and mental activity and with slowing of cardiovascular, gastrointestinal, and neuromuscular function. Hypothyroid patients may complain of lethargy, cold intolerance, weight gain, and constipation. The skin may become coarse, dry, and cold. Eventually, hypothyroidism causes **myxedema,** which is described as a dry, waxy swelling of the skin with nonpitting edema. **Myx-**edema coma is characterized by hypothermia, hypoglycemia, weakness, stupor, and shock and is the end stage of long-standing untreated hypothyroidism.

Many patients with mild hypothyroidism have a T_4 level within the normal range. However, as the disease progresses, the T_4 level usually falls below normal.

The most common cause of hypothyroidism in adults is **autoimmune thyroiditis (Hashimoto's disease).** Other causes include thyroid surgery or radioactive iodine (RAI) treatment for hyperthyroidism; dietary iodine deficiency; and thyroid hypoplasia or enzymatic defects. Pituitary or hypothalamic dysfunction can cause secondary hypothyroidism.

Several types of drugs may induce thyroid disorders. Lithium inhibits the release of thyroid hormones by the thyroid gland (see Fig. 32–1) and may cause hypothyroidism by this mechanism. Amiodarone is an iodine-containing antiarrhythmic drug that may cause either hypothyroidism or hyperthyroidism through a variety of mechanisms that alter multiple thyroid functions.

The treatment for all forms of hypothyroidism is replacement therapy with a thyroid hormone preparation.

Hyperthyroidism

Manifestations of hyperthyroidism, or **thyrotoxicosis,** may include nervousness, emotional lability, weight loss despite an increased appetite, heat intolerance, palpitations, proximal muscle weakness, increased frequency of bowel movements, and irregular menses.

Most cases of hyperthyroidism are associated with overproduction of thyroid hormones by the thyroid gland, as indicated by the finding of increased RAI uptake. Excessive thyroid hormone production may result from excessive TSH, as occurs in patients with **TSH-secreting pituitary adenomas,** or it may result from gland stimulation by thyroid antibodies, as occurs in patients with **Graves' disease.**

Graves' disease results from the formation of antibodies directed against the TSH receptor on the surface of thyroid cells. The antibodies stimulate the receptor in the same manner as TSH, resulting in overproduction of thyroid hormones. Graves' disease is characterized by hyperthyroidism, thyroid enlargement, and exophthalmus (abnormal protrusion of the eyeball). Exophthalmus results from stimulation of orbital muscles by thyroid antibodies.

Excessive thyroid hormone production also occurs in persons with thyroid nodules that are independent of pituitary gland control. **Inflammatory thyroid disease (subacute thyroiditis)** may cause a transient form of hyperthyroidism that is due to the release of preformed thyroid hormone from thyroid follicles.

Three treatment modalities are employed in hyperthyroidism: antithyroid agents, surgery, and RAI treatment. The goals of therapy are to eliminate excessive thyroid hormone production and to control the symptoms of hyperthyroidism. The choice of treatment depends on the type and severity of hyperthyroidism and on the individual characteristics of the patient. Antithyroid agents are primarily used for the short-term treatment of hyperthyroidism, either to induce remission of Graves' disease or to control the symptoms of hyperthyroidism prior to thyroid surgery or RAI treatment. Surgery or RAI treatment can permanently cure hyperthyroidism. However, use of either of these treatment modalities often results in chronic hypothyroidism, which necessitates life-long thyroid hormone replacement therapy.

THYROID HORMONE PREPARATIONS
Natural Hormone Preparations

The natural thyroid hormone preparations include **thyroid [USP]** and **thyroglobulin [USP].** Thy-

roid [USP] is desiccated hog, beef, or sheep thyroid gland that contains a standardized quantity of T_4 and T_3 in each tablet. Thyroglobulin [USP] is a purified hog gland extract that contains a standardized amount of T_4 and T_3 in a ratio of 25:1.

Because the stability of natural thyroid hormone preparations is unpredictable and because some persons are allergic to the animal proteins contained in them, these preparations have been largely replaced by synthetic hormone preparations for the treatment of hypothyroidism.

Synthetic Hormone Preparations

The synthetic thyroid hormone preparations include **levothyroxine** (T_4), **liothyronine** (T_3), and **liotrix** (a mixture containing T_4 and T_3 in a ratio of 4:1). There is little justification for using liotrix to treat hypothyroidism, so it is not discussed further. The pharmacologic and pharmacokinetic properties of levothyroxine and liothyronine are discussed below and compared in Table 32–1.

Levothyroxine

Pharmacokinetics. The oral bioavailability of levothyroxine is about 80%. However, different brands and generic formulations of levothyroxine vary in hormone content and bioavailability, so the substitution of one formulation for another should be undertaken with caution. Because the half-life of levothyroxine is about 7 days, once-daily administration of the drug produces little fluctuation in plasma hormone levels. About 35% of T_4 is converted to T_3 in peripheral tissues. Therefore, exogenous administration of levothyroxine produces physiologic levels of both T_4 and T_3. For this reason, levothyroxine may be considered a prodrug. The exogenously administered hormones are degraded in the same manner as their natural counterparts.

Indications. Levothyroxine is the drug of choice for **thyroid hormone replacement** in patients with **hypothyroidism,** because it is chemically stable, nonallergenic, and can be given orally once a day. Levothyroxine administration produces a stable pool of T_4 that is converted to T_3 at a steady and consistent rate. Levothyroxine tablets are available in a wide range of doses to accommodate individualized therapy based on clinical and laboratory data. Therapy is usually begun with a lower dose, particularly in

TABLE 32–1. Pharmacologic and Pharmacokinetic Properties of Levothyroxine (T_4) and Liothyronine (T_3)

Property	Levothyroxine	Liothyronine
Relative potency	1	4
Oral bioavailability	80% (variable)	95%
Elimination half-life	7 days	1 day
Daily doses	1	1–3

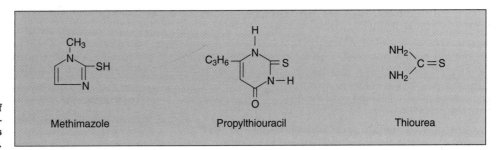

FIGURE 32–2. **Structures of methimazole and propylthiouracil, two antithyroid agents that contain a thiourea moiety.**

elderly patients and those with long-standing hypothyroidism. The dose is then increased at monthly intervals until a full replacement dose is achieved. A gradual increase in the dose prevents excessive stress on the cardiovascular and other organ systems and thereby causes fewer adverse reactions. Children usually require higher doses per kilogram of body weight than do adults.

The steady-state maintenance dose of levothyroxine is determined on the basis of the patient's clinical response, TSH levels, and T_4 levels. Many clinicians consider the TSH level to be the most sensitive test for determining thyroid replacement dosage. An elevated TSH level indicates that the levothyroxine dose is not sufficient. The expected range of T_4 levels in patients receiving thyroid replacement therapy is higher than that in healthy individuals, because a higher level of T_4 is required in patients to maintain adequate T_3 levels in the absence of endogenous T_3 production by the thyroid gland.

Levothyroxine is also the drug of choice for **suppressive therapy** in patients with **thyroid nodules, diffuse goiters,** or **thyroid cancer.** In these conditions, levothyroxine acts to suppress TSH production and reduce stimulation of abnormal thyroid tissue. Suppressive therapy thereby reduces goiter size and thyroid gland volume.

Myxedema coma is a medical emergency that requires intravenous administration of a loading dose of levothyroxine and then requires smaller daily maintenance doses.

Adverse Effects. Thyroid hormone preparations rarely cause adverse reactions if dosing is appropriate and is carefully monitored during the initial treatment of hypothyroidism and periodically thereafter. The effects of excessive doses are similar to the manifestations of hyperthyroidism.

Interactions. Aluminum hydroxide, cholestyramine, ferrous sulfate, and sucralfate are among the drugs that interfere with the absorption of levothyroxine. These drugs should be administered 2 hours before or after levothyroxine is administered. Estrogens, androgens, and glucocorticoids may alter thyroid-binding globulin and total T_4 and T_3 levels, but free T_4 and TSH levels usually remain normal in patients taking these steroid hormones. For this reason, the dosage of levothyroxine usually does not need to be adjusted in persons who are taking steroid hormones.

Liothyronine

As shown in Table 32–1, liothyronine (T_3) is more potent than levothyroxine (T_4) and has a higher oral bioavailability. However, it is seldom used in the treatment of hypothyroidism because it has several disadvantages. Liothyronine has a much shorter half-life than levothyroxine, so multiple daily doses may be needed to obtain a smooth response during hormone replacement therapy. Liothyronine does not increase plasma T_4 levels, so it is difficult to monitor the response to treatment. Liothyronine also causes more adverse cardiac effects and is more expensive than levothyroxine.

ANTITHYROID AGENTS

Antithyroid agents used in the treatment of hyperthyroidism include thiourea drugs, β-adrenergic receptor antagonists (β-blockers), iodide salts, and radioactive iodine.

The thiourea drugs inhibit the synthesis of thyroid hormones, while sufficient doses of iodide salts inhibit the release of these hormones. The β-blockers are used to control the cardiovascular symptoms of hyperthyroidism until definitive treatment becomes effective. The β-blockers, the corticosteroids, some thiourea derivatives (see below), and some iodinated contrast agents, such as **ipodate,** also inhibit the peripheral conversion of T_4 to T_3. Because of this action, ipodate is being investigated for the treatment of acute thyrotoxicosis.

Thiourea Drugs

The thiourea (thioureylene and thioamide) drugs include **methimazole** and **propylthiouracil** (PTU). Their structures are shown in Fig. 32–2.

Drug Properties

Mechanisms. As discussed earlier in this chapter, the synthesis of thyroid hormones requires oxidation of trapped iodide, formation of iodotyrosines, and the coupling of iodotyrosines to form T_3 and T_4. Methimazole and PTU both inhibit peroxidase-catalyzed steps in this process (see Fig. 32–1). In addition, PTU (but not methimazole) inhibits the conversion of T_4 to T_3 in peripheral tissues. However, the contribution of this action to the therapeutic efficacy of PTU is uncertain, since PTU and methimazole appear to be therapeutically equivalent.

Pharmacokinetics. The thiourea drugs are well absorbed from the gut following oral administration. They are actively concentrated in the thyroid gland, which may account for their relatively long duration of action despite having relatively short half-lives. The thiourea drugs are extensively metabolized before undergoing renal excretion.

Indications. In patients with **Graves' disease,** a thiourea drug can be used in an attempt to induce remission or as a means to control symptoms prior to surgery or RAI treatment. The effects of thiourea drugs are delayed because it takes about 4–8 weeks of therapy before the glandular hormone stores are depleted and circulating hormone levels start to return to the normal range. At this time, doses can be gradually tapered at monthly intervals so as to achieve the desired steady-state thyroid hormone level. If the objective is long-term remission of Graves' disease, patients usually remain on the drug for 12–24 months. About 45% of patients will eventually obtain a permanent remission. The mechanisms responsible for remission are uncertain but may involve a reduction in the thyroid-stimulating activity of thyroid antibodies or an alteration of the immunologic defect that stimulated antibody production. Persons with persistent thyroid-stimulating antibodies have a higher incidence of relapse than do persons without persistent antibodies.

Adverse Effects. Arthralgia, pruritic maculo-papular rashes, and fever occur in up to 5% of persons treated with a thiourea drug. Less frequently, a lupus erythematosus–like syndrome, hepatitis, or gastrointestinal distress is reported.

Many patients experience benign and transient leukopenia, with a white blood cell count of less than 4000/μL. This condition does not appear to be associated with the more severe agranulocytosis that sometimes occurs and is characterized by a granulocyte count of less than 250/μL. Severe agranulocytosis usually develops during the first 3 months of therapy and can be prevented by advising patients to stop treatment and immediately contact their physician if they experience fever, malaise, sore throat, or other flu-like symptoms.

Methimazole and PTU exhibit cross-sensitivity in about 50% of patients. For this reason, patients who have experienced a major adverse reaction should not be switched to the other drug.

Specific Drugs

Although methimazole and PTU appear to be clinically equivalent, they have minor differences. The plasma half-lives of methimazole and PTU are about 7 and 2 hours, respectively. However, either drug can be administered once or twice a day. Unlike methimazole, PTU inhibits the peripheral conversion of T_4 to T_3. Nevertheless, the clinical effects of the drugs are primarily related to inhibition of hormone synthesis and depletion of glandular stores.

About 70% of PTU is bound to plasma proteins. Methimazole is not bound to plasma proteins, and it readily crosses the placenta and appears in breast milk. Contrary to older studies, which indicated that PTU crosses the placenta less readily, newer evidence indicates that fetal blood concentrations of PTU are greater than maternal blood concentrations. Hence, both drugs must be used cautiously during pregnancy.

β-Adrenergic Receptor Antagonists

Thyroid hormones and the sympathetic nervous system act synergistically on cardiovascular function. This explains why increased levels of thyroid hormones may cause tachycardia, palpitations, and arrhythmias. β-Adrenergic receptor antagonists, such as **propranolol,** are used to reduce cardiovascular stimulation associated with hyperthyroidism. They act immediately and are particularly useful during **severe acute thyrotoxicosis (thyroid storm).** They are also used to control symptoms of hyperthyroidism in patients awaiting surgery or a response to RAI treatment.

Other Antithyroid Agents
Iodide Salts

Iodide salts are contained in **potassium iodide solutions,** such as **saturated solution of potassium iodide** (SSKI) and **Lugol's solution.** They are used on a short-term basis to treat patients with acute thyrotoxicosis, to prepare patients for thyroid surgery, and to inhibit the release of thyroid hormones following RAI treatment. Iodide salts can also be used to competitively block RAI uptake by the thyroid gland in the event of a nuclear reactor accident or other accidental exposure to toxic levels of RAI.

When administered in sufficient doses, iodide salts act immediately to inhibit the release of thyroid hormones from the thyroid gland. Plasma hormone levels then gradually decline as the circulating hormones are degraded. Patients with hyperthyroidism usually obtain symptomatic improvement within 2–7 days after starting iodide therapy. However, the duration of this effect is limited to several weeks because the thyroid gland eventually escapes from the inhibitory effects of iodide salts. A thiourea drug can be used concurrently with iodide salts to further inhibit thyroid function and to provide a longer-lasting antithyroid effect.

In patients scheduled for thyroid surgery, a potassium iodide solution is usually administered preoperatively for 7–14 days to reduce the size and vascularity of the thyroid gland. As an adjunct to RAI treatment, potassium iodide is given 3–7 days following the administration of RAI.

The adverse effects of iodide salts are usually mild and may include skin rashes and other hypersensitivity reactions, salivary gland swelling, metallic taste, sore gums, and gastrointestinal discomfort.

Radioactive Iodine

Radioactive iodine (RAI) is usually administered as a colorless and tasteless solution of **sodium iodide I 131** (^{131}I). The isotope is rapidly absorbed from the gut and concentrated by the thyroid gland. In the gland, it emits beta particles that destroy thyroid tissue. The particles have a tissue penetration of 2 mm, and the isotope has a half-life of 8 days. As thyroid tissue is destroyed, the circulating thyroid hormone levels gradually return to normal over several weeks.

β-Adrenergic receptor antagonists are usually employed to control symptoms of hyperthyroidism while the patient is awaiting the response to RAI. Methimazole or PTU may be used if β-blockers alone are not adequate to control these symptoms. However, the use of thiourea drugs with RAI appears to cause a higher incidence of posttreatment recurrence or persistence of hyperthyroidism. For this reason, thiourea drugs should be withdrawn several days before RAI and reinstituted several days after RAI.

Iodide salts are used after RAI treatment to inhibit thyroid hormone release. They should not be used before RAI, however, because nonradioactive iodide would compete with ^{131}I for uptake by the thyroid gland.

RAI treatment is absolutely contraindicated in pregnant women, because it destroys fetal thyroid tissue.

Summary of Important Points

- The thyroid gland synthesizes and secretes triiodothyronine (T_3) and tetraiodothyronine (T_4, or thyroxine).
- The steps in thyroid hormone synthesis include active iodide uptake by the thyroid gland, incorporation of iodide into tyrosine residues of thyroglobulin, and coupling of iodotyrosines to form T_3 and T_4. The secretion of T_3 and T_4 is modulated by thyroid-stimulating hormone (TSH, or thyrotropin) and by thyrotropin-releasing hormone (TRH).
- The thyroid hormones activate cytoplasmic receptors and are translocated to the cell nucleus. In the nucleus, they activate gene transcription and thereby increase the metabolic rate and accelerate a wide range of cellular activities that are required for normal growth and development and for the maintenance of normal metabolism.
- Levothyroxine (synthetic T_4) is the drug of choice for all forms of hypothyroidism. It has a long half-life (7 days) and can be administered orally once a day.

- Liothyronine (synthetic T_3) is more potent than levothyroxine and has a higher oral bioavailability. However, it has a shorter half-life and may need to be given several times a day.
- Methimazole and propylthiouracil (PTU) are thiourea drugs that inhibit peroxidase-catalyzed steps in the synthesis of thyroid hormone. PTU also inhibits the peripheral conversion of T_4 to T_3. The onset of action of these drugs is delayed because of the time required to deplete glandular stores of thyroid hormone.
- In patients with Graves' disease, methimazole or PTU is used in an attempt to induce remission or as a means to control symptoms prior to surgery or radioactive iodine (RAI) treatment.
- β-Adrenergic receptor antagonists are used to control the cardiovascular symptoms of hyperthyroidism in patients who are suffering from acute thyrotoxicosis, are awaiting surgery, or are awaiting a response to RAI treatment.
- The iodide salts in potassium iodide solutions act rapidly to inhibit the release of thyroid hormones from the thyroid gland. They produce symptomatic improvement in 2–7 days as circulating levels of thyroid hormones decline. Potassium iodide solutions are used to control symptoms of acute thyrotoxicosis, to reduce the vascularity and size of the thyroid gland prior to surgery, and to inhibit thyroid hormone release following RAI treatment.
- RAI (^{131}I) is concentrated by the thyroid gland and emits beta particles that destroy thyroid tissue. It is used in the treatment of Graves' disease and other forms of hyperthyroidism. RAI treatment is absolutely contraindicated in pregnant women.

Selected Readings

Adlin, V. Subclinical hypothyroidism: deciding when to treat. Am Fam Physician 57:776–780, 1998.

Becker, D. V., and P. Zanzonico. Potassium iodide for thyroid blockade in a reactor accident: administrative policies that govern its use. Thyroid 7:193–197, 1997.

Ecker, J. L., and T. J. Musci. Treatment of thyroid disease in pregnancy. Obstet Gynecol Clin North Am 24:575–589, 1997.

Harjai, K. J., and A. A. Licata. Effects of amiodarone on thyroid function. Ann Intern Med 126:63–73, 1997.

Imseis, R. E., et al. Pretreatment with propylthiouracil but not methimazole reduces the therapeutic efficacy of iodine-131 in hyperthyroidism. J Clin Endocrinol Metab 83:685–687, 1998.

Kannan, C. R., and K. G. Seshadri. Thyrotoxicosis. Dis Mon 43:601–677, 1997.

Kaplan, M. M., et al. Treatment of hyperthyroidism with radioactive iodine. Endocrinol Metab Clin North Am 27:205–223, 1998.

Momotani, N., et al. Effects of propylthiouracil and methimazole on fetal thyroid status in mothers with Graves' hyperthyroidism. J Clin Endocrinol Metab 82:3633–3636, 1997.

Mortimer, R. H., et al. Methimazole and propylthiouracil equally cross the perfused human term placental lobule. J Clin Endocrinol Metab 82:3099–3102, 1997.

CHAPTER THIRTY-THREE

ADRENAL STEROIDS AND

RELATED DRUGS

CLASSIFICATION OF ADRENAL STEROIDS AND RELATED DRUGS

ADRENAL STEROID PREPARATIONS
Mineralocorticoids
- Fludrocortisone

Glucocorticoids
- Betamethasone
- Cortisone
- Dexamethasone
- Hydrocortisone
- Methylprednisolone
- Prednisone
- Triamcinolone

Adrenal androgens
- Dehydroepiandrosterone

ADRENAL STEROID INHIBITORS
Corticosteroid synthesis inhibitors
- Aminoglutethimide
- Ketoconazole
- Metyrapone

Corticosteroid receptor antagonists
- Mifepristone
- Spironolactone

OVERVIEW

Synthesis of Adrenal Steroids

The adrenal cortex occupies about 90% of the adrenal gland, consists of three layers, and produces three types of steroid hormones, or **corticosteroids.** These hormones can be classified as **mineralocorticoids, glucocorticoids,** and **adrenal androgens.** The mineralocorticoids are primarily produced in the outer layer (zona glomerulosa), while the glucocorticoids and adrenal androgens are produced in the middle layer (zona fasciculata) and inner layer (zona reticularis).

The major pathways for mineralocorticoid, glucocorticoid, and androgen biosynthesis are shown in Fig. 33–1. In humans, **aldosterone** is the major mineralocorticoid, **cortisol** is the major glucocorticoid, and **dehydroepiandrosterone** (DHEA) is the major adrenal androgen.

Secretion of Adrenal Steroids

The secretion of adrenal steroids is affected by **physical and mental stress** and by the actions of two hormones: **adrenocorticotropic hormone** (ACTH, or corticotropin), which is secreted by the anterior pituitary, and **corticotropin-releasing hormone** (CRH), which is secreted by the hypothalamus.

The secretion of aldosterone is partly stimulated by ACTH but is chiefly regulated by the **renin-angiotensin system.** In contrast, the secretion of cortisol and adrenal androgens is controlled by ACTH.

Various types of physical and mental stress are powerful activators of CRH secretion, and increased CRH secretion leads to increased ACTH and cortisol production. However, as shown in Fig. 33–2, cortisol and other glucocorticoids act as feedback inhibitors of both CRH and ACTH. This is why exogenously administered glucocorticoids can suppress the hypothalamic-pituitary-adrenal axis and inhibit endogenous cortisol production.

Although exogenously administered glucocorticoids have several actions that increase the body's resistance to stress, people who become dependent on these drugs must receive larger doses of them during periods of stress, including stress caused by surgery, infection, and other trauma or disease states.

Binding of Adrenal Steroids to Receptors

The adrenal steroids act on target tissues by binding to specific cytoplasmic receptors, which are then translocated to the cell nucleus. In the nucleus, the activated receptors stimulate or inhibit the transcription of specific genes and thereby modulate the production of key metabolic enzymes and other proteins. These actions lead to the various metabolic and anti-inflammatory effects of glucocorticoids, which are described below. In the renal tubules, activation of the mineralocorticoid receptor stimulates the synthesis of sodium channels and the sodium-potassium ATPase that are involved in sodium reabsorption. This mechanism is responsible for the salt-retaining effects of mineralocorticoids.

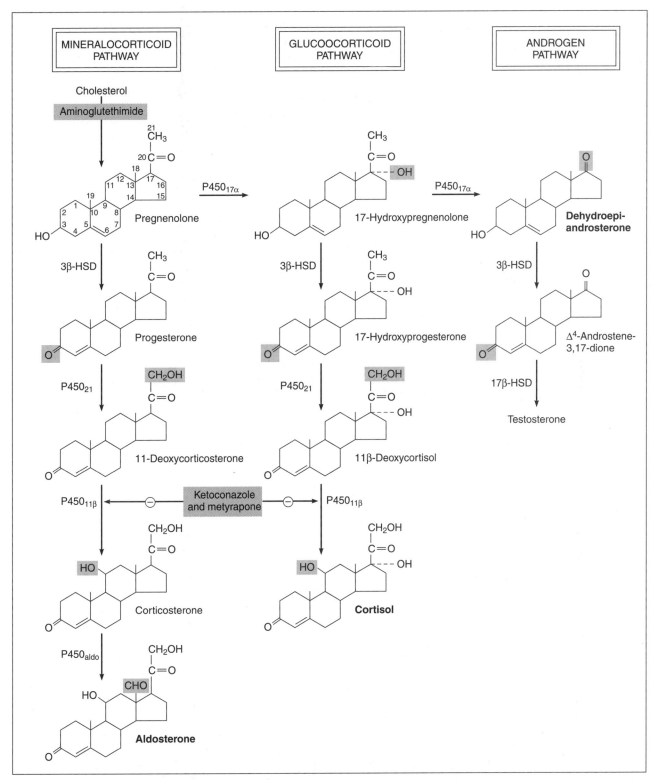

FIGURE 33–1. Biosynthetic pathways for adrenal steroids. Major pathways for mineralocorticoid, glucocorticoid, and androgen biosynthesis are shown. Important enzymes include 3β-hydroxysteroid dehydrogenase (3β-HSD), steroid 21-hydroxylase (P450$_{21}$), steroid 11β-hydroxylase (P450$_{11β}$), aldosterone synthase (P450$_{aldo}$), steroid 17α-hydroxylase (P450$_{17α}$), and 17β-hydroxysteroid dehydrogenase (17β-HSD). The structural changes produced by each reaction are shaded in gray. Aminoglutethimide blocks the synthesis of all adrenal steroids by inhibiting the conversion of cholesterol to pregnenolone. Ketoconazole and metyrapone inhibit P450$_{11β}$. The most common defect causing congenital adrenal hyperplasia is P450$_{21}$ deficiency.

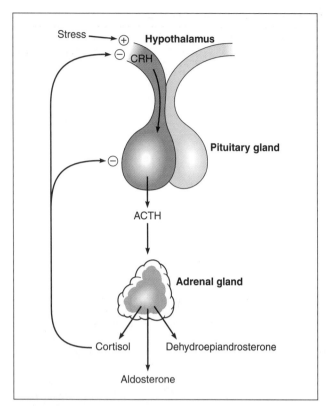

FIGURE 33–2. Regulation of the secretion of cortisol by the adrenal cortex. Stress and other stimuli increase the release of corticotropin-releasing hormone (CRH) from hypothalamic paraventricular nuclei. CRH is carried by hypophysioportal vessels to the anterior pituitary, where it stimulates the release of adrenocorticotropic hormone (ACTH, or corticotropin). ACTH acts on the adrenal cortex to increase the release of adrenal steroids, although the release of aldosterone is primarily regulated by the renin-angiotensin system. Cortisol exerts feedback inhibition on the hypothalamus and pituitary to inhibit the release of CRH and ACTH.

The **glucocorticoid receptor** has a high affinity for cortisol but a much lower affinity for aldosterone, whereas the **mineralocorticoid receptor** has a high affinity for both aldosterone and cortisol. This enables cortisol to exert both glucocorticoid actions and mineralocorticoid actions.

Uses of Adrenal Steroids and Related Drugs

The glucocorticoids are most frequently used clinically because of the anti-inflammatory effects produced by supraphysiologic doses of them. Less commonly, the glucocorticoids and the mineralocorticoids are used as replacement therapy in the treatment of **adrenal insufficiency** and in the treatment of **adrenogenital syndromes** that produce excessive quantities of adrenal androgens and insufficient quantities of other corticosteroids.

Adrenocortical hyperfunction (Cushing's syndrome) is caused by excessive levels of circulating corticosteroids and is treated with surgery, irradiation, and adrenal steroid inhibitors.

ADRENAL STEROID PREPARATIONS

The properties and structures of selected adrenal steroids are shown in Table 33–1 and Fig. 33–3.

Mineralocorticoids

Aldosterone, the major mineralocorticoid in humans, is not available for clinical use.

Fludrocortisone is the mineralocorticoid that is used most frequently. In patients with **primary adrenal insufficiency (Addison's disease),** fludrocortisone is given to supplement the mineralocorticoid effects of hydrocortisone (cortisol) treatment. The need for fludrocortisone is indicated by the continued presence of hyperkalemia after adequate doses of hydrocortisone have been administered. Fludrocortisone is administered orally once a day in the morning. The drug's salt-retaining potency is about 20 times greater than its anti-inflammatory potency.

Glucocorticoids

Numerous glucocorticoids are available for clinical use and are frequently classified on the basis of their duration of action (see Table 33–1). **Cortisol,** the major glucocorticoid in humans, is called **hydrocortisone** when used as a pharmaceutical. Like **cortisone,** hydrocortisone is a short-acting glucocorticoid. **Methylprednisolone, prednisone,** and **triamcinolone** are examples of intermediate-acting glucocorticoids, whereas **betamethasone** and **dexamethasone** are examples of long-acting glucocorticoids.

Drug Properties

Mechanisms and Effects. Although the glucocorticoids were named for their role in the regulation of glucose metabolism, they have a number of other important physiologic actions.

(1) Effects on Carbohydrate, Lipid, and Protein Metabolism. Glucocorticoids induce enzymes involved in gluconeogenesis (the formation of glucose from amino acids), promote glucose formation, and have an anti-insulin effect. This is why glucocorticoid insufficiency may lead to hypoglycemia during stress. Glucocorticoids also activate enzymes involved in protein catabolism, thereby increasing the supply of amino acids needed for gluconeogenesis. Glucocorticoids stimulate lipolysis while inhibiting the uptake of glucose by adipose tissue. For this reason, excessive glucocorticoid levels may lead to abnormal fat distribution and muscle wasting (see below).

(2) Anti-inflammatory Effects. The anti-inflammatory effects of glucocorticoids are primarily attributable to their multiple actions on several types of leukocytes (Fig. 33–4). First, glucocorticoids suppress the activation of T lymphocytes. Second, they suppress the production of cytokines by activated T helper cells. Cytokines normally play a major role in inflammation by recruiting and acti-

TABLE 33–1. Pharmacologic Properties of Adrenal Steroids

Drug*	Route of Administration	Duration of Action (Hours)	Mineralocorticoid (Salt-Retaining) Potency	Glucocorticoid (Anti-inflammatory) Potency
Short-acting drugs				
Hydrocortisone (cortisol)	Oral, parenteral, or topical	8–12	1	1
Cortisone	Oral, parenteral, or topical	8–12	0.8	0.8
Fludrocortisone	Oral	8–12	200	10
Intermediate-acting drugs				
Methylprednisolone	Oral, parenteral, or topical	12–36	0.5	5
Prednisone	Oral	12–36	0.7	3.5
Triamcinolone	Oral, parenteral, or topical	12–36	0	5
Long-acting drugs				
Betamethasone	Oral, parenteral, or topical	24–72	0	30
Dexamethasone	Oral, parenteral, or topical	24–72	0	30

*Fludrocortisone is classified as a mineralocorticoid, while the other drugs are classified as glucocorticoids.

FIGURE 33–3. Structures of selected adrenal steroids. Hydrocortisone (cortisol) is a natural steroid. In the synthetic steroids, glucocorticoid potency is enhanced by the introduction of a double bond at the 1,2 position or the introduction of a hydroxyl or methyl group at the 16 position. These structural modifications are unshaded. Betamethasone and dexamethasone differ only in the configuration of the methyl group at the 16 position: β in betamethasone (solid line) and α in dexamethasone (dashed line). Both glucocorticoid and mineralocorticoid activities are increased by a fluorine substitution at the 9 position.

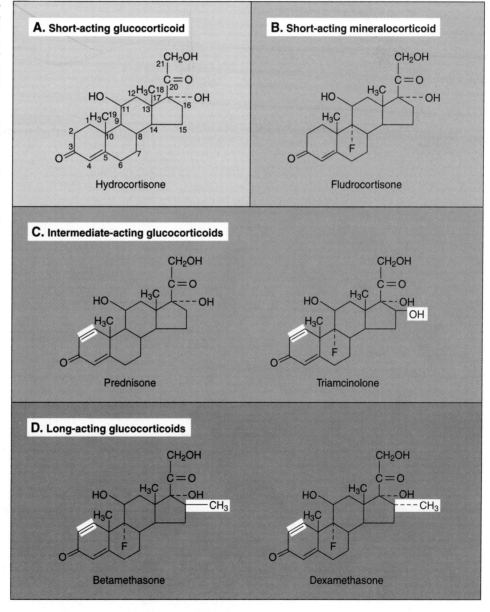

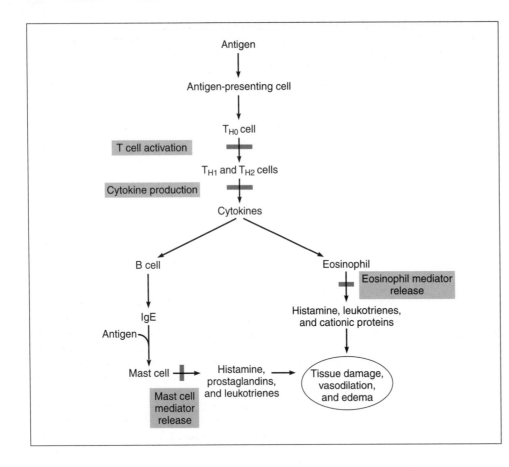

FIGURE 33–4. Anti-inflammatory actions of glucocorticoids. During the inflammatory process, undifferentiated T helper cells (T_{H0}) become activated T cells (T_{H1} and T_{H2}) and produce cytokines. In addition to stimulating antibody production by B cells, cytokines recruit and activate eosinophils. Glucocorticoids act by suppressing T cell activation, suppressing cytokine production, and preventing mast cells and eosinophils from releasing various chemical mediators of inflammation, including histamine, prostaglandins, leukotrienes, and other substances that cause tissue damage, vasodilation, and edema. Glucocorticoids have additional anti-inflammatory effects that are described in the text. IgE = immunoglobulin E.

vating eosinophils and by stimulating antibody production by B cells. Third, glucocorticoids prevent mast cells, basophils, and eosinophils from releasing various chemical mediators of inflammation, including histamine, prostaglandins, leukotrienes, and other substances that cause tissue damage, vasodilation, and edema. Fourth, glucocorticoids stabilize lysosomal membranes and prevent the release of catabolic enzymes from these organelles. Finally, glucocorticoids cause vasoconstriction and decrease capillary permeability by direct actions as well as by inhibiting the actions of kinins, bacterial toxins, and chemical mediators released from mast cells and eosinophils.

Glucocorticoids also have multiple effects on circulating leukocytes. Pharmacologic doses of glucocorticoids suppress lymphoid tissue and reduce the number of circulating lymphocytes. They also reduce the concentration of circulating eosinophils, basophils, and monocytes while at the same time increasing the concentration of erythrocytes, platelets, and polymorphonuclear leukocytes.

(3) Other Effects. Glucocorticoids increase bone catabolism and antagonize the effect of vitamin D on calcium absorption, thereby contributing to the development of osteoporosis (see Chapter 36). Glucocorticoids also have several effects on the central nervous system. They alter the mood in some persons and may cause euphoria or psychosis. Large doses of glucocorticoids stimulate gastric acid and pepsin production and may thereby exacerbate

peptic ulcers. Glucocorticoids can also reduce the secretion of thyroid-stimulating hormone (TSH) and follicle-stimulating hormone (FSH) by the pituitary gland.

Chemistry. In addition to showing the chemical structure of hydrocortisone, Fig. 33–3 shows the structures of several synthetic glucocorticoids that were developed to provide greater glucocorticoid (anti-inflammatory) potency than hydrocortisone. In the synthetic steroids, glucocorticoid potency is enhanced by the introduction of a double bond at the 1,2 position or the introduction of a hydroxyl or methyl group at the 16 position. Both glucocorticoid and mineralocorticoid activities are increased by a fluorine substitution at the 9 position. Table 33–1 shows the ratio of glucocorticoid potency to mineralocorticoid potency in numerous adrenal steroids.

Indications. Glucocorticoids are used for the diagnosis and treatment of adrenal diseases and for the treatment of a diverse group of nonadrenal disorders.

(1) Adrenal Insufficiency. In **primary adrenal insufficiency (Addison's disease),** all regions of the adrenal cortex are destroyed. This gives rise to deficiencies in cortisol and aldosterone and to a reduction in androgen secretion. **Secondary adrenal insufficiency** has several causes, but it most commonly results when steroid drugs are used for a prolonged time, thereby suppressing the hypothalamic-pituitary-adrenal axis. Secondary disease is characterized by low levels of cortisol and androgens but normal levels of aldosterone.

Acute adrenal insufficiency (adrenal crisis, or **addisonian crisis)** is a medical emergency that must be treated promptly with intravenously administered hydrocortisone for up to 48 hours. Once the patient's condition is stabilized, long-term oral hydrocortisone treatment can be instituted.

In the treatment of **chronic adrenal insufficiency,** hydrocortisone is administered orally in a manner that mimics the circadian secretion of cortisol by the normal adrenal gland, with two-thirds of the daily dose given in the morning and one-third given in the evening. If hyperkalemia is still present after the oral hydrocortisone dose is stabilized, the addition of a mineralocorticoid to the treatment regimen is usually required. A single daily dose of fludrocortisone is often employed for this purpose.

Congenital adrenal hyperplasia (CAH) refers to a group of disorders caused by specific enzyme deficiencies that impair the synthesis of cortisol and aldosterone. Impaired synthesis leads to a compensatory increase in ACTH secretion by the pituitary and results in adrenal hyperplasia. Because of the enzyme deficiencies, the steroid biosynthetic pathway is shifted to the production of adrenal androgens, thereby resulting in virilism (masculinization) and hirsutism (excessive hair growth). The most common defect is **21-hydroxylase deficiency,** which accounts for 90% of cases of CAH. The second most common defect is **11β-hydroxylase deficiency,** which accounts for 9% of cases. CAH is treated by giving hydrocortisone to suppress the secretion of ACTH. Fludrocortisone may be given to provide additional mineralocorticoid activity for salt-losing CAH patients.

(2) Cushing's Syndrome. Cushing's syndrome is most often caused by a pituitary adenoma that produces excessive quantities of ACTH, leading to adrenal hyperplasia and excessive cortisol production. Other causes of Cushing's syndrome include adrenal adenomas, adrenal carcinomas, and ectopic ACTH-secreting tumors.

The diagnosis of Cushing's syndrome is often based on the free cortisol level in urine samples and on the results of testing with dexamethasone. In the **low-dose dexamethasone suppression test,** a single dose of dexamethasone is given orally at 11:00 PM, and cortisol levels in plasma are measured at 8:00 AM the following morning. In healthy individuals, dexamethasone will suppress ACTH secretion by the pituitary and cause plasma cortisol levels to be under 5 μg/dL. In persons with Cushing's syndrome, dexamethasone will not suppress ACTH secretion, so the cortisol level will usually exceed 10 μg/dL. The **high-dose dexamethasone suppression test** may be used to differentiate adrenal hyperplasia from other causes of hyperadrenocorticism.

Cushing's syndrome is usually treated by surgical excision of the pituitary adenoma or the hyperplastic adrenal glands. Patients must receive hydro-

cortisone parenterally in large doses during the surgical procedure. The dose is then gradually tapered to normal replacement levels.

(3) Inflammation, Allergy, and Autoimmune Disorders. The glucocorticoids are most frequently employed to suppress inflammation and immune dysfunction associated with diseases affecting almost every organ in the body. Glucocorticoids counteract inflammation evoked by physical trauma, extreme temperatures, noxious chemicals, radiation damage, and microbial pathogens. They also suppress inflammation caused by allergic and autoimmune reactions and other disease states.

(4) Cancer. Because of their lymphotoxic effects, glucocorticoids are used in the treatment of lymphocytic leukemias and lymphomas (see Chapter 45). Dexamethasone is a long-acting glucocorticoid that is employed in combination with other drugs to prevent emesis during cancer chemotherapy.

(5) Respiratory Distress Syndrome. Betamethasone is used to prevent respiratory distress syndrome in premature infants. It acts by promoting fetal lung maturation in the same manner as endogenous cortisol does. Betamethasone is used because it is not highly protein-bound and will readily enter the placental circulation.

(6) Other Disorders. Glucocorticoids are used in the treatment of **hypercalcemia,** and they are the drugs of choice for managing **sarcoidosis.** Glucocorticoids are also used as immunosuppressant drugs to prevent **organ graft rejection** (see Chapter 45).

Pharmacokinetics. Many glucocorticoids are available for oral, parenteral, and topical use. Some are available for inhalational administration.

(1) Oral Preparations. When administered orally, glucocorticoids are extremely lipid-soluble and are well absorbed from the gut. In the circulation, the glucocorticoids are highly bound to corticosteroid-binding globulin and albumin. Glucocorticoids are oxidized by cytochrome P450 enzymes and conjugated with sulfate or glucuronide in the liver before undergoing renal excretion. The biologic half-life and duration of action of glucocorticoids are primarily determined by their potency at the glucocorticoid receptor. The highly potent glucocorticoids evoke a longer-lasting stimulation of gene transcription than do the less potent drugs.

Glucocorticoids are administered orally to treat serious allergic reactions, autoimmune disorders, neoplastic diseases, and many other conditions. Prednisone or another intermediate-acting drug is often used for these purposes. For acute allergic reactions and other acute disorders, glucocorticoids are often more effective when they are given initially in large doses. The dose is then gradually tapered over several days until treatment is discontinued. For severe autoimmune and inflammatory disorders, such as systemic lupus erythematosus and polymyositis with dermatomyositis, large doses of prednisone must be given daily for several months until a remission is achieved, and then the dose is slowly tapered and continued for 1–2 years or longer. In some conditions, it may be possible to convert the patient to alternate-day therapy, in which all or most of the dose is given on alternate days. This dosage schedule appears to reduce the severity of adverse effects and produces less suppression of the hypothalamic-pituitary-adrenal axis by allowing more time for recovery between doses.

(2) Parenteral Preparations. Glucocorticoids are administered parenterally to treat acute adrenal crises, acute allergic reactions, and similar emergencies. In some cases, the drugs are given intravenously. In other cases, they are given intramuscularly, either as a rapidly absorbed solution or as a slowly absorbed drug suspension (depot preparation). Depot preparations are useful in providing a sustained level of the drug for several weeks, as is sometimes necessary in the treatment of a severe allergic reaction.

(3) Topical and Inhalational Preparations. Whenever possible, topical or inhalational administration is preferred because it is usually well tolerated and avoids most systemic adverse effects. Topical administration is widely employed in the treatment of allergic or inflammatory conditions affecting the skin, mucous membranes, or eyes. For example, glucocorticoids are administered topically to treat contact dermatitis, allergic conjunctivitis, and acute uveitis (inflammation of the iris, ciliary body, or choroid). Glucocorticoids are given by inhalation to treat allergic rhinitis, aspiration pneumonia, asthma, and other respiratory conditions (see Chapter 27).

Adverse Effects. The administration of supraphysiologic doses of glucocorticoids for more than 2 weeks produces a series of tissue and metabolic changes that resemble Cushing's syndrome. The face becomes rounded and puffy (moon facies) as fat is redistributed to the face and trunk from the extremities. Fat accumulation in the supraclavicular and dorsocervical areas contributes to the development of a "buffalo hump." Increased hair growth (hirsutism), weight gain, and muscle wasting and weakness are often observed. Dermatologic changes may include acne (steroid acne), bruising, and thinning of the skin.

Other metabolic and physiologic changes caused by glucocorticoid administration include hyperglycemia, glucose intolerance, osteoporosis, and hypertension. Some changes, such as sodium retention, potassium loss, and hypertension, are more common when cortisone or hydrocortisone is used because these drugs have greater mineralocorticoid activity than do other glucocorticoids.

Long-term use of glucocorticoids may cause posterior subcapsular cataracts and glaucoma, may exacerbate the manifestations of peptic ulcer disease, and may mask the symptoms and signs of mycotic and other infections. In children, long-term use may cause growth retardation.

Glucocorticoids are contraindicated or should be used with caution in patients with psychoses, peptic ulcers, heart diseases, hypertension, diabetes, osteoporosis, and certain infections.

Specific Drugs

Short-Acting Glucocorticoids. Hydrocortisone and cortisone have a duration of action of 8–12 hours, have equal glucocorticoid and mineralocorticoid effects, and are the preferred glucocorticoids when replacement therapy is needed for patients with adrenal insufficiency. These drugs are also used as anti-inflammatory agents, but more potent glucocorticoids are often preferred for patients with severe inflammatory, allergic, and autoimmune disorders.

Intermediate-Acting Glucocorticoids. Prednisone, methylprednisolone, and triamcinolone are the glucocorticoids used most often for systemic treatment. In the body, prednisone is rapidly converted to prednisolone, a substance that is itself available as a drug. The intermediate-acting glucocorticoids have a duration of action of 12–36 hours and are often used to treat cancer, inflammation, allergy, and autoimmune disorders.

Long-Acting Glucocorticoids. Betamethasone and dexamethasone are stereoisomers that differ in the configuration of the methyl group at the 16 position. Betamethasone is frequently employed in the topical treatment of a number of skin disorders, including psoriasis, seborrheic or atopic dermatitis, and neurodermatitis. Dexamethasone is used in dexamethasone suppression tests (see above) and in the treatment of a variety of neoplastic, infectious, and other inflammatory conditions that require the use of a potent and long-acting drug.

Inhalational Glucocorticoids. Several glucocorticoids, including **beclomethasone,** are available for nasal inhalation or oral inhalation in the treatment of allergic rhinitis or asthma, respectively. Inhaled glucocorticoids are often first-line therapy for these disorders, and their administration and use are described in Chapter 27.

Adrenal Androgens

Dehydroepiandrosterone (DHEA) is the major androgen secreted by the adrenal cortex. Smaller quantities of androstenedione and testosterone are also secreted by the adrenal gland.

DHEA is an extremely weak androgen, but it is partly converted to testosterone in the body. In humans, studies show that the production of DHEA by the adrenal gland declines in a linear fashion after the age of 20 years. In animals, studies indicate that DHEA protects against the development of diabetes mellitus, immune disorders, and cancer. DHEA also appears to prevent weight gain and prolong life in some species. For these reasons, the use of DHEA supplements has been adopted uncritically by the health food culture. Although there is some evidence for beneficial effects of DHEA in the elderly and other people, much remains to be learned about the clinical utility of this steroid.

Because DHEA is a weak androgen, it should not be used by men with prostate cancer.

ADRENAL STEROID INHIBITORS
Corticosteroid Synthesis Inhibitors

Fig. 33–1 shows the sites of action of three inhibitors of corticosteroid synthesis: aminoglutethimide, metyrapone, and ketoconazole.

Aminoglutethimide

Aminoglutethimide inhibits the conversion of cholesterol to pregnenolone, an early and rate-limiting step in adrenal steroid biosynthesis. Because the synthesis of all steroids is reduced by aminoglutethimide, it has been used in the treatment of **breast cancer** and **malignant adrenocortical tumors.** It also has been used in combination with metyrapone to treat **Cushing's syndrome.**

Metyrapone

Metyrapone inhibits the synthesis of glucocorticoids by inhibiting the 11β-hydroxylase enzyme that catalyzes the final step in the glucocorticoid pathway. As a result of this action, the steroid biosynthetic pathway is shifted to the production of adrenal androgens. Metyrapone is occasionally used to treat **Cushing's syndrome** in patients who are refractory to other treatments and are not candidates for surgery. Metyrapone is also sometimes used in tests of adrenal function.

Ketoconazole

Ketoconazole is an antifungal drug that inhibits several cytochrome P450 enzymes involved in steroid biosynthesis, including 11β-hydroxylase. When used in the treatment of **Cushing's syndrome,** the drug is able to lower the amount of cortisol to the normal range in the majority of patients. However, it also inhibits androgen synthesis and may cause gynecomastia in male patients.

Corticosteroid Receptor Antagonists
Spironolactone

Spironolactone is a synthetic steroid that competes with aldosterone for the mineralocorticoid (aldosterone) receptor in the renal tubules. It is used as a **potassium-sparing diuretic** (see Chapter 13) and as an agent for the treatment of hyperaldosteronism. Spironolactone is the drug of choice for **primary hyperaldosteronism** caused by bilateral adrenal hyperplasia, whereas surgery is the treatment of choice for hyperaldosteronism caused by an aldosterone-producing adenoma. **Secondary hyperaldosteronism** associated with heart failure, Bartter's syndrome, and other causes may also be improved by the administration of spironolactone.

Mifepristone

Mifepristone is an antagonist at both progesterone and glucocorticoid receptors (see Chapter 34). It is undergoing investigation for the treatment of **Cushing's syndrome** and appears to be highly effective in reversing the effects of **hyperadrenocorticism.**

Summary of Important Points

- The adrenal gland secretes mineralocorticoids (primarily aldosterone), glucocorticoids (primarily cortisol), and adrenal androgens (primarily dehydroepiandrosterone).
- Mineralocorticoids have salt-retaining activity. They include fludrocortisone, a short-acting drug that is used to supplement hydrocortisone (cortisol) treatment in patients with adrenal insufficiency.
- Glucocorticoids increase gluconeogenesis, increase protein and lipid catabolism, and increase the body's resistance to stress. They reduce inflammation by inhibiting the migration of leukocytes and the production and release of cytokines, prostaglandins, leukotrienes, and other mediators of inflammation. They also stabilize lysosomal membranes and cause vasoconstriction.
- Glucocorticoids are chiefly used as anti-inflammatory and immunosuppressive drugs in the treatment of a wide range of allergic, inflammatory, and autoimmune disorders. They are also used as replacement therapy in the treatment of primary adrenal insufficiency (Addison's disease) and congenital adrenal hyperplasia.
- Glucocorticoids include short-acting drugs (cortisone and hydrocortisone), intermediate-acting drugs (methylprednisolone, prednisone, and triamcinolone), and long-acting drugs (betamethasone and dexamethasone).
- In comparison with cortisol, most synthetic glucocorticoids have increased glucocorticoid potency and decreased mineralocorticoid potency.
- Glucocorticoids are generally administered topically to treat skin, mucous membrane, and ocular disorders and by inhalation to treat allergic rhinitis and asthma.
- In patients with acute allergic reactions, glucocorticoids are initially given in large doses. The doses are rapidly tapered and eventually discontinued. In patients with severe autoimmune and inflammatory diseases, large doses of prednisone or other glucocorticoids may be required for several months. Alternate-day therapy is preferred for long-term administration.
- Adverse effects of glucocorticoids include fat accumulation in the face and trunk, muscle wasting, skin changes, glucose intolerance, potassium depletion, osteoporosis, hypertension, and cataracts.
- Aminoglutethimide, metyrapone, and ketoconazole inhibit various steps in corticosteroid biosynthesis and are occasionally used to diagnose and treat adrenal hyperplasia.

Selected Readings

Anyaegbuman, W. I., and A. B. Adetona. Use of antenatal corticosteroids for fetal maturation in preterm infants. Am Fam Physician 56:1093–1096, 1997.

Barnes, N. Relative safety and efficacy of inhaled corticosteroids. J Allergy Clin Immunol 101:S460–S464, 1998.

Brown, E. S., and T. Suppes. Mood symptoms during corticosteroid therapy: a review. Harv Rev Psychiatry 5:239–246, 1998.

Dluhy, R. G. Clinical relevance of inhaled corticosteroids and hypothalamic-pituitary-adrenal axis suppression. J Allergy Clin Immunol 101:S447–S450, 1998.

Jones, J. A., et al. Use of dehydroepiandrosterone (DHEA) in a patient with advanced prostate cancer: a case report and review. Urology 50:784–788, 1997.

Keenan, G. F. Management of complications of glucocorticoid therapy. Clin Chest Med 18:507–520, 1997.

Tarantino, M. D., and G. Goldsmith. Treatment of acute immune thrombocytopenic purpura. Semin Hematol 35(supplement 1):28–35, 1998.

van Vollenhoven, R. F. Corticosteroids in rheumatic disease: understanding their effects is key to their use. Postgrad Med 103:137–142, 1998.

Wolkowitz, O. M., et al. Dehydroepiandrosterone (DHEA) treatment of depression. Biol Psychiatry 41:311–318, 1997.

Yates, R. W., and I. J. Doull. A risk-benefit assessment of corticosteroids in the management of croup. Drug Saf 16:48–55, 1997.

CHAPTER THIRTY-FOUR

DRUGS AFFECTING FERTILITY

AND REPRODUCTION

CLASSIFICATION OF DRUGS AFFECTING FERTILITY AND REPRODUCTION

ESTROGENS AND PROGESTINS
Steroidal estrogens
- Conjugated estrogens
- Estradiol
- Ethinyl estradiol
- Mestranol

Nonsteroidal estrogens
- Diethylstilbestrol

Progesterone and its derivatives
- Hydroxyprogesterone caproate
- Medroxyprogesterone acetate
- Megestrol
- Progesterone

Synthetic progestins
- Desogestrel
- Levonorgestrel
- Norethindrone
- Norethynodrel
- Norgestimate

ANTIESTROGENS
- Clomiphene
- Raloxifene
- Tamoxifen

ANTIPROGESTINS
- Mifepristone

ANDROGENS
- Danazol
- Fluoxymesterone
- Methyltestosterone
- Oxandrolone
- Testosterone

ANTIANDROGENS
- Cyproterone
- Finasteride
- Flutamide
- Ketoconazole
- Leuprolide

OVERVIEW

Human reproduction involves a cascade of hormonal secretions, beginning with the secretion of gonadotropin-releasing hormone (GnRH) from the hypothalamus. As described in Chapter 31, GnRH stimulates the pituitary to release two gonadotropins: follicle-stimulating hormone (FSH) and luteinizing hormone (LH). These gonadotropins then stimulate the production of **sex steroids** and gametes by the ovary in the female and by the testis in the male.

There are three categories of sex steroids secreted by the gonads: (1) **estrogens,** which include **estradiol, estrone,** and **estriol;** (2) **progestins,** which include **progesterone;** and (3) **androgens,** which include **testosterone.** Estrogens, progesterone, and testosterone are produced in both males and females, but the relative amounts and patterns of secretion differ markedly between the sexes. Females primarily secrete estrogens and progesterone, whereas males primarily produce testosterone.

Biosynthesis of Sex Steroids

As shown in Fig. 34–1, **pregnenolone** is the precursor to progesterone. It is also the precursor to dehydroepiandrosterone and androstenedione (two androgens secreted by the adrenal gland and discussed in Chapter 33) and to testosterone (the major androgen in males). The adrenal and gonadal androgens are converted to estrogens by **aromatase,** an enzyme that forms the aromatic A ring necessary for the selective high-affinity binding of estradiol, estrone, and estriol to **estrogen receptors.**

In females, ovarian **thecal cells** secrete small quantities of testosterone. In males, about 95% of testosterone is produced by **Leydig cells** in the testes, and the remainder is derived from the **adrenal cortex.** Testosterone is synthesized in the testes by the same pathways as in the ovaries. Testosterone is subsequently converted to **dihydrotestosterone** (DHT) by **5α-reductase** in the prostate, hair follicles, and skin. In the plasma, testosterone is primarily bound to sex steroid–binding globulin. In the liver, it is converted to androstenedione and other metabolites, including sulfate and glucuronide conjugates.

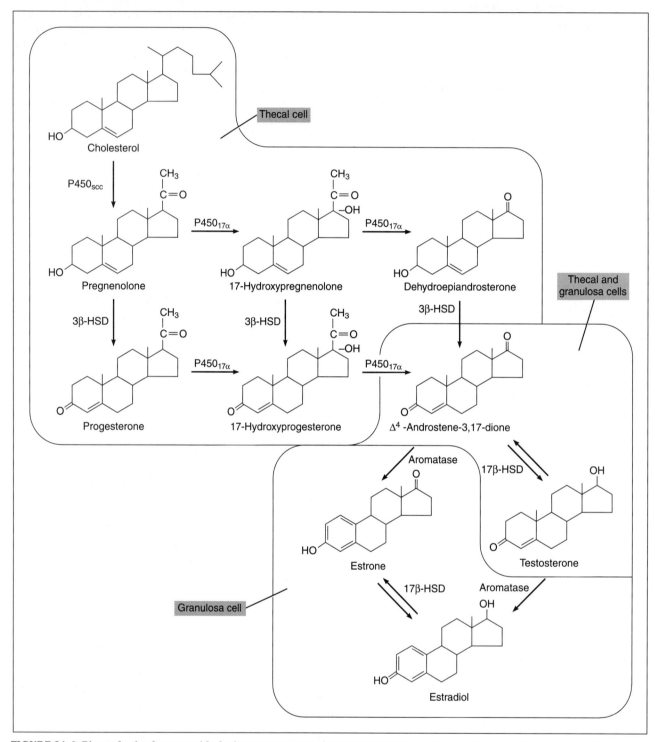

FIGURE 34–1. Biosynthesis of sex steroids. In the ovary, pregnenolone is converted to androstenedione and testosterone in thecal cells. These steroids are then converted to estrone and estradiol in granulosa cells. Enzymes involved in these steps include the cholesterol side-chain cleavage enzyme ($P450_{scc}$), steroid 17α-hydroxylase ($P450_{17α}$), 3β-hydroxysteroid dehydrogenase (3β-HSD), 17β-hydroxysteroid dehydrogenase (17β-HSD), and aromatase. Estrone and estradiol are partly converted to estriol by other enzymes. After ovulation, the major product of thecal cells is progesterone, owing to the development of a relative deficiency of 17α-hydroxylase activity.

About 90% of these metabolites are excreted in the urine.

While both testosterone and DHT activate **androgen receptors,** DHT has greater receptor affinity and forms a more stable receptor-ligand complex than does testosterone. If DHT formation is inhibited, this significantly reduces androgenic stimulation of the prostate gland and hair follicles. The androgen receptor located in the nuclei of target cells interacts with response elements in target genes and thereby stimulates protein synthesis in the same manner as other sex steroids.

Physiologic Actions of Estrogens and Progesterone

In males and females, estrogens are responsible for epiphyseal closure, which halts linear bone growth.

In females, estrogens and progesterone have multiple actions and interactions that are necessary for reproductive activity. Estrogens are formed in the **granulosa cells** of the ovary, while progesterone is primarily produced by the **corpus luteum** in response to LH secretion. Estrogens promote the development and growth of the fallopian tubes, uterus, and vagina, as well as secondary sex characteristics such as breast development, skeletal growth, and axillary and pubic hair patterns.

The pattern of hormonal changes occurring during the **menstrual cycle** is depicted in Fig. 34–2. During the **follicular phase** of the cycle, ovarian follicles are recruited and a dominant estrogen-secreting follicle develops. Estrogen levels gradually increase, whereas progesterone levels remain quite low. A surge of LH is released at midcycle in response to positive estrogen feedback to the pituitary gland, and this LH surge triggers ovulation. During the **luteal phase** of the cycle, the follicle becomes the corpus luteum (yellow body) that secretes both estrogen and progesterone in response to LH. Together, these hormones prepare the uterus for implantation of a fertilized egg as the endometrium becomes more vascular and secretory. If pregnancy does not occur, the corpus luteum ceases to produce estrogen and progesterone, resulting in menstruation. If pregnancy

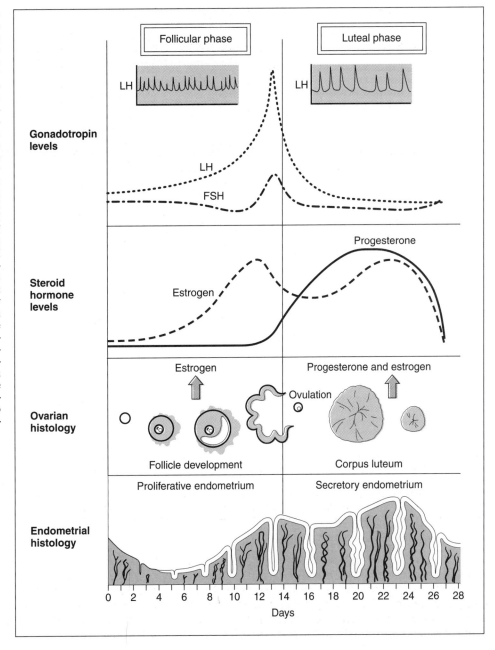

FIGURE 34–2. Hormone secretion during the human menstrual cycle. Luteinizing hormone (LH) and follicle-stimulating hormone (FSH) are released in a pulsatile manner from the pituitary gland in response to the pulsatile secretion of gonadotropin-releasing hormone (GnRH) from the hypothalamus. FSH stimulates ovarian follicle development and the secretion of estrogen during the follicular phase of the cycle. After ovulation, the corpus luteum produces both estrogen and progesterone during the luteal phase. Estrogen decreases FSH and LH secretion during most of the cycle (feedback inhibition) while provoking the midcycle LH and FSH surge that triggers ovulation. Progesterone decreases the frequency of hypothalamic GnRH pulses and the frequency of pulsatile LH and FSH secretion (inset in top panel). During the luteal phase, progesterone increases the amount of LH released (pulse amplitude). Estrogen stimulates the proliferation of the endometrium during the follicular phase, while progesterone causes the endometrium to become more vascular and secretory during the luteal phase.

occurs, the placenta produces human chorionic gonadotropin (hCG), which maintains the production of progesterone by the corpus luteum. After about 3 months, the placenta becomes the predominant source of progesterone. This hormone serves to maintain pregnancy by preventing endometrial sloughing and miscarriage.

Estrogens have a number of other actions that are important in reproduction and other bodily functions. They sensitize the myometrium to oxytocin at parturition, and this facilitates labor. They stimulate protein synthesis in the brain and may thereby affect mood and emotions. Estrogens influence the distribution of body fat and thereby contribute to the development of feminine body contours. They enhance blood coagulation by increasing the synthesis of clotting factors, and they prevent osteoporosis by inhibiting bone resorption.

Progesterone and other progestins increase basal body temperature by 0.5–0.8°C (1.0–1.5°F) at ovulation and throughout the luteal phase. They also affect the emotional state and have mild mineralocorticoid (salt-retaining) properties. Some of the synthetic progestins have other effects that are attributed to their androgenic activity (see below).

Physiologic Actions of Testosterone

LH stimulates testosterone synthesis in **Leydig cells,** while FSH promotes spermatogenesis by **Sertoli cells** in the seminiferous tubules. These cells provide an environment rich in testosterone, which is necessary for germ cell development. Sertoli cells also produce a protein called **inhibin,** which acts in concert with DHT as a feedback regulator of FSH secretion by the pituitary.

Testosterone is responsible for the development of secondary sex characteristics in males during puberty. These include growth of the larynx, thickening of the vocal cords, and growth of facial, axillary, and pubic hair. In addition to stimulating growth of the penis, scrotum, seminal vesicles, and prostate gland, testosterone stimulates and maintains sexual function in males. Testosterone and other androgens also do the following: increase lean body mass; stimulate skeletal growth; accelerate epiphyseal closure; increase sebaceous gland activity and sebum production, thereby contributing to the development of acne in both sexes; increase the production of erythropoietin in the kidneys; and decrease the levels of high-density lipoprotein (HDL) cholesterol.

ESTROGENS AND PROGESTINS

An estrogen or progestin preparation can be used alone for the treatment of various clinical disorders, or the two preparations can be used in combination for **hormone replacement therapy** in postmenopausal women or for **contraception** in women of childbearing age.

Steroidal Estrogens

Chemistry. The natural estrogens include **estradiol** and **conjugated estrogens.** Estradiol is an 18-carbon steroid with an aromatic A ring that is hydroxylated in the 3 position (Fig. 34–3A). **Conjugated estrogens** are sulfate esters of **estrone** and **equilin** and are usually obtained from the urine of pregnant mares. **Ethinyl estradiol** and **mestranol** are synthetic derivatives of estradiol.

Pharmacokinetics. In older formulations of orally administered estradiol, the drug was slowly absorbed and underwent extensive first-pass inactivation by conjugation with sulfate and glucuronide in the liver. As a result, oral bioavailability of these formulations was low. This problem was circumvented in several ways.

First, a small-particle formulation called **micronized estradiol** was developed. This oral formulation is rapidly absorbed and undergoes little first-pass metabolism.

Second, orally administered derivatives of estradiol, such as ethinyl estradiol and mestranol, became available. The addition of an ethinyl group at the C17 position of estradiol (as occurs in these drugs) markedly reduces first-pass metabolism, extends the half-life to about 20 hours, and results in greater oral potency.

Third, several long-acting formulations of estradiol became available for transdermal or intramuscular administration, allowing them to be used instead of an oral drug. **Transdermal estradiol** is available as a skin patch that slowly releases the drug over 3 days or 1 week. **Estradiol cypionate** and **estradiol valerate** are long-acting injectable formulations of estradiol that have been prepared by esterifying the 17-hydroxyl group of estradiol. These esters are slowly absorbed following intramuscular administration and provide effective plasma concentrations of estradiol for several weeks.

Fourth, conjugated estrogens were developed. Following oral administration, the conjugated estrogens are hydrolyzed in the gut prior to absorption. Estrone and equilin undergo relatively little first-pass metabolism, but they are eventually converted in the liver to sulfate and glucuronide conjugates that are primarily excreted in the urine. Estrone is also available in a rapidly absorbed formulation for intramuscular administration.

Following their absorption, the natural estrogens are highly bound to sex steroid–binding globulin, are widely distributed, and are concentrated in fat. They undergo enterohepatic cycling, in which conjugated metabolites are excreted in the bile and converted to free estrogens by intestinal bacteria. The free estrogens are then reabsorbed into the circulation. Like estrone and equilin, estradiol is metabolized in the liver to sulfate and glucuronide conjugates, and these conjugates are primarily excreted in the urine, with small amounts excreted in the feces.

Indications. Estrogen preparations are used in the treatment of **primary hypogonadism,** including

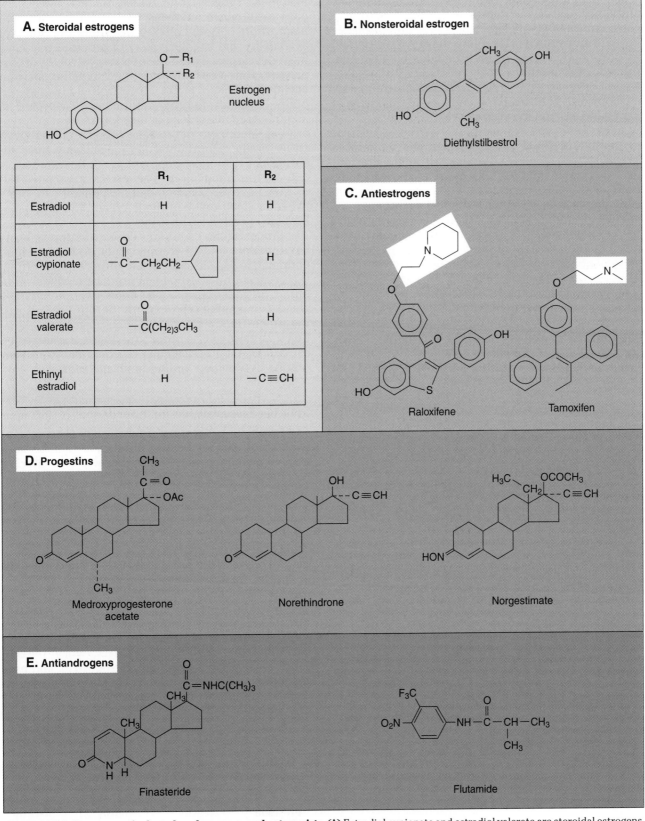

FIGURE 34–3. Structures of selected sex hormones and antagonists. (A) Estradiol cypionate and estradiol valerate are steroidal estrogens that are slowly hydrolyzed to estradiol following intramuscular administration. Ethinyl estradiol is a long-acting estradiol derivative that has good oral bioavailability. **(B)** Diethylstilbestrol is a nonsteroidal compound that has a structural resemblance to estradiol. **(C)** Raloxifene and tamoxifen have estrogen antagonist and partial agonist activity. The antagonist activity is conferred by the unshaded moiety. **(D)** Medroxyprogesterone acetate is the acetate derivative of methylprogesterone (Ac denotes acetate), while norethindrone and norgestimate are derivatives of 19-nortestosterone. Norethindrone has an estrane nucleus, and norgestimate is a gonane derivative. **(E)** Finasteride is a 5α-reductase inhibitor, and flutamide is an androgen receptor antagonist.

cases due to surgical oophorectomy, menopause, and other causes. Micronized estradiol, transdermal estradiol, and conjugated estrogens are primarily used for **hormone replacement therapy** (see below) in postmenopausal women. Combination estrogen-progestin preparations frequently contain ethinyl estradiol or mestranol. These preparations are mainly used for **oral contraception** and for the treatment of **acne vulgaris** and **dysmenorrhea.**

Estrogen preparations have been used to treat inoperable **prostate cancer** in men and inoperable **breast cancer** in men and women. However, they are less commonly employed for these purposes today, because estrogens tend to produce more intolerable side effects than do other hormonal agents that are equally or more effective. Tamoxifen, an estrogen receptor antagonist, is now the most commonly used hormonal therapy for breast cancer, whereas androgen antagonists are more commonly used to treat prostate cancer (see below).

Adverse Effects. When used as hormone replacement to provide physiologic estrogen levels, estrogens produce relatively few adverse effects. Occasionally, they cause breast tenderness, headache, edema, nausea, vomiting, anorexia, and changes in libido. Most of the minor side effects of estrogens can be managed by dosage reduction.

The more serious adverse effects of estrogens include hypertension, thromboembolic disorders, and gallbladder disease. The hypertensive effect of estrogens has been partly attributed to stimulation of angiotensinogen synthesis and subsequent formation of angiotensin II, while thromboembolic complications have been partly attributed to increased synthesis of clotting factors in the liver. Estrogens increase cholesterol excretion in the bile, and this accounts for their tendency to cause gallstones.

Estrogens are contraindicated during pregnancy and should be avoided in women with uterine fibroids. Estrogens should be used with great caution in women with hepatic diseases, endometriosis, thromboembolic diseases, or hypercalcemia.

Nonsteroidal Estrogens

Nonsteroidal estrogens, such as **diethylstilbestrol** (DES), have a structure that resembles that of estradiol and enables them to bind and activate the estrogen receptor (see Fig. 34–3B). DES is well absorbed from the gut and does not undergo first-pass metabolism.

Today, the use of DES is limited to the treatment of inoperable **breast or prostate cancer.** In the past, DES was used to treat threatened miscarriage in pregnant women. Later, it was found that the offspring of these women had a higher incidence of vaginal and cervical cancer.

Progesterone and Its Derivatives

Progesterone, a 21-carbon steroid with a nonaromatic A ring, is the primary natural progestin in

mammals. Progesterone undergoes extensive first-pass metabolism following oral administration and has a short plasma half-life. To extend the oral bioavailability and half-life, esters of progesterone have been developed. These include **megestrol, hydroxyprogesterone caproate,** and **medroxyprogesterone acetate** (see Fig. 34–3D). Megestrol is administered orally, whereas hydroxyprogesterone caproate is administered as a long-acting intramuscular preparation. Medroxyprogesterone acetate can be given either orally or intramuscularly. Following their absorption, the progesterone esters are bound to albumin in the circulation. The esters are converted to several hydroxylated metabolites and to pregnanediol glucuronide in the liver, and these metabolites are excreted in the urine.

Progesterone esters are used to suppress ovarian function in the treatment of **dysmenorrhea, endometriosis,** and **uterine bleeding.** In this setting, the progesterone derivatives produce feedback inhibition of gonadotropin secretion by the pituitary gland. In **hormone replacement therapy** (see below), the progesterone esters are often used in combination with estrogens in order to decrease the incidence of estrogen-induced irregular bleeding and to prevent uterine hyperplasia and endometrial cancer.

Synthetic Progestins

Synthetic progestins are primarily used as **oral contraceptives** (see below), but they are also used to treat **dysmenorrhea, endometriosis,** and **uterine bleeding** in the same manner as the progesterone esters.

The synthetic progestins are derivatives of 19-nortestosterone and have varying degrees of estrogenic, antiestrogenic, and androgenic activity (Table 34–1). The drugs contain a C17 ethinyl substitution that increases their oral bioavailability and duration of action. Their half-lives range from 7 to 24 hours, whereas the half-life of progesterone is only about 5 minutes.

Two classes of 19-norprogestins have been developed: **estranes** and **gonanes.** The estranes include **norethindrone** and **norethynodrel,** while the gonanes include **levonorgestrel, desogestrel,** and **norgestimate** (see Fig. 34–3D). Desogestrel and norgestimate have improved progestational selectivity and less androgenic activity, and they appear to cause

TABLE 34–1. Relative Hormonal Activity of Progestins Used in Oral Contraceptives

Progestin	Estrogenic Activity	Antiestrogenic Activity	Androgenic Activity
Desogestrel	0	0	0
Levonorgestrel	0	+	+
Norethindrone	0	+	+
Norethynodrel	+	0	0
Norgestimate	0	0	0

fewer androgenic side effects than other progestins. Norethynodrel has greater estrogenic activity than other synthetic progestins. These differences enable the clinician to select contraceptives that produce fewer adverse effects in women who experience estrogenic or androgenic side effects when taking oral contraceptives.

Estrogen-Progestin or Estrogen-Only Hormone Replacement Therapy

Although estrogens can be used alone for hormone replacement therapy (HRT) in women who have had a hysterectomy, they are usually used in combination with progestins for HRT in postmenopausal women. This is because giving estrogen alone to women who have not had a hysterectomy increases the risk of endometrial cancer. The association of estrogen-only replacement therapy with breast and ovarian cancer is uncertain; some studies suggest an increased risk, while others do not.

Pharmacologic Effects. Estrogens relieve the vasomotor symptoms of menopause, including the "hot flashes" or flushes that consist of alternating chills and sweating accompanied by nausea, dizziness, headache, tachycardia, and palpitations. Episodes of these symptoms often occur several times a day, but night sweats are particularly common. The vasomotor symptoms are believed to occur in association with surges in GnRH or LH that result from the lack of estrogen feedback inhibition. The hormone surges alter hypothalamic thermoregulatory centers, causing vasomotor instability and the symptoms described above. Estrogens also relieve other symptoms of estrogen deficiency in postmenopausal women, such as atrophic vaginitis.

Epidemiologic studies have established that HRT reduces the incidence of osteoporosis and cardiovascular disease in postmenopausal women. According to a meta-analysis of controlled studies, HRT reduces the risk of osteoporotic hip fractures by 25%. Estrogens also provide a 50% or greater reduction in the rate of cardiovascular disease and mortality in postmenopausal women. The beneficial effects of estrogens in osteoporosis are described in greater detail in Chapter 36. Their protective effects against atherosclerotic cardiovascular disease are primarily due to their beneficial effects on lipoprotein levels.

Estrogens and progestins have different effects on serum lipoprotein levels. Estrogens decrease the levels of **low-density lipoprotein (LDL) cholesterol** and **lipoprotein(a)** while increasing the levels of **high-density lipoprotein (HDL) cholesterol.** These actions are believed to retard the progression of atherosclerosis and reduce the risk of myocardial infarction. In contrast, progestins produce a dose-related increase in LDL levels and a decrease in HDL levels. For this reason, the minimal progestin dose required for endometrial protection should be used in combination with an estrogen for HRT. Studies indicate that when estrogen and progestin are used together, the LDL levels are usually decreased while the HDL levels are either increased or remain unchanged.

Treatment Considerations. Oral, transdermal, intramuscular, and vaginal estrogen preparations may be used for HRT. Each of these preparations has advantages and disadvantages.

Oral estrogen preparations are the ones most widely used for HRT, partly because of their convenience and relatively low cost. However, oral estrogens undergo considerable first-pass metabolism, necessitating the administration of large doses to achieve physiologic serum levels of estradiol. For this reason, oral estrogens induce the synthesis of many hepatic proteins, including angiotensinogen and hepatic drug-metabolizing enzymes. Induction of hepatic protein synthesis may be responsible for some of the adverse effects of estrogens, including hypertension, thromboembolic disorders, and gallbladder disease. Induction of drug-metabolizing enzymes may lead to estrogen tolerance in some women.

Transdermal estradiol preparations are convenient and provide physiologic levels of estradiol without inducing hepatic protein synthesis. These preparations produce consistent blood levels and are more convenient for some women to use because of their long duration of action. Some of the estradiol patches are applied twice a week, while others need only be applied once a week. In some cases, women have mild skin reactions to estrogen patches, which are applied to the trunk or buttock. The effect of transdermal estrogens on serum lipoprotein levels is not as favorable as the effect of oral estrogens, although some studies report increased HDL and decreased LDL levels after long-term administration.

Intramuscular injections of long-acting estrogen preparations may provide effective plasma concentrations for up to 4 weeks. Although a few women prefer these injections over other forms of estrogen therapy, they are not widely used, because of the necessity for the patient to visit a health care professional for each injection.

Two preparations of estradiol are available for vaginal administration: a cream and a vaginal ring. The vaginal ring, which is used as estrogen replacement therapy, slowly releases estradiol for 3 months and is then removed and replaced with another ring. The cream is primarily used for treating atrophic vaginitis. However, sufficient estrogen can be absorbed systemically from the cream to relieve the vasomotor symptoms of menopause.

HRT may be given as cyclic or continuous hormonal therapy. In cyclic therapy, estrogen is given for 25 days, a progestin such as medroxyprogesterone is given for the last 10–13 days of estrogen treatment, and then no therapy is given for 5–6 days. In continuous therapy, estrogen is given every day, and a progestin is added for the first 10–13 days of each month. The addition of a progestin suppresses endometrial hyperplasia and diminishes the risk of endometrial cancer.

CONTRACEPTIVES

Contraceptives are drugs or devices that are used to prevent conception (the onset of pregnancy, as indicated by the implantation of the blastocyst in the endometrium or the formation of a visible zygote). Some contraceptives act locally in the reproductive tract. These include agents that kill sperm **(spermicides)**, devices that prevent sperm from reaching and fertilizing the ovum **(condoms and diaphragms)**, and **intrauterine devices** (IUDs) that kill or prevent implantation of the blastocyst. Other contraceptives are administered orally or parenterally. **Oral contraceptives** contain female sex hormones that act primarily by preventing ovulation. Some of the oral contraceptives contain both an estrogen and a progestin, while others contain only a progestin. Progestin-only products are also available for administration as **long-acting subdermal implants** or as **depot intramuscular injections.**

Estrogen-Progestin Contraceptives

Classification. The combination estrogen-progestin oral contraceptives are classified as monophasic, biphasic, or triphasic, based on their progestin content. **Monophasic contraceptives** contain the same amount of progestin throughout the administration cycle, whereas **biphasic and triphasic contraceptives** increase the amount after the first one-third of the cycle (Fig. 34–4). The amount of progestin is increased in the biphasic and triphasic preparations in order to mimic the naturally occurring ratio of estrogen to progestin during the menstrual cycle. The estrogen content is constant in all monophasic and biphasic contraceptives and in most triphasic contraceptives.

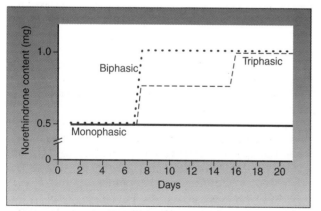

FIGURE 34–4. Progestin (norethindrone) content in typical monophasic, biphasic, and triphasic oral contraceptives. Monophasic preparations contain the same amount of progestin throughout the administration cycle. Biphasic and triphasic preparations increase the progestin content in a stepwise fashion after the initial part of the cycle. The amount of estrogen is constant in all monophasic and biphasic contraceptives and in most triphasic contraceptives. Some triphasic contraceptives contain a slightly greater amount of estrogen in the middle of the cycle.

Mechanisms and Pharmacologic Effects. The oral contraceptives act primarily by feedback inhibition of gonadotropin release from the pituitary gland. Estrogen-progestin contraceptives reduce LH and FSH levels and prevent the midcycle LH surge that stimulates ovulation. These effects are partly attributed to the ability of progestin to decrease the frequency of GnRH pulses and to decrease pituitary responsiveness to GnRH.

Indications. Estrogen-progestin preparations for **oral contraception** are usually packaged as 21 tablets that are administered once a day, beginning on day 5 of the menstrual cycle. Some preparations also include 7 inert pills that can be taken for the remainder of the cycle. The tablets are packaged in a calendar format to facilitate proper utilization. Estrogen-progestin preparations are administered in the same manner for the treatment of **acne vulgaris** and produce a significant improvement in facial acne lesions.

Estrogen-progestin preparations are also useful in managing **dysmenorrhea,** a condition characterized by episodic pain that is believed to result from a local increase in uterine prostaglandins. The release of prostaglandins is a reaction to the ischemia caused by vasoconstriction of small arteries in the uterine wall at the time of menstruation. For this condition, oral contraceptives are started a number of days before the onset of menstruation. Nonsteroidal anti-inflammatory drugs such as ibuprofen and naproxen may be used instead, especially by women desiring to maintain the ovulatory cycle. These drugs act by inhibiting prostaglandin synthesis (see Chapter 30).

A preparation containing ethinyl estradiol and levonorgestrel is available for use as a **postcoital contraceptive** in women who have not been taking another contraceptive. A single dose of this preparation is taken within 72 hours of intercourse and is followed by two doses 12 hours later. When taken after intercourse, these hormones inhibit the transport of ova in the fallopian tubes and alter the endometrium so as to prevent implantation of a fertilized ovum. Use of the postcoital contraceptive routinely causes nausea and vomiting and may require administration of an antiemetic agent such as promethazine. It may also cause headache, dizziness, leg cramps, and abdominal cramps. The postcoital contraceptive is packaged with a urine pregnancy test that can be used to verify the prevention of pregnancy.

Adverse Effects. Table 34–2 lists the common adverse effects resulting from estrogen or progestin excess or deficiency. Less frequent effects of oral contraceptives include hypertension, thromboembolic complications, and gallstones.

Oral contraceptives have been associated with an increased risk of stroke, myocardial infarction, deep vein thrombosis, and other thromboembolic complications. However, the increased risk of thromboembolism in healthy women using preparations containing a low dose of estrogen (<50 μg of ethinyl estradiol) is extremely small. Smokers over 35 years

TABLE 34–2. Common Adverse Effects of Oral Contraceptives

Effects of estrogen excess
Breast enlargement
Dizziness
Dysmenorrhea
Edema
Headache
Irritability
Nausea and vomiting
Weight gain (cyclic)

Effects of progestin excess
Acne
Depression
Fatigue
Hirsutism
Libido change
Oily skin
Weight gain (noncyclic)

Effects of estrogen deficiency
Atrophic vaginitis
Continuous bleeding
Early- or mid-cycle bleeding
Hypomenorrhea
Vasomotor symptoms

Effects of progestin deficiency
Dysmenorrhea
Hypermenorrhea
Late-cycle bleeding

creased risk of deep vein thrombosis. There is some evidence that this increased risk is associated with resistance to the blood's own anticoagulation system, but the significance of these findings is uncertain.

Interactions. Phenytoin, barbiturates, carbamazepine, and other drugs that increase the hepatic metabolism of oral contraceptives may reduce the plasma levels of contraceptive steroids and lead to contraceptive failure. Antibiotics, including penicillins and tetracyclines, can eradicate intestinal flora involved in the enterohepatic cycling of contraceptive steroids and thereby diminish their effectiveness. This interaction is described in greater detail in Chapter 4. Estrogens may inhibit the metabolism and potentiate the effects of cyclosporine, imipramine and other antidepressants, and glucocorticoids. Estrogens increase the synthesis of vitamin K–dependent clotting factors and may thereby antagonize the effect of warfarin. Estrogens also appear to increase the hepatotoxicity of dantrolene.

Progestin-Only Contraceptives

The progestin-only contraceptives include **norethindrone** products that are administered orally (as "minipills"); subdermal implants that slowly release **levonorgestrel** for up to 5 years; long-acting intramuscular injections (depot injections) of **medroxyprogesterone acetate;** and IUDs that release low amounts of **progesterone** locally.

The systemic progestin-only contraceptives may prevent pregnancy through several mechanisms. They act on the hypothalamus to decrease the frequency of the GnRH pulse generator and thereby blunt the midcycle LH surge that produces ovulation. Progestin-only pills thicken and decrease the amount of cervical mucus, making it more difficult for sperm to penetrate. Progestins also create a thin, atrophic endometrium that is hostile to implantation of the blastocyst. The IUD is believed to prevent pregnancy by producing localized effects on the endometrium.

The progestin-only contraceptives are particularly suited for women who smoke, older women, and women in whom an estrogen is contraindicated. However, the estimated failure rates are slightly higher with perfect use of progestin-only contraceptives than with perfect use of estrogen-progestin products (rates of 0.5% and 0.1%, respectively). Progestin-only contraceptives are associated with frequent spotting and amenorrhea and with an increased risk of ectopic pregnancy. Irregular and unpredictable menstrual cycles are one of the most common reasons that women stop using these preparations. Unlike the estrogen-progestin preparations, the progestin-only preparations must be taken daily without interruption in order to prevent pregnancy.

Other Contraceptives

Other types of contraceptives are particularly useful for short-term contraception in women who cannot take oral contraceptives while breast-feeding

of age have a greater risk of thromboembolic complications from oral contraceptives and should use other forms of contraception. Healthy nonsmokers who are 35–44 years old may continue to use oral contraceptives, according to the American College of Obstetricians and Gynecologists.

Contraceptives containing estrogen should be used with caution in women with gallbladder disease. They are contraindicated in women with thromboembolic disease or a history of myocardial infarction or coronary artery disease. They are also contraindicated in women with active liver disease, breast cancer, or carcinoma of the reproductive tract. The relationship between oral contraceptive use and cancer remains controversial. Epidemiologic studies suggest that oral contraceptives decrease the incidence of ovarian and endometrial cancer. Although long-term use of the older high-dose estrogen preparations appears to have been associated with an increased risk of breast cancer, the risk associated with newer low-dose preparations is uncertain. Oral contraceptives have also been associated with a low risk of hepatic adenoma.

The progestin component of oral contraceptives may cause adverse effects that can be attributed to excessive progestational activity or to androgenic activity. The androgenic side effects of progestins include acne, hirsutism, increased libido, and oily skin. Newer progestins, such as norgestimate and desogestrel, appear to cause fewer androgenic side effects than the older progestins. However, some epidemiologic studies have reported that women receiving these newer progestins may have an in-

or for other reasons. These nonhormonal contraceptives include spermicides and barrier devices such as condoms and diaphragms.

Most spermicides contain nonoxynol-9, a detergent that disrupts the cell membrane of the sperm. Spermicides increase the contraceptive efficacy of condoms and other barrier methods. They are moderately effective and well tolerated, although they may cause local irritation in some women.

ANTIESTROGENS

Antiestrogens are nonsteroidal drugs that bind to estrogen receptors and exert tissue-specific antagonist or partial agonist effects. Examples are clomiphene, raloxifene, and tamoxifen. These drugs contain the structural elements required for estrogen receptor binding and weak agonist activity, and they also possess a substituted ethylamine moiety that is responsible for their estrogen antagonist effect (see Fig. 34–3C). Clomiphene and tamoxifen are triphenylethylene compounds, while raloxifene is a benzothiophene derivative. The *trans* isomers of clomiphene and tamoxifen have more antiestrogenic activity than do the *cis* isomers. Tamoxifen is marketed only as the *trans* isomer, whereas clomiphene is available as a racemic mixture.

Clomiphene

Pharmacokinetics. Clomiphene is well absorbed after oral administration. It undergoes hepatic biotransformation and biliary excretion, and it is primarily eliminated in the feces. Its long elimination half-life of about 5 days is due to extensive plasma protein binding, enterohepatic cycling, and accumulation in fatty tissues.

Mechanisms and Indications. Clomiphene is a weak estrogen agonist and a moderate estrogen antagonist. It is used to treat **anovulatory infertility,** including infertility associated with **polycystic ovary disease.** Clomiphene is believed to act by antagonizing estrogen receptors in the hypothalamic-pituitary-ovarian axis (Fig. 34–5). By blocking estrogen's negative feedback inhibition of gonadotropin secretion, clomiphene increases FSH and LH secretion and thereby induces ovarian follicle development and ovulation.

Suitable patients for clomiphene therapy often have an anovulatory disorder dating back to puberty but have a functional hypothalamic-pituitary-ovarian axis. Clomiphene is less successful in women who have reduced estrogen levels, and it is unlikely to benefit women with FSH levels at or above 40 mIU/mL or women with absent or resistant ovarian follicles.

Clomiphene treatment is usually begun on or about the fifth day of the cycle after the start of uterine bleeding and continues for 5 days. Ovulation is expected 5–10 days after the last dose of clomiphene and can be detected by monitoring basal body temperature, urinary LH secretion, plasma progesterone levels, or endometrial histology.

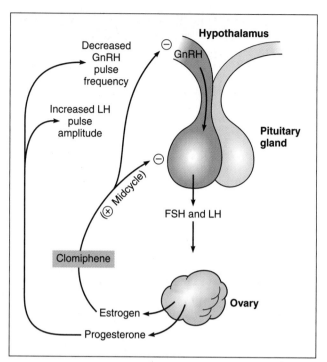

FIGURE 34–5. The hypothalamic-pituitary-ovarian axis. Follicle-stimulating hormone (FSH) and luteinizing hormone (LH) are released from the pituitary gland in response to gonadotropin-releasing hormone (GnRH) produced by hypothalamic neurons. During the follicular phase of the menstrual cycle, FSH stimulates the development of an ovarian follicle and the secretion of estrogen. Estrogen increases the synthesis of LH but inhibits its release until midcycle, when a surge in LH is accompanied by a smaller surge in FSH secretion, leading to ovulation. During the luteal phase, progesterone produced by the corpus luteum feeds back to the hypothalamus to decrease the frequency of GnRH pulses while acting on the pituitary to increase the amplitude of LH secretion. Together, these actions produce less frequent LH pulses of greater amplitude. Clomiphene inhibits estrogen feedback and thereby increases gonadotropin secretion in anovulatory women.

Adverse Effects. From 5% to 12% of women treated with clomiphene have multiple births (twins in the vast majority of cases). The risk of multiple births is reduced if women are started on a lower dose of clomiphene. The dose can then be increased each cycle until ovulation occurs.

Tamoxifen

Pharmacokinetics. Tamoxifen is administered orally, and it is well absorbed from the gut. It is then converted to a number of metabolites in the liver. Some of the minor metabolites, such as 4-hydroxytamoxifen, have greater affinity for the estrogen receptor than tamoxifen does. The terminal elimination half-life of tamoxifen is about 7 days. Tamoxifen undergoes enterohepatic cycling and biliary excretion in the same manner as clomiphene.

Mechanisms and Indications. Tamoxifen has both estrogenic and antiestrogenic properties. In breast tissue, it acts as an estrogen receptor antagonist. It is primarily used to prevent or treat **breast cancer** in patients with tumor cells that are estrogen receptor–positive. In the treatment of breast cancer, it is usually employed as adjuvant therapy in combination with surgery or other chemotherapy. Tamoxifen inhibits the proliferation of breast cancer cells and may thereby contribute to the eradication of micrometastases. In cases of advanced or metastatic breast cancer, tamoxifen may be used alone for palliative treatment.

Adverse Effects. Tamoxifen may cause nausea, vomiting, hot flashes, vaginal bleeding, and menstrual irregularities. It can stimulate proliferation of endometrial cells, and there is some evidence that it increases the risk of endometrial cancer.

Raloxifene

Raloxifene is a new benzothiophene drug that is called a **selective estrogen receptor modulator** (SERM). Its structure is shown in Fig. 34–3C. Raloxifene acts in a manner similar to tamoxifen by producing estrogenlike effects on bone and lipid metabolism while antagonizing the effects of estrogen on breast tissue. However, unlike tamoxifen, raloxifene also acts as an estrogen antagonist in uterine tissue.

Raloxifene is primarily indicated for the prevention of **osteoporosis** in postmenopausal women. The effect of raloxifene on total body bone mineral density is similar to that of conjugated estrogens or alendronate. However, the effect of raloxifene on bone mineral density of the lumbar spine may be less than that of these other drugs. The effect of estrogens on bone metabolism is discussed in greater detail in Chapter 36.

The effect of raloxifene on serum lipoproteins differs from the effect of estrogens. Raloxifene decreases the levels of total cholesterol, LDL cholesterol, and lipoprotein(a). However, unlike estrogens, raloxifene does not increase the level of HDL cholesterol. The effect of raloxifene on cardiovascular disease requires further evaluation.

Studies are being undertaken to compare the ability of raloxifene and tamoxifen to prevent **breast cancer** in postmenopausal women.

ANTIPROGESTINS

Mifepristone is a synthetic steroid compound that acts as a progesterone receptor antagonist when progesterone is present. In the absence of progesterone, it acts as a partial agonist. It is also a competitive antagonist at the glucocorticoid receptor (see Chapter 33). Mifepristone is used in some countries for **medical abortion** in the first trimester of pregnancy. It causes breakdown of the decidua (the endometrium of the pregnant uterus), leading to detachment of the blastocyst from the endometrium. The drug is not approved for this use in the USA.

Mifepristone is administered as a single dose that is followed by a prostaglandin 48 hours later to stimulate uterine contractions (see Chapter 26). Mifepristone has good oral bioavailability. Following absorption, the drug is highly bound to plasma proteins, and this contributes to its long half-life of about 22 hours. Mifepristone is metabolized in the liver and excreted in the bile. It undergoes enterohepatic cycling and is primarily excreted in the feces.

The major adverse effects of mifepristone include anorexia, nausea, vomiting, abdominal pain, fatigue, and heavy uterine bleeding.

ANDROGENS

Several testosterone preparations and synthetic androgens are available for clinical use in the treatment of hypogonadism and a variety of other conditions.

Testosterone and Methyltestosterone

When given orally, testosterone undergoes extensive first-pass metabolism. It must therefore be given parenterally or transdermally instead. Testosterone and several long-acting esters of testosterone, such as testosterone cypionate, are available for intramuscular administration. The testosterone esters are slowly absorbed and provide effective plasma concentrations for several weeks.

Methyltestosterone is a derivative that is resistant to hepatic metabolism, has a longer half-life than testosterone, and is suitable for oral administration. However, prolonged methyltestosterone use is associated with hepatic damage and liver failure, so the drug is inappropriate for long-term treatment of hypogonadism.

Testosterone preparations are primarily used for treating **hypogonadism** that is due to **primary testicular failure** or is secondary to **hypopituitarism.** In patients with hypopituitarism, testosterone should be given in combination with growth hormone in order to obtain a maximal effect on skeletal growth. In these patients, the androgen is added to the treatment regimen at the time of puberty, and the dosage is gradually increased. Either a long-acting injectable preparation or a transdermal testosterone patch can be used.

Testosterone is occasionally employed in **gynecologic disorders.** It is sometimes combined with estrogens for **hormone replacement therapy** in postmenopausal women who experience endometrial bleeding when only an estrogen is used, and it has also been used to treat **osteoporosis.**

Fluoxymesterone and Oxandrolone

Fluoxymesterone and oxandrolone are among the many **synthetic androgens,** or **anabolic steroids,** that have been developed in an attempt to produce a compound with greater anabolic activity and less androgenic activity. The ratio of anabolic activity to androgenic activity for testosterone is 1:1, whereas the ratio for some synthetic androgens is as high as 3:1.

Synthetic androgens such as oxandrolone are occasionally employed as anabolic agents to **promote weight gain** after extensive surgery, chronic infection, or severe trauma. They have also been used to **counteract protein catabolism** associated with prolonged corticosteroid administration. Although they have been used to **treat breast cancer,** they are usually more toxic and less effective than other hormonal therapies.

Anabolic steroids have been used by athletes to **increase body mass, strength, and physical performance.** This type of use has been banned by most sports organizations. The large doses of anabolic steroids that are often employed for this purpose may lead to a number of adverse effects, including hepatic dysfunction or failure, cholestatic jaundice, increased aggressiveness, psychotic symptoms, acne, decreased testicular size and function, and impotence. In women, excessive use of androgens may cause masculinization, hirsutism, deepening of the voice, and menstrual irregularities.

Danazol

Danazol, a synthetic derivative of 17-ethinyl testosterone, has antiestrogenic activity and has weak androgenic and progestational activity. The drug is administered orally, has a half-life of about 5 hours, and is excreted in the urine.

Danazol is primarily used in the treatment of **endometriosis** because it causes atrophy of ectopic endometrial tissue and thereby relieves the symptoms of disease. It also decreases the growth rate of abnormal breast tissue, making it useful in the treatment of **fibrocystic breast disease.** Danazol works primarily by acting on the pituitary gland to reduce the secretion of FSH and LH. These actions indirectly lead to decreased estrogen production.

Danazol is also used to treat **hereditary angioedema.** This disorder is due to a deficiency of C1 esterase inhibitor, a serum inhibitor of the activated first component of complement. Danazol prevents attacks of hereditary angioedema in both males and females by increasing the circulating levels of C1 esterase inhibitor. The mechanisms by which the drug increases these levels are unknown.

Common adverse effects of danazol include mild hirsutism, oily skin, acne, and menstrual irregularities. The drug may also cause hypercholesterolemia, hepatotoxicity, and thromboembolic events, including stroke. Danazol is teratogenic and should not be given to pregnant women.

ANTIANDROGENS

Several types of androgen antagonists have been developed and employed in the treatment of prostate disorders, male pattern baldness, and other conditions. These drugs act through a variety of mechanisms, including inhibition of LH secretion, inhibition of testosterone synthesis, inhibition of DHT synthesis, and antagonism of androgen receptors.

Gonadotropin-Releasing Hormone Analogues

When a gonadotropin-releasing hormone (GnRH) analogue is administered in a continuous rather than a pulsatile fashion, it reduces LH secretion by the pituitary and thereby reduces testosterone production by the testes.

The GnRH analogues include **leuprolide,** an agent discussed in Chapter 31. Leuprolide has been successfully employed in the treatment of inoperable **prostate cancer.** Because leuprolide increases the production of LH and testosterone when it is first administered, the drug is sometimes given in combination with an androgen receptor antagonist such as flutamide. Combined androgen blockade with a GnRH analogue and an androgen receptor antagonist has been shown to significantly prolong the progression-free period and the length of survival in men with advanced prostate cancer.

Androgen Synthesis Inhibitors

Ketoconazole is an antifungal drug that inhibits fungal and human cytochrome P450 enzymes, including those involved in steroidogenesis. When used in the treatment of **fungal infections,** ketoconazole may reduce testosterone synthesis in men and thereby cause gynecomastia.

Ketoconazole appears to be less effective than other androgen inhibitors in the treatment of **prostate cancer.** However, it has been successfully employed to reduce corticosteroid synthesis in patients with **Cushing's syndrome** (see Chapter 33).

Androgen Receptor Antagonists

Flutamide is a nonsteroidal agent that competes with testosterone for the androgen receptor. The drug has been successfully employed alone and in combination with a synthetic GnRH analogue to treat inoperable **prostate cancer.** Adverse effects of flutamide include mild gynecomastia and mild, reversible hepatic toxicity.

Cyproterone is a steroidal androgen receptor antagonist that has orphan drug status in the USA. It is being used to treat **hirsutism** in women and to reduce **excessive sex drive** in men.

Other Antiandrogens

Finasteride is a synthetic testosterone derivative that blocks 5α-reductase and thereby decreases the synthesis of DHT in the prostate gland, skin, and other target tissues. The drug is administered orally, undergoes hepatic metabolism, and is primarily eliminated in the feces. Finasteride has a half-life of about 8 hours, and it reduces DHT synthesis for about 24 hours.

Finasteride is primarily indicated for the treatment of **benign prostatic hyperplasia** but has recently been approved for the treatment of **male pattern baldness.** The drug is moderately effective in reducing the prostate size in men with benign prostatic hyperplasia. However, according to one study, it was not as effective as terazosin (an α-adrenergic receptor blocker) in relieving symptoms of urinary retention.

The adverse effects of finasteride include impotence and decreased libido.

Summary of Important Points

- Estradiol preparations include skin patches for transdermal administration, micronized estradiol for oral administration, and estradiol cypionate and estradiol valerate for intramuscular administration.
- Conjugated estrogens are sulfate esters of estrone and equilin. They are frequently used for hormone replacement therapy in postmenopausal women and for treatment of other forms of hypogonadism.
- In menopausal women, estrogens relieve vasomotor symptoms and protect against osteoporosis and cardiovascular disease. Estrogens decrease low-density lipoprotein (LDL) cholesterol levels and increase high-density lipoprotein (HDL) cholesterol levels.
- Ethinyl derivatives of estradiol (ethinyl estradiol and mestranol) have higher oral bioavailability and longer half-lives than estradiol. They are used primarily in oral contraceptives.
- Diethylstilbestrol is a nonsteroidal estrogen that is occasionally used to treat prostate or breast cancer.
- Progestins include progesterone derivatives and synthetic progestins. Progesterone derivatives such as medroxyprogesterone acetate are primarily used in combination with estrogens in hormone replacement therapy in order to reduce endometrial hyperplasia and the risk of endometrial cancer. They are also used to suppress ovarian function in the treatment of dysmenorrhea, endometriosis, and uterine bleeding. Some progesterone derivatives are used as contraceptives.
- Synthetic progestins are primarily used in contraceptives, including combination estrogen-progestin contraceptives and progestin-only contraceptives. Norethindrone has been the most widely used progestin in oral contraceptives.
- Hormonal contraceptives act primarily by inhibiting gonadotropin secretion and ovulation. They also affect mucus secretion, sperm transport, and endometrial histology.
- Oral contraceptives are classified as monophasic, biphasic, and triphasic, based on the number of stepwise changes in progestin content during an administration cycle. Biphasic and triphasic preparations contain greater amounts of progestin during the last two-thirds of the cycle.
- Synthetic progestins have varying degrees of androgenic, estrogenic, and antiestrogenic activity. Gonanes, such as norgestimate and desogestrel, appear to have less androgenic activity and cause fewer androgenic side effects than other progestins. Norethynodrel has greater estrogenic activity than other progestins.
- Many of the common side effects of oral contraceptives arise from an excess or deficiency of estrogen or progestin activity. These problems can often be managed by using a contraceptive whose hormonal activity is better suited to the particular patient.
- Contraceptives have been associated with an increased risk of hypertension, thromboembolic disorders, and gallstones. The risk of thromboembolism is substantially reduced with preparations containing low doses of estrogen.
- Some progestin-only contraceptives are administered as long-acting implants or injections, and others are given as oral tablets. Adverse effects include frequent spotting and amenorrhea.
- Tamoxifen is an antiestrogen that is primarily used to treat breast cancer and is given in combination with surgery and other chemotherapy.
- Clomiphene is an antiestrogen that is used to treat anovulatory infertility. By reducing estrogen feedback inhibition of gonadotropin secretion, clomiphene increases gonadotropin secretion and stimulates ovulation.
- Raloxifene is a selective estrogen receptor modulator that acts as an estrogen antagonist in breast and uterine tissue. The drug produces estrogenlike effects on bone metabolism and reduces the risk of osteoporosis. Its effects on lipid metabolism are generally favorable, but its long-term effects on cardiovascular disease are uncertain.
- Mifepristone is an antiprogestin that has been used in some countries to produce abortion.
- Testosterone preparations are primarily used to treat hypogonadism and are often administered as a long-acting injectable testosterone ester.
- Anabolic steroids have been used illicitly to increase body mass, strength, and physical performance. They may cause hepatic dysfunction, impotence, aggressiveness, and other adverse effects.
- Danazol is a weak androgen and antiestrogen. It is primarily used to treat endometriosis.
- The continuous administration of a gonadotropin-releasing hormone analogue, such as leuprolide, inhibits testosterone production. Leuprolide is used to treat prostate cancer. Flutamide, an androgen receptor antagonist, has also been used for this purpose.
- Finasteride is a 5α-reductase inhibitor that blocks the formation of dihydrotestosterone. It is used to treat benign prostatic hypertrophy and male pattern baldness.

Selected Readings

Barrett-Connor, E., et al. The postmenopausal estrogen-progestin interventions study: primary outcomes in adherent women. Naturitas 27:261–274, 1997.

Carr, B. R. Reevaluation of oral contraceptive classifications. Int J Fertil Womens Med 42(supplement 1):133–144, 1997.

Favoni, R. E., and A. deCupis. Steroidal and nonsteroidal estrogen antagonists in breast cancer: basic and clinical appraisal. Trends Pharmacol Sci 19:406–415, 1998.

Kaunitz, A. M. Injectable depot medroxyprogesterone acetate contraception: an update for U.S. clinicians. Int J Fertil Womens Med 43:73–83, 1998.

Kuhl, H. Comparative pharmacology of newer progestogens. Drugs 51:188–215, 1996.

Lip, G. Y., et al. Effects of hormone replacement therapy on hemostatic factors, lipid factors, and endothelial function in women undergoing surgical menopause: implications for prevention of atherosclerosis. Am Heart J 134:764–771, 1997.

Lucky, A. W., et al. Effectiveness of norgestimate and ethinyl estradiol in treating moderate acne vulgaris. J Am Acad Dermatol 37:746–754, 1997.

Mahajan, D. K., and S. N. London. Mifepristone (RU486): a review. Fertil Steril 68:967–976, 1997.

Mauck, C. K., et al. A phase I study of Femcap [vaginal contraceptive barrier] used with and without spermicide: postcoital testing. Contraception 56:111–115, 1997.

Mitlak, B. H., and F. J. Cohen. In search of optimal long-term female hormone replacement: the potential of selective estrogen receptor modulators. Horm Res 48:155–163, 1997.

O'Brien, T., and T. T. Nguyen. Lipids and lipoproteins in women. Mayo Clin Proc 72:235–244, 1997.

Piccinino, L. J., and W. D. Mosher. Trends in contraceptive use in the United States: 1982–1995. Fam Plann Perspect 30:4–10, 1998.

Rosenberg, M. J., et al. Estrogen-androgen for hormone replacement therapy: a review. J Reprod Med 42:394–404, 1997.

Simpkins, J. W., et al. Role of estrogen replacement therapy in memory enhancement and the prevention of neuronal loss associated with Alzheimer's disease. Am J Med 103:19S–25S, 1997.

Sullivan, J. M., and L. P. Fowlkes. Estrogens, menopause, and coronary artery disease. Cardiol Clin 14:105–116, 1996.

Zondervan, K. T., et al. Oral contraceptives and cervical cancer: further findings from the Oxford Family Planning Association contraceptive study. Br J Cancer 73:1291–1297, 1996.

CHAPTER THIRTY-FIVE

DRUGS FOR DIABETES MELLITUS

CLASSIFICATION OF DRUGS FOR DIABETES MELLITUS

INSULIN PREPARATIONS
Rapid-acting insulin
- Insulin lispro

Short-acting insulin
- Insulin injection (regular insulin)

Intermediate-acting insulin
- Insulin zinc suspension (lente insulin)
- Isophane insulin suspension (neutral protamine Hagedorn [NPH] insulin)

Long-acting insulin
- Extended insulin zinc suspension (ultralente insulin)

ORAL ANTIDIABETIC DRUGS
Hypoglycemic drugs
Sulfonylurea drugs
- Acetohexamide
- Chlorpropamide
- Glimepiride
- Glipizide
- Glyburide
- Tolazamide
- Tolbutamide

Other hypoglycemic drugs
- Repaglinide

Antihyperglycemic drugs
- Acarbose
- Metformin
- Troglitazone

OVERVIEW
Pancreatic Hormones

The hormones secreted by the endocrine pancreas are produced in clusters of cells called **islets of Langerhans.** These islets contain four types of cells: A (or alpha), B (or beta), D (or delta), and F cells.

The A cells produce **glucagon,** and the B cells secrete **insulin.** These two major hormones of the endocrine pancreas are primarily concerned with regulation of glucose metabolism and blood glucose concentration. Insulin promotes the uptake, utilization, and storage of glucose and thereby lowers the plasma glucose concentration, while glucagon increases the hepatic glucose output and blood glucose concentration. If insulin secretion or insulin activity is not sufficient to maintain normal blood glucose concentrations, diabetes mellitus (DM) results.

The D cells are the source of **somatostatin,** and the F cells produce **pancreatic peptide,** a peptide that appears to facilitate digestive processes. The pancreatic islets also produce **amylin,** a protein that appears to act on the brain to slow gastric churning and to decrease hepatic glucose output when digestion begins. Amylin is currently undergoing investigation as a potential adjunct to insulin therapy for DM.

Insulin

As shown in Box 35–1, **proinsulin** is converted to **insulin** and **C peptide.** Insulin consists of two peptide chains (the A chain and the B chain), which are linked by two disulfide bridges. While both insulin and C peptide are released in response to rising glucose concentrations, the physiologic role of C peptide remains unknown.

Secretion. Insulin secretion has basal and meal-stimulated components. Insulin release is activated by the rise in blood glucose concentration that follows the digestion and absorption of carbohydrates (Fig. 35–1A and 35–1B). The rate of release is 1 U of insulin per 10 g of dietary carbohydrate, and it usually peaks within 1 hour of eating. The released insulin promotes the uptake and storage of glucose and other ingested nutrients, and the postprandial (postmeal) plasma concentrations of both insulin and glucose return to preprandial (premeal) levels within 2 hours. Basal secretion, which usually ranges from 0.5 to 1 U of insulin per hour, serves to retard hepatic glucose output during the postabsorptive state.

Physiologic Effects. Insulin is sometimes referred to as the storage hormone because it promotes anabolism and inhibits catabolism of carbohydrate, fatty acids, and protein.

Insulin has several important actions on the **liver,** the organ that normally serves as the major source of blood glucose to supply the brain in the fasting state. The liver provides blood glucose through the processes of gluconeogenesis (the formation of glucose from amino acids) and glycogenolysis (the breakdown of glycogen). Insulin stimulates the enzymes involved in glycogen synthesis while inhibiting glycogenolytic and gluconeogenetic enzymes. By these actions, insulin significantly inhibits glucose output by the liver.

BOX 35–1. Structures of Proinsulin and Insulin Molecules

Preproinsulin is synthesized in the rough endoplasmic reticulum of pancreatic B cells, and proinsulin is formed by enzymatic cleavage of this precursor molecule. Proinsulin is then transported to the Golgi apparatus and converted to insulin and C peptide (connecting peptide) by the removal of four amino acids (dipeptide linkage). Insulin and C peptide are packaged in storage granules until released in equimolar amounts in response to rising glucose concentrations.

Insulin consists of a 21-amino-acid A chain and a 30-amino-acid B chain linked by two disulfide bridges.

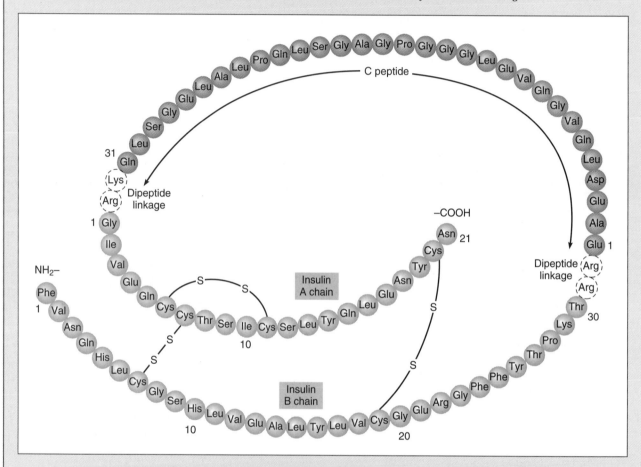

Species differences in the amino acid composition of insulin are shown in the following table. All other amino acids are identical in bovine, porcine, and human insulin. Insulin lispro is a recombinant insulin analogue that has the same structure as human insulin except for the transposition of proline and lysine at positions B28 and B29.

Type of Insulin	A Chain Position		B Chain Position		
	A8	A10	B28	B29	B30
Bovine insulin	Ala	Val	Pro	Lys	Ala
Porcine insulin	Thr	Ile	Pro	Lys	Ala
Human insulin	Thr	Ile	Pro	Lys	Thr
Insulin lispro	Thr	Ile	Lys	Pro	Thr

Insulin promotes the uptake of glucose by **skeletal muscle** and **adipose tissue** via activation of a specific type of glucose transporter that is called GLUT 4 and is located in muscle and adipose tissue. Skeletal muscle and adipose tissue are dependent on insulin for glucose uptake, whereas the brain can obtain glucose in the absence of insulin. By promoting glucose uptake, insulin facilitates the metabolism of glucose to provide energy for skeletal muscle contraction, and it stimulates glycogen synthesis. In adipose tissue, insulin stimulates the conversion of glucose to fatty acids for storage as triglyceride; promotes the uptake and esterification of fatty acids; and inhibits lipolysis (the conversion of triglyceride to fatty acids). In skeletal muscle, insulin inhibits protein catabolism and amino acid output.

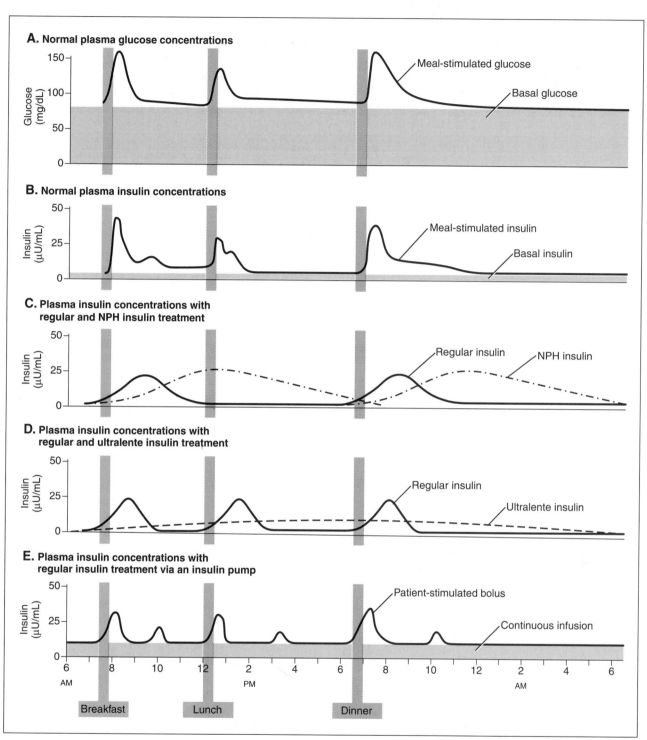

FIGURE 35–1. Time course of plasma glucose concentrations, endogenous insulin secretion, and exogenous insulin action. **(A)** Normal plasma glucose concentrations include a meal-stimulated component and a basal component. **(B)** In healthy individuals, insulin is secreted as the postprandial glucose concentration rises. This acts to increase glucose utilization and return the blood glucose concentration to its basal level. **(C, D, and E)** In patients with diabetes mellitus, insulin treatment seeks to mimic the natural secretion of insulin as closely as possible. Panels A, B, and C compare insulin concentrations obtained with three different treatment regimens. Panel C shows the results of two daily injections of regular insulin and neutral protamine Hagedorn (NPH) insulin. The first injection of each is given before breakfast, and the second injection of each is given before the evening meal. Panel D shows the results of treatment with one daily injection of ultralente insulin, which is given at bedtime, plus three daily injections of regular insulin, each of which is given before a meal. Panel E shows the results obtained with treatment via an insulin pump. The pump delivers a constant infusion of regular insulin to fulfill the basal insulin requirement, and the patient activates small bolus injections of insulin before meals, snacks, and bedtime.

Mechanisms of Action. Insulin binds to specific **insulin receptors** located in the plasma membrane of target cells, which are primarily cells of the liver, skeletal muscle, and adipose tissue. Stimulation of insulin receptors activates **tyrosine kinase** and leads to the phosphorylation of serine residues of target proteins. The phosphorylated proteins then alter the synthesis or activity of enzymes involved in gluconeogenesis, glycogenolysis, and other metabolic processes. Activation of tyrosine kinase also increases the insertion of glucose transporter molecules into cell membranes of muscle and fat tissue.

Glucagon

Glucagon is produced by A cells of the pancreas in response to decreased blood glucose concentrations. It activates glycogenolysis and gluconeogenesis and thereby increases hepatic glucose production. Patients with DM continue to produce glucagon, and the imbalance between glucagon and insulin is one factor that contributes to the metabolic derangements of this disease. Glucagon is available in a formulation for subcutaneous injection that is used to counteract hypoglycemic reactions in patients with DM.

Diabetes Mellitus
Classification

Diabetes mellitus (DM) is a disorder of glucose homeostasis that is characterized by the elevation of both basal and postprandial blood glucose concentrations and affects about 15 million people in the USA. The two major forms of DM are type I and type II, with the latter accounting for about 85% of cases of DM.

Type I diabetes mellitus usually has its onset before the patient reaches 30 years of age, with a median onset of 12 years of age. It is believed to be an autoimmune disease that is triggered by a viral infection or other environmental factor. The resulting destruction of B cells leads to severe insulin deficiency and predisposes patients to **ketonemia** and **ketoacidosis.** Because patients with type I DM require exogenous insulin for survival, this type of disease is also called **insulin-dependent diabetes mellitus** (IDDM).

Type II diabetes mellitus is a heterogenous disease that usually has its onset after the patient reaches 30 years of age and is often associated with a significant degree of **insulin resistance** and **obesity.** Insulin resistance may be due to the presence of insulin antibodies or to defects in insulin receptors and signal transduction mechanisms in target organs. Patients with type II DM are not prone to developing ketonemia. Type II DM is also called **non–insulin-dependent diabetes mellitus** (NIDDM), but the term NIDDM is not always accurate. On the one hand, most patients with type II DM have normal or elevated concentrations of insulin and do not require exogenous insulin for survival. These patients can be effectively managed with oral antidiabetic medications in combination with dietary modifications and exercise. On the other hand, some patients with type II DM do require insulin treatment.

Additional forms of DM include **gestational diabetes** (which has its onset during pregnancy) and **secondary diabetes** (which occurs in association with other endocrine disorders or with exposure to drugs or chemical agents that are toxic to the pancreas).

Pathophysiology

The early manifestations of DM are primarily metabolic abnormalities resulting from the lack of insulin, whereas the long-term complications of DM are believed to result from the glycosylation of proteins. Type I DM is a serious disease that may quickly lead to ketoacidosis, coma, and death if exogenous insulin is not administered. Type II DM is usually less serious because patients are able to continue to secrete some amount of insulin.

The **acute metabolic abnormalities** that occur in untreated DM result from decreased glucose uptake by muscle and adipose tissue, increased hepatic output of glucose, increased catabolism of proteins in muscle tissue, and increased lipolysis and release of fatty acids from adipose tissue. A reduction in glucose utilization combined with an increase in hepatic glucose production leads to hyperglycemia. Hyperglycemia may then cause glycosuria (glucose in the urine), osmotic diuresis, polyuria (excessive urine formation), and polydipsia (excessive water intake). These derangements lead to dehydration and the loss of calories and weight. For these reasons, DM has been described as "starvation in the midst of plenty."

In patients with type I DM, the absence of insulin accelerates lipolysis, and this leads to increased production of ketones (acetoacetic acid, acetone, and β-hydroxybutyric acid) in the liver. When the body becomes unable to metabolize these ketones, the keto acids are excreted in the urine. These derangements ultimately lead to ketoacidosis, acetone breath, abnormal respiration, electrolyte depletion, vomiting, coma, and death. Insulin deficiency also leads to increased catabolism of proteins and increased loss of nitrogen in the urine.

The **long-term complications** of DM include microvascular complications, such as **nephropathy** and **retinopathy;** macrovascular complications, such as **cerebrovascular disease, coronary artery disease,** and **peripheral vascular disease;** and neuropathic complications, such as **sensory, motor, and autonomic neuropathic disorders.**

While all of the complications of DM contribute significantly to morbidity, the most prevalent cause of death is coronary artery disease. Patients with DM often develop **hypertension** and **dyslipidemia** characterized by a decrease in the high-density lipoprotein cholesterol level and an increase in the triglyceride level. Furthermore, DM appears to be a risk factor for coronary artery disease that is independent of other risk factors such as smoking, hypertension, and dyslipidemia. For these reasons, patients with DM should exercise regularly, adhere closely to dietary guidelines, and comply with pharmacologic interventions to control hypertension and dyslipidemia and to achieve near-normal blood glucose concentrations.

INSULIN PREPARATIONS

Insulin preparations are used to treat all patients with type I DM and about one-third of patients with type II DM. Insulin is also used to treat pregnant women with gestational diabetes. A large number of insulin preparations are available today. These preparations can be classified according to the source of insulin and to the onset and duration of action.

Sources

For many years, patients with DM were treated with **bovine and porcine insulin.** In recent years, **human insulin** has become available through recombinant DNA technology, and it is also produced by enzymatic modification of porcine insulin. Recombinant human insulin is produced by *Escherichia coli* strains that have been transfected with the human insulin gene.

The vast majority of diabetics now use human insulin because it has numerous advantages. Clinical studies have demonstrated that those using human insulin have diminished antibody production in comparison with those using animal insulin. Insulin antibodies may bind to insulin and contribute to insulin resistance. Patients with insulin resistance usually show a significant reduction in their insulin requirement when switched from animal insulin to human insulin. Insulin antibodies may also bind to and subsequently release insulin, thereby contributing to less predictable insulin activity. Human insulin is less likely to cause allergic reactions or to produce lipodystrophy (atrophy or hypertrophy of subcutaneous fat at the site of injection). For these reasons, authorities recommend that human insulin be used to treat the following: patients with newly diagnosed type I DM; patients with insulin resistance or insulin allergy; patients with lipodystrophy; pregnant women who already have type II DM or acquire gestational diabetes during their pregnancy; and patients who have type II DM and require intermittent insulin administration, such as during surgery or infection.

Concentration and Purity

The concentration of insulin preparations is expressed as the number of units of insulin per milliliter of solution or suspension. The United States Pharmacopeia (USP) defines 1 U as the amount of insulin needed to decrease the blood glucose concentration by a defined amount in a fasting rabbit. Almost all insulin preparations used by diabetics contain 100 U/mL (U100 insulin). Regular insulin is also available in a concentrated preparation containing 500 U/mL (U500 insulin). This concentrated preparation is used by persons with insulin resistance if they require more than 100 U as a single injection.

The purity of insulin refers to the amount of proinsulin and other contaminants in insulin products. The insulin preparations marketed in the USA today contain fewer than 10 ppm of proinsulin and are classified as highly purified by the Food and Drug Administration (FDA). Human insulin preparations do not contain measurable amounts of proinsulin.

Administration and Absorption

For the treatment of DM in ambulatory patients, insulin is usually injected subcutaneously or is administered by continuous subcutaneous infusion with an insulin pump. Several factors affect the rate of absorption of insulin from subcutaneous sites and thereby contribute to wide variations in the onset and duration of action of insulin preparations in individual patients. These factors include the technique and site of injection, the ambient temperature, the patient's level of exercise, whether the injection site is massaged, and whether subcutaneous lipodystrophy is present. Insulin absorption is fastest from an abdominal injection site and is progressively slower from sites on the arm, thigh, and buttock. Because repeated injections at the same site may contribute to tissue reactions that affect the rate of insulin absorption, patients should be taught to rotate injection sites within a particular anatomic area. The application of heat or massage may increase blood flow and thereby accelerate the rate of absorption of insulin and should generally be avoided.

Regular insulin, which is a clear solution, may also be injected intravenously in situations that require a more rapid response, such as in the treatment of diabetic ketoacidosis. The intermediate-acting and long-acting insulin preparations described below are suspensions of insulin particles that are usually administered subcutaneously and should never be injected intravenously.

Classification and Properties

Based on their onset and duration of action, insulin preparations are classified as rapid-acting, short-acting, intermediate-acting, and long-acting. Table 35–1 compares the pharmacokinetic properties of the four types of insulin.

Rapid-Acting and Short-Acting Insulin

Two insulin preparations are now available for injection prior to meals in order to control postprandial glycemia. **Insulin lispro** is a rapid-acting preparation, while **insulin injection (regular insulin)** is an older, short-acting preparation.

TABLE 35–1. Pharmacokinetic Properties of Insulin Preparations

Type of Preparation	Onset of Action	Peak Effect	Duration of Action
Rapid-acting insulin Insulin lispro	0–15 minutes	30–90 minutes	<5 hours
Short-acting insulin Insulin injection (regular insulin)	30–45 minutes	2–4 hours	5–7 hours
Intermediate-acting insulin Insulin zinc suspension (lente insulin) or isophane insulin suspension (neutral protamine Hagedorn [NPH] insulin)	1–4 hours	6–14 hours	18–24 hours
Long-acting insulin Extended insulin zinc suspension (ultralente insulin)	4–6 hours	18–26 hours	≥30 hours

Regular insulin is a solution that contains insulin hexamers crystallized around a zinc molecule. After subcutaneous injection, the hexamers dissociate into dimers and monomers that are absorbed into the circulation. The dissociation of insulin hexamers occurs as the particles are diluted in body fluids when the insulin diffuses from the injection site into surrounding tissue. Because of the time required for this process, the onset of action of regular insulin occurs about 30–45 minutes after an injection. The peak effect of regular insulin usually occurs 2–4 hours after its administration. Therefore, regular insulin should be injected about 30 minutes before eating in order to provide optimal control of postprandial glycemia.

Insulin lispro is a semisynthetic analogue of human insulin. It is identical to human insulin except for the transposition of proline and lysine at positions B28 and B29 in the B chain (see Box 35–1). Insulin lispro has less capacity for self-association than regular insulin, and it is therefore more rapidly absorbed after subcutaneous injection. Peak plasma concentrations are reached earlier and return to baseline more quickly with insulin lispro than with regular insulin. Consequently, insulin lispro has a more rapid onset of action and a shorter duration of action (see Table 35–1).

Insulin lispro begins to exert its effects within 15 minutes after subcutaneous injection, and patients must eat within this time period. In comparison with the use of regular insulin, the use of insulin lispro may enable patients to more easily coordinate insulin injection times and mealtimes. Insulin lispro provides equal or greater control of postprandial glycemia, and its shorter duration of action allows it to do so without increasing the risk of hypoglycemia between meals. Except when administered by continuous subcutaneous injection with an insulin pump, insulin lispro should be part of a regimen that includes an intermediate- or long-acting insulin.

Intermediate-Acting and Long-Acting Insulin

The intermediate- and long-acting preparations are used to provide basal levels of insulin and to facilitate control of glycemia over an extended period of time. While the plasma half-life of insulin is only about 5–7 minutes, these preparations have been formulated to slowly release the insulin for absorption into the circulation following a subcutaneous injection. The preparations contain suspensions of insulin particles prepared by (1) combining insulin with a large amount of zinc, as in the **insulin zinc suspensions** called **lente insulin** and **ultralente insulin,** or (2) combining insulin with protamine and a smaller amount of zinc, as in the **isophane insulin suspension** called **neutral protamine Hagedorn (NPH) insulin.** Protamine is a basic protein that readily complexes with insulin and zinc to form particles that slowly dissolve in body fluids.

NPH insulin and lente insulin are intermediate-acting preparations. Lente insulin is a mixture of two forms of insulin zinc suspension, the first of which is an amorphous form that dissolves rapidly in body fluids and is absorbed more quickly and the second of which is a crystalline form that is less soluble and is absorbed more slowly. The intermediate-acting insulins have an onset of action of 1–4 hours, a peak effect in 6–14 hours, and a duration of action of 18–24 hours.

Ultralente insulin is the only long-acting insulin currently available in the USA. It consists entirely of crystalline insulin zinc particles that slowly dissolve in body fluids following a subcutaneous injection. Because ultralente insulin has a delayed onset and prolonged duration of action (see Table 35–1), it can be used to provide a basal insulin level that can be supplemented at mealtimes with a shorter-acting insulin.

Two other zinc-containing suspensions of insulin are no longer available in the USA: prompt insulin zinc suspension (semilente insulin) and protamine zinc insulin suspension (PZI).

Treatment Regimens

Regimens for the treatment of DM and its complications are discussed at the end of the chapter.

ORAL ANTIDIABETIC DRUGS

Orally administered antidiabetic drugs are used to treat type II DM and have no role in the treatment of type I DM. The oral drugs can be divided into two

TABLE 35–2. Pharmacologic Properties of Oral Antidiabetic Drugs

Drug	Hypoglycemia	Hyperinsulinemia	Lactic Acidosis	Gastrointestinal Symptoms
Acarbose	No	No	No	Yes (frequent)
Metformin	No	No	Yes (rare)	Yes (frequent)
Repaglinide	Yes	Yes	No	Yes (uncommon)
Sulfonylureas	Yes	Yes	No	Yes (rare)
Troglitazone	No	No	No	No

broad groups, one consisting of hypoglycemic drugs and the other consisting of antihyperglycemic drugs.

Hypoglycemic drugs act primarily by increasing insulin secretion. This action can cause plasma glucose concentrations to fall below the normal range, thereby causing hypoglycemia. The hypoglycemic drugs include the sulfonylurea compounds, as well as a new nonsulfonylurea drug that is called repaglinide and acts more rapidly than the sulfonylureas.

Antihyperglycemic drugs can prevent hyperglycemia, but they do not cause hypoglycemia. They include acarbose, metformin, and troglitazone. Acarbose is an α-glucosidase inhibitor that slows the absorption of glucose and blunts postprandial hyperglycemia. Metformin and troglitazone act in different ways to enhance the action of insulin and decrease the hepatic output of glucose.

The pharmacologic properties, metabolic effects, and therapeutic effects of hypoglycemic and antihyperglycemic drugs are shown in Table 35–2, Table 35–3, and Fig. 35–2.

Hypoglycemic Drugs
Sulfonylurea Drugs

The sulfonylureas are the largest group of oral antidiabetic drugs. The first-generation sulfonylureas include **acetohexamide, chlorpropamide, tolazamide,** and **tolbutamide.** The second-generation sulfonylureas include **glimepiride, glipizide,** and **glyburide.** The first-generation drugs are seldom used today because the second-generation drugs are more potent, are more efficacious, and tend to cause fewer adverse effects.

Drug Properties

Chemistry and Pharmacokinetics. The structures of two sulfonylurea drugs are shown in Fig. 35–3A. The sulfonylureas are administered orally and undergo varying degrees of hepatic metabolism and renal elimination of the parent compound and metabolites. Most of the sulfonylureas are metabolized to inactive or less active compounds in the liver.

Mechanisms and Pharmacologic Effects. Sulfonylureas act primarily by increasing the secretion of insulin and secondarily by decreasing the secretion of glucagon.

Sulfonylureas increase the release of insulin from pancreatic B cells by inhibiting adenosine triphosphate–sensitive potassium channels in the plasma membrane. The potassium channel contains a pore-forming subunit through which potassium moves out of the cell. It also contains a subunit that functions as the receptor for sulfonylureas. When a sulfonylurea drug binds to this subunit, it closes the channel. This prevents potassium efflux and leads to depolarization of the B cell, influx of calcium, and activation of the secretory machinery that releases insulin. According to recent studies, sulfonylureas increase the pulsatile secretion of insulin but have no effect on the basal secretion. The drugs appear to act by increasing the amount of insulin secreted during each pulse, rather than by increasing the frequency of pulses.

The decrease in glucagon secretion appears to result from the increased secretion of insulin and pancreatic somatostatin evoked by sulfonylurea drugs. Both insulin and somatostatin are known to inhibit the release of glucagon from pancreatic A

TABLE 35–3. Metabolic Effects of Oral Antidiabetic Drugs*

Drug	Glycemic Effects			Lipid Effects			Body Weight
	FPG	PPG	HbA$_{1c}$	LDL	HDL	TG	
Acarbose	→ or ↓	↓	↓0.3–1.0%	→	→	↓	→ or ↓
Metformin	↓	↓	↓1.5–2.0%	↓	↑	↓	→ or ↓
Repaglinide	→	↓	Unknown	→	→	→	→
Sulfonylureas	↓	↓	↓1.5–2.0%	→	→	→ or ↓	↑
Troglitazone	↓	↓	↓0.8–1.8%	→	↑	↓	→

*FPG = fasting plasma glucose concentration; PPG = postprandial glucose concentration; HbA$_{1c}$ = glycosylated hemoglobin concentration; LDL = low-density lipoprotein cholesterol level; HDL = high-density lipoprotein cholesterol level; TG = triglyceride level; → = unchanged; ↓ = decreased; and ↑ = increased.

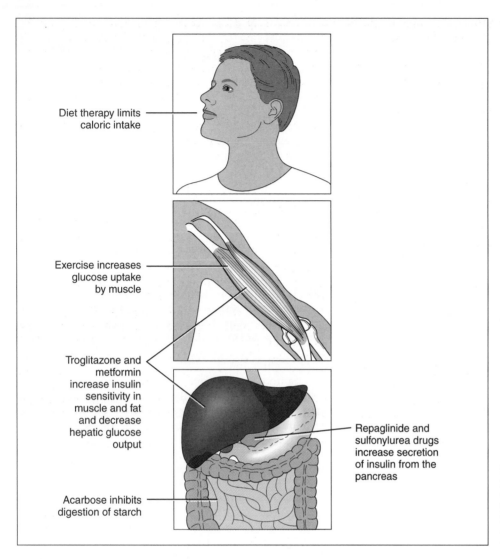

Diet therapy limits
caloric intake

Exercise increases
glucose uptake
by muscle

Troglitazone and
metformin
increase insulin
sensitivity in
muscle and fat
and decrease
hepatic glucose
output

Repaglinide and
sulfonylurea drugs
increase secretion
of insulin from the
pancreas

Acarbose inhibits
digestion of starch

FIGURE 35–2. Therapeutic effects of diet, exercise, and oral drugs used in the treatment of patients with type II diabetes mellitus. If these treatment measures are not adequate, insulin can be used to control glycemia.

cells. This action tends to normalize the ratio of insulin to glucagon in diabetics.

Sulfonylureas have little positive effect on lipoprotein levels, and their use has been associated with weight gain.

The mechanisms responsible for the extrapancreatic effects of sulfonylureas are not completely understood. Most of the experimental evidence indicates that these effects are secondary to the increase in insulin secretion. Because sulfonylureas have not been convincingly shown to improve glucose tolerance or reduce insulin requirements in type I DM, it seems unlikely that the drugs significantly enhance the action of insulin on target tissues. Nevertheless, some investigators claim that a new sulfonylurea, glimepiride, enhances the insulin action more than do other drugs in this class.

Indications. A sulfonylurea drug is often used to treat type II DM that cannot be controlled with dietary restrictions, exercise, and body weight reduction. Although any of the sulfonylureas can be used, most patients are now started on a second-generation drug for reasons cited above. Therapy usually begins with a low dose, which is given once a day and is swallowed 30 minutes before breakfast to maximize absorption. The dose is then gradually increased until adequate glycemic control is achieved, side effects occur, or the maximum dose is reached. A sulfonylurea drug can be given in combination with another antidiabetic drug if glycemia cannot be controlled with the maximum dose. The selection and use of different types of oral antidiabetic drugs are described later in this chapter.

Adverse Effects. Hypoglycemia may result from skipping or delaying meals, inadequate ingestion of carbohydrate, or renal or hepatic disease in patients taking sulfonylureas. Hypoglycemia is the most common adverse effect of every sulfonylurea compound, but it is particularly troublesome with chlorpropamide because this drug has a long duration of action.

Other adverse effects of sulfonylureas include skin rashes (which occur in up to 3% of patients), nausea, vomiting, and cholestasis. Cholestatic jaundice occurs more frequently with chlorpropamide than with other sulfonylureas.

Less commonly, sulfonylureas cause hematologic reactions such as leukopenia, thrombocytopenia, and hemolytic anemia.

Interactions. Health care providers should be aware that sulfonylureas may interact with a large number of other drugs. Although the clinical significance of most of these interactions is usually minimal, dosage adjustments may be required. For example, thiazide diuretics may increase blood glucose concentrations and increase the dosage requirements of sulfonylurea compounds.

Angiotensin-converting enzyme inhibitors, sulfonamides, gemfibrozil, and alcohol (ethanol) are among the agents that may increase the hypoglycemic effect of sulfonylureas. Excessive ingestion of alcohol by patients treated with sulfonylureas or insulin can cause significant hypoglycemia. A disulfiramlike reaction may also result when alcohol is taken with sulfonylureas. Diabetics should be counseled to use alcohol moderately and to limit consumption to about 2 ounces (60 mL) per day.

First-Generation Sulfonylureas

Chlorpropamide and other first-generation sulfonylureas are seldom used today because of their lower potency and their greater tendency to cause side effects. Chlorpropamide has been associated with a higher incidence of adverse effects than other sulfonylurea drugs, especially in patients who are elderly or have renal impairment. Chlorpropamide

can cause significant water retention and hyponatremia, primarily by promoting the release of antidiuretic hormone (vasopressin). This is called the syndrome of inappropriate antidiuretic hormone (SIADH). In addition, chlorpropamide causes a disulfiramlike effect in 30% of patients who ingest alcohol while using the drug. Because chlorpropamide has a longer duration of action than other sulfonylurea compounds, hypoglycemic reactions may be prolonged and severe.

Second-Generation Sulfonylureas

The second-generation sulfonylureas include glimepiride, glipizide, and glyburide. Glyburide is called glibenclamide in some countries. The second-generation drugs are at least 100 times more potent than the first-generation drugs. For this reason, they usually control glycemia without producing as many side effects.

The absorption of second-generation sulfonylureas (particularly glipizide) is slowed by food, so the drugs should be taken at least 30 minutes before breakfast. Glyburide is available in a regular formulation and a micronized one. Because the micronized formulation provides higher plasma concentrations, the recommended doses of it are 60% of those of the regular formulation. Glyburide is completely metabolized by the liver, with half of the metabolites excreted in the urine and the other half eliminated via the bile and gastrointestinal tract. Glipizide is also

FIGURE 35–3. Structures of oral antidiabetic drugs. (A) Most hypoglycemic drugs are sulfonylureas. The sulfonylurea moieties in glimepiride and glyburide are unshaded. **(B)** Metformin is a biguanide drug, and troglitazone is a thiazolidinedione. The biguanide and thiazolidinedione moieties are unshaded.

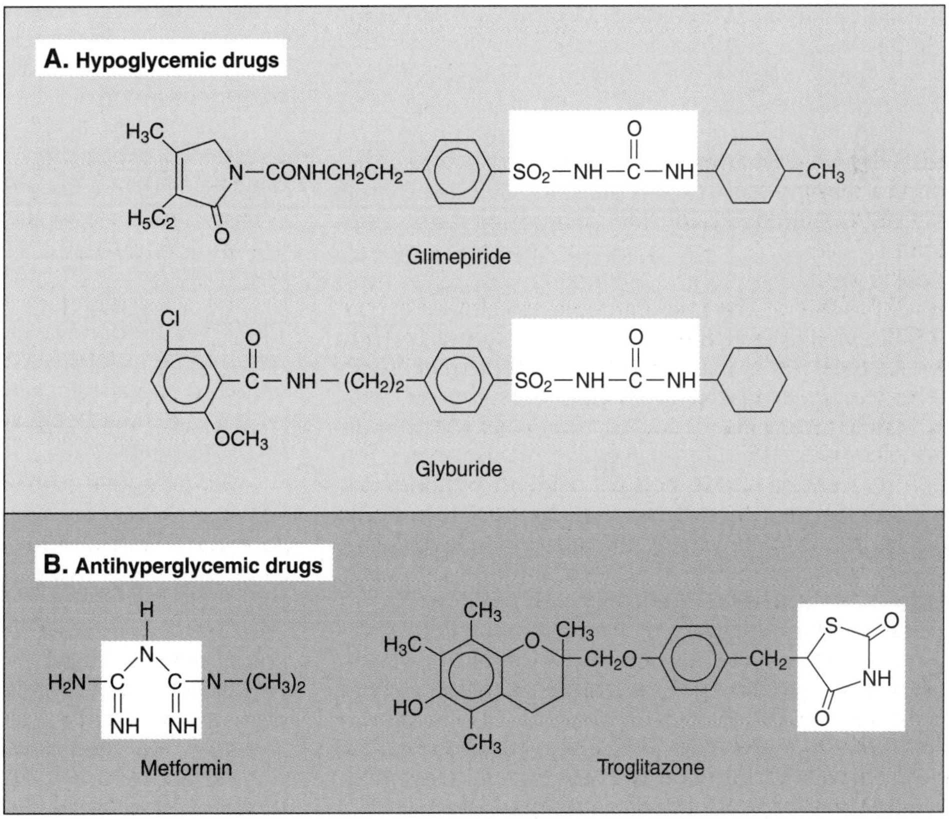

converted to inactive hydroxylated metabolites in the liver, and these are excreted in the urine.

The second-generation sulfonylureas have a duration of action that is considerably longer than the plasma half-life. The duration of action of glyburide is about 24 hours, whereas that of glipizide is about 10–24 hours. Many patients require only one daily dose of these drugs to adequately control glycemia.

Glimepiride is the newest second-generation sulfonylurea, and it is the first one approved for use in combination with insulin. There is some evidence that it increases insulin sensitivity, but this is controversial. The efficacy of glimepiride was found to be similar to that of glipizide and glyburide in a 1-year study. Although glimepiride is well tolerated, it causes hypoglycemia in up to 20% of patients treated with glimepiride alone and in up to 50% of patients treated with glimepiride plus insulin. According to one study, the combination of glimepiride plus insulin was no more effective than insulin alone in achieving target fasting blood glucose concentrations, but control was achieved more rapidly and with lower doses of insulin in patients taking glimepiride.

Other Hypoglycemic Drugs

Repaglinide is a nonsulfonylurea hypoglycemic drug that works quickly and is intended to be taken before meals. Repaglinide increases the amount of insulin released by pancreatic B cells during and immediately after a meal. This results in smaller postprandial increases in the blood glucose concentration and in an overall decline in the average blood glucose concentration over time.

Repaglinide may be taken anytime from 30 minutes before a meal right up to mealtime. It reaches its peak effectiveness in about 1 hour, which coincides with the time when postprandial glucose concentrations are rising toward their peak. Repaglinide is completely metabolized and inactivated by the liver in about 3–4 hours. For this reason, its duration of action is relatively short, and insulin concentrations return to basal levels before the next meal.

Repaglinide is intended as a first-line drug to treat type II DM in conjunction with diet and exercise. It is particularly useful for patients whose meal schedules vary from day to day, a factor that increases their risk of hypoglycemic reactions to sulfonylureas. Repaglinide can be used in combination with metformin when either repaglinide or metformin alone does not adequately control blood glucose concentrations. However, repaglinide should not be used with other oral antidiabetic drugs or with insulin.

The adverse effects of repaglinide include hypoglycemia, headache, nausea, and joint pain. Hypoglycemic reactions to repaglinide have not been serious, but they did cause 1.4% of patients to discontinue their use of repaglinide. This is about half the rate of discontinued drug use attributed to hypoglycemic reactions in patients taking sulfonylureas.

Antihyperglycemic Drugs

Metformin

Chemistry and Pharmacokinetics. Metformin (see Fig. 35–3B) is the only **biguanide** type of oral antidiabetic medication currently available in the USA. Another biguanide, **phenformin,** was removed from the market in the 1970s because of an unacceptable risk of fatal lactic acidosis (see below).

Metformin is administered orally from two to four times a day and is eliminated by renal excretion of the parent compound. Its duration of action is about 18 hours.

Mechanisms and Pharmacologic Effects. Metformin has several mechanisms of action. In patients with type II DM, it alleviates hyperglycemia primarily by decreasing the hepatic glucose output. It also appears to decrease glucose absorption from the gut and increase insulin sensitivity in skeletal muscle and adipose tissue. Unlike sulfonylureas, metformin does not stimulate insulin secretion or cause hypoglycemia, and it does not cause weight gain. Metformin has a favorable effect on plasma lipid levels and may decrease body weight in some patients (see Table 35–3).

Indications. Metformin is now considered a first-line drug for the treatment of type II DM. It may be particularly appropriate for obese patients with insulin resistance and for patients with hyperlipidemia. It may also provide acceptable glycemic control in patients who do not adequately respond to a sulfonylurea drug. Metformin can be used alone, or it can be used in combination with a sulfonylurea for patients who fail to respond appropriately to single-drug therapy. Limited data suggest that metformin may decrease insulin requirements in patients who have type II DM that is uncontrolled by insulin treatment alone.

Adverse Effects. The most common adverse effects of metformin are gastrointestinal disturbances. Diarrhea occurs in up to 30% of patients and causes about 4% of them to stop taking metformin. Unlike phenformin, metformin does not bind to mitochondria or interfere with glucose oxidation, and it causes lactic acidosis rarely (in only 3 cases per 100,000 patient years of use). However, patients with renal or hepatic disease, alcoholism, or a predisposition to metabolic acidosis should not be treated with metformin, because they are at increased risk of lactic acidosis.

Interactions. Metformin has few drug interactions.

Troglitazone and Related Drugs

Chemistry and Pharmacokinetics. Troglitazone (see Fig. 35–3B) was the first of a new class of antidiabetic drugs called **thiazolidinediones.** Two other drugs in this class, **pioglitazone** and **rosiglitazone,** were placed on the market in 1999.

Troglitazone is taken once a day and is administered with food because this increases its absorption by about 50%. The drug is rapidly absorbed from the gut, and more than 99% of it is bound to plasma proteins. Troglitazone is extensively metabolized in the liver, and the metabolites are primarily eliminated in the feces.

Mechanisms and Pharmacologic Effects. Troglitazone acts by increasing the number of GLUT 4 glucose transporters in cell membranes of muscle and adipose tissue. This in turn increases the uptake and utilization of glucose in these tissues. The drug increases the sensitivity of peripheral tissues to insulin by about 60%, and it also suppresses hepatic glucose output. In comparison with metformin, troglitazone appears to have a greater effect on insulin sensitivity, whereas metformin has a greater effect on hepatic glucose output. Troglitazone does not increase insulin secretion.

Troglitazone has beneficial effects on serum lipoprotein levels and may reverse some of the lipid abnormalities that are associated with type II DM. Troglitazone lowers triglyceride levels by about 20% and increases high-density lipoprotein cholesterol levels by about 10%. However, it does not have any consistent effect on low-density lipoprotein cholesterol levels.

Troglitazone routinely increases plasma volume by 6–8%, but the clinical significance of this effect remains uncertain. Red cell mass is not affected by the drug.

Indications. Troglitazone is indicated for the treatment of type II DM in patients who require insulin and whose symptoms are not adequately controlled despite taking over 30 U of insulin a day. Because troglitazone enhances insulin activity, it is particularly useful in patients with insulin resistance. Clinical studies indicate that troglitazone decreases plasma glucose concentrations by 40–80 mg/dL and decreases insulin requirements by 5–30%. In one study, 15% of patients taking troglitazone were able to discontinue their insulin therapy.

Further study is needed to determine the role that troglitazone plays in the treatment of patients who have type II DM and do not require insulin. In one study, use of a combination of troglitazone and metformin was found to be more effective than use of either agent alone in the treatment of these patients.

Adverse Effects and Interactions. Troglitazone may cause hepatic dysfunction or even death due to hepatitis. Patients taking this drug should therefore be closely monitored for signs of hepatitis, particularly during the first several weeks of therapy. Because troglitazone has a low rate of renal elimination, patients with renal dysfunction do not require dosage adjustments. However, troglitazone should not be used in patients with liver disease.

In patients treated with a combination of troglitazone and insulin, hypoglycemia may occur because of enhanced insulin effectiveness. Insulin doses may therefore need to be reduced.

Troglitazone induces CYP3A4, a cytochrome P450 enzyme, and may reduce plasma concentrations of cyclosporine, tacrolimus, some HMG-CoA reductase inhibitors, and some oral contraceptives.

Acarbose

Mechanisms and Pharmacologic Effects. The digestion of dietary starch and disaccharides such as sucrose is dependent on the action of α-**glucosidase,** an enzyme located in the brush border of the intestinal tract. Acarbose is an oligosaccharide compound that competitively inhibits this enzyme. It thereby slows the digestion of starch and disaccharides, decreases the rate of glucose absorption, and lowers the postprandial blood glucose concentration. Studies have demonstrated some reduction in the glycosylated hemoglobin (HbA_{1c}) concentrations of patients treated with acarbose, although the reduction is usually less than that obtained with other oral antidiabetic drugs (see Table 35–3).

Indications and Pharmacokinetics. Acarbose is used in the treatment of type II DM. It is administered with each meal and is particularly effective when given with meals containing large amounts of starch. It is not absorbed systemically, and it is eliminated in the feces.

Adverse Effects and Interactions. The most common side effects of acarbose are increased flatulence and abdominal bloating. These reactions probably result from the delivery of greater amounts of carbohydrate to the lower intestinal tract, where they exert an osmotic attraction for water and are metabolized by bacteria.

Acarbose may increase the oral bioavailability of metformin and cause a decrease in iron absorption.

In patients taking acarbose, if concurrent administration of insulin or a sulfonylurea drug results in hypoglycemia, this complication should be treated with glucose (dextrose), rather than sucrose, because glucose does not require α-glucosidase activity for digestion.

THE MANAGEMENT OF DIABETES MELLITUS AND ITS COMPLICATIONS
Type I Diabetes Mellitus

All patients with type I DM require insulin therapy to achieve a high degree of glycemic control. In 1993, the Diabetes Control and Complications Trial Research Group showed that achieving and maintaining near-normal blood glucose concentrations in patients with type I DM reduced the incidence of nephropathy, neuropathy, and retinopathy. Although there is evidence that poor glycemic control is associated with cardiovascular events, no study has yet shown that aggressive lowering of blood glucose concentrations reduces the incidence of cardiovascular disease.

Objectives of Insulin Therapy

The specific objectives of insulin therapy are to maintain the **fasting plasma glucose concentration** below 140 mg/dL (normal is <115 mg/dL); to maintain the **2-hour postprandial glucose concentration** below 175 mg/dL (normal is <140 mg/dL); and to maintain the **glycosylated hemoglobin (HbA$_{1c}$) concentration** below 8% (normal is 4–6%). The HbA$_{1c}$ concentration provides a cumulative indication of overall glycemic control and may directly relate to the extent to which glycosylation of tissue proteins contributes to the microvascular and other complications of DM.

Insulin Requirements and Dosing Schedules

In patients with type I DM, multiple daily injections of insulin are required to obtain acceptable control of glycemia without causing hypoglycemia. The total amount of insulin required by most of these patients is 0.5–1 U/kg/d. However, this amount usually decreases during the "honeymoon phase" of DM (during the first several months after the initial episode of illness).

Although a number of different insulin treatment regimens are used, each of them seeks to mimic the natural secretion of insulin as closely as possible (see Fig. 35–1B). In most regimens, use of an **intermediate- or long-acting insulin preparation** is supplemented by use of a **rapid- or short-acting insulin** at mealtimes in a dose that matches the quantity of ingested carbohydrate. Three examples of insulin dosing schedules that are used to treat type I DM are illustrated in Fig. 35–1C, 35–1D, and 35–1E.

A commonly used regimen consists of injecting an intermediate-acting insulin (NPH or lente insulin) plus a short-acting insulin (regular insulin) twice a day. Two-thirds of the total daily dose is given in the morning 30 minutes before breakfast, and the remainder is given 30 minutes before the evening meal. The morning injection usually consists of a 2:1 or 70:30 ratio of intermediate-acting insulin to regular insulin, whereas the evening injection typically consists of a 50:50 ratio. The specific doses of intermediate-acting and regular insulin can be adjusted on the basis of self-monitored glucose readings taken at the time of the peak action of each insulin injection. For regular insulin, the morning dose and evening dose are evaluated on the basis of blood glucose measurements before lunch and at bedtime, respectively. For the intermediate-acting insulin, the morning dose and evening dose are evaluated on the basis of blood glucose measurements obtained just prior to the evening insulin injection and just prior to the morning insulin injection, respectively. If these blood glucose measurements are too high or too low, the subsequent doses of insulin can be adjusted appropriately.

Two preparations of a mixture of NPH and regular insulin are available for use in the above treatment regimen. One mixture contains NPH and regular insulin in a ratio of 70:30, and the other contains the two insulins in a ratio of 50:50. These preparations offer greater convenience and reliability to patients and obviate the need for them to mix the drugs before each injection. There is no premixed preparation of lente and regular insulin; patients must mix these drugs immediately before administering them, because the mixture is not stable for long periods of time.

Another regimen that has been developed in an attempt to provide better glycemic control consists of the following: one daily injection of long-acting insulin (ultralente insulin), given at bedtime; plus three daily injections of a rapid- or short-acting insulin (either insulin lispro or regular insulin), with each injection given before a meal. In this regimen, the injection of ultralente insulin provides a basal level of insulin that controls hepatic glucose output during the nighttime hours and between meals, and the other three injections control postprandial glycemia.

Similar results can be obtained with an alternative regimen that provides continuous subcutaneous insulin infusion (CSII) via an insulin pump. The insulin pump delivers a constant infusion of regular insulin to fulfill the basal insulin requirement, and the patient activates small bolus injections of insulin prior to meals and snacks. Although CSII can theoretically provide greater glycemic control than other regimens, it has been associated with a significant incidence of hypoglycemia and mechanical problems. This is why the American Diabetes Association recommends restricting use of the insulin pump to highly knowledgeable and motivated patients who are under the care of physicians properly trained in the use of these pumps.

Diabetic Ketoacidosis

Diabetic ketoacidosis is a common and life-threatening complication of type I DM, with a mortality rate as high as 6–10%. Therapy must be individualized, based on the clinical and laboratory status of the patient. Intravenous fluids are given to alleviate dehydration, and continuous intravenous infusion of insulin is given to decrease the plasma glucose concentration at a rate of at least 75–100 mg/dL/h. Intravenous administration of potassium chloride is usually required to counteract hypokalemia that results from the correction of dehydration and acidosis. Dextrose (glucose) is often needed as therapy progresses, because hyperglycemia is usually corrected more rapidly than is acidosis. Insulin should be continued until acidosis is resolved. Bicarbonate is not routinely used and should be reserved for the treatment of patients who have severe acidosis after hypokalemia is corrected.

Type II Diabetes Mellitus

The treatment of type II DM rests on the foundation of a nutritious diet and appropriate exercise. Dietary recommendations should attempt to limit calories and saturated fat. Overweight patients should be encouraged to exercise and lose weight in an attempt to improve glycemic control, reduce insulin resistance, and lower plasma lipid levels. If nonpharmacologic measures are inadequate, as indicated by fasting blood glucose concentrations exceeding 140 mg/dL or HbA$_{1c}$ concentrations exceeding 8%, the next step is usually to add an oral antidiabetic medication.

Acarbose, metformin, and sulfonylureas are considered first-line drugs for type II DM. There is no clear drug of choice for all patients. Acarbose is generally less effective than the other drugs, but it is sometimes used to treat patients who have mild DM or cannot tolerate other oral medications. It is also used as "booster therapy" in patients who have borderline control when they use either oral hypoglycemic agents or insulin. In patients who have insulin resistance or hyperlipidemia, metformin is a logical choice to begin drug therapy for type II DM. Until recently, sulfonylureas were the only available oral antidiabetic drugs, and many clinicians still prefer to initiate drug therapy with one of these agents. However, unlike acarbose or metformin, the sulfonylurea drugs may cause hypoglycemia, hyperinsulinemia, and weight gain.

If single-drug therapy is inadequate to control glycemia, the clinician is faced with the difficult choice of using combination therapy or switching to insulin. The most frequently used drug combination is metformin plus a sulfonylurea. However, recent studies indicate that metformin and troglitazone can be extremely effective in patients not controlled by a single drug.

The insulin regimens used to treat type II DM are usually less complicated than those used to treat type I. Patients with type II disease are usually not prone to ketoacidosis, and most of them have significant endogenous insulin production. For these reasons, the initial insulin requirement is often less than 20 U/d. Insulin therapy is usually started with a single daily dose of intermediate- or long-acting insulin. Giving the single dose at bedtime may be adequate for patients who experience only early morning hyperglycemia. If multiple daily doses of insulin are needed or if insulin requirements are greater than 30 U/d, troglitazone can be added to the regimen to improve insulin sensitivity and decrease insulin requirements. Metformin is sometimes used to treat type II DM in patients who wish to wean themselves from insulin, although this indication is not approved by the FDA.

Summary of Important Points

- Insulin increases glucose uptake by muscle and fat, decreases hepatic glucose output, and controls postprandial glycemia.
- Insulin preparations can be classified on the basis of their onset and duration of action. Insulin lispro is rapid-acting; insulin injection (regular insulin) is short-acting; insulin zinc suspension (lente insulin) and isophane insulin suspension (neutral protamine Hagedorn, or NPH, insulin) are intermediate-acting; and extended insulin zinc suspension (ultralente insulin) is long-acting.
- There are two main types of diabetes mellitus (DM). Type I is also called insulin-dependent DM (IDDM). Type II is also called non–insulin-dependent DM (NIDDM). All patients with type I DM require insulin. Most patients with type II DM can be managed with diet, exercise, and oral antidiabetic drugs, but some require insulin. Oral antidiabetic drugs have no role in the treatment of type I DM.
- The long-term complications of DM include nephropathy, retinopathy, and coronary artery and other vascular diseases. The Diabetes Control and Complications Trial Research Group showed that maintaining near-normal glucose concentrations in patients with type I DM reduces the incidence of most of these complications.
- In patients with type I DM, multiple daily doses of insulin are required for optimal control of blood glucose concentrations. In a commonly used regimen, insulin is given in two daily doses, with each dose consisting of an intermediate-acting insulin plus regular insulin. In another regimen, patients are treated with a single daily injection of ultralente insulin plus three preprandial injections of regular insulin or insulin lispro.
- Oral antidiabetic drugs include hypoglycemic agents (sulfonylureas and repaglinide) and antihyperglycemic agents (acarbose, metformin, and troglitazone).
- Sulfonylureas and repaglinide act by increasing insulin release from pancreatic B cells. Second-generation sulfonylureas (glipizide, glyburide, and glimepiride) are preferable to first-generation sulfonylureas because they have greater potency and clinical efficacy and are associated with fewer adverse effects. Hypoglycemia is the main side effect of these drugs.
- Acarbose inhibits α-glucosidase and slows digestion and absorption of glucose.
- Metformin primarily acts by decreasing hepatic glucose output but also increases insulin sensitivity. Troglitazone primarily acts by enhancing insulin sensitivity while reducing hepatic glucose output. Both drugs have favorable effects on plasma lipid levels. Unlike sulfonylureas, they do not cause weight gain.
- Acarbose, metformin, and sulfonylureas are first-line drugs for the treatment of type II DM. Troglitazone was initially approved for patients whose symptoms could not be controlled by insulin, but studies suggest it may be useful alone or in combination with metformin in patients who are not taking insulin.

Selected Readings

Ashcroft, F. M. Mechanisms of the glycemic effects of sulfonylureas. Horm Metab Res 28:456–463, 1996.
Bressler, R., and D. G. Johnson. Pharmacologic regulation of blood glucose levels in non–insulin-dependent diabetes mellitus. Arch Intern Med 157:836–848, 1997.

Davidson, M. B., and A. L. Peters. An overview of metformin in the treatment of type II diabetes mellitus. Am J Med 102:99–110, 1997.

The Diabetes Control and Complications Trial Research Group. The effect of intensive treatment of diabetes on the development and progression of long-term complications in insulin-dependent diabetes mellitus. N Engl J Med 329:977–986, 1993.

Langtry, H. D., and J. A. Balfour. Glimepiride: a review of its use in the management of type II diabetes mellitus. Drugs 55:563–584, 1998.

McFarland, K. F. Type II diabetes: stepped-care approach to patient management. Geriatrics 52:22–26, 1997.

Melander, A. Oral antidiabetic drugs: an overview. Diabet Med 13:S143–S147, 1996.

Noble, S. L., et al. Insulin lispro: a fast-acting insulin analog. Am Fam Phys 57:279–286, 1998.

Repaglinide for type II diabetes mellitus. Med Lett Drugs Ther 40:55–56, 1998.

Shorr, R. I., et al. Incidence and risk factors for serious hypoglycemia in older persons using insulin or sulfonylureas. Arch Intern Med 157:1681–1686, 1997.

Spencer, C. M., and A. Markham. Troglitazone. Drugs 54:89–101, 1997.

Yee, H. S., and N. T. Fong. A review of the safety and efficacy of acarbose in diabetes mellitus. Pharmacotherapy 16:792–805, 1996.

CHAPTER THIRTY-SIX

DRUGS AFFECTING CALCIUM

AND BONE

CLASSIFICATION OF DRUGS AFFECTING CALCIUM AND BONE

Calcium and vitamin D supplements
- Calcitriol
- Calcium carbonate
- Calcium citrate
- Cholecalciferol

Bisphosphonates
- Alendronate
- Pamidronate
- Tiludronate

Other agents
- Calcitonin
- Estrogen
- Fluoride
- Plicamycin
- Raloxifene

OVERVIEW

Calcium and Bone Metabolism

The strength and the structure of bone depend on the presence of **calcium salts** deposited on bone matrix proteins. Normal bone is constantly undergoing remodeling via demineralization and mineralization processes. During remodeling, bone calcium is in a dynamic equilibrium with ionized calcium in extracellular fluid. Bone **mineralization** tends to increase as the extracellular calcium concentration rises, and **demineralization** tends to increase as this concentration falls. The proper extracellular calcium concentration is required for normal function of nerves and muscles, blood coagulation, enzyme activities, and other physiologic functions.

Control of the extracellular calcium concentration depends on hormonal regulation of the absorption and excretion of calcium, as well as on the exchange of ionized calcium with bone. As shown in Fig. 36–1, the hormones involved in regulation include **vitamin D, parathyroid hormone** (PTH), and **calcitonin.**

Vitamin D stimulates calcium absorption by increasing the synthesis of a calcium-binding protein that mediates the gastrointestinal absorption of calcium. Vitamin D also stimulates bone resorption and the closely coupled process of bone formation.

PTH has four actions that increase the extracellular calcium concentration. First, it stimulates resorption of calcium by renal tubules. Second, it decreases resorption of phosphate by renal tubules. This decreases the extracellular phosphate concentration, which in turn tends to increase the extracellular calcium concentration. Third, PTH stimulates the hydroxylation of vitamin D in the kidneys (Fig. 36–2). Fourth, PTH increases bone resorption by stimulating osteoclast activity, which enables bone calcium to enter the extracellular pool. PTH does not have any clinical use as a drug at the present time.

Calcitonin is released in response to increased plasma calcium levels, and it acts to inhibit bone resorption and thereby decrease plasma calcium levels. The physiologic significance of calcitonin is unclear, since normal calcium balance is maintained in the absence of calcitonin in persons who undergo thyroidectomy.

Bone remodeling consists of a sequence of events involving the dynamic interaction of **osteoclasts** (bone-resorbing cells) and **osteoblasts** (bone-forming cells). The recruitment and activation of osteoclasts are mediated by compounds that are released from osteoblasts and peripheral leukocytes and are called **bone cell cytokines.** The cytokines include **interleukins, tumor necrosis factor,** and **colony-stimulating factors.** After the osteoclasts are activated, they adhere to the bone surface and release hydrogen ions and proteases to break down the bone. The destroyed bone releases growth factors that increase osteoblast production and decrease osteoclast activity. The osteoblasts then lay down new bone in the cavity created by osteoclasts. The entire remodeling process takes about 100 days on average. Trabecular bone undergoes more remodeling than cortical bone (25% versus 3% annually).

The balance between **bone resorption** and **bone formation** is usually maintained until the third or fourth decade of life, when a slow, age-related imbalance begins and favors resorption over formation. Hormonal and nutritional deficiencies can also contribute to this imbalance.

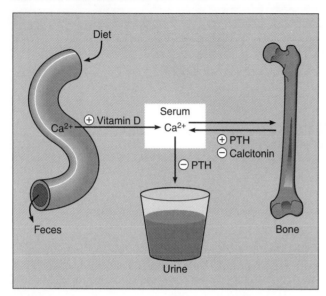

FIGURE 36–1. Calcium and bone metabolism. Vitamin D facilitates calcium absorption from the gut. Parathyroid hormone (PTH) decreases calcium excretion in the urine but increases phosphorus excretion (not shown). PTH also increases bone resorption, while calcitonin decreases bone resorption.

Bone Disorders

Osteoporosis, the most common bone disorder, is characterized by a gradual reduction in bone mass that weakens the bone and leads to the occurrence of fractures with minimal trauma. The disorder is frequently classified as postmenopausal, senile, or secondary to other diseases. **Vertebral fractures** are the most frequent type of fractures seen in patients with **postmenopausal osteoporosis,** a disorder that is primarily due to estrogen deficiency. **Hip, humerus, pelvis, and vertebral fractures** occur in patients with **senile osteoporosis,** a disorder that is primarily due to advanced age and is a major cause of immobility, morbidity, and mortality in the elderly. In the USA, the annual cost of osteoporotic hip fractures alone is currently about $10 billion, and the cost is projected to rise to $240 billion by the year 2040 if more effective methods of prevention and treatment are not discovered and implemented.

Paget's disease of bone, or **osteitis deformans,** is the second most common bone disorder. Its manifestations include bone deformities, pain, and fractures. Its cause is unknown.

Osteomalacia is characterized by abnormal mineralization of new bone matrix. The condition has numerous causes, the most common of which include vitamin D deficiency, abnormal vitamin D metabolism, phosphate deficiency, and osteoblast dysfunction. In children, osteomalacia is usually due to vitamin D deficiency and is called **rickets.** This disorder is uncommon today because of vitamin D–supplemented foods and sun exposure. In adults, factors such as aging, malabsorption, chronic renal impairment, and use of phenytoin or other anticonvulsant drugs may interfere with vitamin D absorption, metabolism, or target organ response and result in osteomalacia.

DRUGS
Calcium and Vitamin D Supplements

An adequate intake of calcium and vitamin D is essential for optimal bone formation in children and for the prevention of osteoporosis in adults.

In the USA, two-thirds of women 18–30 years old and three-fourths of women over 30 years old have an inadequate calcium intake, and this predisposes them to osteoporosis. All persons, regardless of age or gender, should meet the recommendations of the National Institutes of Health for daily calcium intake (Table 36–1). These recommendations can be met by ingesting calcium-rich foods, which are primarily dairy products, and taking oral calcium supplements if dietary intake is inadequate. By ingesting optimal amounts of calcium and vitamin D, young adults may be able to increase their bone mass, and older adults can decrease the rate of bone loss.

In one clinical study, nursing-home residents who were given 800 IU of vitamin D_3 and 1200 mg of calcium were found to have an increase in bone density and a decrease in the incidence of hip and nonvertebral fractures in comparison with nursing-home residents who were given placebos. In another study, administration of vitamin D_3 was found to decrease the incidence of vertebral and peripheral fractures in women with previous fractures.

Calcium

Pharmacokinetics. Calcium absorption from the gut is incomplete, even in the presence of adequate amounts of vitamin D. Only about 30% of calcium is absorbed from milk and other dairy products, and calcium absorption from supplements is often less than 30%. To enhance absorption, calcium tablets should be taken between meals.

The absorption of **calcium carbonate** requires stomach acid, whereas the absorption of **calcium citrate** does not. Because elderly persons may have decreased stomach acid secretion, they tend to benefit more from using calcium citrate.

Indications. In addition to their role in the prevention and treatment of **osteoporosis,** calcium and vitamin D are also the primary treatment for **hypocalcemia.** For this purpose, calcium may be given orally or intravenously.

Adverse Effects and Interactions. The most common adverse effect of calcium supplements is constipation. This is best managed by ingesting adequate amounts of fruits and vegetables. Calcium should not be taken with fiber laxatives, because they decrease calcium absorption. Calcium can decrease the absorption of ciprofloxacin, fluoride, phenytoin, and tetracycline, so calcium supplements should be taken at least 2 hours before or after taking these drugs.

Vitamin D

Chemistry and Pharmacokinetics. Vitamin D is a fat-soluble substance similar to cholesterol. The

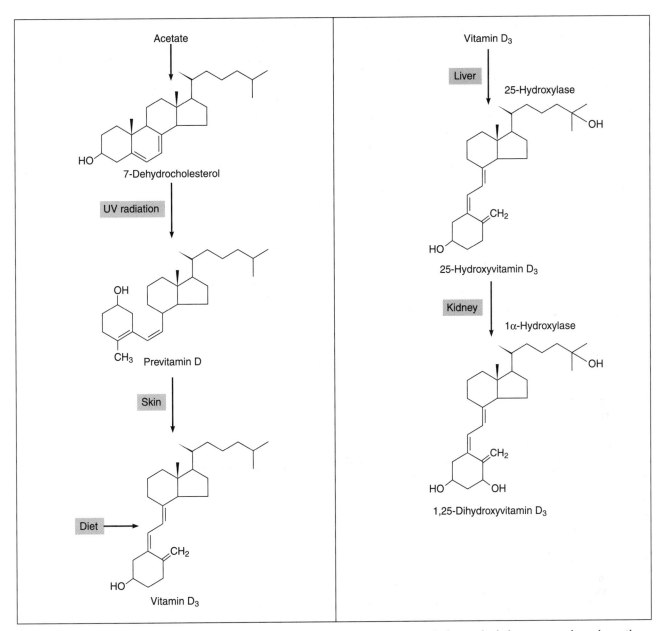

FIGURE 36–2. Synthesis of vitamin D. Vitamin D_3 (cholecalciferol) can be synthesized in the human body from acetate through a pathway that requires ultraviolet (UV) radiation. Diet and vitamin supplements also provide vitamin D_3, which is activated by specific hydroxylation steps in the liver and kidneys to form 1,25-dihydroxyvitamin D_3 (calcitriol).

form of the vitamin that is obtained from the diet and can be synthesized in skin exposed to ultraviolet radiation is called **vitamin D_3** or **cholecalciferol.** It is a relatively inactive precursor of **1,25-dihydroxyvitamin D_3,** which is also called **calcitriol** and is the most active form of the vitamin. The formation of calcitriol involves hydroxylation of vitamin D_3 at the 25 position in the liver and at the 1 position in the kidneys (see Fig. 36–2). PTH stimulates the renal hydroxylation of vitamin D. The roles of PTH and vitamin D in calcium metabolism and homeostasis are described above.

Indications. Persons with inadequate dietary vitamin D intake and low sun exposure should take oral vitamin D supplements. Vitamin D_3 is used to prevent **osteoporosis** and to treat **rickets** and other types of **osteomalacia.** Patients with **chronic renal impairment** must be treated with calcitriol (the active form of the vitamin) because they are unable to synthesize it.

Adverse Effects and Interactions. Excessive doses of vitamin D may cause hypercalcemia and hypercalciuria. Cholestyramine inhibits vitamin D absorption, and phenytoin and barbiturates can induce enzymes that metabolize vitamin D.

Bisphosphonates

Several bisphosphonate compounds are used today to treat disorders of calcium metabolism and bone. These compounds include **alendronate, pamidronate,** and **tiludronate.** The original bisphospho-

TABLE 36–1. Calcium Intake Recommended by the National Institutes of Health Consensus Panel

Age Group	Daily Calcium Intake (mg)
Infants	
0–6 months	400
7–12 months	600
Children	
1–5 years	800
6–10 years	800–1200
Adolescents and young adults	
11–24 years	1200–1500
Men	
25–65 years	1000
>65 years	1500
Women	
25–50 years	1000
>50 years (postmenopausal)	
Taking estrogens	1000
Not taking estrogens	1500
>65 years	1500
Pregnant and nursing	1200–1500

nate, **etidronate,** is no longer used extensively, because it is a less potent inhibitor of bone resorption than these newer compounds and because its long-term administration has been associated with the development of osteomalacia.

Drug Properties

Chemistry. Bisphosphonate drugs are organic pyrophosphate compounds in which the P–O–P group is replaced with a nonhydrolyzable P–C–P moiety (Fig. 36–3).

Pharmacokinetics. Pamidronate is usually given intravenously, whereas alendronate and tiludronate are administered orally. Less than 5% of the oral drug is absorbed when taken on an empty stomach, and absorption is further reduced by food, certain drugs, and liquids other than water. Hence, patients should be advised to take alendronate or tiludronate with a full glass of water 30 minutes before ingesting anything else in the morning. Once absorbed, about half of the drug is deposited in bone, and the remainder is excreted in the urine.

The bisphosphonates adsorb to hydroxyapatite and become a permanent part of the bone structure. They are slowly released from bone during bone remodeling, and their half-life in bone is estimated to be 1–10 years.

Mechanisms and Pharmacologic Effects. Bisphosphonates prevent bone resorption by inhibiting osteoclast activity through a variety of mechanisms. The most important mechanism appears to be prevention of the attachment of osteoclast precursor cells to bone. Bisphosphonates also decrease the metabolic activity of osteoclasts and their ability to resorb bone. There is experimental evidence that tiludronate inhibits tyrosine phosphatase activity in osteoclasts and thereby causes their de-

tachment from bone surfaces. It may also inhibit the proton pump through which osteoclasts secrete hydrogen ions that participate in bone resorption.

Indications. Bisphosphonate compounds are used in the management of a variety of disorders, including **osteoporosis, Paget's disease of bone, hypercalcemia,** and **osteolytic bone lesions of metastatic cancer.** As discussed below, the various compounds have different uses.

Adverse Effects. Orally administered bisphosphonates can cause esophageal erosion, but this can be prevented by advising the patient to remain upright after swallowing these drugs. The bisphosphonate compounds produce varying degrees of gastrointestinal distress. Pamidronate causes more gastric irritation than other bisphosphonates and is not available in an oral formulation at this time. Alendronate seldom causes gastric distress except when high doses are used to treat Paget's disease. Occasionally, alendronate causes mild and transient nausea, dyspepsia, constipation, or diarrhea. Unlike etidronate, alendronate does not cause osteomalacia during long-term use.

Interactions. The bisphosphonates have few interactions with other drugs. Calcium supplements and antacids decrease the bioavailability of alendronate and tiludronate and should be taken at least 2 hours before or after the bisphosphonate compound is taken.

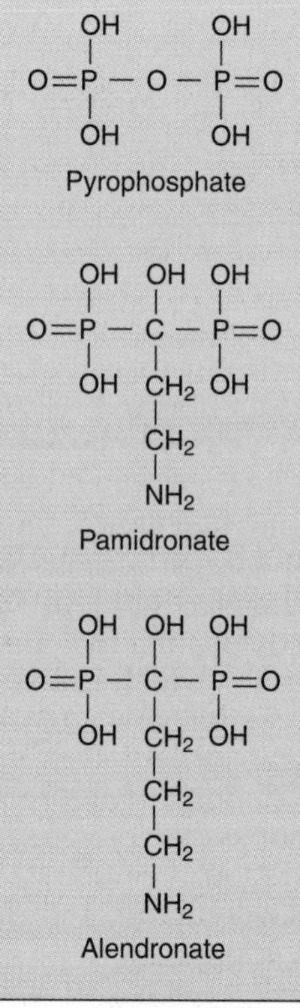

FIGURE 36–3. Structures of selected bisphosphonates. Pamidronate and alendronate are analogues of pyrophosphate.

Specific Drugs

Alendronate is the first bisphosphonate to be approved for the treatment of osteoporosis, and it appears to be effective in all forms of this disorder, including glucocorticoid-induced osteoporosis. Clinical trials in women with postmenopausal osteoporosis indicate that alendronate prevents bone loss and is more effective than calcium supplements or calcitonin therapy in producing a sustained increase in bone mass. A study of women with low bone mass and preexisting vertebral fractures has shown that alendronate treatment resulted in a 47% reduction in the risk of new vertebral fractures over a 3-year period.

Alendronate, pamidronate, and tiludronate are all approved for the treatment of Paget's disease. Before treatment, imaging and laboratory studies usually show evidence of increased bone turnover (remodeling), bone hypertrophy, and abnormal bone structure. By inhibiting abnormal osteoclast activity in patients with this disease, the bisphosphonates help to normalize biochemical indices of bone remodeling and restore normal bone structure. Patients who are symptomatic or who require orthopedic surgery are candidates for bisphosphonate therapy. Treatment should be initiated as early as possible to halt disease progression. Tiludronate given once daily is usually effective in 3 months, whereas other bisphosphonate compounds may require 6 months to be effective. If a relapse occurs, another course of treatment can be given after a 6-month interval.

In patients with cancer, bisphosphonates have been found to be useful in the management of hypercalcemia and metastatic bone disease. Intravenous administration of a bisphosphonate such as pamidronate is the most effective treatment for hypercalcemia associated with cancer. Bisphosphonate treatment has been found to inhibit bone resorption, reduce the tumor burden in bone, decrease bone pain, and reduce the risk of fractures in patients whose cancer has metastasized to the bone. For example, pamidronate was shown to significantly reduce the incidence and prolong the median time to skeletal complications in women who had stage IV breast cancer with bone metastases. In addition, monthly pamidronate infusions were found to significantly decrease the incidence of osteolytic bone lesions in women with metastatic breast cancer. In men, pamidronate was found to inhibit the adhesion of prostate carcinoma cells to bone, and this suggests a potential prophylactic role for bisphosphonate drugs in patients who have other forms of cancer that are known to preferentially metastasize to the bone.

Other Agents for Calcium and Bone Disorders
Estrogen and Raloxifene

Estrogen is considered a first-line therapy for the prevention of **osteoporosis** in postmenopausal women. Raloxifene, a selective estrogen receptor modulator, can also be used for this purpose. Estrogen preparations and raloxifene are discussed in Chapter 34.

Estrogen reduces bone resorption by regulating various bone cell cytokines. Estrogen inhibits the production of interleukin-1, tumor necrosis factor, and granulocyte-macrophage colony-stimulating factor by peripheral blood monocytes, and it also inhibits the secretion of interleukin-6 and colony-stimulating factors by osteoblasts. These actions lead to a decrease in osteoclast differentiation and activation, which in turn slows the bone loss that occurs in postmenopausal women.

Calcitonin

Chemistry and Pharmacokinetics. Calcitonin is a peptide hormone secreted by the parafollicular cells of the thyroid gland. It is not reliably absorbed from the gut and must be administered parenterally or by nasal inhalation. **Salmon calcitonin** has been available for a number of years, and **recombinant human calcitonin** is also available. Salmon calcitonin is 50–100 times more potent than human calcitonin.

Mechanisms and Effects. Calcitonin binds directly to receptors on osteoclasts and increases cyclic adenosine monophosphate (cAMP) levels. When given on a short-term basis, calcitonin inhibits osteoclast activity, decreases bone resorption, lowers serum calcium concentrations, and reduces bone pain. When given on a long-term basis, calcitonin also reduces the number of osteoclasts and decreases bone formation. The long-term effects of calcitonin on bone mass are uncertain.

Indications. Because of its ability to inhibit osteoclast activity and decrease bone turnover, calcitonin is used in the treatment of **osteoporosis, Paget's disease of bone,** and **hypercalcemia.**

In patients with osteoporosis, calcitonin treatment has been shown to increase bone mass at multiple sites in the body during a period of up to 2 years, but there is some uncertainty about whether these changes are maintained over longer periods of time. Calcitonin treatment is usually reserved for women who cannot take estrogen and have been in menopause for over 5 years. In these women, studies indicate that calcitonin increases the bone mineral density (BMD) in the spine but has variable effects on the BMD in the hips. Patients with osteoporosis can be treated with either subcutaneous or intranasal calcitonin. In those who have had fractures, treatment in the immediate postfracture period appears to be particularly useful because of the drug's analgesic effect. Patients taking calcitonin should be advised of the importance of adequate calcium and vitamin D intake.

In patients with Paget's disease, calcitonin is administered subcutaneously or intramuscularly every 1–3 days. The nasal spray is not used. When treatment inhibits osteoclast activity and slows the rate of bone turnover, this causes reductions in markers of abnormal bone turnover, such as serum alkaline phosphatase activity and urine hydroxyproline levels. Alleviation of bone pain usually occurs 2–8 weeks after calcitonin therapy has begun.

Hypercalcemia can be treated with subcutaneous or intramuscular injections of calcitonin. The injections are administered every 12 hours until a satisfactory response occurs.

Fluoride

In some countries, fluoride is approved for the treatment of osteoporosis. In the USA, a sodium fluoride preparation is available but is approved only for the prevention of tooth decay. Fluoride is of considerable interest as a therapeutic agent for osteoporosis because it is capable of stimulating new bone formation. All other substances currently used in the treatment of osteoporosis act by inhibiting bone resorption. Fig. 36–4 compares the effects that fluoride and other treatments have on BMD measurements over time.

Mechanisms and Pharmacologic Effects. Fluoride is rapidly and almost completely absorbed from the gut, and it is primarily stored in bone and teeth. Fluoride replaces the hydroxyl group in the calcium phosphate salts (hydroxyapatite) of bone and teeth and thereby forms fluorapatite. Fluoride increases bone crystal size and decreases solubility so as to render bone more resistant to resorption. At the same time, fluoride prolongs the bone remodeling cycle by increasing the amount of time between new bone formation and subsequent mineralization. In this way, fluoride increases the BMD and may markedly increase bone mass.

Indications and Pharmacokinetics. Fluoride is used for the prevention of **dental caries,** a condition in which localized destruction of calcified tissue on the tooth surface is followed by enzymatic lysis of organic material and by the subsequent development of cavities. Minerals deposited on the tooth surface as fluorapatite are more resistant to erosion than is hydroxyapatite.

Fluoride has been added to the drinking water supply in many localities as a method of caries prevention. It can also be administered orally as a liquid or chewable tablet, and it can be applied directly to the tooth surface as a dental gel or rinse. The oral liquid formulation is usually employed (in drops) to provide fluoride to infants and young children.

A sustained-release fluoride preparation is currently being evaluated by the Food and Drug Administration for the treatment of **osteoporosis.** Monofluorophosphate products are also under development. The latter compounds can be administered with calcium, and they may cause fewer adverse effects than other fluoride preparations.

Adverse Effects. Sodium fluoride may cause considerable gastrointestinal distress, including nausea, vomiting, and bleeding. Skin rashes and arthralgia are also fairly common. These side effects can usually be prevented by using a lower dose or a sustained-release formulation and by taking the drug with food.

Excessive doses of fluoride can cause osteosclerosis (excessive hardness of bone) and mottling of tooth enamel.

Fluoride increases trabecular bone volume, but it may either decrease or have no effect on cortical bone volume. The use of lower doses and sustained-release fluoride products, along with the ingestion of sufficient calcium and vitamin D, may prevent the negative effect on cortical bone.

The type of bone formed in the presence of fluoride is more resistant to compressive forces but less resistant to torsional strain. Compressive strain tends to cause vertebral fractures, whereas torsional strain causes hip fractures. These factors probably explain why fluoride reduces vertebral fractures but may increase fractures at other sites. Intermittent fluoride regimens with a 2-month drug-free interval may decrease some of the problems associated with continuous fluoride therapy.

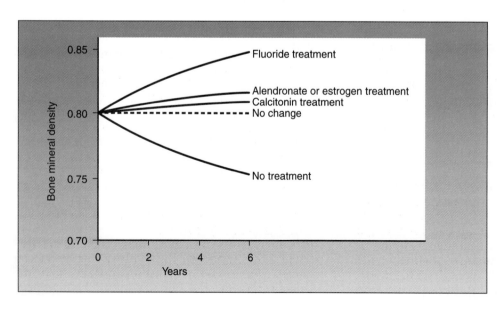

FIGURE 36–4. Effects of different treatments on bone mineral density (BMD) in postmenopausal women. In the absence of treatment, BMD steadily declines and may eventually reach the fracture threshold (0.70). Treatment with alendronate (a bisphosphonate), calcitonin, or estrogen may reduce bone resorption and increase BMD slightly. Fluoride increases bone formation and produces a greater and more sustained increase in BMD.

Interactions. Fluoride forms a complex with calcium and magnesium and thereby reduces the absorption of these cations. Hence, calcium and magnesium supplements or antacids should not be taken at the same time as fluoride. However, adequate calcium and vitamin D intake is essential in persons taking fluoride, because studies have shown that the use of fluoride without calcium supplementation may lead to osteomalacia.

Plicamycin

Plicamycin is a cytotoxic antibiotic that is a potent osteoclast inhibitor and may block the action of PTH. Plicamycin inhibits bone resorption and is used to treat **hypercalcemia** and **hypercalciuria** that are caused by malignant tumors and are not responsive to conventional therapy. It is also used to treat **Paget's disease of bone.**

Plicamycin is administered by intravenous infusion and causes numerous adverse effects, including myelosuppression, coagulation disorders, and frequent nausea and vomiting.

THE MANAGEMENT OF CALCIUM AND BONE DISORDERS
Osteoporosis

The prevention of osteoporosis rests on a foundation of life-long calcium and vitamin D intake in an amount that is sufficient to maximize bone formation during development and to sustain bone mass during adulthood. Weight-bearing exercise reduces bone loss and helps improve strength and balance. Endogenous estrogen in women and testosterone in men also reduce bone resorption. After menopause, the absence of estrogen accelerates bone loss in women. While all postmenopausal women are at risk of developing osteoporosis, BMD measurements are being increasingly used to identify those who are at greatest risk.

In most postmenopausal women, osteoporosis can be prevented by ensuring an adequate intake of calcium and vitamin D, exercising, and taking either estrogen replacement therapy or raloxifene. Other agents may be employed in women who exhibit decreased or accelerated BMD measurements, women who have had fractures or other signs of osteoporosis, and women who are at an increased risk of developing osteoporosis because they require chronic corticosteroid therapy or because they underwent natural or surgical menopause at an early age. In these groups of women, alendronate can be used in place of or in addition to estrogen. Alendronate is a particularly attractive drug because it can be taken orally, is efficacious, and has a low incidence of adverse effects. Moreover, clinical trials comparing alendronate and calcitonin showed that only alendronate produced a sustained increase in bone mass in postmenopausal women with evidence of osteoporosis. The introduction of new fluoride preparations is anticipated and may provide another therapeutic modality for the prevention and treatment of osteoporosis.

Paget's Disease of Bone

The goals of treating patients with Paget's disease are to control bone pain and to prevent progressive bone deformity and other manifestations of the disease. Calcitonin is usually the first-line treatment, and it can be given alone or in combination with a bisphosphonate such as alendronate, pamidronate, or tiludronate. Alternatively, a bisphosphonate can be used alone. Plicamycin is reserved for the treatment of patients who fail to respond to other drugs.

Hypercalcemia

The treatment of hypercalcemia depends on the etiology and severity of the condition. The major causes of hypercalcemia are hyperparathyroidism and cancer.

Saline diuresis is usually the preferred method of managing hypercalcemia that is severe enough to cause symptoms. A saline infusion is used for this purpose and serves to increase renal calcium excretion and to counteract the dehydration that often accompanies hypercalcemia. A loop diuretic such as furosemide can be added to the saline infusion, and this will further enhance calcium excretion.

Pamidronate and other bisphosphonates are useful in the treatment of hypercalcemia associated with cancer. Calcitonin is usually employed to supplement other treatments for hypercalcemia, and plicamycin is useful if other therapeutic agents and procedures fail. As a last resort, intravenous phosphate infusions can be used to control hypercalcemia, but these infusions place the patient at considerable risk for acute hypocalcemia, hypotension, renal failure, and tissue calcification.

Summary of Important Points

- The extracellular calcium concentration is regulated by vitamin D, parathyroid hormone (PTH), and calcitonin. Vitamin D increases calcium absorption from the gut; PTH increases calcium reabsorption from renal tubules and increases bone resorption; and calcitonin decreases bone resorption.
- Vitamin D is converted to its most active form, 1,25-dihydroxyvitamin D_3 (calcitriol), by hydroxylation in the liver and kidneys. This active form must be supplied to patients with renal impairment. Dietary vitamin D is essential for prevention of rickets in children.
- Osteoporosis is the most common bone disorder and is characterized by a gradual loss of bone mass that leads to skeletal weakness and increased fractures.

- In most postmenopausal women, osteoporosis can be prevented by ensuring an adequate intake of calcium and vitamin D, exercising, and taking either estrogen replacement therapy or raloxifene.
- Osteoporosis can be treated with alendronate (a bisphosphonate), calcitonin, or fluoride (not yet approved for this indication in the USA). Alendronate reduces osteoclast activity and can increase bone mass and reduce fractures in postmenopausal women. It is taken orally and is effective and well tolerated.
- In addition to alendronate, the bisphosphonate compounds include pamidronate and tiludronate. These agents are used to treat Paget's disease of bone, hypercalcemia, and osteolytic bone lesions associated with cancer.
- Calcitonin is also used to treat Paget's disease and hypercalcemia.

Selected Readings

Boissier, S., et al. Bisphosphonates inhibit prostate and breast carcinoma cell adhesion to unmineralized and mineralized bone extracellular matrices. Cancer Res 57:3890–3894, 1997.

Castelo-Branco, C. Management of osteoporosis: an overview. Drugs Aging 12(supplement 1):25–32, 1998.

Chesnut, C. H. Tiludronate: development as an osteoporosis therapy. Bone 17:517S–519S, 1995.

Coukell, A. J., and A. Markham. Pamidronate: a review of its use in the management of osteolytic bone metastases, tumor-induced hypercalcemia, and Paget's disease of bone. Drugs Aging 12:149–168, 1998.

Delmas, P. D. Bisphosphonates in the treatment of bone diseases. N Engl J Med 335:1836–1837, 1996.

Jeal, W., et al. Alendronate: a review of its pharmacologic properties and therapeutic efficacy in postmenopausal osteoporosis. Drugs 53:415–434, 1997.

Lipton, A. Bisphosphonates and breast carcinoma. Cancer 80: 1668–1673, 1997.

Meunier, P. J., and E. Vignot. Therapeutic strategy in Paget's disease of bone. Bone 17:489S–491S, 1995.

SECTION VII

CHEMOTHERAPY

CHAPTER THIRTY-SEVEN

PRINCIPLES OF ANTIMICROBIAL

CHEMOTHERAPY

ANTIBIOTICS AND CHEMOTHERAPY

Overview

Chemotherapy can be defined as the use of drugs to eradicate pathogenic organisms or neoplastic cells in the treatment of infectious diseases or cancer. Chemotherapy is based on the principle of **selective toxicity.** According to this principle, chemotherapeutic drugs inhibit functions in invading organisms or neoplastic cells that differ qualitatively or quantitatively from functions in normal host cells. The chemotherapeutic drugs include antimicrobial drugs (introduced in this chapter and discussed further in Chapters 38–43), antiparasitic drugs (discussed in Chapter 44), and antineoplastic drugs (discussed in Chapter 45).

The **antimicrobial drugs** can be subclassified as **antibacterial, antifungal, and antiviral agents.** These agents include natural compounds, called antibiotics, as well as synthetic compounds produced in laboratories. An **antibiotic** is a substance that is produced by one microbe and inhibits the growth or viability of other microbes. The earliest use of antibiotics was probably in the treatment of skin infections with **moldy bean curd** by the ancient Chinese. The development of modern antibiotics can be traced to the work of **Louis Pasteur,** who observed that the in vitro growth of one microbe was inhibited when another microbe was added to the culture. Pasteur called this phenomenon **antibiosis** and predicted that substances derived from microbes would someday be used to treat infectious diseases.

Several decades later, **Alexander Fleming** observed that the growth of his staphylococcal cultures was inhibited by a *Penicillium* contaminant. Fleming postulated that the fungus produced a substance which he called **penicillin** and that this substance inhibited the growth of staphylococci. His observations eventually led to the isolation and use of penicillin for treating bacterial infections. The discovery of penicillin stimulated the discovery and development of a large number of other antibiotics, the use of which has revolutionized the treatment of infectious diseases.

Synthetic drugs have also provided major advances in the treatment of infectious diseases and cancer. During the Renaissance, **Paracelsus** used

mercury compounds for the treatment of syphilis. In the late 19th and early 20th centuries, **Paul Ehrlich** pioneered the search for selectively toxic compounds. After many failed attempts, he discovered **arsphenamine (salvarsan),** an arsenical compound for the treatment of syphilis. Ehrlich, who became known as the father of chemotherapy, also studied bacterial stains as potential antimicrobial agents. He reasoned that a stain's selective affinity for bacteria could be coupled with an inhibitory action to halt microbial metabolism and thereby destroy invading organisms. This concept led to the discovery of **sulfonamides,** drugs that were originally derived from a bacterial stain called **Prontosil.** The sulfonamides were the first effective drugs for the treatment of systemic bacterial infections, and their development accelerated the search for other antimicrobial agents.

Classification of Antimicrobial Drugs

Antimicrobial drugs are usually classified on the basis of their site and mechanism of action and are subclassified on the basis of their chemical structure. The antimicrobial drugs include **cell wall synthesis inhibitors, protein synthesis inhibitors, metabolic and nucleic acid inhibitors,** and **cell membrane inhibitors.** The sites of action of these drugs are depicted in Fig. 37–1, and their mechanisms of action, pharmacologic properties, and clinical uses are described in subsequent chapters.

ANTIMICROBIAL ACTIVITY

The antimicrobial activity of a drug can be characterized in terms of its bactericidal or bacteriostatic effect, its spectrum of activity against important groups of pathogens, and its concentration- and time-dependent effects on sensitive organisms.

Bactericidal or Bacteriostatic Effect

A **bactericidal drug** kills sensitive organisms so that the number of viable organisms falls rapidly after exposure to the drug (Fig. 37–2). In contrast, a **bacteriostatic drug** inhibits the growth of bacteria but does not kill them. For this reason, the number of

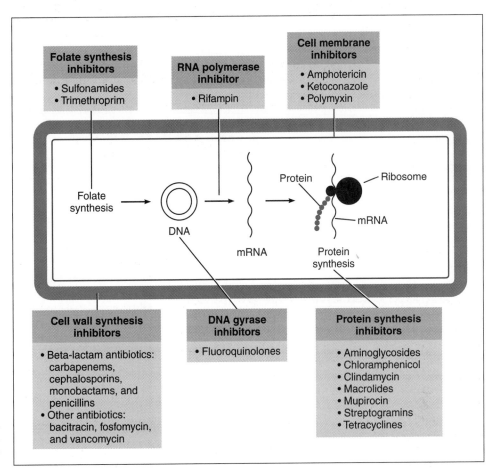

FIGURE 37–1. Sites of action of antimicrobial drugs. Antimicrobial drugs include cell wall synthesis inhibitors, protein synthesis inhibitors, metabolic and nucleic acid inhibitors (such as inhibitors of folate synthesis, DNA gyrase, and RNA polymerase), and cell membrane inhibitors.

bacteria remains relatively constant in the presence of a bacteriostatic drug, and immunologic mechanisms are required to eliminate organisms during treatment of an infection with this type of drug. (The same principle applies to a drug that kills or inhibits the growth of fungi and is referred to as a **fungicidal drug** or a **fungistatic drug,** respectively.)

A bactericidal drug is usually preferable to a bacteriostatic drug for the treatment of most bacterial infections. This is because bactericidal drugs

FIGURE 37–2. In vitro effects of bactericidal and bacteriostatic drugs. In the absence of an antimicrobial drug, bacteria exhibit logarithmic growth in a broth culture. The addition of a bacteriostatic drug (tetracycline) inhibits further growth but does not reduce the number of bacteria. The addition of a bactericidal drug (penicillin) reduces the number of viable bacteria.

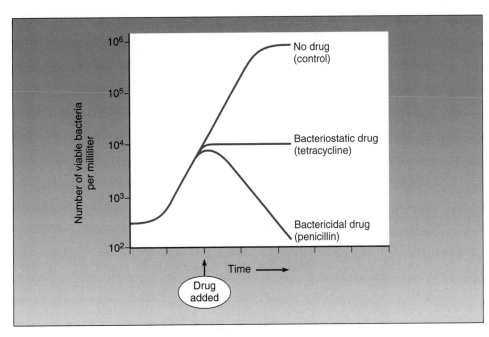

usually produce more rapid microbiologic response and clinical improvement and are less likely to elicit microbial resistance. Bactericidal drugs have actions that induce lethal changes in microbial metabolism or block activities that are essential for microbial viability. For example, drugs that inhibit the synthesis of the bacterial cell wall, such as **penicillins,** prevent the formation of a structure that is required for the survival of bacteria. At the same time, penicillins activate autolytic enzymes that destroy bacteria. In contrast to bactericidal drugs, bacteriostatic drugs usually inhibit a metabolic reaction that is needed for bacterial growth but is not necessary for cell viability. For example, **sulfonamides** block the synthesis of folic acid, which is a cofactor for enzymes that synthesize DNA components and amino acids. A reduction in folic acid synthesis may prevent bacterial growth, but it does not kill bacteria.

Drugs that reversibly inhibit bacterial protein synthesis, such as **tetracyclines,** are also bacteriostatic, whereas drugs that irreversibly inhibit protein synthesis, such as **streptomycin,** are usually bactericidal.

Some drugs may be either bactericidal or bacteriostatic, depending on their concentration and the bacterial species against which they are used.

Antimicrobial Spectrum

The spectrum of antimicrobial activity of a drug is the primary determinant of its clinical use. Antimicrobial agents that are active against a single species or a limited group of pathogens, such as gram-positive bacteria, are called **narrow-spectrum drugs,** whereas agents that are active against a wide range of pathogens are called **broad-spectrum drugs.** Agents that have an intermediate range of activity are sometimes called **extended-spectrum drugs.**

If the specific pathogen that is responsible for an infection is known, use of a narrow-spectrum drug is the logical choice for treatment of the infection. This is because a broad-spectrum drug is more likely to cause superinfection by eradicating organisms that make up the normal flora of the gut or respiratory tract. However, in cases in which an infection is serious and the responsible pathogen is not yet known, a broad-spectrum bactericidal drug, such as imipenem, is often used for initial treatment.

Concentration- and Time-Dependent Effects

Antimicrobial drugs exhibit various concentration- and time-dependent effects that influence their clinical efficacy, dosage, and frequency of administration. Examples of these effects are the **minimum inhibitory concentration** (MIC), the **concentration-dependent killing rate** (CDKR), and the **postantibiotic effect** (PAE).

The MIC is the lowest concentration of a drug that inhibits bacterial growth. Based on the MIC, a particular strain of bacteria can be classified as susceptible or resistant to a particular drug (see below).

An example of a CDKR is shown in Fig. 37–3A. Some **aminoglycosides** (such as tobramycin) and some **fluoroquinolones** (such as ciprofloxacin) exhibit a CDKR against a large group of gram-negative bacteria, including *Pseudomonas aeruginosa* and members of the family Enterobacteriaceae. In contrast, **penicillins and other beta-lactam antibiotics** usually do not exhibit a CDKR.

After an antibacterial drug is removed from a bacterial culture, there may be evidence of a persis-

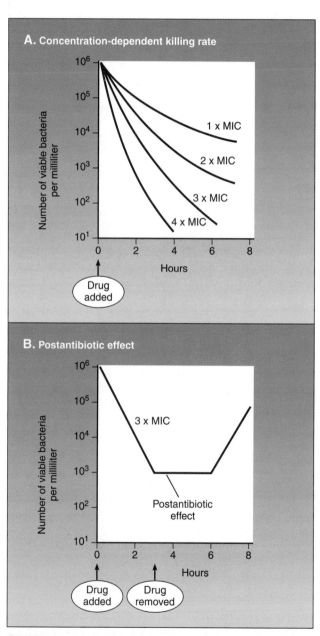

FIGURE 37–3. Concentration- and time-dependent effects of antimicrobial drugs. (A) When an aminoglycoside, such as tobramycin, is added to a culture of a gram-negative bacterium, such as *Escherichia coli*, it will exhibit a concentration-dependent killing rate. In this example, 10^6 bacteria were incubated with different concentrations of tobramycin, ranging from 1 to 4 times the minimum inhibitory concentration (MIC). **(B)** When tobramycin is removed from the culture, bacterial growth continues to be inhibited for several hours.

tent effect on bacterial growth. This effect (see Fig. 37–3B) is called the PAE. Most bactericidal antibiotics exhibit a PAE against susceptible pathogens. For example, penicillins show a PAE against gram-positive cocci, and aminoglycosides show a PAE against gram-negative bacilli. While a PAE is usually cited as a desirable characteristic of antimicrobial drugs, its clinical relevance is uncertain. Because aminoglycosides exhibit both a CDKR and a PAE, treatment regimens have been developed in which the entire daily dose of an aminoglycoside is given at one time. Theoretically, the high rate of bacterial killing produced by these regimens would more rapidly eliminate bacteria, and the PAE would prevent any remaining bacteria from replicating for several hours after the drug has been eliminated from the body.

MICROBIAL SENSITIVITY AND RESISTANCE

Laboratory Tests for Microbial Sensitivity

Microbial sensitivity to drugs can be determined by various means, including the **broth dilution test,** the **disk diffusion method (Kirby-Bauer test),** and the **Etest method.**

Either the broth dilution test or the Etest method can be used to determine the MIC of a drug, which is the lowest drug concentration that prevents visible growth of bacteria. On the basis of the MIC, the organism is classified as having **susceptibility, intermediate sensitivity,** or **resistance** to the drug tested. These categories are based on the relationship between the MIC and the peak serum concentration of the drug after administration of typical doses. In general, the peak serum concentration of a drug should be 2–4 times greater than the MIC in order for a pathogen to be susceptible to a drug (see below). Pathogens with intermediate sensitivity may respond to treatment with maximum doses of an antimicrobial drug.

The disk diffusion method is a less time-consuming and more convenient method of determining microbial susceptibility, intermediate sensitivity, or resistance to drugs.

The three laboratory procedures are described in Box 37–1. The results of these procedures enable the clinician to select the most effective drug for treating a particular infection and thereby improve the patient's outcome and prevent the development of microbial resistance.

Microbial Resistance to Drugs

Patterns of Resistance

Resistance may be innate or acquired. Acquired drug resistance arises from mutation and selection or from the transfer of plasmids that confer drug resistance.

Mutation and Selection. Microbes may spontaneously mutate to a form that is resistant to a particular antimicrobial drug. These mutations occur at a relatively constant rate, such as 1 in 10^{12} organisms per unit of time. If the organisms are exposed to an antimicrobial drug during this time period, the sensitive organisms may be eradicated, enabling the resistant mutant to multiply and become the dominant strain (Fig. 37–4A).

The probability that mutation and selection of a resistant mutant will occur is increased during the exposure of an organism to suboptimal concentrations of an antibiotic, and it is also increased during prolonged exposure to an antibiotic. This observation has obvious implications for antimicrobial therapy. Laboratory tests should be used to guide the selection of an antimicrobial drug, and the dosage and duration of therapy should be appropriate for the type of infection being treated. Whenever possible, the bacteriologic response to drug therapy should be verified by culturing samples of appropriate body fluids.

Transferable Resistance. Transferable resistance usually results from bacterial conjugation and the transfer of plasmids (extrachromosomal DNA) that confer drug resistance (see Fig. 37–4B). However, transferable resistance may also be mediated by transformation (uptake of naked DNA) or transduction (transfer of bacterial DNA by a bacteriophage). Bacterial conjugation enables a bacterium to donate a plasmid containing genes that encode proteins responsible for resistance to an antibiotic. These genes are called **resistance factors (R factors).** The R factors can be transferred not only within a particular species but also between different species, so they often confer **multidrug resistance.** The various species need not all be present during the period in which the antibiotic is administered. Studies have shown that resident microflora of the human body can serve as reservoirs for resistance genes, allowing the transfer of these genes to organisms that later invade and colonize the host.

Several genes responsible for drug resistance have been cloned, and the factors that control their expression are being studied. In the future, drugs that block the expression of these genes may find use as adjunct therapy for infectious diseases. For example, it may be possible to develop antisense nucleotides that block the transcription or translation of genes that encode proteins responsible for drug resistance.

Mechanisms of Resistance

The three primary mechanisms of microbial resistance to an antibiotic are (1) inactivation of the drug by microbial enzymes, (2) decreased accumulation of the drug by the microbe, and (3) reduced affinity of the target macromolecule for the drug. Examples of drugs affected by these mechanisms are provided in Table 37–1.

Inactivation of the drug by enzymes is an important mechanism of resistance to beta-lactam antibiotics, including the penicillins. This form of resistance results from bacterial elaboration of beta-lactamase enzymes that destroy the beta-lactam ring. Resistance to aminoglycosides, such as gentamicin, is partly due to the elaboration of drug-inactivating enzymes that acetylate, adenylate, or phosphorylate these antibiotics.

Decreased accumulation of an antibiotic may result from **increased efflux** or **decreased uptake** of the drug. Both of these mechanisms contribute to the resistance of microbes to tetracyclines and fluoroquinolones. Increased drug efflux is often mediated by membrane proteins that transport antimicrobial drugs out of bacterial cells. Some of these transport proteins are similar to or indistinguishable from human **P-glycoprotein,** a glycoprotein that transports antineoplastic drugs out of human cancer cells and thereby confers resistance to the drugs (see Chapter 45). Compounds that inhibit these transport proteins are being investigated as potential therapeu-

---

BOX 37–1.   Laboratory Determination of Microbial Sensitivity to Antibiotics

Microbial sensitivity to drugs can be determined by various means, including the broth dilution test, the disk diffusion method, and the Etest method.

Broth Dilution Test

Tubes that contain a nutrient broth are inoculated with equal numbers of bacteria and serially diluted concentrations of an antibiotic. After incubation, the minimum inhibitory concentration (MIC) is identified as the lowest antibiotic concentration that prevents visible growth of bacteria. On the basis of the MIC, the organism is classified as having susceptibility, intermediate sensitivity, or resistance to the drug tested. In the following example, the MIC is 1 µg/mL, and the organism is susceptible to the drug.

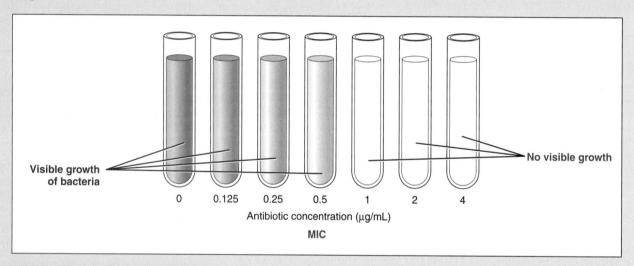

Disk Diffusion Method (Kirby-Bauer Test)

Each disk used in the disk diffusion method is impregnated with a different antibiotic. The disks are placed on agar plates seeded with the test organism. During the incubation period, the antibiotic diffuses from the disk and inhibits bacterial growth. After incubation, the zone inhibited by each antibiotic is measured. The zone diameter for each antibiotic is compared with standard values for that particular antibiotic. The organism is thereby determined to be susceptible, intermediate, or resistant to the various antibiotics tested.

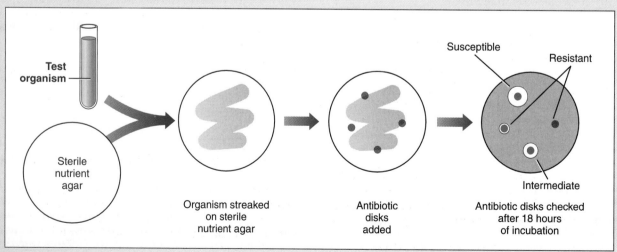

Continued

Etest Method

The Etest strip is a proprietary device that uses a diffusion method to determine the MIC of an organism. The device is a plastic strip that is impregnated with a gradient of antibiotic concentrations. After the strip is placed on an agar culture of the organism, the culture is incubated. During incubation, a tear-shaped zone of inhibition is formed. The point of intersection between the zone of inhibition and the scale displayed on the strip is the MIC. In the following example, the MIC is 0.125 µg/mL.

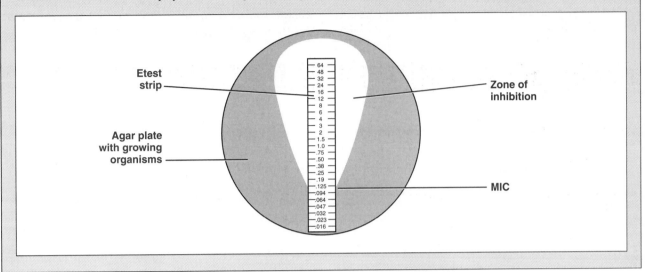

tic agents to reduce drug resistance. Decreased uptake of antimicrobial drugs may result from altered bacterial **porins.** Porins are membrane proteins containing channels through which drugs and other compounds enter bacteria. Resistance to penicillins by gram-negative bacilli is partly due to altered porin channels that do not permit penicillin entry.

Reduced affinity of target macromolecules for antimicrobial drugs is a common mechanism of drug resistance. It is partly responsible for resistance to cell wall synthesis inhibitors, protein synthesis inhibitors, DNA gyrase inhibitors, and RNA polymerase inhibitors (see Table 37–1). This type of drug resistance is often due to bacterial mutation followed by the selection of resistant mutants during exposure to an antimicrobial drug. Altered target affinity has been the most difficult form of drug resistance to counteract by pharmacologic agents.

SELECTION OF ANTIMICROBIAL DRUGS

The selection of an antimicrobial agent for the treatment of a particular infection is based on consideration of the type of infection, the status of the patient, and the pharmacologic properties of the available drugs.

Host Factors

Host factors that influence the choice of a drug include pregnancy, drug allergies, age and immune status, and the presence of renal impairment, hepatic insufficiency, abscesses, or indwelling catheters and similar devices.

Most antimicrobial drugs cross the placenta and may thereby affect the fetus. For example, administering tetracyclines to a woman during **pregnancy** may cause permanent staining of her offspring's teeth. However, penicillins and cephalosporins cause very little fetal toxicity and may be safely administered to pregnant women who are not allergic to these drugs.

Many individuals are allergic to one or more antimicrobial drugs, so clinicians should always ask patients if they have **drug allergies** before prescribing or administering drugs. Penicillins are the most common cause of drug allergy. Penicillin allergy and its detection and management are discussed in Chapter 38.

The patient's **immune status** is an important factor determining the success of antimicrobial therapy, because the immune system is ultimately responsible for eliminating the invading organisms. **Advanced age, diabetes, cancer chemotherapy,** and **human immunodeficiency virus (HIV) infection** are among the more common causes of impaired immunity. Immunocompromised individuals should be treated with larger doses of bactericidal drugs and may require a longer duration of therapy than do immunocompetent individuals.

Antibiotic access to **abscesses** is poor, so the concentration of an antibiotic in an abscess is usually lower than normal. Moreover, immune responses to abscesses are impaired. For these reasons, abscesses must be surgically drained before they can be cured.

Foreign bodies, such as **indwelling catheters,** provide sites where microbes may become covered with a glycocalyx coating that protects them from antibiotics and immunologic destruction.

Many antibiotics are excreted unchanged by the kidneys, and lower doses must be used if the patient has significant **renal impairment.** Less commonly,

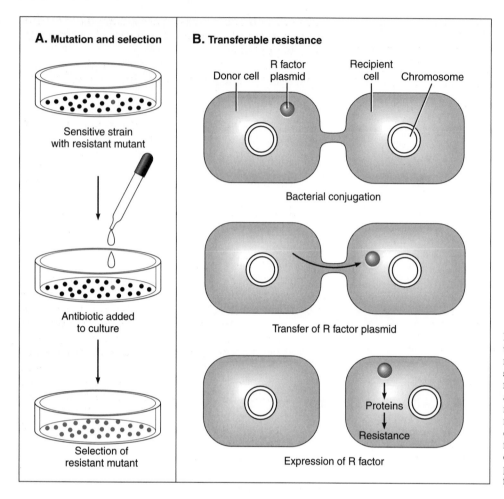

A. Mutation and selection

Sensitive strain
with resistant mutant

Antibiotic added
to culture

Selection of
resistant mutant

B. Transferable resistance

Donor cell

R factor
plasmid

Recipient
cell

Chromosome

Bacterial conjugation

Transfer of R factor plasmid

Proteins

Resistance

Expression of R factor

FIGURE 37–4. Acquired resistance to antimicrobial drugs may arise by mutation and selection or by transferable resistance. **(A)** Exposure of an organism to an antibiotic may result in the selection of a resistant mutant. **(B)** The most common mechanism of transferable resistance is bacterial conjugation and exchange of plasmids containing resistance factors (R factors).

hepatic insufficiency may require dosage adjustment for antimicrobial drugs that are extensively metabolized in the liver. For example, neonates cannot metabolize chloramphenicol, so their dosage of this drug per kilogram of body weight must be lower than the dosage given to older children or adults. Tables showing appropriate drug dosages for individuals with different degrees of renal insufficiency, as indicated by the creatinine clearance or creatine levels, can be found in prescribing compendiums and clinical pharmacology references.

Drug Characteristics

An ideal antimicrobial drug would be bactericidal to the causative pathogen, distributed to the site of infection in adequate concentrations, devoid of serious adverse effects, and convenient and inexpensive.

Antimicrobial Activity

Antimicrobial agents may be selected on the basis of laboratory test results (described above) or knowledge of the most common organisms causing various types of infections and the drugs of choice for these organisms (empiric considerations). Empiric therapy is often used for the initial treatment of

serious infections until test results are available. Empiric therapy is also used for the treatment of minor upper respiratory tract infections and urinary tract infections because of the predictability of causative organisms and their sensitivity to drugs. In these situations, the cost of microbial culture and drug sensitivity testing is not usually justified.

The current drugs of choice for the treatment of infections caused by specific bacterial pathogens are listed in Table 37–2. Additional tables listing drugs of choice for various types of infection can be found in medical texts and at numerous sites on the Internet (see, for example, the site for Medical College of Wisconsin/Froedtert Memorial Lutheran Hospital).

Pharmacokinetic Properties

The pharmacokinetic parameters of antibiotics that influence their selection for a particular use include their oral bioavailability, peak serum concentration, distribution to particular sites of infection, routes of elimination, and elimination half-life. An ideal antimicrobial drug for ambulatory patients would have good oral bioavailability and a long plasma half-life so that it would need to be taken only once or twice a day.

As described above, the peak serum concentration of an antimicrobial drug should generally be

TABLE 37–1.   Mechanisms of Microbial Resistance

Mechanism	Examples
Inactivation of the drug by microbial enzymes	Inactivation of aminoglycosides by acetylase, adenylase, and phosphorylase enzymes. Inactivation of penicillins and other beta-lactam antibiotics by beta-lactamase enzymes.
Decreased accumulation of the drug by the microbe	Decreased uptake of beta-lactam antibiotics due to altered porins in gram-negative bacteria. Decreased uptake and increased efflux of fluoroquinolones. Decreased uptake and increased efflux of tetracyclines.
Reduced affinity of the target macromolecule for the drug	Reduced affinity of DNA gyrase for fluoroquinolones. Reduced affinity of folate synthesis enzymes for sulfonamides and trimethoprim. Reduced affinity of ribosomes for aminoglycosides, chloramphenicol, clindamycin, macrolides, or tetracyclines. Reduced affinity of RNA polymerase for rifampin. Reduced affinity of transpeptidase and other penicillin-binding proteins for penicillins and other beta-lactam antibiotics.

2–4 times greater than the MIC of the pathogenic organism in order for the drug to be effective in eliminating the organism. This is partly because the tissue concentrations of a drug are often lower than the plasma concentration. The relationship between the plasma concentration of a typical antimicrobial drug and the drug's MIC for several organisms is shown in Fig. 37–5. The urine concentration of an antimicrobial drug may be 10–50 times the peak serum concentration. For this reason, infections of the urinary tract may be easier to treat than are infections at other sites.

Sites of infection that are not readily penetrated by many antimicrobial drugs include the central nervous system, bone, prostate gland, and ocular tissues. The treatment of meningitis requires that drugs achieve adequate concentrations in the cerebrospinal fluid (CSF). Some antibiotics, such as penicillin G, penetrate the blood-CSF barrier when the meninges are inflamed, but the aminoglycosides do not. For this reason, aminoglycosides may be given intrathecally for the treatment of meningitis. Because antimicrobial drug concentrations are low in bone, patients with osteomyelitis must usually be treated with antibiotics for several weeks to effect a cure. The prostate gland restricts the entry of some antimicrobial drugs because the drugs have difficulty crossing the prostatic epithelium and because prostatic fluid has a low pH. These characteristics favor the entry

and accumulation of weak bases, such as trimethoprim, and tend to exclude the entry of weak acids, such as penicillin.

The route of elimination affects both the selection and the use of antimicrobial drugs. Drugs that are eliminated by renal excretion are more effective for urinary tract infections than are drugs that are largely metabolized or undergo biliary excretion. However, antibiotics that are eliminated by the kidneys, such as the aminoglycosides, may accumulate in patients whose renal function is compromised, so their dosage must be reduced in these patients. Other antibiotics, such as doxycycline, do not depend on renal excretion for their elimination and may be safer for use in patients with renal impairment.

Adverse Effect Profile

Any antimicrobial drug may cause mild to severe adverse effects, but the incidence of these effects varies greatly among different classes of drugs. For this reason, it is important to consider the probable risk-benefit ratio when selecting drugs for treatment. The beta-lactam and macrolide antibiotics cause a relatively low incidence of organ system toxicity and are often used for the treatment of minor infections, including infections in pregnant women. In contrast, the aminoglycosides cause a relatively high incidence of severe adverse effects and are usually reserved for the treatment of serious or life-threatening infections.

Cost and Convenience

The total cost of drug treatment is determined by adding the cost of each dose of a drug plus the cost of administering each dose and then multiplying the sum by the total number of doses. For hospitalized patients, a drug that costs more for each dose but is administered less frequently or for a shorter duration of time may be less expensive than a drug that costs less per dose but requires more frequent administration or a longer duration of treatment.

The convenience of a drug regimen for ambulatory patients is an important factor because it affects whether the patients will take their prescribed antimicrobial agents as directed. Patient compliance is usually greater with a drug that is taken once or twice a day for a few days than with a drug that must be taken several times a day for a week or longer.

COMBINATION DRUG THERAPY

When antimicrobial drugs are given in combination, they may exhibit antagonistic, additive, synergistic, or indifferent effects against a particular microbe (Fig. 37–6). The relationship between two drugs and their combined effect is as follows: **antagonistic** if the combined effect is less than the effect of either drug alone; **additive** if the combined effect is equal to the sum of the independent effects; **synergistic** if the combined effect is greater than the sum of the independent effects; and **indifferent** if the

TABLE 37–2. Antimicrobial Drugs of Choice for the Treatment of Infections Caused by Bacteria*

Bacteria	Primary Drugs	Alternative Drugs
Gram-positive cocci		
Enterococcus species		
Endocarditis and other serious infections	Penicillin G/gentamicin; ampicillin/ gentamicin.	Vancomycin/gentamicin; teicoplanin; quinupristin/dalfopristin.
Urinary tract infections	Amoxicillin; ampicillin.	A fluoroquinolone.
Staphylococcus aureus or *Staphylococcus epidermidis*		
Methicillin-resistant strains	Vancomycin/gentamicin/rifampin; vancomycin/gentamicin; vancomycin/ rifampin; gentamicin/rifampin; vancomycin; gentamicin; rifampin.	A fluoroquinolone; minocycline; clindamycin; quinupristin/dalfopristin.
Non–penicillinase-producing strains	Penicillin G; penicillin V.	A cephalosporin; vancomycin; clindamycin; imipenem; a fluoroquinolone.
Penicillinase-producing strains	Nafcillin; oxacillin.	A cephalosporin; vancomycin; clindamycin; imipenem; a fluoroquinolone; penicillin/ beta-lactamase inhibitor.
Streptococcus pneumoniae	Penicillin G; penicillin V.	A cephalosporin; a macrolide; clindamycin; vancomycin/rifampin; vancomycin; quinupristin/dalfopristin.
Streptococcus pyogenes	Penicillin G; penicillin V.	Clindamycin; vancomycin; a macrolide; a cephalosporin.
Other *Streptococcus* species		
Anaerobic strains	Penicillin G.	A cephalosporin; clindamycin; vancomycin.
Viridans group	Penicillin G/gentamicin; penicillin G.	A cephalosporin; vancomycin.
Gram-positive bacilli		
Bacillus anthracis	Penicillin G.	A macrolide; a tetracycline.
Clostridium difficile	Metronidazole.	Vancomycin.
Clostridium perfringens	Penicillin G.	Clindamycin; metronidazole; imipenem.
Clostridium tetani	Penicillin G.	A tetracycline.
Corynebacterium diphtheriae	A macrolide.	Penicillin G.
Listeria monocytogenes	Ampicillin/gentamicin; ampicillin.	TMP/SMX.
Gram-negative cocci		
Moraxella catarrhalis	TMP/SMX.	A cephalosporin (II or III); a macrolide; a fluoroquinolone; amoxicillin/ clavulanate.
Neisseria gonorrhoeae	Ceftriaxone; cefixime.	Spectinomycin; a fluoroquinolone.
Neisseria meningitidis	Penicillin G.	A cephalosporin (III); chloramphenicol.
Enteric gram-negative bacilli		
Bacteroides species		
Gastrointestinal strains	Metronidazole.	Clindamycin; chloramphenicol; penicillin/ beta-lactamase inhibitor; a cephalosporin.
Oropharyngeal strains	Penicillin G; clindamycin.	Metronidazole; cefoxitin; cefotetan; chloramphenicol.
Campylobacter fetus	Imipenem.	Gentamicin.
Campylobacter jejuni	A fluoroquinolone; erythromycin.	A tetracycline; gentamicin.
Enterobacter species	Imipenem.	A cephalosporin (III); an aminoglycoside; an extended-spectrum penicillin; a fluoroquinolone.
Escherichia coli	Cefotaxime; ceftizoxime; ceftriaxone; ceftazidime.	Ampicillin/gentamicin; ampicillin; an aminoglycoside; penicillin/beta- lactamase inhibitor; imipenem; aztreonam; a fluoroquinolone; TMP/SMX.
Helicobacter pylori	Tetracycline/metronidazole/bismuth subsalicylate.	Tetracycline/clarithromycin/bismuth subsalicylate; amoxicillin/ metronidazole/bismuth subsalicylate.
Klebsiella pneumoniae	A cephalosporin (III).	Imipenem; an aminoglycoside; penicillin/ beta-lactamase inhibitor; TMP/SMX; aztreonam; a fluoroquinolone.
Proteus mirabilis	Ampicillin.	A cephalosporin; an aminoglycoside; an extended-spectrum penicillin; TMP/ SMX; imipenem; aztreonam; a fluoroquinolone.
Proteus vulgaris	A cephalosporin (III).	Imipenem; an aminoglycoside; extended- spectrum penicillin/beta-lactamase inhibitor; TMP/SMX; a fluoroquinolone.

Continued

TABLE 37–2. Antimicrobial Drugs of Choice for the Treatment of Infections Caused by Bacteria* *(Continued)*

Bacteria	Primary Drugs	Alternative Drugs
Enteric gram-negative bacilli *(continued)*		
Providencia stuartii	A cephalosporin (III).	Imipenem; an aminoglycoside; extended-spectrum penicillin/beta-lactamase inhibitor; aztreonam; TMP/SMX; a fluoroquinolone.
Salmonella species	A fluoroquinolone; ceftriaxone.	Chloramphenicol; TMP/SMX; ampicillin.
Serratia species	A cephalosporin (III).	An aminoglycoside; imipenem; aztreonam; TMP/SMX; an extended-spectrum penicillin; a fluoroquinolone.
Shigella species	A fluoroquinolone.	TMP/SMX; ampicillin.
Yersinia enterocolitica	TMP/SMX.	A fluoroquinolone; an aminoglycoside; a cephalosporin (III).
Other gram-negative bacteria		
Acinetobacter species	Imipenem.	An aminoglycoside; a cephalosporin (III); an extended-spectrum penicillin; a fluoroquinolone; doxycycline; minocycline.
Bordetella pertussis (whooping cough)	A macrolide.	Doxycycline.
Brucella species	A tetracycline/gentamicin.	A tetracycline/rifampin.
Calymmatobacterium granulomatis (granuloma inguinale)	A tetracycline.	Gentamicin; TMP/SMX.
Eikenella corrodens	Ampicillin.	A tetracycline; a macrolide; penicillin/beta-lactamase inhibitor; ceftriaxone.
Francisella tularensis (tularemia)	Streptomycin.	Gentamicin; a tetracycline; chloramphenicol.
Gardnerella vaginalis	Metronidazole.	Clindamycin.
Haemophilus ducreyi (chancroid)	Erythromycin; azithromycin; ceftriaxone.	A fluoroquinolone.
Haemophilus influenzae		
Meningitis and other serious infections	Cefotaxime; ceftriaxone.	Chloramphenicol.
Upper respiratory tract infections	TMP/SMX.	A cephalosporin (II or III); azithromycin; amoxicillin/clavulanate; a fluoroquinolone.
Legionella species	Erythromycin/rifampin; erythromycin.	Another macrolide; ciprofloxacin.
Pasteurella multocida	Penicillin G.	A tetracycline; a cephalosporin.
Pseudomonas aeruginosa		
Urinary tract infections	A fluoroquinolone.	An aminoglycoside; ticarcillin; piperacillin; aztreonam; ceftazidime.
Other infections	Ticarcillin/aminoglycoside; piperacillin/aminoglycoside.	Ceftazidime; imipenem; aztreonam/aminoglycoside; ciprofloxacin.
Vibrio cholerae (cholera)	A tetracycline.	A fluoroquinolone; TMP/SMX.
Yersinia pestis (plague)	Streptomycin.	A tetracycline; chloramphenicol; gentamicin.
Acid-fast bacilli		
Mycobacterium avium-intracellulare	Clarithromycin/ethambutol; clarithromycin/rifabutin; clarithromycin/ciprofloxacin; azithromycin/ethambutol; azithromycin/rifabutin; azithromycin/ciprofloxacin.	Rifampin; clofazimine; amikacin.
Mycobacterium kansasii	Isoniazid/rifampin/ethambutol; isoniazid/rifampin/streptomycin; isoniazid/rifampin.	Clarithromycin; ethionamide; cycloserine.
Mycobacterium leprae (leprosy)	Dapsone/rifampin/clofazimine; dapsone/rifampin.	Minocycline; a fluoroquinolone; clarithromycin.
Mycobacterium tuberculosis	Isoniazid/rifampin/pyrazinamide/ethambutol; isoniazid/rifampin/pyrazinamide/streptomycin; isoniazid/rifampin/pyrazinamide.	A fluoroquinolone; an aminoglycoside; ethionamide; cycloserine; clofazimine; capreomycin; aminosalicylic acid.
Actinomycetes		
Actinomyces israelii	Penicillin G.	A tetracycline; erythromycin; clindamycin.
Nocardia asteroides	TMP/SMX.	A sulfonamide; imipenem; amikacin.
Chlamydiae		
Chlamydia pneumoniae	A tetracycline.	A macrolide.
Chlamydia psittaci	A tetracycline.	Chloramphenicol.
Chlamydia trachomatis		
Cervicitis or urethritis	Doxycycline; azithromycin.	Ofloxacin.
Pneumonia	Erythromycin.	A sulfonamide.
Trachoma	Azithromycin.	A tetracycline; a sulfonamide.

Continued

**TABLE 37–2. Antimicrobial Drugs of Choice for the Treatment of Infections
Caused by Bacteria*** *(Continued)*

Bacteria	Primary Drugs	Alternative Drugs
Ehrlichiae		
Ehrlichia chaffeensis	A tetracycline.	Rifampin.
Mycoplasmas		
Mycoplasma pneumoniae	Erythromycin; a tetracycline.	Azithromycin; clarithromycin.
Ureaplasma urealyticum	Erythromycin.	A tetracycline; clarithromycin.
Rickettsiae		
Rickettsia species	A tetracycline.	Chloramphenicol; a fluoroquinolone.
Spirochetes		
Borrelia burgdorferi (Lyme disease)	Doxycycline; amoxicillin.	A cephalosporin (II or III); azithromycin; clarithromycin; penicillin G.
Borrelia recurrentis (relapsing fever)	A tetracycline.	Penicillin G.
Leptospira species	Penicillin G.	A tetracycline.
Treponema pallidum		
subspecies *pallidum* (syphilis)	Benzathine penicillin G.	A tetracycline; ceftriaxone.
subspecies *pertenue* (yaws)	Penicillin G.	A tetracycline.

*Antibiotics are listed in their general order of recommended use, with the drug or drug combination used most often listed first. Antibiotics used in combination are separated by the symbol /, such as the combination of vancomycin and gentamicin, which is listed as vancomycin/gentamicin. The combination of trimethoprim and sulfamethoxazole is listed as TMP/SMX. For cephalosporins, I = first-generation drug; II = second-generation drug; and III = third-generation drug.

combined effect is similar to the greatest effect produced by either drug alone.

Treatment of Infections Caused by a Single Microbial Species

Some bacteriostatic drugs, such as chloramphenicol or tetracycline, are antagonistic to bactericidal drugs. Bactericidal drugs are usually more effective against rapidly dividing bacteria, and their effect is reduced if bacterial growth is slowed by a bacteriostatic drug. Therefore, for an infection caused by a single species, combination therapy with a bactericidal drug and a bacteriostatic drug is usually avoided.

Most infections caused by a single microbial species are treated with a single drug. This is because monotherapy usually is less expensive, equally or more effective, and less toxic than is combination therapy. However, as discussed below, there are a few situations in which combination therapy is preferable.

If two bactericidal drugs that act by two different mechanisms are given in combination, they tend to exhibit additive or synergistic effects against susceptible bacteria (Table 37–3). For example, penicillins

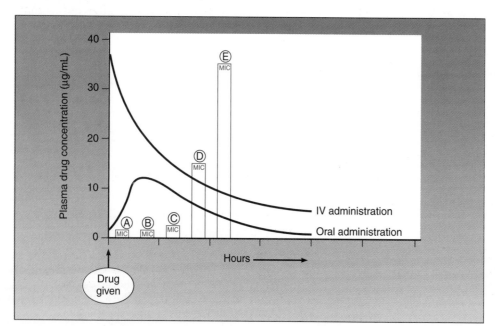

FIGURE 37–5. Relationship between the plasma concentration of a typical antimicrobial drug and the drug's minimum inhibitory concentration (MIC) for five bacterial organisms. The curves represent typical plasma concentrations over time after intravenous (IV) or oral administration of the drug. Each bar represents the MIC of a particular organism: *Streptococcus pneumoniae, Staphylococcus aureus,* and *Escherichia coli* (shown as A, B, and C, respectively, in this example) are susceptible to the drug; *Enterobacter* species (shown as D) are intermediate in sensitivity; and *Pseudomonas aeruginosa* (shown as E) is resistant.

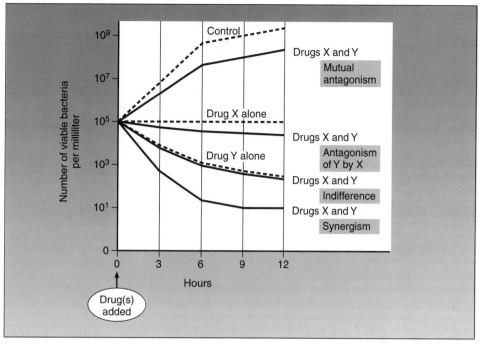

FIGURE 37–6. **Comparison of several possible interactions of two antimicrobial drugs combined in vitro.** Curves show the results when cultures containing 10^5 bacteria per milliliter are incubated with no drug (control), with drug X alone, with drug Y alone, and with a combination of drugs X and Y. In this example, drug X is bacteriostatic, whereas drug Y is bactericidal. In an antagonistic interaction, the combined effect is less than the effect of either drug alone. In an indifferent interaction, the combined effect is similar to the greatest effect produced by either drug alone. In a synergistic interaction, the combined effect is greater than the sum of the independent effects.

(which are cell wall synthesis inhibitors) often show additive or synergistic effects with aminoglycosides (which are protein synthesis inhibitors) when they are used in combination against a gram-negative bacillus such as *P. aeruginosa.* These drugs also show additive or synergistic effects against many enterococci and staphylococci.

A few antimicrobial agents exhibit synergistic activity against some or all of the bacteria that are sensitive to the drugs. For example, sulfamethoxazole and trimethoprim inhibit sequential steps in bacterial folate synthesis and exhibit synergistic activity against many strains of organisms that are resistant

TABLE 37–3.   **In Vitro Activity of Antimicrobial Drug Combinations**

Synergistic combinations
- Aminoglycoside plus ampicillin used against enterococci
- Aminoglycoside plus penicillin G used against enterococci
- Aminoglycoside plus broad-spectrum penicillin used against gram-negative bacilli
- Aminoglycoside plus cephalosporin used against gram-negative bacilli
- Amphotericin B plus flucytosine used against *Cryptococcus neoformans*
- Antistaphylococcal penicillin plus aminoglycoside used against staphylococci
- Antistaphylococcal penicillin plus rifampin used against staphylococci
- Reverse transcriptase inhibitor plus protease inhibitor used against human immunodeficiency virus

Antagonistic combinations
- Aminoglycoside plus chloramphenicol used against members of the family Enterobacteriaceae
- Broad-spectrum penicillin plus chloramphenicol used against *Streptococcus pneumoniae*
- Broad-spectrum penicillin plus imipenem used against gram-negative bacilli

to either drug alone. The treatment of HIV infection also employs drugs that exhibit a synergistic effect when used in combination. These drugs are described in Chapter 43.

Treatment of Mixed Infections

Mixed infections are infections that are caused by more than one microbial species and are usually treated with more than one drug. For example, an intra-abdominal infection may be caused by the combination of an aerobic gram-negative bacillus and an anaerobic gram-negative bacillus, such as *Escherichia coli* and *Bacteroides fragilis,* respectively. This type of infection may be treated with an aminoglycoside (active against aerobic bacilli) plus either metronidazole or clindamycin (active against anaerobic bacilli). Urethritis due to a mixed infection with *Neisseria gonorrhoeae* and *Chlamydia trachomatis* may be treated with a cephalosporin such as ceftriaxone (active against gonococci) plus a tetracycline (active against chlamydiae). In this example, because each drug is active against a different organism, it does not matter that the cephalosporin is bactericidal and the tetracycline is bacteriostatic.

Empiric Treatment of Serious Infections

More than one antibiotic is often used to treat patients with a serious infection until the causative organism can be identified and its sensitivity to antimicrobial drugs can be determined. For example, the initial treatment of serious nosocomial (hospital-acquired) infections may include the use of penicillin or vancomycin (active against staphylococci) in combination with an aminoglycoside or a cephalosporin (active against gram-negative bacilli).

Prevention of Antibiotic Resistance

As discussed in Chapter 40, tuberculosis is always treated with more than one drug. This is because about 1 in 10^6 *Mycobacterium tuberculosis* organisms will mutate to a resistant form during treatment with a single drug. The rate of mutation to a form that is resistant to two drugs is the product of the individual drug resistant rates, or about 1 in 10^{12} organisms. Because fewer than 10^{12} organisms are usually present in a patient with tuberculosis, it is unlikely that a resistant mutant will emerge during combination therapy.

PROPHYLACTIC THERAPY

The prevention of infections requires the sterilization of diagnostic and surgical instruments, the use of disinfectants to reduce environmental pathogens in hospitals and clinics, and the disinfection of skin and mucous membranes prior to invasive procedures. In some cases, antimicrobial drugs are also administered prophylactically either to reduce the incidence of infections associated with surgical and other invasive procedures or to prevent disease transmission to close contacts of infected persons. Recommendations for prophylaxis are summarized in Table 37–4.

Prevention of Infection During Invasive Procedures

Antibiotics are used to prevent **endocarditis** in persons with a history of valvular heart disease, including mitral valve prolapse and rheumatic heart disease. These individuals are at risk of developing acute bacterial endocarditis due to viridans and other streptococci that may be acquired during routine dental, oral, or upper respiratory tract procedures and surgery. Amoxicillin is currently considered the drug of choice, but endocarditis can be prevented by using an alternative drug such as clindamycin, cephalexin, azithromycin, or clarithromycin.

TABLE 37–4. Prophylactic Use of Antimicrobial Drugs

Prevention of infection during invasive procedures
- To prevent **endocarditis** in persons with a history of valvular heart disease, administer amoxicillin or other antibiotic prior to dental, oral, or upper respiratory tract procedures.
- To prevent **wound and tissue infections** in persons who will undergo surgery, administer a single dose of cefazolin (active against staphylococci and oral anaerobic organisms) or a single dose of cefoxitin or cefotetan (active against aerobic or anaerobic enteric bacilli).

Prevention of disease transmission in persons at increased risk
- To prevent **influenza type A,** give amantadine or rimantadine.
- To prevent **malaria,** give chloroquine or mefloquine.
- To prevent **meningococcal disease,** give rifampin.
- To prevent **tuberculosis,** give isoniazid.

Antibiotics are routinely used to prevent **wound and tissue infections** that may be acquired during a wide range of surgical procedures. The choice of antibiotic depends on the most likely sources of bacterial pathogens during a particular procedure. The skin is the most common source of pathogens, especially staphylococci, during most types of surgery. The gastrointestinal tract is also an important source of pathogens when surgical procedures involve the gastrointestinal system. Surgery to repair contaminated wounds, such as gunshot or knife wounds, presents the most severe requirements for prophylaxis because of the greater number and variety of bacteria that are often associated with this type of trauma.

Prevention of Disease Transmission

Antimicrobial drugs are occasionally used to prevent the transmission of a highly contagious disease, such as **meningococcal infection,** from an infected person or insect vector to an exposed individual. Drugs are also used to prevent **malaria** in persons who are traveling to regions of the world where malaria is endemic and to prevent **influenza type A** and **tuberculosis** in certain groups at increased risk for these diseases. Prophylactic drugs are discussed more thoroughly in subsequent chapters.

Summary of Important Points

- Antibiotics are substances that are produced by one microbe and are capable of inhibiting the growth or viability of other microbes. Antimicrobial drugs include cell wall synthesis inhibitors, protein synthesis inhibitors, metabolic and nucleic acid inhibitors, and cell membrane inhibitors.
- Antimicrobial drugs can be characterized as bactericidal (able to kill microbes) or bacteriostatic (able to slow the growth of microbes). They can also be characterized as narrow-spectrum, broad-spectrum, or extended-spectrum, based on their range of antimicrobial activity.
- Laboratory tests used to determine microbial sensitivity to drugs include the disk diffusion method (Kirby-Bauer test) and the broth dilution test. The latter test is used to determine the minimum inhibitory concentration (MIC), which is the lowest drug concentration that inhibits microbial growth in vitro.
- Acquired microbial resistance arises by mutation and selection or by transfer of genes encoding resistance factors (R factors). The most common mechanism of transferable resistance is bacterial conjugation and exchange of plasmids containing R factors.
- The mechanisms responsible for microbial resistance to a drug include inactivation of the drug by microbial enzymes, decreased accumulation of the drug by the microbe, and reduced affinity of the target macromolecule for the drug.

- The selection of an antimicrobial drug for treating a particular infection requires consideration of host factors (pregnancy, drug allergies, age and immune status, and the presence of concomitant diseases) and drug characteristics (antimicrobial activity, pharmacokinetic properties, adverse effect profile, cost, and convenience).
- Combination drug therapy is generally used for the treatment of mixed infections, the empiric treatment of serious infections, and the prevention of antibiotic resistance. In some cases, combination therapy with synergistic drugs is used for the treatment of infections caused by a single microbial species.
- Antibiotic prophylaxis is used to prevent infections during surgical and other invasive procedures and to prevent the transmission of infectious diseases to persons at increased risk.

Selected Readings

Baquero, F. Gram-positive resistance: challenge for the development of new antibiotics. J Antimicrob Chemother 39(supplement A):1–6, 1997.

Courvalin, P. Evasion of antibiotic action by bacteria. J Antimicrob Chemother 37:855–869, 1996.

Marchese, A., et al. Multidrug-resistant gram-positive pathogens. Drugs 54(supplement 6):11–20, 1997.

Nieman, R. E., et al. Antimicrobial Therapy in Primary Care Medicine. West Chester, Pa., Medical Surveillance, Inc., 1997.

Rybak, M. J., and B. J. McGrath. Combination antimicrobial therapy for bacterial infections. Drugs 52:390–405, 1996.

CHAPTER THIRTY-EIGHT

INHIBITORS OF BACTERIAL

CELL WALL SYNTHESIS

CLASSIFICATION OF INHIBITORS OF BACTERIAL CELL WALL SYNTHESIS

BETA-LACTAM ANTIBIOTICS
Narrow-spectrum penicillins
- Penicillin G
- Penicillin V

Penicillinase-resistant penicillins
- Dicloxacillin
- Nafcillin

Extended-spectrum penicillins
- Amoxicillin
- Ampicillin
- Piperacillin
- Ticarcillin

Beta-lactamase inhibitors
- Clavulanate
- Sulbactam
- Tazobactam

First-generation cephalosporins
- Cefazolin
- Cephalexin

Second-generation cephalosporins
- Cefotetan
- Cefoxitin
- Cefprozil
- Cefuroxime

Third-generation cephalosporins
- Cefixime
- Cefotaxime
- Ceftazidime
- Ceftriaxone

Fourth-generation cephalosporins
- Cefepime

Monobactams
- Aztreonam

Carbapenems
- Imipenem
- Meropenem

OTHER BACTERIAL CELL WALL SYNTHESIS INHIBITORS
- Bacitracin
- Cycloserine
- Fosfomycin
- Vancomycin

OVERVIEW

A large group of antimicrobial drugs, including the penicillins and other beta-lactam antibiotics, act by inhibiting the synthesis of the bacterial cell wall. The penicillins were the first true antibiotics to be discovered, and their development inaugurated the modern era of antimicrobial chemotherapy.

Cell Envelope

Two components of the cell envelope that are found in both gram-positive and gram-negative bacteria are the **cytoplasmic membrane** and the **cell wall.** The envelope of each gram-negative bacterium also has an **outer membrane** that is not found in other types of bacteria. The cell envelope components are illustrated in Fig. 38–1.

Cytoplasmic and Outer Membranes

The cytoplasmic membrane is a trilaminar membrane. It contains various types of **transport proteins,** which facilitate the uptake of a wide variety of substrates used by bacteria, and it also contains several enzymes required for the synthesis of the cell wall. These enzymes, whose functions are described below, are collectively known as **penicillin-binding proteins** (PBPs).

The outer membrane of gram-negative bacteria is also a trilaminar membrane. It contains species-specific forms of a complex **lipopolysaccharide** (LPS) and various types of protein channels called **porins.** One portion of LPS (the lipid A portion) is the **endotoxin** responsible for gram-negative sepsis. This endotoxin activates immunologic mechanisms that lead to fever, platelet aggregation, increased vascular permeability, and other adverse effects on tissues. Porins allow ions and other small hydrophilic molecules to pass through the outer membrane, and they are responsible for the entry of several types of antibiotics. Acquired alterations in porin structure may lead to microbial antibiotic resistance.

The bacterial cytoplasmic and outer membranes are the target of a minor group of polypeptide antibiotics called **polymyxins.** The polymyxins act as detergents that increase the permeability of these

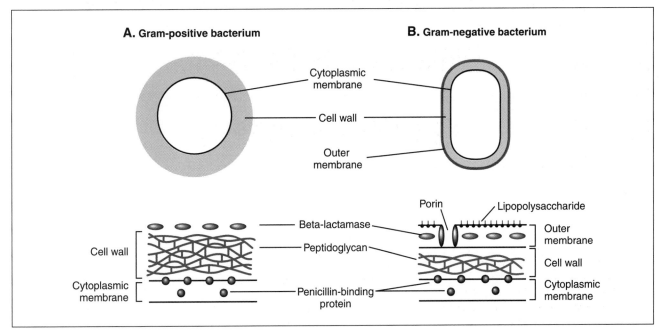

FIGURE 38–1. Comparison of the cell envelopes of gram-positive and gram-negative bacteria. (A) The gram-positive bacterium has a thick cell wall but does not have an outer membrane. Beta-lactamases are located in the outer portion of the cell wall. Penicillin-binding proteins are found in the cytoplasmic membrane. **(B)** The gram-negative bacterium has a thin cell wall. It also has an outer membrane that contains lipopolysaccharide and protein channels called porins.

membranes and thereby enable the cytoplasmic contents to leak out of the cell. The properties and uses of polymyxins are discussed in Chapter 41.

Cell Wall

The cell wall consists primarily of **peptidoglycan,** a polymer constructed from repeating disaccharide units of **N-acetylglucosamine** (GlcNAc) and **N-acetylmuramic acid** (MurNAc). Each disaccharide is attached to others through glycosidic bonds. Each molecule of MurNAc has a peptide containing two molecules of D-alanine and a pentaglycine side chain (Fig. 38–2). The strands of peptidoglycan in the cell wall are cross-linked by a transpeptidase reaction in which the glycine pentapeptide of one strand is attached to the penultimate D-alanine molecule of another strand. During this reaction, the terminal D-alanine is removed.

The cell wall is much thicker in gram-positive bacteria than it is in gram-negative bacteria. Because a cell wall is not found in higher organisms, antimicrobial drugs can inhibit its formation without harming host cells. The cell wall maintains the shape of the bacterium and protects it from osmotic lysis if it is placed in a hypotonic medium. Without a cell wall, the bacterium is unprotected. This is why inhibition of cell wall synthesis by antimicrobial drugs is usually bactericidal. Because the cell wall is synthesized during bacterial replication, drugs that inhibit cell wall synthesis are more active against rapidly dividing bacteria than they are against bacteria in the resting or stationary phase. For the same reason, the effectiveness of cell wall inhibitors is usually reduced

by concurrent administration of bacteriostatic antibiotics that slow the growth of bacteria.

Sites of Drug Action
Beta-Lactam Drugs

The beta-lactam antibiotics bind to a diverse group of bacterial enzymes known as the **penicillin-binding proteins** (PBPs). These enzymes are anchored in the cytoplasmic membrane and extend into the periplasmic space. The PBPs are responsible for the assembly, maintenance, and regulation of the peptidoglycan portion of the bacterial cell wall. Some of the PBPs have transpeptidase activity, while others have carboxypeptidase and transglycosylase activity.

Table 38–1 outlines the functions of the three major types of PBPs, referred to as PBP-1, PBP-2, and PBP-3. The beta-lactam antibiotics form a covalent bond with PBPs and thereby inhibit the catalytic activity of these enzymes. Inhibition of some PBPs prevents **cross-linking of peptidoglycan** (see Fig. 38–2), whereas inhibition of other PBPs leads to the bacterium's **autolysis** or to its change to a **spheroplast** or a **filamentous form.**

Bacterial species have different types of PBPs, and specific beta-lactam antibiotics selectively bind to the different types. This partly accounts for the variation in the sensitivity of different organisms to beta-lactam antibiotics.

Other Drugs

Bacitracin, vancomycin, and **fosfomycin** inhibit cell wall peptidoglycan synthesis by blocking specific

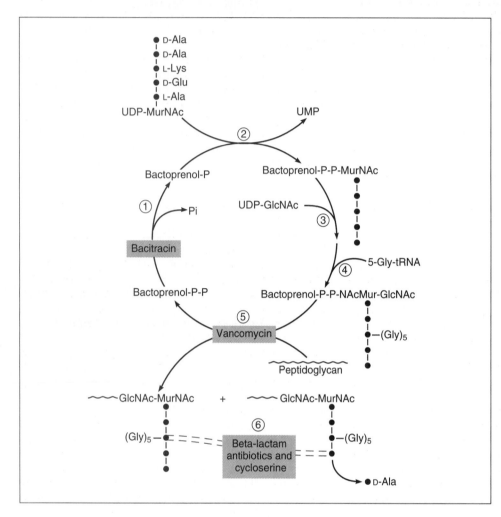

FIGURE 38–2. Sites of action of bacterial cell wall synthesis inhibitors. The bacterial cell wall consists primarily of peptidoglycan, a polymer constructed from repeating disaccharide units of *N*-acetylglucosamine (GlcNAc) and *N*-acetylmuramic acid (MurNAc). Numbers indicate the steps involved in the synthesis of the cell wall. In step 1, bactoprenol pyrophosphate (bactoprenol-P-P) is dephosphorylated to regenerate the carrier molecule, bactoprenol phosphate (bactoprenol-P). In step 2, uridine diphosphate–MurNAc (UDP-MurNAc) is added. Uridine monophosphate (UMP) is a by-product. In steps 3 and 4, UDP-GlcNAc and a glycine penta-peptide (5-Gly-tRNA) are added. In step 5, the disaccharide pep-tide is transferred to the pep-tidoglycan growth point. In step 6, the cross-linking of pepti-doglycan strands is catalyzed by transpeptidase, a type of penicillin-binding protein. In this reaction, a glycine in one strand forms a new peptide bond with a D-alanine in the adjacent strand, and the terminal D-alanine is released from the adjacent strand. Bacitracin blocks step 1; vancomycin blocks step 5; and beta-lactam antibiotics and cycloserine block step 6. Fos-fomycin (not shown) inhibits enolpyruvyl transferase, the en-zyme that catalyzes the con-densation of UDP-GlcNAc with phosphoenolpyruvate in order to synthesize UDP-MurNAc.

steps in the formation of the disaccharide precursor, MurNAc-GlcNAc. As shown in Fig. 38–2, bacitracin inhibits the dephosphorylation of bactoprenol pyro-phosphate, which is the carrier lipid required for regeneration of bactoprenol phosphate, the active carrier of the disaccharide precursor. Vancomycin inhibits the step in which the disaccharide precur-sor is added to the growing peptidoglycan chain. Fosfomycin inhibits enolpyruvyl transferase, the en-zyme that catalyzes the condensation of uridine diphosphate–GlcNAc (UDP-GlcNAc) with phospho-enolpyruvate in order to synthesize UDP-MurNAc.

Cycloserine is a second-line antitubercular drug that is structurally similar to D-alanine. It inhibits two enzymes, L-alanine racemase and D-alanine synthe-tase, both of which are involved in the incorporation of D-alanine into the peptidoglycan structure of the bacterial cell wall. The absence of D-alanine prevents cross-linking of peptidoglycan strands and results in a weak cell wall that is easily lysed.

BETA-LACTAM ANTIBIOTICS

The beta-lactam drugs include penicillins, beta-lactamase inhibitors, cephalosporins, monobactams, and carbapenems.

Penicillins

The penicillins were the first antibiotics to be isolated from microorganisms and used to treat systemic bacterial infections. Alexander Fleming is credited with the discovery of penicillin, but he was unable to isolate the substance in sufficient purity

TABLE 38–1. Major Types of Penicillin-Binding Proteins (PBPs)

Type	Function	Effect of PBP Inhibition on Bacterium
PBP-1	Elongation of bacterial cell wall.	Rapid autolysis of bacterium.
PBP-2	Maintenance of rod shape of bacterium.	Change of bacterium to a spheroplast.
PBP-3	Formation of septa.	Change of bacterium to a filamentous form.

and quantity for clinical use. Later, E. B. Chain and H. W. Florey, working in England, obtained enough penicillin to establish its clinical effectiveness. The production of sufficient quantities of penicillin for widespread use around the world was made possible by advances in microbial fermentation technology in the USA.

Classification

The penicillins can be grouped according to their antimicrobial spectrum of activity. Narrow-spectrum penicillins include **penicillin G** and **penicillin V**. Penicillinase-resistant penicillins include **dicloxacillin** and **nafcillin**. Extended-spectrum penicillins include **amoxicillin, ampicillin, piperacillin,** and **ticarcillin.**

Drug Properties

Chemistry. The penicillins consist of a beta-lactam ring fused to a thiazolidine ring, with an R group side chain that is unique for each drug (Fig. 38–3). The **original (natural) penicillins** were isolated from strains of *Penicillium* and were assigned letter designations because their chemical structures could not be identified at that time. Of the original penicillins, only penicillin G and penicillin V are still used today, and they are classified as narrow-spectrum drugs. The **semisynthetic penicillins** are produced from 6-aminopenicillanic acid, a building block obtained by removing the R group of a natural penicillin. A different R group is then substituted to prepare each of the various penicillinase-resistant and extended-spectrum penicillins that are available today. The penicillinase-resistant penicillins have a large, bulky R group that protects them from hydrolysis by staphylococcal beta-lactamase.

Pharmacokinetics. The route of administration of penicillins depends on the stability of the drugs in gastric acid. **Acid-stable penicillins,** which include amoxicillin, dicloxacillin, and penicillin V, are effective when given orally. In contrast, **acid-labile penicillins,** which include piperacillin and ticarcillin, must be administered parenterally. Penicillin G has intermediate sensitivity to gastric acid and may be given orally in large doses, but penicillin V has better acid stability and oral bioavailability, so it is usually preferable when an oral narrow-spectrum penicillin is indicated.

The penicillins are widely distributed to organs and tissues except the central nervous system. However, because penicillins readily penetrate the cerebrospinal fluid when the meninges are inflamed (Fig. 38–4A), they may be administered intravenously for the treatment of meningitis.

Most penicillins are eliminated primarily by active renal tubular secretion and have short half-lives of about 0.5–1.3 hours (Table 38–2). A few penicillins, such as ampicillin and nafcillin, are excreted primarily in the bile. The renal tubular secretion of penicillins is inhibited by **probenecid,** a drug that competes with penicillins for the organic acid transporter located in the proximal tubule. Probenecid has been used to slow the excretion and prolong the half-life of penicillin G (see Fig. 38–4B).

Penicillin G is available in two long-acting forms for intramuscular administration, **procaine penicillin G** and **benzathine penicillin G.** Penicillin G is slowly released from these two preparations for absorption into the circulation following an intramuscular injection. Benzathine penicillin G is hydrolyzed slowly over a period of several weeks and provides low plasma concentrations of the drug for an extended period of time. In contrast, procaine penicillin G is hydrolyzed more rapidly and produces significant plasma concentrations of penicillin for about 24 hours (see Fig. 38–4B).

Spectrum and Indications. Table 38–3 outlines the spectrum and major clinical uses of penicillins.

The **narrow-spectrum penicillins,** penicillins G and V, were traditionally used to treat infections due to streptococci (including pneumococci), staphylococci, gonococci, meningococci, and spirochetes (such as *Treponema pallidum*). For example, benzocaine penicillin G was used to prevent streptococcal infections and to treat syphilis, and procaine penicillin G was used to treat acute respiratory tract infections and gonorrhea. However, many strains of the bacteria responsible for these diseases are now resistant, necessitating the use of more toxic or expensive antibiotics.

The **penicillinase-resistant penicillins,** such as dicloxacillin and nafcillin, were developed to treat penicillin-resistant strains of staphylococci that elaborate penicillinase (beta-lactamase). The penicillinase-resistant penicillins are not active against most other species of penicillinase-producing bacteria. Dicloxacillin is a member of the isoxazole group of penicillins, which also includes oxacillin and cloxacillin. Dicloxacillin is often employed when an orally administered drug is needed, whereas nafcillin is usually preferred when parenteral administration is required.

The penicillinase-resistant drugs are used to treat serious staphylococcal infections, such as acute endocarditis and osteomyelitis, as well as skin and soft tissue infections due to susceptible staphylococci. Staphylococci that are resistant to these penicillins are often designated **methicillin-resistant *Staphylococcus aureus*** (MRSA) because methicillin was the original drug in this class. However, methicillin is seldom used today, because of its greater toxicity and tendency to cause interstitial nephritis. Bacteria that are resistant to methicillin are also cross-resistant to nafcillin and all other penicillinase-resistant penicillins. Most strains of MRSA are also resistant to cephalosporins and other beta-lactam drugs.

The **extended-spectrum penicillins** can be subdivided into the **aminopenicillins** (amoxicillin and ampicillin) and the **antipseudomonal penicillins** (piperacillin, ticarcillin, and others).

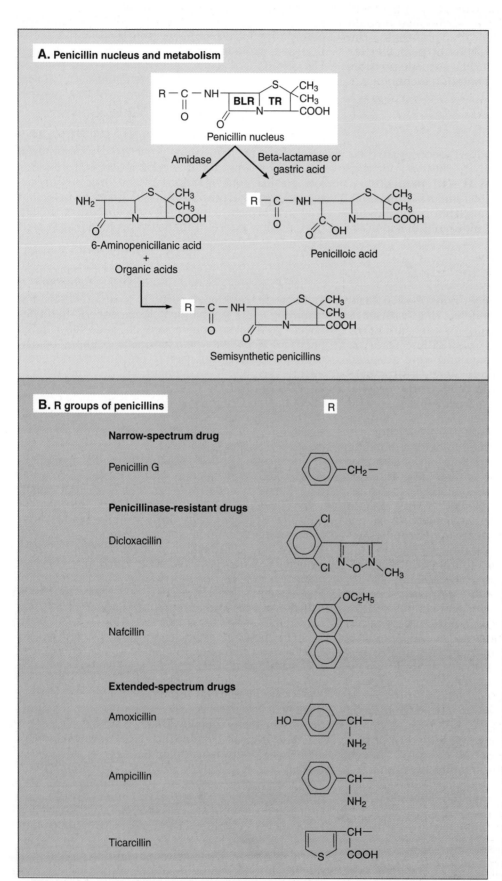

FIGURE 38–3. Metabolism and structure of penicillins. (A) The penicillin nucleus contains a beta-lactam ring (BLR) fused with a thiazolidine ring (TR). Amidase enzymatically removes the R group from penicillins and thereby forms 6-aminopenicillanic acid, the building block for semisynthetic penicillins. Beta-lactamases hydrolyze the beta-lactam ring and thereby inactivate penicillins and other beta-lactam drugs. Some penicillins are also degraded by gastric acid. (B) Each penicillin has a unique R group that determines the antimicrobial activity of the drug and its susceptibility to beta-lactamase and acid hydrolysis. The narrow-spectrum drugs are natural penicillins, whereas the other drugs shown are semisynthetic penicillins.

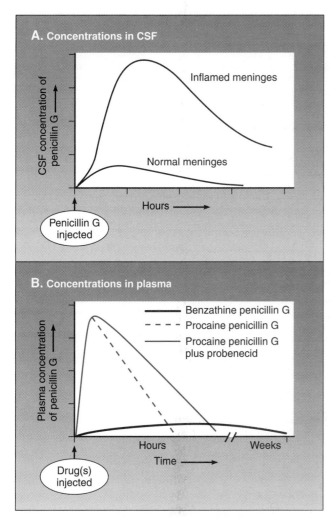

A. Concentrations in CSF

CSF concentration of penicillin G

Inflamed meninges

Normal meninges

Hours

Penicillin G injected

B. Concentrations in plasma

Plasma concentration of penicillin G

——— Benzathine penicillin G
- - - - Procaine penicillin G
——— Procaine penicillin G plus probenecid

Hours   Weeks

Time

Drug(s) injected

FIGURE 38–4. Pharmacokinetics of penicillin G preparations. **(A)** When penicillin G is administered to patients with normal meninges, the concentration in cerebrospinal fluid (CSF) remains low. When it is administered to patients with meningitis, the concentration increases. This is because meningitis increases the permeability of meninges to penicillin G. **(B)** Administration of benzathine penicillin G produces low plasma concentrations of the drug for several weeks. Administration of procaine penicillin G produces therapeutic plasma concentrations for about 24 hours. Probenecid inhibits the renal excretion of penicillin G, prolongs its half-life, and increases its plasma concentrations.

The aminopenicillins are active against many streptococci and some gram-negative bacteria, including *Escherichia coli, Haemophilus influenzae,* and *Proteus* species. Amoxicillin is often used to treat otitis media, and it may be combined with **clavulanate** (a beta-lactamase inhibitor) for the treatment of otitis media due to penicillinase-producing strains of *H. influenzae* and other organisms. Additional uses of amoxicillin are listed in Table 38–3. Ampicillin is highly active against *Listeria monocytogenes* and is used to treat meningitis and other infections caused by this organism. It is often employed in combination with **sulbactam** (a beta-lactamase inhibitor) for the treatment of infections due to penicillinase-producing strains of bacteria, including bite wounds and diabetic foot ulcers. Ampicillin may be combined

with an **aminoglycoside,** such as gentamicin, for the treatment of serious enterococcal infections, such as enterococcal endocarditis.

The antipseudomonal penicillins are active against infections caused by *Pseudomonas aeruginosa* and a number of other aerobic gram-negative bacilli. In some cases, they are given in combination with an aminoglycoside. They are often combined with a beta-lactamase inhibitor for the treatment of mixed infections, such as nosocomial pneumonia involving gram-positive and anaerobic organisms.

Bacterial Resistance.   As shown in Table 38–4, there are three primary mechanisms by which bacteria become resistant to penicillins and other beta-lactam antibiotics: inactivation of the drugs by beta-lactamase enzymes, reduced affinity of PBPs for the drugs, and decreased entry of the drugs into bacteria through outer membrane porins. In some bacteria, resistance may be due to a combination of these effects.

There are several classes of beta-lactamase enzymes. One class is produced by gram-positive bacteria. Six major classes (classes I through VI) are produced by gram-negative bacteria. The beta-lactamases are synthesized under the control of both chromosomal and plasmid DNA. Some beta-lactamases are induced by beta-lactam drugs, and this may represent an important mechanism of acquired resistance.

Beta-lactamases are found in the bacterial cell wall and outer membrane, and they may also be excreted by bacteria into the environment. The staphylococci were the first major group of bacterial pathogens to acquire beta-lactamases that rendered them resistant to penicillin G. Later, many gonococci and other gram-negative bacteria acquired beta-lactamases. Resistance of *H. influenzae* to amoxicillin and other penicillins is primarily due to the presence of these enzymes.

Gram-positive bacteria are innately resistant to aztreonam because their PBPs do not bind to this drug. Resistance of other bacteria to penicillins can be acquired when the structure of PBPs is altered in a manner that reduces the affinity of PBPs for the drugs. This mechanism has been responsible for much of the recent emergence of pneumococci that are resistant to penicillin G and of staphylococci that are resistant to methicillin.

Many gram-negative bacteria are innately resistant to penicillins because porins in their outer membrane are impermeable to these drugs. This is also an important mechanism of acquired resistance to penicillins, as in the case of *P. aeruginosa* resistance to imipenem.

Adverse Effects.   The penicillins are the most common cause of **drug-induced hypersensitivity reactions.** Hypersensitivity reactions are evoked when penicillin in the body is degraded to penicilloic acid and other compounds. These compounds subsequently combine with body proteins to form antigens that elicit antibody formation.

Immediate hypersensitivity reactions, which are

TABLE 38–2. Pharmacokinetic Properties of Bacterial Cell Wall Synthesis Inhibitors*

Drug	Route of Administration	Elimination Half-Life (Hours)	Primary Route of Elimination
Beta-lactam antibiotics			
Narrow-spectrum penicillins			
Penicillin G	Oral or parenteral	0.5	Renal (TS)
Penicillin V	Oral	1.0	Renal (TS)
Penicillinase-resistant penicillins			
Dicloxacillin	Oral	0.6	Renal (TS)
Nafcillin	Oral or parenteral	0.5	Biliary
Extended-spectrum penicillins			
Amoxicillin	Oral	1.0	Renal (TS)
Ampicillin	Oral or parenteral	1.0	Renal (TS) and biliary
Piperacillin	Parenteral	1.3	Renal (TS)
Ticarcillin	Parenteral	1.2	Renal (TS)
First-generation cephalosporins			
Cefazolin	Parenteral	2.0	Renal (TS)
Cephalexin	Oral	0.5	Renal (TS)
Second-generation cephalosporins			
Cefotetan	Parenteral	4.0	Renal (TS)
Cefoxitin	Parenteral	0.8	Renal (TS)
Cefprozil	Oral	1.3	Renal (TS)
Cefuroxime	Oral or parenteral	1.7	Renal (TS)
Third-generation cephalosporins			
Cefixime	Oral	3.5	Renal (TS)
Cefotaxime	Parenteral	1.6†	Renal (TS)
Ceftazidime	Parenteral	1.8	Renal (GF)
Ceftriaxone	Parenteral	8.0	Biliary
Fourth-generation cephalosporins			
Cefepime	Parenteral	2.0	Metabolized
Monobactams			
Aztreonam	Parenteral	1.7	Metabolized
Carbapenems			
Imipenem	Parenteral	1.0	Renal (TS)
Meropenem	Parenteral	1.2	Renal (TS)
Other bacterial cell wall synthesis inhibitors			
Bacitracin	Topical	NA	NA
Cycloserine	Oral	10.0	Renal (GF)
Fosfomycin	Oral	6.0	Renal (GF)
Vancomycin	Oral or parenteral	6.0	Renal (GF)

*Values shown are the mean of values reported in the literature. TS = tubular secretion; GF = glomerular filtration; and NA = not applicable.
†For cefotaxime, the value shown is the half-life of the metabolite.

a type of reaction mediated by immunoglobulin E (IgE), may lead to urticaria (hives) or anaphylactic shock. Other types of hypersensitivity reaction may lead to serum sickness, interstitial nephritis, hepatitis, and various skin rashes. Hepatitis is more common with antistaphylococcal and extended-spectrum penicillins and is usually reversible when use of the drug is discontinued. Ampicillin is particularly prone to cause a maculopapular skin rash in patients with certain viral infections, such as mononucleosis. This reaction is mediated by sensitized lymphocytes, and its incidence in ampicillin-treated patients with mononucleosis is over 90%.

Penicillin allergy can be confirmed by the use of a commercial preparation of penicillin antigens. This preparation is injected intradermally and will cause erythema at the injection site if allergy is present. The preparation should be administered only by personnel who are prepared to provide treatment for anaphylactic shock in the event that the patient develops a severe hypersensitivity reaction following the injection.

Except for hypersensitivity reactions, the penicillins are remarkably nontoxic to the human body and produce very few other adverse effects. High concentrations of penicillins may be irritating to the central nervous system and elicit seizures in patients who have received very large doses of these drugs. Like other antibiotics, penicillins may disturb the normal flora of the gut and produce diarrhea and superinfections with penicillin-resistant organisms, such as staphylococci and *Clostridium difficile*. Pseudomembranous colitis may occur in association with *C. difficile* superinfections.

Beta-Lactamase Inhibitors

Clavulanate, sulbactam, and **tazobactam** are drugs that inhibit class II through class VI beta-lactamase enzymes. When one of these drugs is given alone, it has no antimicrobial activity. When it is given in combination with a beta-lactam antibiotic, it will act as a suicide inhibitor of these classes of beta-lactamase enzymes by serving as a surrogate sub-

TABLE 38–3. Major Clinical Uses of Bacterial Cell Wall Synthesis Inhibitors

Drug	Major Clinical Uses
Beta-lactam antibiotics	
Narrow-spectrum penicillins	
Penicillin G	Treatment of endocarditis due to viridans group streptococci; meningitis due to meningococci or pneumococci; necrotizing fasciitis; pneumonia due to pneumococci; serious group A streptococcal infections; and syphilis and other spirochetal infections.
Penicillin V	Treatment of pharyngitis due to streptococci.
Penicillinase-resistant penicillins	
Dicloxacillin	Treatment of skin and soft tissue infections due to staphylococci.
Nafcillin	Treatment of endocarditis, osteomyelitis, skin and soft tissue infections, and other infections due to staphylococci.
Extended-spectrum penicillins	
Amoxicillin	Prevention of endocarditis in persons at risk.
	Empiric treatment (with clavulanate) of bite wound infections.
	Empiric treatment (with or without clavulanate) of otitis media and sinusitis.
	Treatment of urinary tract infections due to enterococci, *Escherichia coli,* or *Proteus* species.
Ampicillin	Empiric treatment (with sulbactam) of bite wound infections.
	Treatment of urinary tract infections due to enterococci, *E. coli,* or *Proteus* species.
	Treatment (with an aminoglycoside) of endocarditis due to enterococci.
	Treatment (with sulbactam) of intra-abdominal, skin, and soft tissue infections due to gram-positive and anaerobic organisms, including decubitus ulcers and diabetic foot ulcers.
	Treatment (with sulbactam) of meningitis due to *Listeria monocytogenes.*
Piperacillin	Treatment (with an aminoglycoside or with both an aminoglycoside and a beta-lactamase inhibitor) of infections due to *Pseudomonas aeruginosa.*
	Treatment (with or without a beta-lactamase inhibitor) of intra-abdominal, skin, and soft tissue infections due to aerobic and anaerobic organisms.
	Treatment (with or without a beta-lactamase inhibitor) of nosocomial pneumonia due to aerobic and anaerobic organisms.
Ticarcillin	Same as piperacillin.
First-generation cephalosporins	
Cefazolin	Prevention of infections due to staphylococci and aerobic enteric bacilli during surgical procedures.
	Treatment of skin infections due to staphylococci or streptococci.
	Treatment of urinary tract infections due to *E. coli* or other enteric bacilli.
Cephalexin	Treatment of skin infections due to staphylococci or streptococci.
	Treatment of urinary tract infections due to *E. coli* or other enteric bacilli.
Second-generation cephalosporins	
Cefotetan	Prevention of infections due to aerobic and anaerobic gram-negative bacilli during surgical procedures.
	Treatment of diverticulitis, pelvic inflammatory disease, and other infections due to aerobic and anaerobic organisms.
Cefoxitin	Same as cefotetan.
Cefprozil	Empiric treatment of skin and urinary tract infections.
	Treatment of respiratory tract and other infections due to *Moraxella catarrhalis,* penicillinase-producing *Haemophilus influenzae,* or streptococci.
Cefuroxime, oral	Same as cefprozil.
Cefuroxime, parenteral	Empiric treatment of community-acquired pneumonia.
	Treatment of pneumonia due to *Klebsiella pneumoniae.*
	Treatment of respiratory tract infections due to *M. catarrhalis* or penicillinase-producing *H. influenzae.*
Third-generation cephalosporins	
Cefixime	Treatment of otitis media due to *M. catarrhalis* or penicillinase-producing *H. influenzae.*
	Treatment (single-dose therapy) of gonococcal urethritis.
Cefotaxime	Empiric treatment of community-acquired pneumonia.
	Empiric treatment of intra-abdominal infections, meningitis, osteomyelitis, otitis media, skin and soft tissue infections, and urinary tract infections.
	Treatment of Lyme disease, especially with cardiac, neurologic, or rheumatic involvement.
	Treatment (single-dose therapy) of gonorrhea.
Ceftazidime	Treatment of infections with *P. aeruginosa.*
Ceftriaxone	Same as cefotaxime.
Fourth-generation cephalosporins	
Cefepime	Treatment of infections due to multidrug-resistant aerobic gram-negative bacilli.
Monobactams	
Aztreonam	Treatment of infections due to *P. aeruginosa.*
Carbapenems	
Imipenem	Empiric treatment of nosocomial infections.
	Treatment of infections due to multidrug-resistant gram-negative bacilli.
	Treatment of intra-abdominal infections due to aerobic and anaerobic organisms.
Meropenem	Same as imipenem.

Continued

TABLE 38–3. Major Clinical Uses of Bacterial Cell Wall Synthesis Inhibitors (Continued)

Drug	Major Clinical Uses
Other bacterial cell wall synthesis inhibitors	
Bacitracin	Treatment (topical) of staphylococcal and streptococcal infections.
Cycloserine	Treatment of multidrug-resistant tuberculosis.
Fosfomycin	Treatment (single-dose therapy) of uncomplicated urinary tract infections due to *E. coli* or *Enterococcus faecalis.*
Vancomycin	Treatment of enterocolitis due to *Clostridium difficile,* infections due to methicillin-resistant staphylococci, infections due to penicillin-resistant enterococci, and infections due to penicillin-resistant streptococci.

strate for them. It will not inhibit class I beta-lactamase enzymes. Structures of beta-lactamase inhibitors are shown in Fig. 38–5A.

Drug combinations and their routes of administration are as follows: **amoxicillin plus clavulanate** is given orally; **ampicillin plus sulbactam** is given parenterally; **piperacillin plus tazobactam** is given parenterally; and **ticarcillin plus clavulanate** is given parenterally. The major uses of these combinations are listed in Table 38–3.

Cephalosporins
Classification

The cephalosporins are one of the largest and most widely used groups of antibiotics. Based on differences in their antimicrobial spectrum, they have been divided into four generations. Table 38–2 lists examples of each. The first-generation cephalosporins are primarily active against gram-positive cocci and a limited number of gram-negative bacilli. Subsequent generations of cephalosporins have in-

TABLE 38–4. Bacterial Resistance to Beta-Lactam Antibiotics

Mechanism	Examples
Inactivation of the drug by beta-lactamase enzymes	Resistance of gonococci and staphylococci to penicillin G. Resistance of gram-negative bacteria to carbapenems, extended-spectrum penicillins, cefoxitin, and other cephalosporins. Resistance of *Haemophilus influenzae* to amoxicillin and other penicillins.
Reduced affinity of penicillin-binding proteins (PBPs) for the drug	Resistance of enterococci to cephalosporins. Resistance of gram-positive bacteria to aztreonam. Resistance of meningococci, pneumocococci, and strepto-cocci to penicillin G. Resistance of staphylococci to methicillin.
Decreased entry of the drug into bacteria through outer membrane porins	Resistance of gram-negative bacteria to various beta-lactam antibiotics. Resistance of *Pseudomonas aeruginosa* to imipenem.

creased activity against gram-negative bacilli and less activity against some species of gram-positive cocci. With the large number of cephalosporin drugs that are available, it is important to recognize that the members of each generation share many common characteristics.

Drug Properties

Chemistry. The cephalosporins comprise a large group of semisynthetic drugs, most of which are derived from cephalosporin C, a substance obtained from a species of *Cephalosporium* discovered near a sewage outlet off the coast of Sardinia. Cephalosporins have a beta-lactam ring and a dihydrothiazine ring (Fig. 38–6). Unlike the penicillins, the cephalosporins have at least two R groups attached to the molecule, thereby enabling the synthesis of a greater number of derivatives with potentially useful properties. In **cephamycins,** a subcategory of cephalosporins that includes **cefotetan** and **cefoxitin,** there is a third R group that is attached to the beta-lactam ring. By manipulating the structure of cephalosporins, it has been possible to obtain drugs with greater resistance to bacterial beta-lactamases and with a wider range of antimicrobial activity.

Pharmacokinetics. In comparison with penicillins, the cephalosporins are more stable when administered to patients and are less likely to form antigens that evoke hypersensitivity reactions.

The route of administration depends on the particular cephalosporin being used. Some of the cephalosporins are given only orally; others are given only parenterally. **Cefuroxime** is one of the few cephalosporins available for use by both routes (as cefuroxime axetil for oral administration and cefuroxime sodium for parenteral administration). Some of the parenterally administered cephalosporins are used only intravenously; others are given either intravenously or intramuscularly. **Ceftriaxone,** for example, is administered as a single intramuscular injection for the treatment of gonococcal infections.

The orally administered cephalosporins are well absorbed from the gut, and their bioavailability usually is not significantly affected by food.

Most cephalosporins are excreted primarily by renal tubular secretion, but ceftriaxone is excreted primarily in the bile. For this reason, ceftriaxone has a much longer half-life than other cephalosporins.

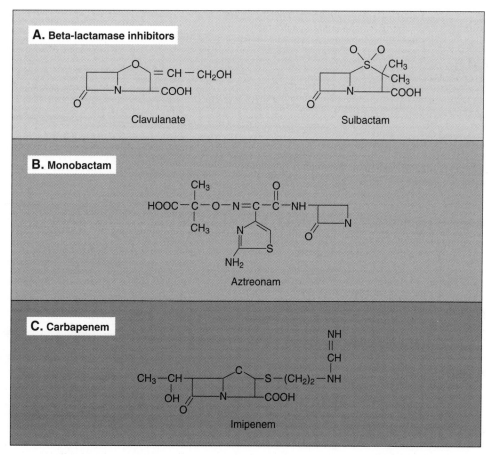

FIGURE 38–5. Structures of selected beta-lactamase inhibitors, monobactams, and carbapenems. (A) Each beta-lactamase inhibitor has a beta-lactam ring that is fused with a unique heterocyclic structure. (B) Each monobactam has a beta-lactam ring that is not fused with another ring structure. (C) Each carbapenem has a carbon substituted for the sulfur atom in the ring that is fused with the beta-lactam ring.

Spectrum and Indications. Table 38–3 outlines the spectrum and major clinical uses of cephalosporins.

The **first-generation cephalosporins** have good activity against most streptococci and methicillin-sensitive staphylococci. They are also active against a few gram-negative enteric bacilli, including *E. coli* and *Klebsiella pneumoniae.* The orally administered drugs, such as **cephalexin,** are primarily used to treat skin and soft tissue infections caused by gram-positive cocci and to treat uncomplicated urinary tract infections caused by susceptible organisms. The parenterally administered drugs, such as **cefazolin,** are used to treat more serious infections caused by these organisms. Cefazolin is also widely employed for surgical prophylaxis of infections due to staphylococci and aerobic gram-negative enteric bacilli.

In comparison with first-generation cephalosporins, the **second-generation cephalosporins** have similar activity against gram-positive cocci while demonstrating increased activity against gram-negative bacilli. In addition, the second-generation drugs are active against many strains of *H. influenzae* and have been used to treat respiratory tract and other infections due to this organism. Many oral second-generation drugs, including **cefprozil** and **cefuroxime axetil,** are used to treat otitis media, particularly when it is due to *H. influenzae* strains that are resistant to amoxicillin and other drugs. **Cefuroxime**

sodium, a parenteral preparation, has been used as empiric therapy for patients with community-acquired pneumonia. Some second-generation drugs, such as **cefotetan** and **cefoxitin,** have activity against anaerobic gram-negative bacilli, including *Bacteroides fragilis,* and are used to treat pelvic inflammatory disease and other infections due to aerobic and anaerobic gram-negative bacilli.

In comparison with second-generation cephalosporins, the **third-generation cephalosporins** have greater activity against a wider range of gram-negative organisms, including enteric gram-negative bacilli, *H. influenzae,* and *Moraxella catarrhalis.* A few third-generation drugs, such as **ceftazidime,** are active against *P. aeruginosa.* Several third-generation drugs, including **cefixime, cefotaxime,** and **ceftriaxone,** are active against gonococci and have been used as a single-dose treatment for gonorrhea. Other clinical indications for third-generation drugs include otitis media, pneumonia, meningitis, intra-abdominal or urinary tract infections, and Lyme disease.

Cefepime is a new cephalosporin that has been classified as a **fourth-generation cephalosporin,** based on its broad antimicrobial activity. In comparison with other cephalosporins, cefepime is active against a greater percentage of gram-negative enteric bacteria. Cefepime is also active against many drug-resistant strains of streptococci. Cefepime is primarily indicated for the treatment of infections due to multidrug-resistant bacteria. The superior activity of

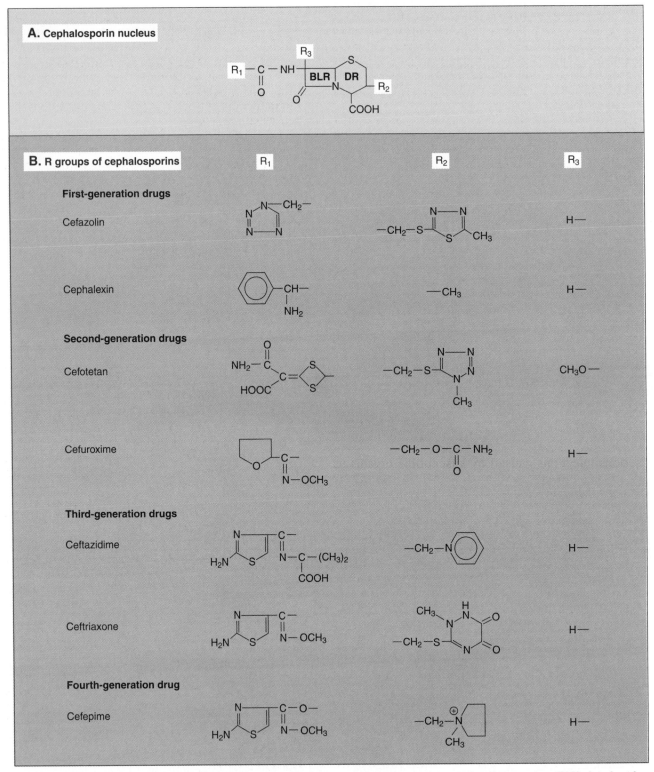

FIGURE 38–6. Structures of selected cephalosporins. (A) Each cephalosporin contains a beta-lactam ring (BLR) fused with a dihydrothiazine ring (DR). **(B)** All cephalosporins are semisynthetic drugs with a unique group at the R_1 and R_2 positions. Cefotetan contains a methoxy substitution at the R_3 position and is therefore called a cephamycin antibiotic. The R_1 groups of third- and fourth-generation drugs are quite similar, whereas the R_2 groups of these drugs differ markedly.

cefepime appears to be related to its ability to inhibit organisms that either produce an excessive amount of cephalosporinase or produce a more active beta-lactamase enzyme.

Bacterial Resistance. Bacteria acquire resistance to cephalosporins through the same three mechanisms by which they acquire resistance to penicillins (see Table 38–4). The cephalosporins are more resistant to beta-lactamases than are the penicillins, and resistance to gram-negative beta-lactamases increases with successive generations of cephalosporins. However, many cephalosporins are susceptible to certain types of beta-lactamases, and some cephalosporins (including cefoxitin) induce these enzymes.

Adverse Effects. The cephalosporins cause little toxicity to the host and have an excellent safety record. Although they can elicit hypersensitivity reactions, the incidence of this is lower for cephalosporins than for most penicillins. Cephalosporins exhibit some cross-sensitivity with penicillins. On the one hand, a person who has had a mild hypersensitivity reaction to a penicillin will usually not cross-react to a cephalosporin. On the other hand, a person who has had a severe hypersensitivity reaction to a penicillin, such as an anaphylactic reaction, has a greater risk of cross-reacting and should usually not be given a cephalosporin.

A few cephalosporins can cause platelet dysfunction and bleeding. Some cephalosporins may produce a disulfiramlike reaction if they are taken with alcohol.

Monobactams

Aztreonam is a monocyclic beta-lactam (monobactam) antibiotic (see Fig. 38–5B). It is active against many gram-negative bacilli, including about 90% of strains of *P. aeruginosa*. Aztreonam is used to treat serious infections caused by susceptible organisms and is particularly useful for infections caused by multidrug-resistant strains of *P. aeruginosa*. The drug is administered intravenously and is extensively metabolized before undergoing renal excretion. Aztreonam sometimes causes nausea, vomiting, and diarrhea. Its most common serious adverse effects are seizures and leukopenia. The latter is due to bone marrow suppression.

Carbapenems

Imipenem and **meropenem** are penicillinlike antibiotics in which the sulfur atom of the thiazolidine ring is replaced with a carbon atom (see Fig. 38–5C). These antibiotics, called carbapenems, are bactericidal to a wide range of gram-positive and gram-negative bacteria, including many aerobic and anaerobic gram-negative bacilli. Imipenem has high affinity for PBP-2, whereas meropenem binds to both PBP-2 and PBP-3. The greater affinity of meropenem for PBP-3 appears to account for its superior activity against many Enterobacteriaceae, *P. aeruginosa,* and other gram-negative organisms. Imipenem and meropenem are primarily used for the empiric treatment of serious nosocomial infections, for infections caused by multidrug-resistant organisms, and for mixed intra-abdominal infections caused by aerobic and anaerobic enteric bacilli.

Imipenem and meropenem are administered intravenously. Unlike meropenem, imipenem is rapidly inactivated by renal dehydropeptidase. For this reason, imipenem is coadministered with a dehydropeptidase inhibitor called **cilastatin.** Imipenem and meropenem are primarily eliminated in the urine by the process of renal tubular secretion. Dosage adjustments are required when either drug is given to persons with renal impairment. Probenecid interacts with imipenem and meropenem, causing inhibition of their renal excretion.

The carbapenems exhibit cross-sensitivity with penicillins, cephalosporins, and other beta-lactam antibiotics and should not be administered to patients who are allergic to these drugs. The carbapenems are generally well tolerated, but they can cause seizures in patients with epilepsy, so they should be used cautiously in these patients. Imipenem and meropenem sometimes cause hematologic reactions, including anemia, leukopenia, thrombocytopenia, and altered bleeding time.

OTHER BACTERIAL CELL WALL SYNTHESIS INHIBITORS

Vancomycin

Vancomycin is a glycopeptide antibiotic. Because it has activity against various gram-positive cocci and bacilli, including some strains that are resistant to penicillin, it is often used to treat staphylococcal or enterococcal endocarditis, staphylococcal osteomyelitis, streptococcal necrotizing fasciitis, and other serious infections that are caused by penicillin-resistant organisms. Nevertheless, some strains of staphylococci and streptococci have acquired resistance to vancomycin. This resistance is conferred by chromosomal or plasmid genes, which alter the structure of the cell wall pentapeptide component containing D-alanine.

Vancomycin is also active against some *Bacillus, Clostridium,* and *Corynebacterium* species. Although it is occasionally used to treat diarrhea and pseudomembranous colitis due to *C. difficile,* metronidazole is usually preferred for this indication because of its much lower cost.

Vancomycin is poorly absorbed from the gut and must be administered parenterally for the treatment of systemic infections. It is administered orally, however, for the treatment of gastrointestinal infections. Vancomycin is distributed to most body fluids and tissues, and it is excreted in the urine by the process of glomerular filtration. The half-life of vancomycin is normally about 6 hours (see Table 38–2), but the half-life is markedly prolonged in patients with renal failure.

Improvements in the manufacturing of vancomycin preparations have reduced the incidence of nephrotoxicity and ototoxicity associated with their use. Even though vancomycin-induced nephrotoxicity is now rare, vancomycin should be used cautiously with other nephrotoxic drugs, including aminoglycosides and amphotericin B. Ototoxic effects of vancomycin may include both vestibular dysfunction (ataxia, vertigo, nystagmus, and nausea) and cochlear dysfunction (tinnitus and hearing loss). Ototoxicity is usually due to excessive serum concentrations and is reversible when these concentrations are reduced.

Bacitracin

Bacitracin is an antibiotic derived from a *Bacillus subtilis* strain isolated from a girl named Tracy. The drug inhibits cell wall peptidoglycan synthesis by blocking the regeneration of bactoprenol phosphate, the lipid carrier molecule (see Fig. 38–2). Bacitracin is active against gram-positive cocci, including staphylococci and streptococci, and it is primarily used for the topical treatment of minor skin and ocular infections. It is often combined with polymyxin or neomycin in ointments and creams. Bacitracin is quite nephrotoxic, so it is no longer used systemically.

Cycloserine

Cycloserine is a moderately toxic antibiotic that is primarily used to treat multidrug-resistant tuberculosis. It can be used for this purpose because it does not exhibit cross-resistance with other antitubercular drugs.

Cycloserine is a structural analogue of D-alanine. It inhibits the transpeptidase enzyme that breaks the bond between D-alanine residues during cross-linking of the peptidoglycan portion of the cell wall (see Fig. 38–2). It also inhibits L-alanine racemase and D-alanine synthetase, which are two enzymes required for incorporation of D-alanine into the peptidoglycan pentapeptide.

Cycloserine is administered orally and is mostly excreted unchanged in the urine. The drug causes central nervous system side effects, including sedation, headache, tremor, vertigo, confusion, and psychotic states. For this reason, it is used only when other antitubercular drugs are ineffective or are not tolerated.

Fosfomycin

Fosfomycin is a newer antibiotic that blocks one of the first steps in cell wall peptidoglycan synthesis, the formation of UDP-MurNAc. Fosfomycin is structurally similar to phosphoenolpyruvate. By irreversibly inhibiting the enzyme enolpyruvyl transferase, fosfomycin blocks the addition of phosphoenolpyruvate to UDP-GlcNAc and thereby prevents the synthesis of UDP-MurNAc.

Fosfomycin is active against enterococci and many gram-negative enteric bacilli, including *E. coli*, *Citrobacter* species, *Klebsiella* species, *Proteus* species, and *Serratia marcescens*. The drug is specifically approved by the Food and Drug Administration for the treatment of uncomplicated urinary tract infections due to *E. coli* or *Enterococcus faecalis*. For this purpose, fosfomycin is administered orally as a single dose. The drug is excreted unchanged in the urine and feces and has a half-life of about 6 hours. Fosfomycin sometimes causes diarrhea but is otherwise well tolerated and is associated with few adverse effects.

Summary of Important Points

- Beta-lactam antibiotics, vancomycin, bacitracin, cycloserine, and fosfomycin are drugs that inhibit bacterial cell wall synthesis.
- The beta-lactam antibiotics inhibit the transpeptidase reaction that cross-links the peptidoglycan component of the cell wall. These antibiotics include penicillins, cephalosporins, monobactams, and carbapenems.
- A beta-lactamase inhibitor, such as clavulanate, sulbactam, or tazobactam, is administered in combination with a beta-lactam antibiotic to prevent degradation of the antibiotic by bacteria.
- Narrow-spectrum penicillins (such as penicillin G) are primarily active against gram-positive cocci and spirochetes; penicillinase-resistant penicillins (such as dicloxacillin and nafcillin) are used to treat staphylococcal infections; and extended-spectrum penicillins (such as amoxicillin and ticarcillin) are active against various gram-negative bacilli.
- Acid-stable penicillins (such as penicillin V, amoxicillin, and dicloxacillin) can be given orally, whereas acid-labile drugs (such as piperacillin and ticarcillin) must be given parenterally.
- Most penicillins are eliminated primarily by renal tubular secretion, a process that is inhibited by probenecid. Two long-acting forms of penicillin G (procaine and benzathine penicillin G) are available for intramuscular administration.
- Penicillins may elicit any of the four types of hypersensitivity reactions, including anaphylactic shock and other immediate hypersensitivity reactions mediated by IgE.
- Cephalosporins are semisynthetic antibiotics that are subdivided into four generations on the basis of their antimicrobial spectrum. The activity against gram-negative organisms increases from the first to the fourth generation.
- Some cephalosporins (such as cefazolin) are eliminated by renal tubular secretion, whereas others (such as ceftriaxone) are eliminated in the bile. Ceftriaxone has a much longer half-life than other cephalosporins, enabling it to be used as single-dose treatment for certain infections, including gonorrhea.
- Vancomycin is a glycopeptide antibiotic that is active against gram-positive organisms, including methicillin-sensitive and methicillin-resistant staphylococci, enterococci, and *Clostridium*.
- Bacitracin is used topically for infections due to gram-positive cocci. Cycloserine is primarily employed in the treatment of multidrug-resistant tuberculosis. Fosfomycin is administered as a single-dose treatment for uncomplicated urinary tract infections due to *E. coli* or enterococci.

Selected Readings

Canafax, D. M., et al. Amoxicillin middle ear fluid penetration and pharmacokinetics in children with acute otitis media. Pediatr Infect Dis J 17:149–156, 1998.

Flores, P. A., and S. M. Gordon. Vancomycin-resistant *Staphylococcus aureus:* an emerging public health threat. Cleve Clin J Med 64:527–532, 1997.

Gentry, C. A. Retrospective evaluation of therapies for *Staphylococcus aureus* endocarditis. Pharmacotherapy 17:990–997, 1997.

Iaconis, J. P., et al. Comparison of antibacterial activities of meropenem and six other antimicrobials against *Pseudomonas aeruginosa* isolates from North American studies and clinical trials. Clin Infect Dis 24(supplement 2):S191–S196, 1997.

Manduru, M., et al. Comparative bactericidal activity of ceftazidime against isolates of *Pseudomonas aeruginosa* as assessed in an in vitro pharmacodynamic model versus the traditional time-kill method. Antimicrob Agents Chemother 41:2527–2532, 1997.

Murray, B. E. Vancomycin-resistant enterococci. Am J Med 102:284–293, 1997.

Nicas, T. I., et al. Beyond vancomycin: new therapies to meet the challenge of glycopeptide resistance. Trends Microbiol 5:240–249, 1997.

Pichichero, M. E., et al. Cefprozil treatment of persistent and recurrent acute otitis media. Pediatr Infect Dis J 16:471–478, 1997.

Stein, G. E. Single-dose treatment of acute cystitis with fosfomycin. Ann Pharmacother 32:215–219, 1998.

Varsana, I., et al. Intramuscular ceftriaxone compared with oral amoxicillin-clavulanate for treatment of acute otitis media in children. Eur J Pediatr 156:858–863, 1997.

Walton, M. A., et al. The use of aztreonam as an alternative therapy for multi-resistant *Pseudomonas aeruginosa.* Burns 23:225–227, 1997.

CHAPTER THIRTY-NINE

INHIBITORS OF BACTERIAL

PROTEIN SYNTHESIS

CLASSIFICATION OF INHIBITORS OF BACTERIAL PROTEIN SYNTHESIS

DRUGS THAT AFFECT THE 30S RIBOSOMAL SUBUNIT
  Aminoglycosides
  - Amikacin
  - Gentamicin
  - Neomycin
  - Streptomycin
  - Tobramycin

  Tetracyclines
  - Doxycycline
  - Minocycline
  - Tetracycline

  Other antibiotics
  - Spectinomycin

DRUGS THAT AFFECT THE 50S RIBOSOMAL SUBUNIT
  Macrolides
  - Azithromycin
  - Clarithromycin
  - Dirithromycin
  - Erythromycin

  Other antibiotics
  - Chloramphenicol
  - Clindamycin
  - Quinupristin-dalfopristin

OTHER BACTERIAL PROTEIN SYNTHESIS INHIBITORS
  - Mupirocin

OVERVIEW

After the introduction of penicillin, scientists began an extensive search for antibiotics that could inhibit penicillin-resistant bacteria. A number of *Streptomyces* species were isolated from soil samples collected from all over the world, and these species eventually yielded several new classes of antibiotics, including the aminoglycosides, tetracyclines, and macrolides. Streptomycin, an aminoglycoside, was the first new antibiotic to be introduced through these efforts.

Bacterial Protein Synthesis

In the new classes of antibiotics, most of the drugs act by selectively blocking one or more steps in the protein synthesis of bacteria (prokaryotes) while having relatively little effect on the protein synthesis of humans (eukaryotes). The selectivity for bacterial protein synthesis appears to result from differences in the structure and function of ribosomes in prokaryotic versus eukaryotic organisms.

Each ribosome has two subunits. The **ribosome in prokaryotes** is composed of a 30S subunit and a 50S subunit (with S denoting the Svedberg unit of flotation, which forms the basis for the separation and isolation of ribosomal subunits from cell homogenates). In contrast, the **ribosome in eukaryotes** is composed of a 40S and a 60S subunit, and the proteins that initiate and carry out translation of messenger RNA (mRNA) in eukaryotic systems are more complex and function differently than the proteins of bacterial systems.

The basic steps in bacterial protein synthesis are illustrated in Fig. 39–1. These steps include the binding of aminoacyl transfer RNA (tRNA) to the ribosome, the formation of a peptide bond, and translocation. Aminoacyl tRNA binds to the 30S ribosomal subunit, whereas peptide bond formation and translocation involve components of the 50S ribosomal subunit.

Sites of Drug Action

As shown in Fig. 39–1, each type of antibiotic discussed in this chapter acts at a specific site on the ribosome to inhibit one or more particular steps in protein synthesis. Tetracyclines, aminoglycosides, and spectinomycin act at the **30S ribosomal subunit.** Macrolides, chloramphenicol, dalfopristin, and clindamycin act at the **50S ribosomal subunit.**

Tetracyclines competitively block binding of tRNA to the 30S subunit and thereby prevent the addition of new amino acids to the growing peptide chain. This reversible effect is responsible for the bacteriostatic action of tetracyclines.

Aminoglycosides and **spectinomycin** bind primarily to the 30S subunit, where they interfere with the initiation of protein synthesis. They also cause

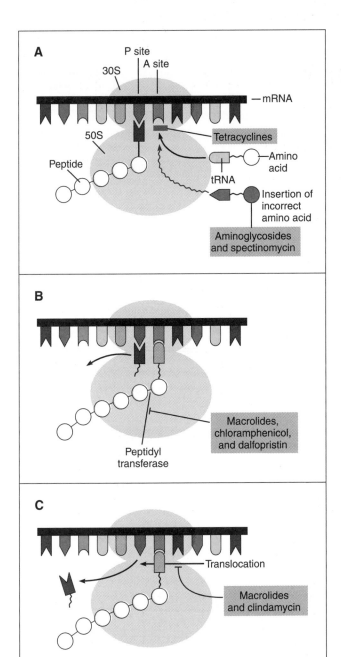

FIGURE 39–1. Bacterial protein synthesis and sites of drug action. The bacterial ribosome is composed of a 30S subunit and a 50S subunit. The steps in protein synthesis and translation of messenger RNA (mRNA) include the binding of aminoacyl transfer RNA (tRNA) to the ribosome, the formation of a peptide bond, and translocation. **(A)** Under normal circumstances, the nascent peptide is attached to the ribosome at the peptidyl site (P site), and the next aminoacyl tRNA binds to the acceptor or aminoacyl site (A site). Tetracyclines block aminoacyl tRNA from binding to the A site. Aminoglycosides and spectinomycin cause misreading of the genetic code, which leads to binding of the wrong aminoacyl tRNA and insertion of the wrong amino acid into the nascent peptide. **(B)** Macrolides, chloramphenicol, and dalfopristin block peptidyl transferase, the enzyme that catalyzes the formation of a peptide bond between the nascent peptide and the amino acid attached to the A site. **(C)** Macrolides and clindamycin block the translocation step in which the nascent peptide is transferred from the A site to the P site following the formation of a new peptide bond.

misreading of the genetic code so that the wrong amino acid is inserted into the protein structure. These irreversible actions account for the bactericidal effects of aminoglycosides and spectinomycin.

Macrolides, chloramphenicol, and **dalfopristin** block peptidyl transferase, the enzyme that catalyzes the formation of a peptide bond between the new amino acid and the nascent peptide. **Macrolides** and **clindamycin** prevent translocation of the nascent peptide from the acceptor or aminoacyl site (A site) to the peptidyl site (P site) on the ribosome, and this in turn prevents binding of the next aminoacyl tRNA to the ribosome.

DRUGS THAT AFFECT THE 30S RIBOSOMAL SUBUNIT

Aminoglycosides

The aminoglycosides include **amikacin, gentamicin, neomycin, streptomycin,** and **tobramycin.** The properties and major clinical uses of these drugs are compared in Tables 39–1 and 39–2.

Drug Properties

Chemistry and Pharmacokinetics. All aminoglycosides are composed of amino sugars linked through glycosidic bonds (Fig. 39–2A). The amino groups are highly basic and become extensively protonated and ionized in body fluids. Their highly ionized structure determines many of their pharmacokinetic properties, including their absorption, distribution, and excretion.

The aminoglycosides are poorly absorbed from the gut and must be administered parenterally for the treatment of systemic infections. Occasionally, they are administered orally to treat gastrointestinal infections such as neonatal necrotizing enterocolitis. They are also administered topically to treat infections of the skin, mucous membranes, and ocular tissues.

Because of their highly ionized nature, aminoglycosides do not penetrate body cells. As a result, their volumes of distribution are similar to the extracellular fluid volume. Aminoglycosides do not penetrate the meninges very well, even when the meninges are inflamed, so intrathecal administration may be required to treat meningitis.

The aminoglycosides are not metabolized. They are excreted primarily by the process of renal glomerular filtration, with little tubular reabsorption. The renal clearance of aminoglycosides is approximately equal to the creatinine clearance, since creatinine is also filtered at the glomerulus but is not secreted or reabsorbed significantly by the tubules. Because the clearance of aminoglycosides is proportional to the glomerular filtration rate, the dosage of aminoglycosides must be reduced in patients with renal impairment. In most cases, this is accomplished by increasing the interval between doses.

The plasma concentrations of aminoglycosides are routinely measured to ensure adequate dosage

TABLE 39-1. Pharmacokinetic Properties of Bacterial Protein Synthesis Inhibitors*

Drug	Route of Administration	Oral Bioavailability	Elimination Half-Life (Hours)	Primary Route of Elimination
Drugs that affect the 30S ribosomal subunit				
Aminoglycosides				
Amikacin	IV	NA	2.5	Renal excretion.
Gentamicin	IV or topical	NA	1.5	Renal excretion.
Neomycin	Topical	NA	NA	NA.
Streptomycin	IM	NA	2.0	Renal excretion.
Tobramycin	IV or topical	NA	2.5	Renal excretion.
Tetracyclines				
Doxycycline	Oral or IV	90%	20.0	Fecal and renal excretion.
Minocycline	Oral or IV	95%	20.0	Biliary and renal excretion.
Tetracycline	Oral or IV	70%	10.0	Renal excretion.
Other antibiotics				
Spectinomycin	IM	NA	2.0	Renal excretion.
Drugs that affect the 50S ribosomal subunit				
Macrolides				
Azithromycin	Oral	37%	12.0	Biliary excretion.
Clarithromycin	Oral	62%	5.0	Biliary and renal excretion.
Dirithromycin	Oral	10%	44.0	Fecal excretion of active metabolite.
Erythromycin	Oral, IV, or topical	35% ± 25%	2.0	Biliary excretion.
Other antibiotics				
Chloramphenicol	Oral, IV, or topical	95%	3.0	Hepatic metabolism; renal excretion.
Clindamycin	Oral, IV, or topical	95%	2.5	Hepatic metabolism; renal, biliary, and fecal excretion.
Quinupristin-dalfopristin	IV	NA	0.8/0.4†	Hepatic metabolism; biliary excretion.
Other bacterial protein synthesis inhibitors				
Mupirocin	Topical	NA	NA	NA.

*Values shown are the mean of values reported in the literature. IV = intravenous; IM = intramuscular; and NA = not applicable.
†The half-lives for quinupristin and dalfopristin are 0.8 and 0.4 hours, respectively. The drugs are given in combination.

and to minimize toxicity. The peak concentration is usually found about 30 minutes after completing an intravenous infusion of an aminoglycoside, whereas the trough concentration is found prior to administration of the next dose. Optimal peak and trough concentrations have been established and can be used to guide dosage adjustments for individuals receiving the standard regimen of three daily doses given at 8-hour intervals. For example, therapeutic concentrations of gentamicin and tobramycin are usually between 4 and 8 mg/L. A peak concentration above 12 mg/L or a trough concentration above 2 mg/L is considered toxic and indicates the need to reduce the dosage of gentamicin or tobramycin. Therapeutic concentrations of amikacin are between 16 and 32 mg/L, and the toxic peak and trough concentrations are above 35 mg/L and above 10 mg/L, respectively.

Spectrum and Indications.   In comparison with other classes of drugs, the aminoglycosides have greater activity against aerobic gram-negative bacilli but are often more toxic. While the less toxic classes of drugs are preferred for management of patients whenever possible, aminoglycosides continue to be

extensively used for prophylaxis and treatment of serious infections. As discussed below, the specific aminoglycoside drugs differ in terms of their antimicrobial spectrum.

Bacterial Resistance.   Resistance to aminoglycosides is primarily due to inactivation of the drugs by bacterial acetylase, adenylase, and phosphorylase enzymes (Table 39–3). These enzymes attach acetyl, adenyl, or phosphoryl moieties to the amino groups on the antibiotics, thereby preventing inhibition of bacterial protein synthesis. Resistance to aminoglycosides may also be due to decreased binding of the drugs to the 30S ribosomal subunit or to decreased uptake of the drugs via porins in bacterial membranes. Both plasmid and chromosomal genes may be involved in resistance that is due to enzymatic inactivation of the antibiotics, whereas only chromosomal genes are involved in resistance that is due to decreased binding or decreased uptake.

Adverse Effects.   The major adverse effects of aminoglycosides are nephrotoxicity and ototoxicity. The risk of toxicity is related to the dosage and duration of treatment and varies with the specific drug. Irreversible toxicity may occur, even after use of the drug is discontinued, but serious toxicity is less likely if the offending drug is discontinued at the earliest sign of dysfunction.

Aminoglycosides are the most common cause of drug-induced renal failure. When the drugs accumulate in proximal tubule cells, they can cause acute tubular necrosis. This reduces the level of renal function and leads to a rise in plasma concentrations of the aminoglycosides. The elevated drug concentrations may further impair renal function and contribute to ototoxicity. For this reason, it is important to monitor renal function and plasma aminoglycoside concentrations and to adjust the aminoglycoside dosage accordingly.

Ototoxicity is associated with the accumulation of aminoglycosides in the labyrinth and in the hair cells of the cochlea. Patients may suffer from both vestibular and cochlear toxicity. Manifestations of vestibular toxicity include dizziness, impaired vision, nystagmus, vertigo, nausea, vomiting, and problems with postural balance and walking. Cochlear toxicity is characterized by tinnitus and hearing impairment and may lead to irreversible deafness. There is often a delay between the beginning of drug administration and the onset of symptoms, so many hospitalized patients are ambulatory before signs of toxicity appear.

Specific Drugs

The aminoglycosides differ in their potential to cause toxicity and in their antimicrobial activity.

TABLE 39–2. Major Clinical Uses of Bacterial Protein Synthesis Inhibitors

Drug	Major Clinical Uses
Drugs that affect the 30S ribosomal subunit	
Aminoglycosides	
Amikacin	Treatment of serious infections due to aerobic gram-negative bacilli, including *Pseudomonas aeruginosa.* Treatment (with a penicillin or other appropriate antibiotic) of serious infections due to enterococci, staphylococci, or viridans group streptococci.
Gentamicin	Same as amikacin.
Neomycin	Empiric treatment (usually with bacitracin and polymyxin) of superficial infections of the skin and mucous membranes.
Streptomycin	Treatment of plague, tularemia, and multidrug-resistant tuberculosis.
Tobramycin	Same as amikacin.
Tetracyclines	
Doxycycline	Treatment of brucellosis, cholera, ehrlichiosis, granuloma inguinale, Lyme disease, or relapsing fever. Treatment of infections due to *Chlamydia* species, *Helicobacter pylori, Mycoplasma pneumoniae, Propionibacterium acnes,* or *Rickettsia* species.
Minocycline	Same as doxycycline.
Tetracycline	Same as doxycycline.
Other antibiotics	
Spectinomycin	Treatment of gonorrhea due to penicillinase-producing gonococci.
Drugs that affect the 50S ribosomal subunit	
Macrolides	
Azithromycin	Treatment of infections due to *Chlamydia* species or *Mycobacterium avium-intracellulare.* Treatment of otitis media due to *Haemophilus influenzae* or *Moraxella catarrhalis.*
Clarithromycin	Treatment of infections due to *M. avium-intracellulare.* Treatment of respiratory tract and other infections due to *Chlamydia* species, *M. pneumoniae,* or streptococci. Treatment (with other drugs) of peptic ulcers due to *H. pylori.*
Dirithromycin	Treatment of acute bronchitis due to gram-positive cocci, *H. influenzae,* or *M. catarrhalis.* Treatment of community-acquired pneumonia due to *Legionella pneumophila, M. pneumoniae,* or pneumococci.
Erythromycin	Treatment of community-acquired pneumonia due to *Chlamydia pneumoniae, L. pneumophila, M. pneumoniae,* or pneumococci. Treatment of *Corynebacterium diphtheriae* infections or carrier state.
Other antibiotics	
Chloramphenicol	Treatment of *Bacteroides* infections, *Salmonella* infections, or meningitis due to organisms that are resistant to other antibiotics.
Clindamycin	Treatment of infections due to anaerobic streptococci or *Bacteroides* species. Treatment of streptococcal infections that are resistant to penicillins or other antibiotics.
Quinupristin-dalfopristin	Treatment of bacteremia, pneumonia, and skin and soft tissue infections due to enterococci, staphylococci, or streptococci that are resistant to vancomycin or other antibiotics.
Other bacterial protein synthesis inhibitors	
Mupirocin	Treatment of impetigo and other skin infections due to staphylococci or streptococci.

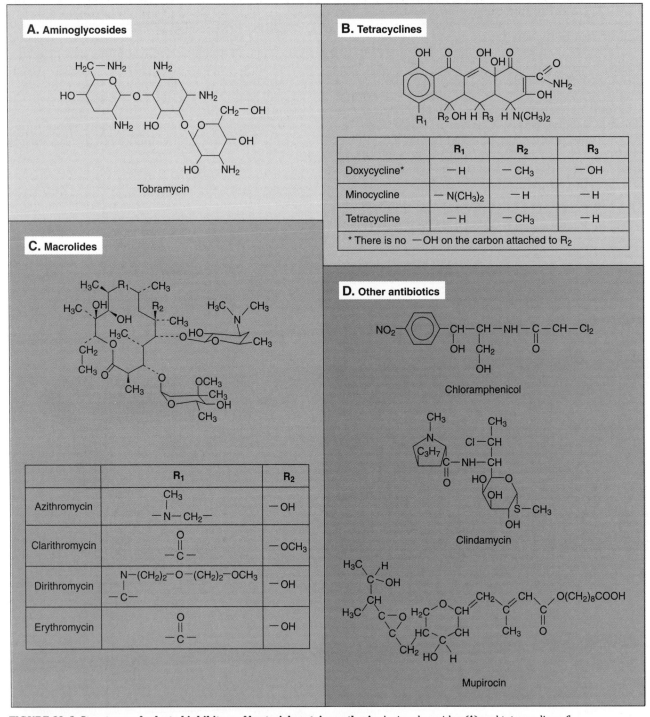

FIGURE 39–2. Structures of selected inhibitors of bacterial protein synthesis. Aminoglycosides **(A)** and tetracyclines (
affect the 30S ribosomal subunit. Macrolides **(C)** and chloramphenicol and clindamycin **(D)** are drugs that affect the 50S ril
Mupirocin competes with isoleucine and prevents the addition of isoleucine to nascent peptides during protein synth

Of the five aminoglycosides listed in Table 39–2, streptomycin is the least toxic, but it is also the least active against *Pseudomonas aeruginosa* and other gram-negative bacilli. Streptomycin is primarily used to treat multidrug-resistant tuberculosis and infections due to *Yersinia pestis* (plague) and *Francisella tularensis* (tularemia).

Amikacin, gentamicin, and tobramycin have superior activity against most members of the family Enterobacteriaceae and against *P. aeruginosa*. Tobra-

mycin has the greatest activity against most strains of *P. aeruginosa,* whereas gentamicin is usually more active against *Serratia* species than are other aminoglycosides. Gentamicin is also used in combination with a penicillin or other appropriate antibiotic for the treatment of serious enterococcal, staphylococcal, or viridans group streptococcal infections. Amikacin is more resistant to inactivation by acetylases, adenylases, and phosphorylases than are gentamicin and tobramycin, so it can be used to treat infections

TABLE 39–3. Bacterial Resistance to Protein Synthesis Inhibitors

Mechanism	Examples
Inactivation of the drug by bacterial enzymes	Inactivation of aminoglycosides by acetylase, adenylase, and phosphorylase enzymes. Inactivation of chloramphenicol by acetyltransferase.
Decreased binding of the drug	Decreased binding of aminoglycosides to the 30S ribosomal subunit. Decreased binding of macrolides and clindamycin to the 50S ribosomal subunit.
Decreased accumulation of the drug by bacteria	Active removal of macrolides from bacteria via membrane proteins. Decreased uptake of aminoglycosides via porins in bacterial membranes. Decreased uptake of tetracyclines via porins in bacterial membranes.

due to organisms that are resistant to these drugs. Because amikacin is the most expensive aminoglycoside, it is generally reserved for use against organisms that are resistant to other aminoglycosides.

The aminoglycosides vary in their propensity to cause cochlear or vestibular toxicity. Amikacin produces more cochlear toxicity, whereas gentamicin and streptomycin cause more vestibular toxicity. Tobramycin appears to cause similar degrees of cochlear and vestibular toxicity.

Neomycin is the most nephrotoxic aminoglycoside, so its use is limited to topical treatment of superficial infections. Neomycin is available in ointments and creams and is usually combined with bacitracin and polymyxin in triple antibiotic preparations. Bacitracin provides gram-positive coverage, polymyxin provides gram-negative coverage, and neomycin is active against both gram-positive and gram-negative organisms. Neomycin can elicit hypersensitivity reactions, especially with long-term topical administration. Partly for this reason, products containing only bacitracin and polymyxin are also available and may be used by individuals who are allergic to neomycin.

Tetracyclines

The tetracyclines include **doxycycline, minocycline,** and **tetracycline.** The properties and major clinical uses of these drugs are outlined in Tables 39–1 and 39–2.

Drug Properties

Chemistry and Pharmacokinetics. The tetracycline antibiotics are anthracene derivatives, some of which are produced by various *Streptomyces* species. Doxycycline, minocycline, and tetracycline (see Fig. 39–2B) are semisynthetic derivatives of two older tetracycline antibiotics, chlortetracycline and oxytetracycline. As discussed below, the various drugs in the tetracycline class are primarily distinguished by their pharmacokinetic properties.

Spectrum and Indications. The tetracyclines are broad-spectrum, bacteriostatic drugs that have similar antimicrobial activities and inhibit the growth of many gram-positive and gram-negative organisms, rickettsiae, spirochetes, mycoplasmas, and chlamydiae.

Tetracyclines are the drugs of choice for Rocky Mountain spotted fever and other infections caused by *Rickettsia* species. They are also the drugs of choice for the treatment of two spirochetal infections, Lyme disease and relapsing fever, which are caused by *Borrelia burgdorferi* and *Borrelia recurrentis,* respectively. Tetracyclines can be used as alternatives to macrolides for the treatment of infections caused by *Mycoplasma pneumoniae.* For most genital infections caused by *Chlamydia trachomatis,* the Centers for Disease Control and Prevention recommends a 7-day course of oral doxycycline. For pelvic inflammatory disease caused by chlamydiae, intravenous doxycycline may be necessary.

Tetracyclines (especially minocycline) are used in the management of acne vulgaris and are usually the most effective drugs for the treatment of moderately severe acne. Tetracyclines and other antibiotics are used to treat acne because they suppress the growth of *Propionibacterium acnes,* an organism that is found on the skin and may infect sebaceous glands. This organism converts sebum triglycerides to fatty acids, which then cause skin irritation and contribute to sebaceous gland inflammation and the formation of comedones.

Tetracyclines are used in the treatment of brucellosis, ehrlichiosis, and granuloma inguinale. While oral rehydration therapy is the most important treatment modality for persons suffering from severe diarrhea caused by *Vibrio cholerae,* a tetracycline may be used to shorten the course of cholera and reduce the risk of disease transmission to other persons. A tetracycline is included in some regimens for the treatment of peptic ulcers due to *Helicobacter pylori.*

Although tetracyclines continue to inhibit the growth of a wide range of bacteria, they are infrequently used today to treat infections caused by many gram-positive cocci and gram-negative bacilli because strains of these organisms have become resistant.

Bacterial Resistance. Resistance to tetracyclines is widespread and is due to the transmission of R factors by bacterial conjugation. The R factors usually confer resistance to tetracyclines via altered bacterial porins that prevent bacterial uptake of the drugs. The practice of including tetracyclines in animal feeds for the purpose of promoting weight gain probably contributed significantly to the development and transmission of tetracycline resistance around the world.

Adverse Effects. Tetracyclines can cause a large number of adverse effects, including several that are potentially life-threatening. However, these effects can be avoided in most cases by careful screening of patients before the drugs are administered.

Tetracyclines are concentrated in growing teeth and bone. Their use by pregnant women or children under 8 years of age may cause discoloration of the teeth and hypoplasia of the enamel. In affected children, marked yellow-brown or gray mottling of a significant portion of the enamel of the front teeth occurs and is cosmetically unattractive.

Tetracyclines may cause potentially severe nephrotoxicity and hepatotoxicity in the form of fatty degeneration. Both of these reactions are rare, but the fact that pregnant women are at increased risk of hepatotoxicity is another reason for not administering tetracyclines to this population. Use of tetracyclines potentiates the nephrotoxicity of aminoglycosides and other nephrotoxic drugs and should be avoided in patients undergoing treatment with these other drugs. Tetracyclines are slowly degraded in pharmaceutical preparations to products that are more nephrotoxic than the parent drug. For this reason, tetracycline preparations must be used or discarded by their expiration date.

Tetracyclines sometimes cause phototoxicity in individuals who are exposed to the sun during therapy. This adverse effect appears to result from the absorption of ultraviolet radiation by the tetracycline following its accumulation in the skin. The activated drug then emits energy at a lower frequency that damages skin tissue, leads to erythema, and either exacerbates sunburn or causes a reaction that appears similar to sunburn.

Specific Drugs

Doxycycline, minocycline, and tetracycline have similar chemical structures, spectrums, and uses. They are primarily distinguished by their pharmacokinetic properties.

The oral bioavailability of the drugs varies from about 70% for tetracycline to 90% or more for doxycycline and minocycline. All tetracyclines bind divalent and trivalent cations, including calcium, aluminum, and iron. For this reason, their oral bioavailability is reduced if they are taken with foods or drugs containing these cations. Dairy products reduce the oral bioavailability of tetracycline but have little effect on the bioavailability of doxycycline and minocycline. However, none of the tetracyclines should be taken with antacids or iron supplements containing these cations.

The tetracycline drugs undergo minimal biotransformation and are excreted primarily in the urine and feces. Unlike most other tetracyclines, doxycycline is not dependent on renal elimination, and doses do not need to be adjusted in persons with renal insufficiency. It is therefore the preferred tetracycline for patients with renal failure. Minocycline is more lipophilic than are other tetracyclines, and it reaches higher concentrations in the central nervous system. This is why minocycline occasionally causes

mild vestibular toxicity, an adverse effect that is usually manifested as dizziness and ataxia. Elderly persons appear to be more susceptible to this effect than are younger individuals. Doxycycline is more frequently associated with phototoxicity than are tetracycline and minocycline.

In general, minocycline and doxycycline exhibit pharmacokinetic properties that are superior to those of tetracycline, so they are often preferred for the treatment of infections. Minocycline is preferred for the treatment of acne because of its excellent penetration of the skin. As discussed above, doxycycline is particularly useful in patients with renal disease because doxycycline doses do not need to be adjusted in these patients.

Other Antibiotics

Spectinomycin has an aminocyclitol structure that is similar to but chemically distinct from the structure of aminoglycoside drugs. Like the aminoglycosides, spectinomycin acts at the 30S ribosomal subunit. Although spectinomycin can be used to treat gonorrhea caused by penicillinase-producing gonococci, this type of infection is usually treated with ceftriaxone or another third-generation cephalosporin. Spectinomycin may cause nausea and produce pain at the site of injection.

DRUGS THAT AFFECT THE 50S RIBOSOMAL SUBUNIT
Macrolides

The macrolides include **azithromycin, clarithromycin, dirithromycin,** and **erythromycin.** The properties and major clinical uses of these drugs are compared in Tables 39–1 and 39–2.

Drug Properties

Chemistry and Pharmacokinetics. Each macrolide antibiotic consists of a large, 14-atom lactone ring with two sugars attached to the ring (see Fig. 39–2C). Erythromycin is produced by *Saccharopolyspora erythraea* (formerly *Streptomyces erythreus*). The newer macrolides, such as azithromycin, clarithromycin, and dirithromycin, are semisynthetic derivatives of erythromycin. As discussed below, the derivatives offer considerably improved pharmacokinetic properties.

Spectrum and Indications. The macrolides are active against several bacteria that cause upper respiratory tract infections and pneumonia. They are most active against group A streptococci, pneumococci, chlamydiae, *M. pneumoniae,* and *Legionella pneumophila.* They are less active against gram-negative bacteria, such as *Klebsiella pneumoniae,* which most often cause pneumonia in neonates, elderly individuals, and chronic alcoholics.

The newer macrolides are also active against important pathogens responsible for otitis media, bronchitis, and other infections, and this significantly extends their clinical use. However, unlike erythromycin, the newer macrolides are not yet available in parenteral formulations for the treatment of patients with severe infections.

Bacterial Resistance. Although most staphylococci were sensitive to macrolides in the past, many strains of staphylococci are now resistant. Nevertheless, the problem of resistance has not been as significant with macrolides as it has been with some other classes of antibiotics. Acquired resistance to macrolides is primarily due to active transport of the drugs out of bacteria via specialized transport systems. Resistance is also caused by decreased binding of macrolides to the ribosome.

Adverse Effects. The macrolides are largely devoid of serious toxicity. Their most common adverse effects are stomatitis, heartburn, nausea, anorexia, abdominal discomfort, and diarrhea. These are the result of their stimulating and irritating effects on the gastrointestinal tract when they are given orally. Their less common adverse effects are associated with intravenous administration. Large intravenous doses cause ototoxicity in the form of tinnitus or impaired hearing. The ototoxic effects usually subside when use of the macrolide is discontinued. Intravenously administered erythromycin is quite irritating to veins and may cause thrombophlebitis. Rarely, use of a macrolide causes cholestatic hepatitis, which is probably a form of hypersensitivity and is reversible. The estolate form of erythromycin causes this reaction more frequently than do other esters or erythromycin base.

Specific Drugs

Azithromycin, clarithromycin, and dirithromycin are administered orally. Erythromycin can be administered orally, intravenously, or topically. When given orally, erythromycin has a relatively low and highly variable degree of bioavailability (see Table 39–1), whereas azithromycin and clarithromycin are more reliably absorbed from the gut, have a greater degree of bioavailability, and achieve higher tissue concentrations.

Erythromycin has a shorter half-life than the newer macrolides and is usually administered four times a day. Clarithromycin is administered twice a day, and azithromycin and dirithromycin are given once a day. Because the newer drugs can be administered less frequently and for shorter durations of time, patients are more likely to take their medication as directed. Patient compliance in turn reduces the risk of developing bacterial resistance.

The macrolides undergo variable degrees of hepatic metabolism and are primarily excreted in the bile and urine. Dirithromycin is rapidly hydrolyzed in the plasma to erythromycylamine, an active metabolite that is responsible for the antimicrobial effects of the drug and is excreted in feces. Erythromycin and clarithromycin inhibit cytochrome P450 isozyme 3A4 (CYP3A4) and may thereby elevate the plasma concentration of drugs metabolized by this isozyme. In contrast, azithromycin and dirithromycin appear to have little effect on P450 drug metabolism. Concurrent administration of erythromycin or clarithromycin with astemizole, cisapride, or terfenadine may lead to cardiac arrhythmias in susceptible individuals. Concurrent administration of carbamazepine, disopyramide, or triazolam also results in adverse effects. Doses of these drugs should be decreased, or the drug combination should be avoided.

As shown in Table 39–2, several macrolides are active against chlamydiae and are effective in treating pneumonia and genitourinary tract infections due to *Chlamydia pneumoniae* and *C. trachomatis*, respectively. Indeed, azithromycin is an effective single-dose treatment for uncomplicated chlamydial urethritis. Azithromycin also has good activity against *Haemophilus influenzae* and may be used to treat otitis media and other respiratory tract infections due to this organism. Either azithromycin or clarithromycin can be used to treat *Mycobacterium avium-intracellulare* infections, such as those occurring in patients with acquired immunodeficiency syndrome (AIDS). Clarithromycin is the most active macrolide against *H. pylori*, an organism that is frequently associated with peptic ulcer disease. As discussed in Chapter 28, clarithromycin is used in combination with amoxicillin and a gastric acid inhibitor for the treatment of this condition.

Other Antibiotics
Clindamycin

Clindamycin (see Fig. 39–2D) is a semisynthetic derivative of lincomycin, an antibiotic that was isolated from a *Streptomyces* species found in soil near Lincoln, Nebraska. The two drugs are aminosugar compounds that are structurally unrelated to other antibiotics. Because lincomycin is less active than clindamycin against most bacteria and appears to offer no advantage over clindamycin, it is seldom used today.

Clindamycin is primarily active against grampositive cocci and anaerobic organisms, such as *Bacteroides fragilis*. It has gained importance as a treatment for infections caused by penicillin-resistant streptococci, including necrotizing fasciitis due to *Streptococcus pyogenes*.

Clindamycin can be administered orally, parenterally, or topically. It is generally well tolerated, but the use of clindamycin is associated with a higher incidence of gastrointestinal superinfections due to *Clostridium difficile* than is the use of other antibiotics. These superinfections may lead to severe diarrhea and life-threatening pseudomembranous colitis. In affected patients, the pseudomembrane can be observed during proctoscopic examination and consists of mucous, desquamated epithelial cells, and inflammatory cells. Persons who develop diarrhea during clindamycin therapy should discontinue use of the drug and be closely monitored for superinfection and colitis.

Chloramphenicol

Chemistry. Chloramphenicol is a nitrobenzene derivative that is structurally unrelated to other antibiotics. The chemical structure is shown in Fig. 39–2D.

Pharmacokinetics and Adverse Effects. Because chloramphenicol is highly lipophilic, it is well absorbed from the gut and achieves high concentrations in the central nervous system, even in the absence of inflamed meninges. This property contributes to the drug's effectiveness in the treatment of meningitis.

Chloramphenicol is metabolized partly by glucuronate conjugation, and the parent drug and metabolites are excreted in the urine. In neonates, the ability to conjugate the drug is decreased because of low levels of glucuronosyltransferase. If doses of chloramphenicol are not reduced in neonates, plasma drug concentrations become excessive, and this leads to "gray baby" syndrome. The syndrome is characterized by ashen gray cyanosis, weakness, respiratory depression, hypotension, and shock.

Other adverse effects of chloramphenicol include two distinct forms of anemia. One form is a predictable, dose-dependent anemia that is due to blockade of iron incorporation into heme. The blockade occurs when high plasma concentrations of the drug are reached and the activity of the enzyme ferrochelatase is inhibited. Another form of anemia is a potentially fatal aplastic anemia. This form of anemia is rare, affecting 1 of 20,000–40,000 individuals who are exposed to the drug. Although the exact mechanism responsible for the anemia is unknown, a hypersensitivity mechanism is suspected. There is epidemiologic evidence that prolonged or repeated exposure to the drug increases the incidence of chloramphenicol-induced aplastic anemia, so such exposure should be avoided. In addition, clinical reports indicate that aplastic anemia can occur after only a single topical ocular administration of chloramphenicol. Because safer antibiotics are now available, there is little justification for the use of chloramphenicol for trivial infections.

Spectrum and Indications. Chloramphenicol is a broad-spectrum antibiotic that is active against pneumococci, meningococci, and *H. influenzae,* which are the most common pathogens causing meningitis. Chloramphenicol has also been used to treat *Salmonella* and *Bacteroides* infections. The drug may be either bacteriostatic or bactericidal, depending on the organisms and the drug concentration. Today, chloramphenicol treatment is usually reserved for infections caused by organisms that are resistant to other drugs and for infections in persons who are allergic to other, less toxic antibiotics.

Quinupristin-Dalfopristin

Chemistry and Pharmacokinetics. Quinupristin and dalfopristin are members of a new class of antibacterial agents called **streptogramins.** Both of these antibiotics are semisynthetic derivatives of pristinamycin. Dalfopristin is designated a group A streptogramin, whereas quinupristin is designated a group B streptogramin. These drugs are administered intravenously, are partly converted to active metabolites, and are extensively distributed to tissues except those in the central nervous system. About 75% of the drugs are excreted in the bile.

Quinupristin and dalfopristin act synergistically to inhibit bacterial protein synthesis when they are administered in a ratio of 30 parts of quinupristin to 70 parts of dalfopristin. Quinupristin and dalfopristin bind to separate sites on the 50S ribosomal subunit and form a ternary complex with the ribosome. Quinupristin prevents the addition of new amino acids to the nascent peptide chain, partly by inhibiting the synthesis of tRNA. Dalfopristin directly blocks peptide bond formation by inhibiting peptidyl transferase in the same manner as chloramphenicol and erythromycin inhibit this enzyme.

Spectrum and Indications. Quinupristin and dalfopristin are bactericidal against susceptible strains of staphylococci and streptococci, but they are usually bacteriostatic against *Enterococcus faecium.* They do not appear to exhibit synergism with beta-lactam or aminoglycoside antibiotics against most strains of bacteria.

The combination quinupristin-dalfopristin is active against a wide range of gram-positive bacteria, including staphylococci that are resistant to methicillin, quinolones, and vancomycin; pneumococci that are resistant to penicillin; and *E. faecium* strains that are resistant to vancomycin. The combination has been used primarily for the treatment of bacteremia, pneumonia, and skin and soft tissue infections due to drug-resistant gram-positive cocci. For example, it has been successfully employed in cases of bacteremia, peritonitis, endocarditis, or aortic graft infections that are caused by vancomycin-resistant organisms. Quinupristin-dalfopristin is also highly active against viridans group streptococci, *L. pneumophila,* and *Moraxella catarrhalis,* but its role in treating infections caused by these organisms has not been established.

Adverse Effects. Quinupristin-dalfopristin is generally well tolerated but may cause inflammation of veins, arthralgia, myalgia, diarrhea, and nausea. A few cases of elevated serum transaminase levels have been reported.

OTHER BACTERIAL PROTEIN SYNTHESIS INHIBITORS

Mupirocin, an antibiotic obtained from *Pseudomonas fluorescens,* is structurally unrelated to all other antibiotics.

Mupirocin contains an epoxide side chain that is similar in structure to isoleucine. The drug competes with isoleucine for binding to bacterial isoleucyl tRNA synthetase, an enzyme that catalyzes the formation of isoleucyl tRNA from isoleucine and tRNA. In this manner, mupirocin prevents the addition of isoleucine to nascent peptides during protein synthesis. Because of its unique mechanism of action, it does not exhibit cross-resistance with other antimicrobial drugs.

Mupirocin is active against most staphylococci, including many strains that are resistant to methicillin. It inhibits the majority of β-hemolytic streptococci, including most strains of *S. pyogenes.* Mupirocin is the first effective topical therapy for impetigo caused by streptococci or staphylococci. In cases of impetigo, it is applied as a cream to affected areas three times a day for 5 days. Mupirocin is also used to eradicate nasal colonization of methicillin-resistant staphylococci in infected adult patients and in health-care workers. This reduces the risk of spreading infection during institutional outbreaks of this pathogen.

Summary of Important Points

- Inhibitors of bacterial protein synthesis act by selectively binding to components of the 30S or 50S ribosomal subunits. Aminoglycosides, tetracyclines, and spectinomycin inhibit 30S ribosomal function. Macrolides, clindamycin, chloramphenicol, and dalfopristin inhibit 50S ribosomal function.
- Aminoglycosides exist as positively charged cations in body fluids. They are poorly absorbed from the gut and do not penetrate the central nervous system. They are excreted unchanged in the urine. Aminoglycosides are active against many aerobic gram-negative bacilli, including *P. aeruginosa.*
- Tetracyclines are broad-spectrum, bacteriostatic drugs that are primarily used to treat infections caused by rickettsiae, chlamydiae, and mycoplasmas. They are concentrated in growing teeth and bone and may cause permanent staining of

teeth if administered during pregnancy or in children under 8 years of age.
- Most tetracyclines are excreted primarily in the urine, but doxycycline is excreted by other routes and may be used without dosage adjustment in patients with renal failure.
- Macrolides are active against most pathogens causing respiratory tract infections and are used to treat otitis media and pneumonia due to pneumococci, chlamydiae, *M. pneumoniae,* and *L. pneumophila.* Azithromycin is particularly effective against *H. influenzae,* whereas clarithromycin is active against *H. pylori* and may be used in the treatment of peptic ulcer disease.
- Clindamycin is active against gram-positive cocci and is useful in treating infections caused by organisms that are resistant to penicillin and other drugs. It causes a higher incidence of pseudomembranous colitis than do other antibiotics.

Selected Readings

Ali, M. Z., and M. B. Goetz. A meta-analysis of the relative efficacy and toxicity of single daily dosing versus multiple daily dosing of aminoglycosides. Clin Infect Dis 24:796–809, 1997.

Bryson, H. M., and C. M. Spencer. Quinupristin-dalfopristin. Drugs 52:406–414, 1996.

Griswold, M. W., et al. Quinupristin-dalfopristin: an injectable streptogramin combination. Am J Health-Syst Pharm 53:2045–2053, 1996.

McManus, M. C. Mechanisms of bacterial resistance to antimicrobial agents. Am J Health-Syst Pharm 54:1420–1432, 1997.

Ridgway, G. L. Treatment of chlamydial genital infection. J Antimicrob Chemother 40:311–314, 1997.

Rubinstein, E., and F. Bompart. Activity of quinupristin-dalfopristin against gram-positive bacteria: clinical applications and therapeutic potential. J Antimicrob Chemother 39(supplement A):139–143, 1997.

Thomas, R. J. Neurotoxicity of antibacterial therapy. South Med J 87:869–874, 1994.

Westphal, J. F., et al. Hepatic side effects of antibiotics. J Antimicrob Chemother 33:387–401, 1994.

CHAPTER FORTY

ANTIMYCOBACTERIAL DRUGS

CLASSIFICATION OF ANTIMYCOBACTERIAL DRUGS*

Drugs for tuberculosis
- Ethambutol
- Isoniazid
- Pyrazinamide
- Rifabutin
- Rifampin
- Streptomycin

Drugs for *Mycobacterium avium-intracellulare* infections
- Azithromycin
- Ciprofloxacin
- Clarithromycin
- Clofazimine
- Ethambutol
- Rifabutin

Drugs for leprosy
- Clofazimine
- Dapsone
- Rifampin
- Thalidomide

*Note that some drugs are listed more than once.

MYCOBACTERIAL INFECTIONS

Mycobacteria are acid-fast bacilli that cause a variety of diseases, including tuberculosis, leprosy, and localized or disseminated *Mycobacterium avium-intracellulare* infections.

Tuberculosis is usually caused by *Mycobacterium tuberculosis.* However, atypical mycobacteria, such as *Mycobacterium kansasii* and members of the *M. avium-intracellulare* complex (MAC), are responsible for a significant number of cases. It is estimated that about one-third of the world's population is infected with *M. tuberculosis.* In the USA, the incidence of tuberculosis underwent a steady decline from the 1960s through the mid 1980s, owing to public health measures and the availability of effective drug therapy. However, this trend was reversed, at least temporarily, during the late 1980s, partly because the incidence of acquired immunodeficiency syndrome (AIDS) was rising and tuberculosis was frequently found in patients with AIDS. At the same time, an increased incidence of tuberculosis occurred among economically disadvantaged persons and immigrants, and this increase was associated with

the development of widespread drug resistance by tubercular organisms. Today, the treatment of tuberculosis poses a greater challenge to clinicians than it did a few decades ago.

M. avium-intracellulare **infections** are seen most frequently in immunocompromised patients, such as those with AIDS, and often take the form of **pulmonary disease, lymphadenitis,** or **bacteremia.** In immunocompetent persons with chronic bronchitis or emphysema, exposure to *M. avium-intracellulare* may result in **pulmonary tuberculosis.**

Leprosy is relatively common in many parts of the world. Also called **Hansen's disease,** leprosy results from infection of the skin and peripheral nervous system with *Mycobacterium leprae.* Because *M. leprae* grows so slowly, the disease exhibits a slow, progressive course over several decades. Contrary to popular opinion, leprosy is not highly contagious, and transmission of infection usually requires prolonged close contact with an infected individual. The disease occurs in two primary forms, **lepromatous leprosy** and **tuberculoid leprosy,** each of which has a characteristic pathophysiology and clinical presentation. If leprosy is not treated, it ultimately causes severe deformities and disabilities. Treatment of leprosy often requires years of therapy with antimycobacterial agents, although the introduction of newer drugs has enabled the use of shorter courses of therapy for some patients.

DRUGS FOR MYCOBACTERIAL INFECTIONS
Drugs for Tuberculosis

Drugs that are initially used to treat most patients with tuberculosis are referred to as **first-line drugs.** They include the following: **isoniazid, ethambutol,** and **pyrazinamide** (which are synthetic drugs); **rifampin** and **rifabutin** (which are semisynthetic derivatives of the antibiotic rifamycin); and **streptomycin** (which is an antibiotic). The first-line drugs are discussed below, and some of their properties and structures are shown in Table 40–1 and Fig. 40–1.

The **second-line drugs** are either less active or more toxic than the first-line drugs. Therefore, they are usually reserved for the treatment of patients who are infected with organisms that are resistant to first-line drugs and for the treatment of patients in whom drug-resistant organisms emerge during treatment. Drug resistance is more likely to develop in patients who do not take their medicine

TABLE 40–1.   **Pharmacokinetic Properties of Antimycobacterial Drugs***

Drug	Route of Administration	Oral Bioavailability	Elimination Half-Life	Routes of Elimination
Azithromycin	Oral	37%	12 hours	Biliary excretion.
Ciprofloxacin	Oral or IV	75%	4 hours	Metabolism; renal excretion.
Clarithromycin	Oral	62%	5 hours	Biliary and renal excretion.
Clofazimine	Oral	55%	70 days	Biliary and fecal excretion.
Dapsone	Oral	≈100%	28 hours†	Metabolism; renal excretion.
Ethambutol	Oral	≈100%	3.5 hours	Metabolism; renal and fecal excretion.
Isoniazid	Oral or IM	≈100%	2.5 hours†	Metabolism; renal excretion.
Pyrazinamide	Oral	≈100%	9.5 hours	Metabolism; renal excretion.
Rifabutin	Oral	16%	45 hours	Metabolism; renal and biliary excretion.
Rifampin	Oral or IV	≈100%	2.75 hours	Metabolism; renal and biliary excretion.
Streptomycin	IM	NA	2 hours	Renal excretion.
Thalidomide	Oral	≈90%	6 hours	Metabolism; renal excretion.

*Values shown are the mean of values reported in the literature. IM = intramuscular; IV = intravenous; and NA = not applicable.
†The half-lives of dapsone and isoniazid exhibit genetic variation.

as directed or are not treated for a long enough period.

The second-line drugs include the following: **rifapentine** (which, like rifampin and rifabutin, is a derivative of rifamycin); **cycloserine** (which is discussed in Chapter 38); and **capreomycin, ethionamide,** and **aminosalicylic acid.** The second-line drugs are not discussed further in this chapter.

Isoniazid

After in vitro studies showed that nicotinic acid had a weak antitubercular effect, investigators began to synthesize and test a large number of nicotinic acid derivatives. Isoniazid, also known as **isonicotinic acid hydrazide** (INH), was found to be the most active derivative and subsequently became available for clinical use. Isoniazid is often considered the

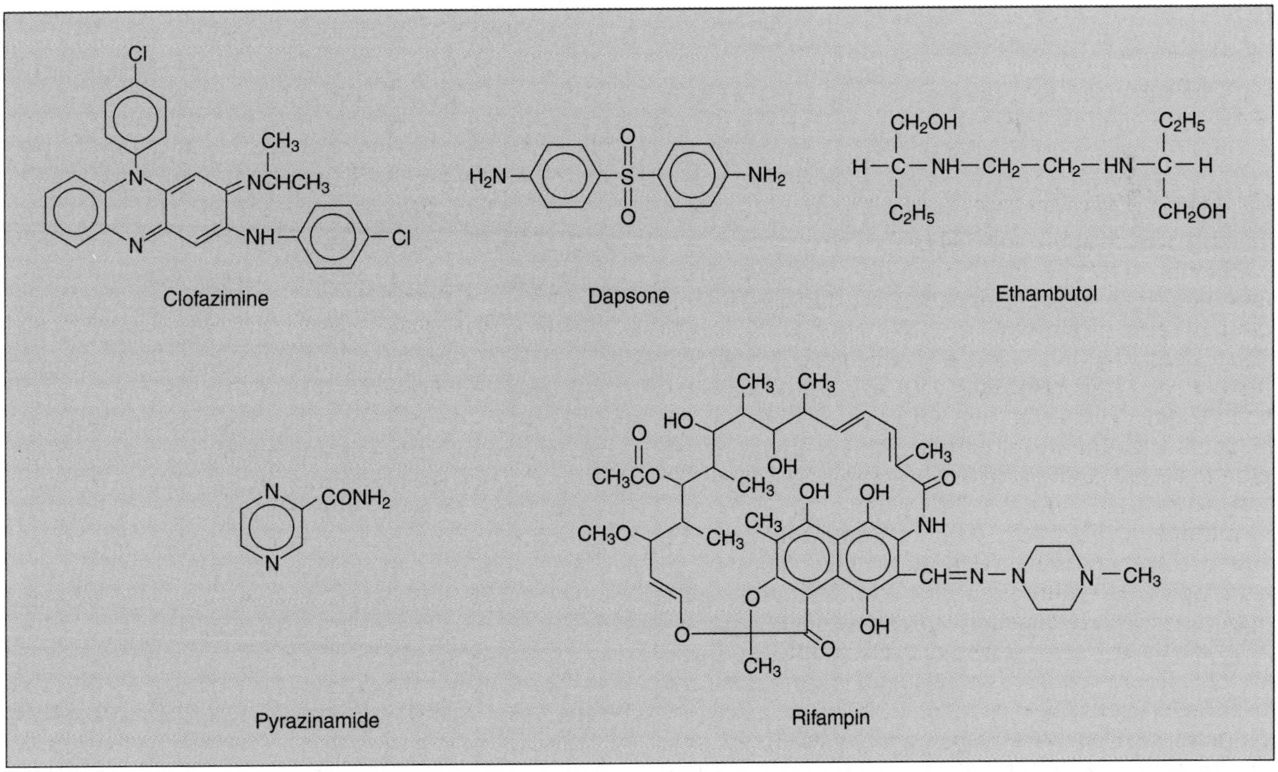

FIGURE 40–1. **Structures of selected antimycobacterial drugs.** Drugs for the prevention or treatment of tuberculosis include ethambutol, which is a butanol derivative; isoniazid (see Fig. 40–2) and pyrazinamide, both of which are nicotinic acid derivatives; and rifampin, which is a semisynthetic antibiotic. Drugs for the treatment of leprosy include clofazimine, which is a phenazine dye; dapsone, which is a sulfone; and rifampin.

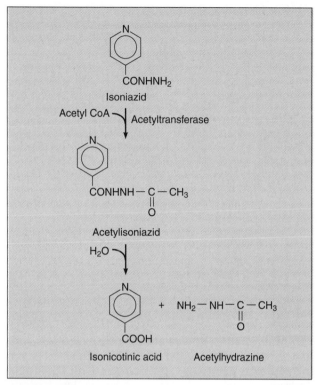

FIGURE 40-2. Structures of isoniazid and its metabolites. Isoniazid conjugates with acetyl CoA and is converted to acetylisoniazid in a reaction catalyzed by acetyltransferase. A small amount of acetylisoniazid is hydrolyzed to isonicotinic acid and acetylhydrazine.

premier drug for the management of tuberculosis. The introduction of isoniazid in the early 1960s revolutionized the treatment of this disease.

Chemistry and Mechanisms. The structures of isoniazid and its metabolites are shown in Fig. 40-2.

Isoniazid acts by inhibiting the synthesis of **mycolic acid.** This acid is the mycobacterial cell wall component that is responsible for the acid-fast staining property of mycobacteria.

Isoniazid is activated by mycobacterial catalase-peroxidase, an enzyme encoded by the *kat*G gene. The hydrazine moiety of isoniazid reduces the ferric component of catalase-peroxidase, and the reduced (ferrous) enzyme combines with oxygen to form an oxyferrous enzyme complex. This complex ultimately interacts with the target enzyme, a long-chain enoyl reductase that is involved in the synthesis of mycolic acid.

Pharmacokinetics. Although isoniazid is available for oral and intramuscular administration, it is usually given orally and is well absorbed from the gut. The drug is widely distributed to tissues and reaches intracellular concentrations that are high enough to act effectively against organisms inside cells and caseous lesions.

Isoniazid is extensively metabolized. The primary metabolite, acetylisoniazid, is formed by conjugation of acetyl CoA with isoniazid (see Fig. 40-2). The reaction is catalyzed by acetyltransferase, an enzyme whose rate of activity is genetically deter-

mined. Slow acetylation is an autosomal recessive trait, and persons with the slow phenotype are homozygous for the slow allele. Persons with the fast phenotype can be either heterozygous or homozygous dominant. The prevalence of phenotypes varies from population to population. The slow phenotype predominates in some Middle Eastern populations, whereas the fast phenotype predominates in Japanese populations. In the USA, about half the population exhibits each phenotype. Because of the different rates of acetylation of isoniazid, persons with the fast phenotype have lower plasma isoniazid concentrations than do persons with the slow phenotype (Fig. 40-3).

A small amount of acetylisoniazid is converted to isonicotinic acid and acetylhydrazine (see Fig. 40-2). Investigators believe that acetylhydrazine is responsible for the hepatic toxicity of the drug.

Isoniazid and its metabolites are excreted in the urine.

Spectrum and Indications. Isoniazid is active against sensitive strains of *M. tuberculosis* and sensitive strains of some atypical mycobacteria, such as *M. kansasii.* It has limited activity against *M. avium-intracellulare.* It is not active against *M. leprae* or against most other bacteria, and its use is limited to the prevention and treatment of tuberculosis.

Isoniazid is given to prevent tuberculosis in individuals whose results in the tuberculin skin test have recently converted from negative to positive. Typically, the drug is administered once a day for 6 months. Isoniazid is also given to prevent tuberculosis in close contacts of patients in whom active tuberculosis was recently diagnosed. Rifampin may be used for prophylaxis if isoniazid is contraindicated or if the mycobacterial strain is known to be resistant to isoniazid.

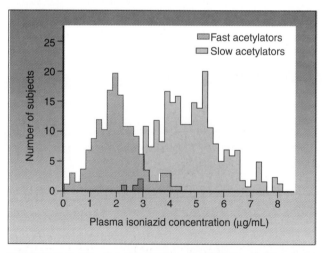

FIGURE 40-3. Bimodal distribution of plasma isoniazid concentrations. Plasma concentrations of isoniazid were measured 2 hours after the administration of a single 300-mg dose of isoniazid to each member of a general population of human subjects. Subjects with the fast acetylation phenotype showed lower plasma drug concentrations than did subjects with the slow acetylation phenotype.

Isoniazid is used to treat persons with newly diagnosed tuberculosis unless they are known to be infected with a strain that is resistant to the drug. In persons who have had a relapse of tuberculosis after earlier treatment, the choice of drugs is guided by in vitro susceptibility of the infecting mycobacterial strain.

Bacterial Resistance. Resistance to isoniazid is not yet common in the USA but is increasing. In some cases, immigrants to the country have tuberculosis and harbor organisms that are resistant to isoniazid and other first-line drugs. Resistance to isoniazid appears to be mediated primarily by mutations of the *kat*G gene, which result in loss of the catalase-peroxidase enzyme required for activation of isoniazid in bacteria.

Adverse Effects. Isoniazid is well tolerated by most patients. However, it causes elevation of serum transaminase levels and potentially life-threatening hepatitis in some individuals. The risk of developing hepatitis during isoniazid therapy is low in persons under 35 years of age, is moderate in persons between 35 and 50, and is highest in persons over 50. The fact that the risk is age-related should be kept in mind when choosing a drug to prevent tuberculosis in older persons. Patients who have tuberculosis and are being treated with isoniazid should have their serum transaminase levels monitored periodically and should be told to inform their health care provider if they develop symptoms of hepatitis.

Isoniazid may also cause peripheral neuritis, with symptoms including paresthesias and numbness of the fingers and toes. This adverse effect is more likely to occur in individuals with the slow acetylator phenotype, because they have higher plasma concentrations of isoniazid. Peripheral neuritis is due to a pyridoxine (vitamin B_6) deficiency resulting from inactivation of pyridoxine by the drug. It can be prevented or treated by administering pyridoxine supplements to patients who are taking isoniazid.

In rare circumstances, isoniazid causes toxic encephalopathy or seizures. Hematologic abnormalities, such as granulocytosis, anemia, or thrombocytopenia, may occur.

Ethambutol

Ethambutol is a butanol derivative that has bacteriostatic activity against mycobacterial organisms. As shown in Table 40–2, it is used to treat tuberculosis or *M. avium-intracellulare* infections in persons who are resistant to other drugs or who have concomitant human immunodeficiency virus (HIV) infection.

Ethambutol is administered orally, undergoes hepatic biotransformation, and is excreted in the urine and feces. The drug is generally well tolerated, but it may produce dose-dependent optic neuritis and impaired red-green color discrimination. It may also cause hyperuricemia, gout, hepatitis, and thrombocytopenia.

Pyrazinamide

Pyrazinamide is a nicotinamide derivative that is converted to pyrazinoic acid by susceptible mycobacteria. Pyrazinoic acid inhibits the growth of *M. tuberculosis,* partly by lowering the ambient pH to a level at which the organism can no longer grow.

Pyrazinamide was considered a second-line drug until investigators found that giving it in combination with other antimycobacterial drugs made it possible to reduce the duration of treatment of tuberculosis. Pyrazinamide is usually given for the first 2 months of treatment in combination with isoniazid and rifampin. Then when pyrazinamide treatment is stopped, the other drugs are administered for an additional period of time (see Table 40–2).

Pyrazinamide is given orally, is widely distributed to tissues, and is largely converted to pyrazinoic acid in the liver. A small amount of the drug is excreted unchanged in the urine, along with its metabolite.

Adverse reactions to pyrazinamide include hyperuricemia, gout, hematologic toxicity, fever, hepatitis, and an increase in the serum iron concentration.

Rifampin

Chemistry and Pharmacokinetics. Rifampin is a rifamycin derivative whose structure is shown in Fig. 40–1. Also called **rifampicin,** rifampin is rapidly absorbed after oral administration and is converted in the liver to an active metabolite, desacetyl-rifampicin. The drug and its metabolite are widely distributed to tissues and fluids, including lung tissue, saliva, and peritoneal and pleural fluids. Rifampin undergoes significant enterohepatic cycling. It is primarily excreted in the feces via biliary elimination, but up to 30% is excreted in the urine. The half-life of rifampin decreases with long-term administration, owing to increased biliary excretion.

Mechanisms, Spectrum, and Indications. Rifampin is a broad-spectrum antibiotic that has significant activity against many gram-positive, gram-negative, and acid-fast bacilli, including *M. tuberculosis, M. avium-intracellulare, M. kansasii,* and *M. leprae.* The drug acts by binding to the β subunit of DNA-dependent RNA polymerase. This prevents the enzyme from binding to DNA and thereby prevents subsequent DNA transcription. The drug does not bind to the RNA polymerase of eukaryotic cells.

Rifampin is given prophylactically to prevent several types of diseases. It is used as an alternative to isoniazid for the prevention of tuberculosis in HIV-positive persons, especially when resistance to isoniazid is known or suspected. It is used to prevent meningococcal disease in individuals who have had close contact with a *Neisseria meningitidis*–infected person or an asymptomatic meningococcal carrier. It is also given to individuals who have been exposed to *Haemophilus influenzae* type b (Hib) and are at risk of

TABLE 40–2. The Management of Mycobacterial Infections*

Indication	Characteristics of Persons to Be Treated	Initial Drug Treatment	Subsequent Drug Treatment
Prevention of tuberculosis	Negative for HIV; no known or suspected resistance to isoniazid.	Isoniazid for 6 months.	None.
	Negative for HIV; resistant to isoniazid.	Rifampin for 6 months.	None.
	Positive for HIV; no known or suspected resistance to isoniazid.	Isoniazid for 6 months.	None.
	Positive for HIV; resistant to isoniazid.	Rifampin or rifabutin for 12 months.	None.
Treatment of tuberculosis	Negative for HIV; no known resistance to isoniazid.	Combination of isoniazid, rifampin, and pyrazinamide for 2 months.	Combination of isoniazid and rifampin for 4 more months.
	Negative for HIV; suspected resistance to isoniazid.	Combination of isoniazid, rifampin, pyrazinamide, and either ethambutol or streptomycin for 6 months.	Individualized therapy based on microbial susceptibility testing.
	Positive for HIV; no known resistance to isoniazid.	Combination of isoniazid, rifampin, and pyrazinamide for 2 months.	Combination of isoniazid and rifampin for 7 more months.
	Positive for HIV; suspected resistance to isoniazid.	Combination of isoniazid, rifampin, pyrazinamide, and ethambutol for 6 months.	Individualized therapy based on microbial susceptibility testing.
	Suspected or known resistance to multiple drugs.†	Combination of at least four drugs believed to be active in the patient's demographic population and given for 6 months.	Individualized therapy based on microbial susceptibility testing.
Prevention of *Mycobacterium avium-intracellulare* diseases	Positive for HIV or evidence of immunosuppression.	Azithromycin, clarithromycin, or rifabutin.	None.
Treatment of *M. avium-intracellulare* diseases	All patients.	Various combinations of several of the following: azithromycin, ciprofloxacin, clarithromycin, clofazimine, ethambutol, and rifabutin.	Same as initial therapy.
Treatment of leprosy	All patients.	Combination of dapsone and rifampin, with or without clofazimine.	Same as initial therapy, depending on drug tolerability.

*HIV = human immunodeficiency virus.
†Patients suspected of multidrug resistance include those from certain demographic populations, those who have failed to respond to previous treatment, and those who have experienced a relapse of tuberculosis.

transmitting infection to children 4 years of age or under.

Rifampin is usually combined with isoniazid and pyrazinamide for the initial treatment of tuberculosis, and it may be combined with a sulfone, such as dapsone, or with clofazimine for the treatment of leprosy (see below). Rifampin penetrates inflamed meninges and reaches levels in the cerebrospinal fluid that are 10–20% of levels in the serum. Hence, it can be used in the treatment of tubercular meningitis.

Rifampin is used in combination with vancomycin and gentamicin for the treatment of staphylococcal endocarditis. It is occasionally used to treat *Legionella pneumophila* infections, usually in combination with a macrolide or a quinolone drug.

Bacterial Resistance. The major drawback of rifampin is the tendency for microbes to acquire resistance during exposure to the drug. Resistance is usually caused by the decreased affinity of RNA polymerase for rifampin. Because of the potential for the emergence of resistance during treatment, rifampin is usually given in combination with other drugs for the treatment of active infections.

Adverse Effects and Interactions. The adverse effects of rifampin are usually mild, but the drug may impair liver function, elevate serum bilirubin and transaminase levels, and cause hepatitis. Liver function tests should be conducted every 2–4 weeks during treatment, and rifampin should be discontinued if signs or symptoms of hepatic dysfunction become evident.

A hypersensitivity reaction, manifested as a flu-like illness with chills, fever, fatigue, and headache, develops in as many as 50% of persons taking rifampin. This reaction is more common in those who take large doses once or twice a week than in those who take smaller doses every day. High-dose intermittent therapy may also cause renal disease, leukopenia, and thrombocytopenia. Rifampin should be discontinued if purpura develops in persons taking the drug.

The consumption of alcohol by individuals who are taking rifampin appears to increase the risk of hepatitis. Rifampin can cause a reddish-orange to reddish-brown discoloration of saliva, tears, and urine. It can also cause permanent staining of soft contact lenses. Patients should be informed of these potential reactions.

Rifampin induces cytochrome P450 isozymes CYP1A2, CYP2C9, and CYP3A4 and may thereby accelerate the metabolism of other drugs and reduce their serum concentrations and therapeutic effectiveness. The affected drugs include macrolide antibiotics, benzodiazepines, calcium channel blockers, digoxin, estrogens, sulfonylureas, theophylline, and warfarin.

Rifabutin

Like rifampin, rifabutin is a derivative of rifamycin. Rifabutin inhibits DNA-dependent RNA polymerase in *Escherichia coli,* and there is evidence that it interferes with DNA synthesis in *M. tuberculosis.* The drug is active against *M. avium-intracellulare,* but its mechanism of action is unknown.

Rifabutin is primarily used to prevent *M. avium-intracellulare* diseases in individuals who are HIV-positive or immunosuppressed and to treat these and other individuals who have diseases due to *M. avium-intracellulare.* Rifabutin is also used as an alternative to rifampin for the prevention of tuberculosis in HIV-positive persons.

For the treatment of *M. avium-intracellulare* infections, rifabutin is administered in combination with azithromycin, clarithromycin, or ethambutol for a period of at least 16 weeks. Rifabutin is administered orally once a day with food in order to reduce gastrointestinal irritation. The drug is highly lipophilic, is widely distributed to tissues, and reaches substantial intracellular concentrations. Rifabutin undergoes hydroxylation and deacetylation to active metabolites that contribute about 10% of the drug's antimicrobial activity.

Streptomycin and Other Aminoglycosides

Streptomycin was the first effective drug for the treatment of tuberculosis. The drug must be administered parenterally and is often less active than other first-line drugs, so it is less commonly used today than in the past. However, it is still used for the initial treatment of patients with risk factors for multidrug-resistant tuberculosis, as well as for the re-treatment of patients whose tuberculosis has relapsed following therapy with other antibiotics.

Amikacin is another aminoglycoside that is occasionally used to treat tuberculosis. It is more active than streptomycin against some strains of mycobacteria.

Drugs for *Mycobacterium avium-intracellulare* Infections

The drugs that are active against *M. avium-intracellulare* include **ethambutol** and **rifabutin** (described above); **azithromycin** and **clarithromycin** (described in Chapter 39); **ciprofloxacin** and other fluoroquinolones (described in Chapter 41); and **clofazimine** (described below).

Azithromycin, clarithromycin, or rifabutin can be used to prevent *M. avium-intracellulare* diseases in HIV-positive or immunosuppressed patients.

Multiple-drug therapy involving various combinations of azithromycin, ciprofloxacin, clarithromycin, ethambutol, and rifabutin are usually used to treat *M. avium-intracellulare* diseases in all patients, including those who are HIV-positive or immunosuppressed. Clofazimine has been used as an alternative drug in regimens for HIV-positive or immunosuppressed patients with *M. avium-intracellulare* diseases.

Drugs for Leprosy

The treatment of leprosy requires the administration of antimycobacterial drugs for long periods of time, ranging from several months to a person's lifetime. The World Health Organization now recommends multidrug therapy for most persons with leprosy. Multidrug therapy has been shown to hasten the eradication of bacteria, to reduce the duration of active disease, and to prevent worsening of disabilities in persons with leprosy. In addition, multidrug therapy appears to reduce overall costs, increase patient compliance, and increase the motivation and availability of leprosy workers.

Dapsone and Other Sulfones

The sulfones have served as the foundation of drug therapy for leprosy for several decades. These compounds are structurally related to the sulfonamides and have a similar mechanism of action. They inhibit the synthesis of folic acid by *M. leprae,* and they exhibit a bacteriostatic action against this organism.

Dapsone, or **diaminodiphenylsulfone,** is the sulfone that is most commonly used in the treatment of leprosy. It is given orally in combination with other drugs (see Table 40–2), is metabolized by acetylation, and is excreted in the urine. Adverse reactions are usually minimal, but dapsone may cause gastrointestinal disturbances, peripheral neuropathy, optic neuritis and blurred vision, proteinuria and nephrotic syndrome, lupus erythematosus–like syndrome, and hematologic toxicity. Individuals who have glucose-6-phosphate dehydrogenase deficiency may exhibit hemolytic anemia resulting from the oxidation of erythrocyte membranes by dapsone.

Rifampin

Rifampin (described above) is the drug that exhibits the greatest bactericidal activity against

M. leprae. For the treatment of leprosy, rifampin is usually combined with dapsone or with dapsone plus clofazimine. It is never used alone, because of the risk that organisms will become resistant to it during treatment.

Clofazimine

Clofazimine is a phenazine dye that has antimycobacterial and anti-inflammatory effects. The drug is bactericidal against *M. tuberculosis,* is bacteriostatic against *M. leprae,* and is active against *M. avium-intracellulare.* Clofazimine has little activity against other bacteria. In addition to its antimicrobial effects, the drug enhances the phagocytic activity of neutrophils and macrophages while reducing the motility of neutrophils and the ability of lymphocytes to transform.

The anti-inflammatory and immunologic effects of clofazimine may contribute to the drug's efficacy in the prevention and treatment of **erythema nodosum leprosum,** a type II hypersensitivity reaction that is sometimes seen during or after the treatment of patients with lepromatous leprosy. This reaction is characterized by tender erythematous skin nodules that occur with inflammation of subcutaneous fat and acute vasculitis. Clofazimine appears to reduce the incidence of the reaction.

In patients with lepromatous leprosy, clofazimine is approved for use in combination with dapsone and rifampin. Clofazimine is usually combined with corticosteroids for the treatment of leprosy that is complicated by erythema nodosum leprosum.

Clofazimine is slowly and incompletely absorbed from the gut, with an average bioavailability of about 55%. The highly lipophilic drug is primarily distributed to adipose tissue and reticuloendothelial cells, but it is accumulated by macrophages and may also concentrate in the liver, lungs, lymph nodes, spleen, and other tissues. The drug has a long half-life (about 70 days), and some of it remains in the body for years after therapy is discontinued. It is primarily excreted unchanged in the feces following biliary excretion.

Adverse effects of clofazimine include various forms of gastrointestinal distress (such as anorexia, nausea, vomiting, abdominal pain, and diarrhea); photosensitivity; skin discoloration or other dermatologic reactions; and discoloration of body secretions (sweat, tears, sputum, feces, and urine) during therapy. Because clofazimine may elevate hepatic enzyme levels and cause hepatitis, use of the drug is generally avoided in persons with hepatic disease.

Thalidomide

Thalidomide is a drug that was once banned because it caused phocomelia (congenital abnormalities of the limbs) in the offspring of women who took it during pregnancy. Subsequent investigations have shown that the drug has immunomodulating actions (see Chapter 45) that are beneficial in the management of several conditions. Thalidomide currently has orphan drug status in the USA and can be used for the treatment of tuberculosis, leprosy, or erythema nodosum leprosum. The drug is often effective in alleviating the manifestations of erythema nodosum leprosum, possibly because of its ability to stimulate human T cells (particularly the CD8$^+$ cell subset of T cells).

Other Drugs for Leprosy

Other drugs that are used in combination with dapsone, rifampin, and clofazimine for the treatment of leprosy include **ethionamide** and **prothionamide.** Information concerning these drugs can be found in texts that focus on leprosy treatment.

Summary of Important Points

- Tuberculosis and leprosy are chronic mycobacterial infections that often require treatment with multiple drugs for months or years. Combination drug therapy accelerates the eradication of bacteria and reduces the emergence of microbial drug resistance during therapy.
- Most patients with tuberculosis are initially treated with a combination of isoniazid, rifampin, and pyrazinamide. If patients are suspected or known to be infected with drug-resistant organisms, ethambutol or streptomycin may be added to the treatment regimen.
- Most patients with leprosy are treated with a combination of dapsone and rifampin or a combination of dapsone, rifampin, and clofazimine.
- Isoniazid (isonicotinic acid hydrazide, or INH) acts partly by inhibiting mycolic acid synthesis. The rate of acetylation of the drug exhibits genetic polymorphism, with some persons showing fast acetylation and some showing slow acetylation.
- Isoniazid sometimes causes hepatitis; the risk is age-related. The drug may also cause peripheral neuritis, an effect that results from drug-induced pyridoxine deficiency and can be prevented or treated with pyridoxine supplementation.
- Rifampin is a semisynthetic antibiotic with broad-spectrum activity. It is used in the management of tuberculosis and leprosy, in the prevention of meningococcal and *H. influenzae* type b infections, and in the treatment of serious staphylococcal and *L. pneumophila* infections. Adverse effects of rifampin include hepatitis and discoloration of body fluids.
- Pyrazinamide is a synthetic drug that shortens the total duration of therapy for patients with tuberculosis. When pyrazinamide is given in combination with isoniazid and rifampin, treatment with pyrazinamide is stopped after 2 months.

Treatment with the other drugs continues for an additional period.

- Rifabutin is a semisynthetic antibiotic that is primarily used for the prevention and treatment of *M. avium-intracellulare* diseases in individuals who are infected with human immunodeficiency virus (HIV) or are immunosuppressed. Rifabutin is often given in combination with azithromycin, clarithromycin, or other drugs.
- Dapsone is a sulfone drug that forms the foundation of therapy for leprosy. It is used in combination with other drugs, such as rifampin and clofazimine.
- Clofazimine is a synthetic dye that has antimycobacterial and anti-inflammatory activity. Like rifampin, it may discolor body fluids.

Selected Readings

Barry, C. E. New horizons in the treatment of tuberculosis. Biochem Pharmacol 54:1165–1172, 1997.

Burrish, G., et al. Leprosy (Hansen's disease) in South Dakota. S D J Med 49:185–187, 1996.

DeCarsalade, G. Y., et al. Daily multidose therapy for leprosy: results of a fourteen-year experience. Int J Lepr Other Mycobact Dis 65:37–44, 1997.

Kritski, A. L., et al. Re-treatment tuberculosis cases: factors associated with drug resistance and adverse outcomes. Chest 111:1162–1167, 1997.

Moore, M., et al. Trends in drug-resistant tuberculosis (TB) in the United States, 1993–1996. JAMA 278:833–837, 1997.

Moreno, S., et al. Isoniazid preventive therapy in human immunodeficiency virus–infected persons: long-term effect on development of tuberculosis and survival. Arch Intern Med 157:1729–1734, 1997.

Willcox, M. L. The impact of multiple drug therapy on leprosy disabilities. Lepr Rev 68:350–366, 1997.

CHAPTER FORTY-ONE

MISCELLANEOUS ANTIBACTERIAL DRUGS

CLASSIFICATION OF MISCELLANEOUS ANTIBACTERIAL DRUGS

ANTIFOLATE DRUGS
Sulfonamides
- Sulfacetamide
- Sulfadiazine
- Sulfamethoxazole
- Sulfasalazine
- Sulfisoxazole

Folate reductase inhibitors
- Trimethoprim
- Trimethoprim-sulfamethoxazole

FLUOROQUINOLONES
- Ciprofloxacin
- Levofloxacin
- Norfloxacin
- Ofloxacin
- Sparfloxacin

OTHER ANTIBACTERIAL DRUGS
- Nitrofurantoin
- Polymyxin B

ANTIFOLATE DRUGS

There are two basic groups of antifolate drugs. Members of the first group, the **sulfonamides,** selectively inhibit the synthesis of dihydrofolate in bacteria. Members of the second group, the **folate reductase inhibitors,** block the action of dihydrofolate reductase and the formation of tetrahydrofolate in various organisms. This second group includes the following: **pyrimethamine,** which inhibits folate reduction in some protozoa, is primarily used to treat toxoplasmosis and malaria, and is discussed in Chapter 44; **trimetrexate,** which inhibits folate reduction in mammalian cells as well in some protozoa, can be used to treat *Pneumocystis carinii* infections, and is discussed in Chapter 44; **methotrexate,** which inhibits folate reduction in mammalian cells, is used in the treatment of neoplastic and autoimmune diseases, and is discussed in Chapter 45; and **trimethoprim,** which selectively blocks folate reduction in bacteria and is discussed below.

Mechanisms of Action

Bacterial synthesis of folate begins with the fusion of pteridine and *p*-aminobenzoic acid (PABA) to form **dihydrofolate.** This step involves the enzyme **dihydropteroate synthase.** Dihydrofolate is then converted to **tetrahydrofolate** in a reaction involving **folate reductase.**

In bacteria, the sulfonamides and trimethoprim inhibit sequential steps in the synthesis of folate (Fig. 41–1). The sulfonamides are structural analogues of PABA. They act by competitively inhibiting dihydropteroate synthase, and their effects can be counteracted by the administration of PABA. Trimethoprim acts by inhibiting folate reductase.

In mammalian cells, dihydrofolate synthesis does not occur, so humans must obtain folic acid as a vitamin in food. However, as discussed in Chapter 17, folate reduction is a necessary step in the formation of active folate derivatives (methyl, formyl, and methylene tetrahydrofolate) that donate single-carbon atoms during the synthesis of purine bases and other components of DNA. Although folate reductase is found in microbial and mammalian cells, the affinity of trimethoprim for the enzyme in bacteria is about 100,000 times greater than the affinity of the drug for the enzyme in mammalian cells.

Trimethoprim is often administered in combination with sulfamethoxazole. One reason is that their inhibition of sequential steps in bacterial folate synthesis produces a synergistic effect against susceptible organisms. Another reason is that together the drugs sometimes exhibit bactericidal activity against organisms that are not susceptible to either drug when given alone.

Sulfonamides

In the 1930s, sulfanilamide was found to be the active metabolite of Prontosil, a dye that had been developed in the search for bacterial stains with antimicrobial properties. This discovery led to the synthesis and development of a large number of sulfonamide compounds that are used to treat human infections. Examples include **sulfacetamide, sulfadiazine, sulfamethoxazole, sulfasalazine,** and **sulfisoxazole.**

Drug Properties

Chemistry and Pharmacokinetics. The structures of various sulfonamides are shown in Fig. 41–2A. Each drug is a substituted benzene sulfonic acid amide derivative.

Some sulfonamides are available in topical preparations, and others are administered orally or

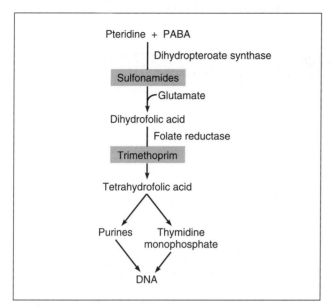

FIGURE 41–1. Mechanisms of action of antifolate drugs. Sulfonamides inhibit the action of dihydropteroate synthase and thereby block the synthesis of dihydrofolate. Trimethoprim inhibits the action of dihydrofolate reductase and thereby blocks the formation of tetrahydrofolate. PABA = *p*-aminobenzoic acid.

parenterally. Most oral compounds are adequately absorbed from the gut and are widely distributed to tissues and fluids throughout the body, including the cerebrospinal fluid. The half-lives of sulfonamides vary greatly (Table 41–1), but the most widely used compounds for treating human infections have half-lives ranging from 6 to 10 hours.

Sulfonamides are converted to inactive compounds by *N*-acetylation, and the parent drug and its metabolites are excreted in the urine. The acetylated metabolites are less soluble than the parent compound in urine, and they may precipitate in the renal tubules, causing crystalluria. Therefore, it is important for patients who are being treated with a sulfonamide to consume adequate quantities of water. The earlier sulfonamides, such as sulfanilamide, have a greater tendency to cause crystalluria than do the newer drugs, such as sulfamethoxazole.

Spectrum, Indications, and Bacterial Resistance. The sulfonamides were the first drugs used in the treatment of systemic bacterial infections. They were once active against a wide variety of organisms, including streptococci, gonococci, meningococci, many gram-negative bacilli, and chlamydiae. Over the years, however, significant resistance to sulfonamides has developed in many species, and the effective clinical spectrum of these drugs has been greatly curtailed. Today, sulfonamides are primarily used to prevent or treat urinary tract and upper respiratory tract infections (Table 41–2).

Adverse Effects. In some patients, sulfonamides cause skin rashes, which are hypersensitivity reactions that may remain mild or may progress to a serious or life-threatening form, such as erythema multiforme or Stevens-Johnson syndrome. Other adverse effects of sulfonamides include crystalluria

(discussed above), gastrointestinal reactions, headaches, hepatitis, and hematopoietic toxicity. In persons with glucose-6-phosphate dehydrogenase deficiency, sulfonamides may cause hemolytic anemia.

Specific Drugs

Sulfisoxazole or sulfamethoxazole can be used to prevent urinary tract infections or to treat uncomplicated infections of the urinary tract. Sulfisoxazole is also used in the management of otitis media. To prevent this ear infection, sulfisoxazole is used alone. To treat otitis media in pediatric patients, a liquid preparation containing sulfisoxazole and erythromycin is available. Sulfamethoxazole is often administered in combination with trimethoprim (see below).

Sulfadiazine is available in the form of silver sulfadiazine ointment for the prevention or treatment of burn infections and other superficial skin infections. The silver ions in this preparation have antibacterial activity and contribute to its utility. Sulfadiazine is given orally for the treatment of urinary tract infections.

Sulfacetamide is administered topically to treat blepharitis and conjunctivitis, ocular infections that are common throughout the world. It is also effective in treating trachoma, a highly contagious ocular infection that is caused by *Chlamydia trachomatis* and is prevalent in Asia and the Middle East.

Sulfasalazine is used in the treatment of ulcerative colitis (see Chapter 28). Unlike most sulfonamides, sulfasalazine is not absorbed significantly from the gut. It is hydrolyzed to sulfapyridine and 5-aminosalicylic acid by colonic bacteria, and its therapeutic benefit is mostly due to the anti-inflammatory effects of 5-aminosalicylic acid.

Folate Reductase Inhibitors
Trimethoprim

Trimethoprim is a synthetic aminopyrimidine drug (see Fig. 41–2C). It is well absorbed from the gut and is widely distributed to tissues. After it undergoes extensive hepatic metabolism, the parent compound and metabolites are excreted in the urine.

Trimethoprim is a weak base. It is concentrated in prostatic tissues and vaginal fluids because they are more acidic than plasma. This makes trimethoprim useful in the treatment of bacterial prostatitis and vaginitis.

Trimethoprim is active against a wide variety of aerobic gram-negative bacilli and a few gram-positive organisms. It is usually administered in combination with sulfamethoxazole for the prevention and treatment of urinary tract infections (see below), but it may be used alone for these purposes.

The adverse effects of trimethoprim include nausea, vomiting, and epigastric distress; rashes and other hypersensitivity reactions; hepatitis; and thrombocytopenia, leukopenia, and other hematologic disorders.

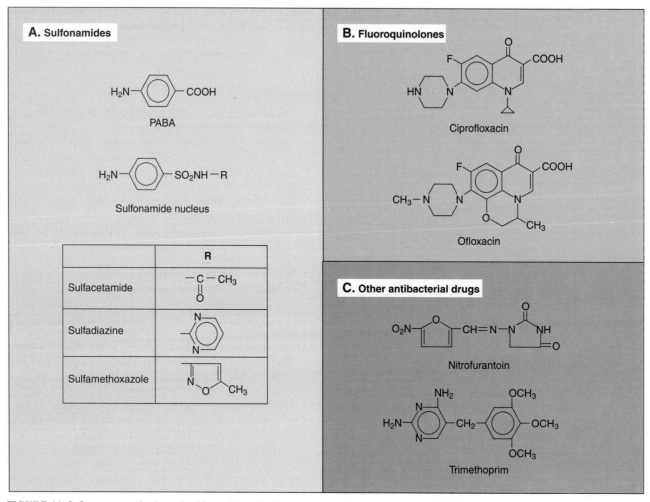

FIGURE 41–2. Structures of selected sulfonamides (A), fluoroquinolones (B), and other antibacterial drugs (C). The sulfonamides are analogues of *p*-aminobenzoic acid (PABA). Sulfamethoxazole (a sulfonamide) is often given in combination with trimethoprim (a folate reductase inhibitor).

TABLE 41–1. Pharmacokinetic Properties of Antifolate Drugs, Fluoroquinolones, Nitrofurantoin, and Polymyxin B*

Drug	Route of Administration	Oral Bioavailability	Elimination Half-Life (Hours)	Routes of Elimination
Antifolate drugs				
Sulfacetamide	Topical	NA	10	Metabolism; renal excretion.
Sulfadiazine	Oral or topical	≈100%	10	Metabolism; renal excretion.
Sulfamethoxazole	Oral	≈100%	10	Metabolism; renal excretion.
Sulfasalazine	Oral	12%	10	Metabolism; renal excretion.
Sulfisoxazole	Oral	≈100%	6	Metabolism; renal excretion.
Trimethoprim	Oral	≈100%	10	Metabolism; renal excretion.
Trimethoprim-sulfamethoxazole	Oral or IV	≈100%	10	Metabolism; renal excretion.
Fluoroquinolones				
Ciprofloxacin	Oral, IV, or topical	75%	4	Metabolism; renal excretion.
Levofloxacin	Oral or IV	99%	8	Metabolism; renal excretion.
Norfloxacin	Oral	35%	3.5	Metabolism; renal excretion.
Ofloxacin	Oral, IV, or topical	98%	6	Metabolism; renal excretion.
Sparfloxacin	Oral	Unknown	20	Metabolism; renal excretion.
Other antibacterial drugs				
Nitrofurantoin	Oral	87%	0.5	Metabolism; renal excretion.
Polymyxin B	IV or topical	NA	5	NA.

*Values shown are the mean of values reported in the literature. IV = intravenous; and NA = not applicable.

**TABLE 41–2. Major Clinical Uses of Antifolate Drugs,
Fluoroquinolones, Nitrofurantoin, and Polymyxin B**

Drug	Major Clinical Uses
Antifolate drugs	
Sulfacetamide	Empiric treatment of blepharitis and conjunctivitis.
	Treatment of ocular infections due to *Chlamydia trachomatis.*
Sulfadiazine	Prevention and empiric treatment of burn infections and other superficial skin infections.
	Empiric treatment of uncomplicated urinary tract infections.
Sulfamethoxazole	Prevention of urinary tract infections.
	Empiric treatment of uncomplicated urinary tract infections.
Sulfasalazine	Empiric treatment of ulcerative colitis.
Sulfisoxazole	Prevention of otitis media and urinary tract infections.
	Empiric treatment of uncomplicated urinary tract infections.
	Empiric treatment (with erythromycin) of otitis media.
Trimethoprim	Prevention of urinary tract infections.
	Empiric treatment of prostatitis, uncomplicated urinary tract infections, and vaginitis.
Trimethoprim-sulfamethoxazole	Prevention and empiric treatment of upper respiratory tract and urinary tract infections.
	Prevention and treatment of infections due to *Pneumocystis carinii.*
	Empiric treatment of bronchitis and otitis media.
	Treatment of infections due to *Moraxella catarrhalis, Nocardia asteroides,* or sensitive strains of *Salmonella* or *Shigella.*
Fluoroquinolones	
Ciprofloxacin	Empiric treatment of ophthalmic infections.
	Empiric treatment (with other drugs) of diseases in patients who have febrile neutropenia or intra-abdominal infections.
	Treatment of bronchitis, sinusitis, and community-acquired pneumonia due to *Chlamydia pneumoniae, Haemophilus influenzae, Klebsiella pneumoniae, Legionella pneumophila, M. catarrhalis, Mycoplasma pneumoniae,* or *Streptococcus pneumoniae.*
	Treatment of diarrhea due to *Campylobacter jejuni, Escherichia coli, Salmonella* species, or *Shigella* species.
	Treatment of infections due to *Mycobacterium avium-intracellulare.*
	Treatment of prostatitis and urinary tract infections due to enterococci, *Pseudomonas aeruginosa,* members of the family Enterobacteriaceae, and other sensitive organisms.
Levofloxacin	Same as ciprofloxacin.
Norfloxacin	Empiric treatment of lower urinary tract infections (cystitis).
Ofloxacin	Same as ciprofloxacin.
Sparfloxacin	Same as ciprofloxacin.
Other antibacterial drugs	
Nitrofurantoin	Prevention and empiric treatment of lower urinary tract infections (cystitis).
Polymyxin B	Empiric treatment (with bacitracin, neomycin, or trimethoprim) of skin and ocular infections.
	Treatment of serious infections due to gram-negative bacilli.

Trimethoprim-Sulfamethoxazole

Pharmacokinetics. Sulfamethoxazole is the sulfonamide that is commonly used in combination with trimethoprim because it has a similar half-life (10 hours). In vitro tests have shown that the maximal synergistic activity of the two drugs against microbes occurs when the concentration of sulfamethoxazole is 20 times greater than the concentration of trimethoprim. In order to obtain plasma drug concentrations in a ratio of 20:1, the drugs are administered in a ratio of 5 parts of sulfamethoxazole to 1 part of trimethoprim. The 5:1 dose ratio produces a 20:1 plasma concentration ratio because trimethoprim has a greater volume of distribution than does sulfamethoxazole.

Spectrum and Indications. Trimethoprim-sulfamethoxazole (TMP-SMX) is active against many members of the family Enterobacteriaceae, including *Escherichia coli, Klebsiella pneumoniae, Proteus* species, *Enterobacter* species, and other enteric organisms. Thus, the drug combination is often used for the prevention and treatment of urinary tract infections

caused by these organisms. Unfortunately, TMP-SMX is not active against *Pseudomonas aeruginosa,* a common cause of urinary tract infections in hospitalized patients.

TMP-SMX is active against *Haemophilus influenzae, Moraxella catarrhalis, P. carinii,* and *Streptococcus pneumoniae* and is used to prevent or treat otitis media, bronchitis, and other infections caused by these organisms. Because TMP-SMX has variable activity against β-hemolytic streptococci, including *Streptococcus pyogenes,* it is not usually employed to treat streptococcal pharyngitis and other streptococcal infections.

Some authorities consider TMP-SMX to be the drug of choice for treating *M. catarrhalis* infections. TMP-SMX is also one of the drugs of choice for treating *Nocardia asteroides* infections.

TMP-SMX is active against many strains of *Salmonella* and *Shigella,* but other strains are resistant. Currently, a fluoroquinolone (see below) is usually preferred for treating most infections caused by these organisms.

Adverse Effects. The adverse effects of TMP-SMX are similar to those of the individual drugs. TMP-SMX can cause megaloblastic anemia in persons who have a low dietary intake of folic acid, but this adverse effect is uncommon.

FLUOROQUINOLONES

The fluoroquinolones are a newer group of synthetic antibacterial drugs that include **ciprofloxacin, levofloxacin, norfloxacin, ofloxacin,** and **sparfloxacin.** These drugs have greater antimicrobial activity than do older quinolone drugs, such as nalidixic acid.

Drug Properties

Chemistry and Mechanisms. Structures of representative fluoroquinolones are depicted in Fig. 41–2B.

The fluoroquinolones are examples of **DNA topoisomerase inhibitors.** DNA topoisomerases are a group of enzymes involved in the repair and replication of DNA. Although type II topoisomerases are found in both prokaryotic and eukaryotic organisms, their structures and functions are different enough to enable selective inhibition of bacterial topoisomerase by fluoroquinolone drugs.

Bacterial type II topoisomerase is often called **DNA gyrase** because of its role in promoting supercoiling of DNA in bacteria. DNA gyrase has the unique ability to introduce negative superhelical twists (coils) into closed circular bacterial DNA. In addition to being required for supercoiling of DNA, the enzyme is required for initiation and propagation of the DNA replication fork during DNA replication and transcription. As shown in Fig. 41–3, DNA supercoiling is accomplished by nicking, moving, and resealing both strands of double-stranded DNA. DNA gyrase is a tetramer composed of two A and two B subunits. Fluoroquinolones selectively bind to the A subunits, which contain the catalytic site for the nicking and resealing reaction.

Mammalian cell type II DNA topoisomerase removes positive supercoils from DNA to prevent the DNA from tangling during replication. Only very high concentrations of fluoroquinolones can inhibit mammalian topoisomerase. However, the enzyme is blocked by normal concentrations of etoposide and other drugs that are used in the treatment of cancer (see Chapter 45). These anticancer drugs do not have antibacterial activity.

Pharmacokinetics. Fluoroquinolones have several attractive pharmacokinetic properties that enable their oral administration for the treatment of infections that formerly required parenteral therapy with other antibacterial drugs (see Table 41–2).

When given orally, fluoroquinolones are well absorbed from the gut and are widely distributed to tissues. In addition to being available for oral use, some fluoroquinolones are available for intravenous or topical ocular administration. Fluoroquinolone concentrations in many tissues, including the lungs, kidneys, liver, gallbladder, prostate, endometrium, fallopian tubes, and ovaries, are greater than concentrations in the plasma. For example, levofloxacin concentrations in lung tissue are 2–5 times greater than those in the plasma. Fluoroquinolones have relatively long elimination half-lives and a long postantibiotic effect, with some organisms failing to resume growth for 2–6 hours after drug levels are no longer detectable. For these reasons, they are usually administered once or twice a day.

Like the tetracyclines, the fluoroquinolones chelate divalent and trivalent cations, including calcium, iron, magnesium, and zinc. Therefore, fluoroquinolones should be taken 2 hours before or 2 hours after ingesting dairy products, drugs, or nutritional supplements containing these cations.

Fluoroquinolones undergo varying degrees of hepatic biotransformation, and they are excreted unchanged in the urine, along with their metabolites. Some metabolites have low levels of antimicrobial activity, but these metabolites probably do not contribute significantly to the clinical efficacy of the drugs. Fluoroquinolones inhibit the hepatic metabolism of caffeine and theophylline and may thereby increase their serum levels (see below).

Spectrum and Indications. Fluoroquinolones exhibit bactericidal activity against a broad spectrum of aerobic gram-positive and gram-negative bacteria, including many gram-positive cocci, gram-negative bacilli, and acid-fast bacilli.

The drugs are highly effective in eradicating organisms that cause urinary tract infections and prostatitis, including *P. aeruginosa* and many members of the family Enterobacteriaceae. Some fluoroquinolones are also active against enterococci. Fluoroquinolones can kill several bacterial species that cause diarrhea, including *Campylobacter, Salmonella,* and *Shigella* species. The drugs are also effective in treating traveler's diarrhea, which is often due to enterotoxigenic strains of *E. coli.* Fluoroquinolones are used in combination with other drugs to treat patients with intra-abdominal infections and patients with febrile neutropenia.

Fluoroquinolones appear to have a growing role in the treatment of respiratory tract infections. They are used to treat sinusitis and bronchitis due to pneumococci, *H. influenzae,* or *M. catarrhalis.* Some fluoroquinolones, such as levofloxacin, are approved for the treatment of community-acquired pneumonia caused by pneumococci, *Chlamydia pneumoniae, K. pneumoniae,* or *Mycoplasma pneumoniae.* Fluoroquinolones are used as alternatives to macrolides for the treatment of infections caused by *Legionella pneumophila* and other *Legionella* species. They are active against mycobacteria and are used in the treatment of *Mycobacterium avium-intracellulare* infections (see Chapter 40). Fluoroquinolones achieve high concentrations in neutrophils, and this contributes to their effectiveness in patients with mycobacterial infections.

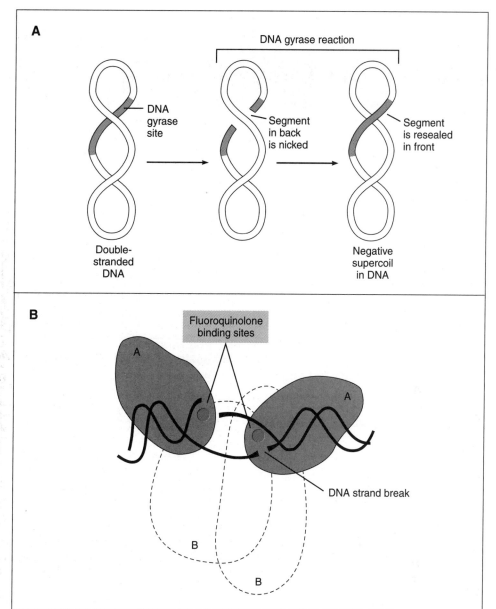

FIGURE 41–3. Effect of fluoroquinolones on DNA gyrase. **(A)** In the absence of fluoroquinolones, DNA gyrase catalyzes the formation of negative supercoils in the double-stranded DNA of bacteria. After both strands of one segment are nicked, the broken strands are passed across the other strands of DNA and then are resealed. This reaction requires energy in the form of adenosine triphosphate (ATP). **(B)** DNA gyrase is a tetramer composed of two A subunits and two B subunits. Fluoroquinolones inhibit DNA gyrase by binding to the catalytic sites on the A subunits. ATP binds to the B subunits.

Bacterial Resistance. Resistance to fluoroquinolones is most prevalent among staphylococci, mycobacteria, and strains of *P. aeruginosa*. Resistance is usually caused by decreased affinity of the A subunit of DNA gyrase for the drugs, but it may also result from decreased uptake or increased efflux of the drugs. Resistance to fluoroquinolones is conferred by mutations in chromosomal DNA. Plasmid R factors have not been implicated.

Adverse Effects and Interactions. Fluoroquinolones are generally well tolerated. Because they have been found to cause arthropathy and osteochondrosis in juvenile animals, the drugs are usually not administered to persons under 18 years of age. However, the drugs have been used safely to treat serious *P. aeruginosa* infections in children with cystic fibrosis.

Fluoroquinolones inhibit the metabolism of caffeine and theophylline. In a few cases, seizures have occurred in persons who consumed large quantities of caffeine while taking a fluoroquinolone. Patients undergoing fluoroquinolone therapy should be advised to reduce their intake of caffeine to avoid excessive central nervous system stimulation. Because serum levels of theophylline may rise during fluoroquinolone therapy, doses of theophylline may need to be reduced.

Specific Drugs

The individual fluoroquinolone drugs differ in their antimicrobial activity and pharmacokinetic profile (see Table 41–1).

Norfloxacin has a relatively short half-life and is indicated only for the treatment of urinary tract infections. Some fluoroquinolones, such as ciprofloxacin and ofloxacin, can be administered by several routes and are used to treat a wide variety of infections, including superficial ocular infections. In comparison with other fluoroquinolones in current use, levofloxacin is more active against many gram-negative bacteria, including *P. aeruginosa,* and it has better oral bioavailability. It also has a relatively long half-life, so it is often administered once a day.

OTHER ANTIBACTERIAL DRUGS
Nitrofurantoin

Like norfloxacin (a fluoroquinolone discussed above), nitrofurantoin is an example of a **urinary tract antiseptic.** The antibacterial activity of these antiseptics is localized to the urinary bladder.

Nitrofurantoin is a synthetic nitrofuran derivative (see Fig. 41–2C). It is administered orally, and ingesting it with food enhances its absorption and reduces the risk of gastrointestinal irritation. Once absorbed from the gut, the drug is rapidly excreted in the urine.

Nitrofurantoin is bactericidal against gram-positive and gram-negative bacteria that commonly cause acute lower urinary tract infections, including *E. coli, Enterococcus faecalis, K. pneumoniae,* and *Staphylococcus saprophyticus.* However, nitrofurantoin is not active against *Proteus* species, *Serratia* species, or *P. aeruginosa.* Acquired microbial resistance to nitrofurantoin has generally not been a significant clinical problem.

Nitrofurantoin is usually well tolerated, but it may cause gastrointestinal irritation, nausea, vomiting, and diarrhea. To avoid these adverse effects, a macrocrystalline formulation of the drug is usually administered. The large crystals of drug in this formulation dissolve slowly in the gut, producing less gastrointestinal distress than do other formulations. Less common adverse effects of nitrofurantoin include pulmonary fibrosis, hepatitis, and hematologic toxicity.

Polymyxin B

Polymyxin B is a drug that is often found in creams or ointments containing bacitracin, neomycin, or trimethoprim. The preparations are applied topically for skin and ocular infections.

Like other **polymyxins,** polymyxin B is a polypeptide antibiotic that interacts with the phospholipid component of bacterial cell membranes to disrupt cell membrane integrity and permit cytoplas-mic components to leak out of the cell. The polymyxins are active against almost all gram-negative bacilli except *Proteus* species, but they produce considerable nephrotoxicity when given parenterally. Although they have been used in the past to treat systemic infections caused by these organisms, safer drugs are now available for parenteral use.

Summary of Important Points

- Sulfonamides and trimethoprim inhibit sequential steps in bacterial folic acid synthesis. Sulfonamides inhibit dihydropteroate synthase and the synthesis of dihydrofolate, whereas trimethoprim inhibits folate reductase and the formation of tetrahydrofolate.
- The combination of sulfamethoxazole and trimethoprim (TMP-SMX) is primarily used to treat urinary tract infections, upper respiratory tract infections, and infections caused by *P. carinii* or *N. asteroides.*
- Fluoroquinolones inhibit DNA gyrase and have bactericidal activity against a wide range of pathogens. They are primarily used to treat infections of the urinary, gastrointestinal, and respiratory tracts. Because of the risk of arthropathy and osteochondrosis, fluoroquinolones are usually not used in children.
- Nitrofurantoin is a urinary tract antiseptic that is effective in the treatment of uncomplicated urinary tract infections.
- Polymyxin B is primarily used in combination with other drugs to treat superficial ocular and skin infections.

Selected Readings

Brook, I., and A. E. Gober. Prophylaxis with amoxicillin or sulfisoxazole for otitis media: effect on the recovery of penicillin-resistant bacteria from children. Clin Infect Dis 22:143–145, 1996.

Ernst, M. E., et al. Levofloxacin and trovafloxacin: the next generation of fluoroquinolones? Am J Health-Syst Pharm 54:2569–2584, 1997.

Mizuki, Y., et al. Pharmacokinetic interactions related to the chemical structures of fluoroquinolones. J Antimicrob Chemother 37(supplement A):41–55, 1997.

Nicolle, L. E. A practical guide to the management of complicated urinary tract infection. Drugs 53:583–592, 1997.

Reid, G., and L. Howard. Effect on uropathogens of prophylaxis for urinary tract infection in spinal cord–injured patients. Spinal Cord 35:605–607, 1997.

Tabet, S. R., et al. Bacterial infections in adult patients hospitalized with AIDS: case-control study of prophylactic efficacy of trimethoprim-sulfamethoxazole versus aerosolized pentamidine. Int J STD AIDS 8:563–569, 1997.

CHAPTER FORTY-TWO

ANTIFUNGAL DRUGS

CLASSIFICATION OF ANTIFUNGAL DRUGS

Polyene antibiotics
- Amphotericin B
- Natamycin
- Nystatin

Azole derivatives
- Clotrimazole
- Econazole
- Fluconazole
- Itraconazole
- Ketoconazole

Allylamine drugs
- Naftifine
- Terbinafine

Other antifungal drugs
- Ciclopirox
- Flucytosine
- Griseofulvin
- Tolnaftate

OVERVIEW

Fungal Infections

Fungal infections can be divided into three main groups: systemic mycoses, subcutaneous mycoses, and superficial mycoses.

Patients with **systemic mycoses** may present with signs and symptoms of **soft tissue infection, urinary tract infection, pneumonia, meningitis,** or **septicemia.** The diseases may be chronic and indolent or may be invasive and life-threatening. The systemic mycoses are most commonly caused by members of the genera *Aspergillus, Blastomyces, Candida, Coccidioides, Cryptococcus,* and *Histoplasma.* Some infections, such as **blastomycosis, coccidioidomycosis,** and **histoplasmosis,** are endemic to certain geographic regions and are found in both immunocompetent and immunocompromised individuals. Other infections, such as **aspergillosis, candidiasis, cryptococcosis,** and **mucormycosis** are more likely to occur in immunocompromised or debilitated patients, such as those receiving immunosuppressive drugs, those with indwelling catheters or prostheses, or those with acquired immunodeficiency syndrome (AIDS), diabetes, or chronic renal, hepatic, or cardiac diseases. These conditions either suppress cellular immunity or facilitate colonization and infection by fungi.

Subcutaneous mycoses are often caused by puncture wounds contaminated with soil fungi. Examples of these infections are **chromomycosis, pseudallescheriasis,** and **sporotrichosis.**

Superficial mycoses are infections of the nails, skin, and mucous membranes and are usually caused by dermatophytes or yeasts. The most common dermatophytes are *Epidermophyton, Microsporum,* and *Trichophyton.* Dermatophyte infections of the nails are referred to as **tinea unguium** or **onychomycosis.** Other dermatophyte infections include **tinea pedis** (athlete's foot), **tinea capitis** (ringworm of the scalp), **tinea corporis** (ringworm of the body), and **tinea cruris** ("jock itch"). These infections usually present as a rash with pruritus (itching) and erythema. **Ringworm** is described as an annular, scaling rash with a clear center.

The most common yeasts causing superficial mycoses are *Candida albicans* and other *Candida* species. Affected patients may present with **thrush** (oral candidiasis), **vaginal candidiasis,** or *Candida* **infections of the axilla, groin, and gluteal folds** (including **diaper rash** in infants). Less common yeasts causing superficial mycoses include *Malassezia furfur* (also called *Pityrosporum orbiculare*) and *Pityrosporum ovale* (also called *Malassezia ovalis*). *M. furfur* causes **tinea versicolor,** or **pityriasis versicolor,** a skin infection characterized by hypo- and hyperpigmented macules, typically in the shoulder girdle area. *P. ovale* and *M. furfur* cause **seborrheic dermatitis,** characterized by scaling and erythema on the ears, eyebrows, nose, and chest.

Clinical Uses and Mechanisms of Antifungal Drugs

Fungi are eukaryotic organisms whose growth is not inhibited by antibacterial drugs. However, drugs that are selectively toxic to fungi have been discovered and used to treat fungal infections in humans.

As shown in Table 42–1, drugs used in the treatment of systemic and subcutaneous mycoses include a polyene antibiotic (amphotericin B), several azole derivatives (fluconazole, itraconazole, and ketoconazole), and flucytosine. The other drugs listed are used only in the treatment of superficial mycoses. Amphotericin B is the premier drug used to treat the most severe systemic and subcutaneous mycoses, whereas the azoles are used for less severe forms of these infections. Flucytosine is usually administered in combination with amphotericin B for

TABLE 42–1. **Clinical Uses and Mechanisms of Antifungal Drugs**

Drug	Clinical Uses			Mechanisms
	Systemic and Subcutaneous Mycoses	Dermatophyte Infections	Superficial *Candida* Infections	
Polyene antibiotics				
Amphotericin B	Yes	No	Yes	Binds ergosterol in fungal cell membrane; increases membrane permeability.
Natamycin	No	No	Yes	Same as amphotericin B.
Nystatin	No	No	Yes	Same as amphotericin B.
Azole derivatives				
Clotrimazole	No	Yes	Yes	Inhibits ergosterol synthesis.
Econazole	No	Yes	Yes	Same as clotrimazole.
Fluconazole	Yes	No	Yes	Same as clotrimazole.
Itraconazole	Yes	Yes	Yes	Same as clotrimazole.
Ketoconazole	Yes	Yes	Yes	Same as clotrimazole.
Allylamine drugs				
Naftifine	No	Yes	No*	Inhibits ergosterol biosynthesis.
Terbinafine	No	Yes	No*	Same as naftifine.
Other antifungal drugs				
Ciclopirox	No	Yes	Yes	Increases fungal cell membrane permeability.
Flucytosine	Yes	No	No	Inhibits nucleic acid synthesis.
Griseofulvin	No	Yes	No	Inhibits microtubule function and mitosis.
Tolnaftate	No	Yes	No	Unknown.

*Naftifine and terbinafine have fungistatic activity against *Candida* but are not approved for the treatment of candidiasis.

the treatment of systemic *Cryptococcus* or *Candida* infections.

Many antifungal drugs act by impairing plasma membrane function in fungal cells. The selective toxicity of these drugs is due to the difference in the sterols found in fungal and mammalian cell membranes. Fungal cell membranes contain **ergosterol,** whereas mammalian cell membranes contain **cholesterol.** Some antifungal drugs bind to ergosterol and thereby increase plasma membrane permeability, whereas other drugs inhibit the synthesis of ergosterol (Fig. 42–1 and Table 42–1).

Polyene antibiotics selectively bind to ergosterol in fungal membranes. This action increases fungal membrane permeability and allows the cytoplasmic contents to escape from the cell. The polyene drugs can also bind to cholesterol in mammalian cells, and this may account for their ability to produce kidney damage. **Ciclopirox** increases fungal cell membrane permeability by a different mechanism. It prevents amino acid transport into fungal cells, thereby altering membrane structure and allowing the escape of intracellular material.

The **allylamine drugs** and the **azole derivatives** block distinct steps in ergosterol biosynthesis, but these groups of drugs have little effect on cholesterol biosynthesis in humans. The allylamine drugs inhibit **squalene monooxygenase,** which converts squalene to squalene-2,3 oxide, the immediate precursor of lanosterol. The azoles inhibit **14-α-demethylase,** a cytochrome P450 enzyme that converts lanosterol to ergosterol.

Flucytosine is a pyrimidine antimetabolite, and it is the only antifungal drug that affects nucleic acid. Flucytosine is converted to **5-fluorouracil** (5-FU) in fungal cells by cytosine deaminase, an enzyme not found in mammalian cells. 5-FU is then incorporated into fungal RNA, and this inhibits fungal protein synthesis.

Griseofulvin acts by binding to fungal microtubules and thereby inhibiting microtubule function and mitosis. The mechanism of action of **tolnaftate** is unknown.

DRUGS
Polyene Antibiotics

The polyene antibiotics are produced by various soil organisms of the family Streptomycetaceae. Examples are amphotericin A and B, natamycin, and nystatin. Each of these compounds consists of a macrolide (lactone) ring containing conjugated double bonds (polyene), with acidic and basic side groups. Because the acidic group and basic group are capable of donating or accepting a proton, respectively, the polyene drugs are **amphoteric.**

Amphotericin B has greater antifungal activity than does amphotericin A, which is not used clinically. Amphotericin B is the only polyene drug used to treat systemic and subcutaneous mycoses. The other polyene drugs are limited to topical application for the treatment of superficial mycoses.

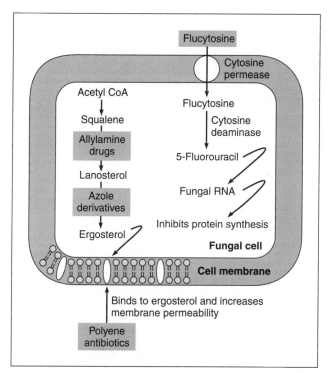

FIGURE 42–1. Mechanisms of action of antifungal drugs. The synthesis of ergosterol is inhibited by allylamine drugs and by azole derivatives. Amphotericin B and other polyene antibiotics bind to ergosterol in fungal cell membranes and increase membrane permeability. Ciclopirox increases membrane permeability by another mechanism (not shown). Flucytosine is accumulated by fungal cells and converted to 5-fluorouracil. When 5-fluorouracil is incorporated into fungal RNA, protein synthesis is inhibited. Griseofulvin interferes with microtubule function and blocks mitosis (not shown).

Amphotericin B

Chemistry and Pharmacokinetics. The structure and pharmacokinetic properties of amphotericin B are shown in Fig. 42–2A and Table 42–2.

Because amphotericin B is not absorbed from the gut, it is not available in oral formulations. The drug is available in topical preparations for the treatment of superficial infections. It is also available in two parenteral formulations for the treatment of systemic or subcutaneous infections: a deoxycholate complex and a new phospholipid complex. The **amphotericin B lipid complex** appears to protect the kidney and other organs from the drug's toxicity while retaining its antifungal activity.

The dosage and route of parenteral treatment depend on the site and severity of the infection and on the immune status of the patient. In general, higher doses of amphotericin B are employed to treat infections with more resistant fungi, especially *Aspergillus* species, and lower doses are used to treat esophageal and urinary tract infections. Concentrations of the drug in cerebrospinal fluid are only 2–3% of those in plasma, reflecting the fact that amphotericin B does not penetrate the blood-brain barrier very well. Nevertheless, the drug is usually administered intravenously for the treatment of fungal meningitis

and other systemic mycoses. Intrathecal administration or intraventricular administration with an Ommaya reservoir is generally reserved for extremely ill patients and those who do not respond to intravenous therapy.

Amphotericin B is extensively metabolized in the liver, and the metabolites are slowly excreted in the urine. The biotransformation pathways are not well understood. Amphotericin B has a biphasic half-life, with an initial half-life of about 24 hours and a terminal half-life of about 15 days.

Spectrum and Indications. Amphotericin B is active against a wide variety of fungi (Table 42–3). In addition, it is active against *Naegleria fowleri,* a freshwater ameba that causes a rare but often fatal form of meningoencephalitis (see Chapter 44).

Fungal Resistance. Although polyene antibiotics have been used to treat fungal infections for nearly 50 years, there have been few reports of fungal resistance to these drugs. Fungi that do become resistant to polyenes have a reduced content of ergosterol in their cell membranes.

Adverse Effects. Amphotericin B is often called "amphoterrible" and is probably the most toxic antibiotic in use today. It has been reported to cause some degree of renal toxicity in about 80% of patients who are treated with it, although the incidence appears to be reduced when the lipid complex formulation of amphotericin B is used. Renal toxicity reduces the glomerular filtration rate and contributes to azotemia (accumulation of nitrogenous compounds in the blood), hypokalemia, and hypomagnesemia. Therefore, electrolytes (especially sodium, potassium, and magnesium) should be monitored weekly during treatment with amphotericin B, and replacements should be administered as needed.

In addition to causing nephrotoxicity, amphotericin B may cause acute liver failure, cardiac arrhythmias, and hematopoietic disorders such as anemia, leukopenia, and thrombocytopenia. The drug frequently causes less severe but unpleasant effects, including chills, fever, headache, nausea, and vomiting. The severity of these minor adverse effects may be lessened by pretreatment with corticosteroids, antipyretic drugs such as acetaminophen, and antihistamine drugs.

Nystatin and Natamycin

Nystatin is active against *Candida* species and is available in various formulations, including the following: creams, ointments, and powders for mucocutaneous candidiasis; lozenges (troches) for oral candidiasis; orally administered tablets and suspensions for intestinal candidiasis; and vaginal tablets for vaginal candidiasis.

Natamycin is active against *Aspergillus, Candida, Fusarium,* and *Penicillium* species and is available as an ophthalmic suspension for the treatment of fungal blepharitis, conjunctivitis, or keratitis.

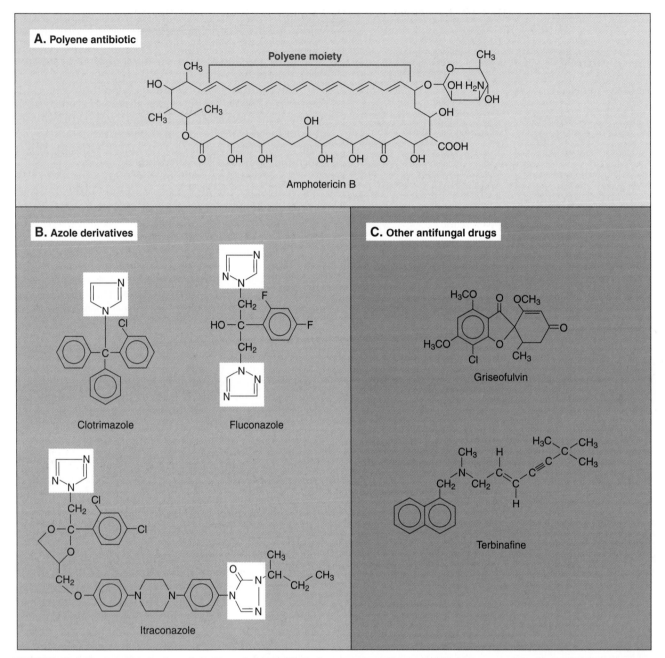

FIGURE 42–2. Structures of selected antifungal drugs. (A) Each polyene antibiotic consists of a macrolide (lactone) ring containing conjugated double bonds (polyene), with acidic and basic side groups. **(B)** Some azole derivatives, such as clotrimazole, are diazole (imidazole) compounds. Others, such as fluconazole and itraconazole, are triazole congeners. The diazole and triazole structures are unshaded. **(C)** Griseofulvin is a fungistatic antibiotic derived from *Penicillium griseofulvum*. Terbinafine is an allylamine drug.

Azole Derivatives

The azole derivatives are synthetic drugs that are used in the treatment of various mycoses (see Table 42–1). One group, the diazole (imidazole) compounds, includes **clotrimazole, econazole,** and **ketoconazole.** Another group, the triazole congeners, includes **fluconazole** and **itraconazole.**

Drug Properties

Chemistry and Pharmacokinetics. Representative structures of azole derivatives are shown in

Fig. 42–2B, and pharmacokinetic properties are compared in Table 42–2.

Some azoles are applied topically to treat superficial fungal infections, while others are given orally to treat the more stubborn superficial mycoses (such as onychomycosis). Azoles are usually given orally to treat systemic or subcutaneous mycoses, although fluconazole can also be administered intravenously.

Azole drugs are well absorbed from the gut. The absorption of ketoconazole and itraconazole requires the presence of gastric acid, so other drugs that reduce gastric acid should not be administered concurrently. Azoles are widely distributed to tissues

TABLE 42–2. Pharmacokinetic Properties of Antifungal Drugs*

Drug	Route of Administration	Oral Bioavail- ability	Elimination Half-Life	Routes of Elimination
Polyene antibiotics				
Amphotericin B	Topical, IV, intrathecal, or intraventricular	NA	24 hours or 15 days†	Metabolism; renal excretion.
Natamycin	Topical ocular	NA	NA	NA.
Nystatin	Oral or topical	None	NA	NA.
Azole derivatives				
Clotrimazole	Topical	NA	NA	NA.
Econazole	Topical	NA	NA	NA.
Fluconazole	Oral or IV	95%	35 hours	Renal excretion.
Itraconazole	Oral	55%	60 hours	Biliary, fecal, and renal excretion.
Ketoconazole	Oral or topical	Highly variable	8 hours	Biliary and fecal excretion.
Allylamine drugs				
Naftifine	Topical	NA	2.5 days	Renal and fecal excretion.
Terbinafine	Oral or topical	40%	12.5 days	Metabolism; renal excretion.
Other antifungal drugs				
Ciclopirox	Topical	NA	NA	NA.
Flucytosine	Oral	82%	3.5 hours	Renal excretion.
Griseofulvin	Oral	Variable	16 hours	Metabolism; renal excretion.
Tolnaftate	Topical	NA	NA	NA.

*Values shown are the mean of values reported in the literature. IV = intravenous; and NA = not applicable.
†For amphotericin B, the values represent the initial and terminal half-life, respectively.

and body fluids, but only fluconazole achieves significant concentrations in the cerebrospinal fluid (about 50% of concentrations in the plasma). For this reason, only fluconazole is used in the prophylaxis and treatment of fungal meningitis.

The azole derivatives undergo considerable hepatic biotransformation, and the parent compound and metabolites are excreted in the urine and feces. Itraconazole has an active metabolite, hydroxyitraconazole.

Spectrum and Indications.   Azole drugs may be either fungistatic or fungicidal, depending on the particular organism and the drug concentration. The drugs are active against a wide range of fungi that cause systemic and subcutaneous mycoses (see Table 42–3) and frequently serve as alternatives to amphotericin B for the treatment of these mycoses. Azoles are active against most dermatophytes that cause tinea infections, including *Epidermophyton floccosum*, *Microsporum canis*, *Microsporum gypseum*, *Trichophyton mentagrophytes*, *Trichophyton rubrum*, and *Trichophyton tonsurans*. Azoles also inhibit the growth of yeasts, including *Candida* and *Malassezia* species.

TABLE 42–3. Causes and Management of Systemic and Subcutaneous Mycoses

Mycosis	Most Common Pathogens	Treatment for Severe Infection	Treatment for Mild or Moderate Infection
Aspergillosis	*Aspergillus fumigatus.*	Amphotericin B.	Itraconazole or fluconazole.
Blastomycosis	*Blastomyces dermatitidis.*	Amphotericin B.	Itraconazole or ketoconazole.
Candidiasis	*Candida albicans.*	Amphotericin B, with or without flucytosine.	Fluconazole, ketoconazole, or itraconazole.
Chromomycosis	*Cladosporium, Fonsecaea,* and *Phialophora* species.	Amphotericin B.	No recommendation.
Coccidioidomycosis	*Coccidioides immitis.*	Amphotericin B for non-meningeal infection; fluconazole for meningeal infection.	Fluconazole, ketoconazole, or itraconazole.
Cryptococcosis	*Cryptococcus neoformans.*	Amphotericin B, with or without flucytosine; or amphotericin B followed by fluconazole.	Fluconazole or itraconazole.
Histoplasmosis	*Histoplasma capsulatum.*	Amphotericin B.	Itraconazole or ketoconazole.
Mucormycosis	*Absidia, Mucor,* and *Rhizopus* species.	Amphotericin B.	No recommendation.
Pseudallescheriasis	*Pseudallescheria boydii.*	Itraconazole.	No recommendation.
Sporotrichosis	*Sporothrix schenckii.*	Amphotericin B.	Itraconazole for disseminated infection; or iodide for cutaneous lesions.

Fungal Resistance. Resistance to azoles has emerged during treatment of systemic candidiasis with fluconazole, but the mechanisms have not been clearly defined.

Adverse Effects and Interactions. Azole derivatives are usually well tolerated, but systemic administration may cause skin rash, elevated hepatic enzyme levels, hepatic injury, hematopoietic toxicity, or gastrointestinal distress (nausea, vomiting, and diarrhea). Because azoles inhibit CYP3A4, a cytochrome P450 isozyme, their concurrent use with other drugs sometimes results in drug interactions. Ketoconazole is the most potent cytochrome inhibitor, and it may interfere with the biotransformation of other drugs and with the biosynthesis of testosterone. In fact, ketoconazole has been used to suppress testosterone synthesis in the treatment of prostate cancer and other conditions. Fluconazole, itraconazole, and ketoconazole may inhibit the biotransformation of astemizole and cisapride and thereby lead to elevated plasma concentrations and cardiac arrhythmias. Other drugs whose metabolism is inhibited by the azoles include HMG-CoA reductase inhibitors, some benzodiazepines, quinidine, and warfarin. The dosage of these drugs may need to be reduced during concurrent azole therapy.

Specific Drugs

Itraconazole is particularly useful in the treatment of blastomycosis and histoplasmosis, and it is widely used to treat onychomycosis. For onychomycosis, the drug is often administered orally three times a week. This procedure is called pulse dosing.

Fluconazole achieves excellent penetration of the cerebrospinal fluid. It is useful in the prevention of cryptococcal meningitis in patients with AIDS, and it is effective as follow-up therapy in patients whose cryptococcal meningitis has been successfully treated with amphotericin B. Based on the results of clinical studies, fluconazole is probably the drug of choice to prevent the relapse of cryptococcal meningitis. Fluconazole is also used to treat mucocutaneous (oropharyngeal and esophageal) and disseminated candidiasis. Because the drug is excreted in the urine, it is effective in patients with urinary tract infections caused by *Candida.* A single dose of fluconazole can eradicate acute vaginal candidiasis.

Ketoconazole is available in oral and topical formulations. The oral drug is less widely used than itraconazole or fluconazole, because it has a greater potential for drug interactions, does not effectively penetrate the cerebrospinal fluid, and has lower activity against most fungi. It is sometimes useful, however, in the treatment of nonmeningeal coccidioidomycosis and other mycoses (see Table 42-3). Topical formulations are useful for treating seborrheic dermatitis.

Clotrimazole is available in topical formulations for treatment of the following: *Candida* infections of the mouth, throat, vagina, and vulva; *M. furfur* infection of the skin (tinea versicolor); and dermatophyte infections of the skin (such as tinea pedis and tinea cruris). Econazole is also available in topical formulations for the treatment of *Candida* and dermatophyte infections of the skin. However, these and other topical drugs are not effective for the treatment of dermatophyte infections of the scalp (tinea capitis) or nails (tinea unguium, or onychomycosis).

Other azole derivatives not discussed in this chapter are available for the treatment of vaginal candidiasis and other superficial fungal infections.

Allylamine Drugs

Naftifine and **terbinafine** are allylamines that inhibit ergosterol synthesis (see Figs. 42-1 and 42-2C). Although they are primarily used to treat superficial dermatophyte infections, they are also fungistatic against *Candida.*

Both drugs are available in topical formulations, and terbinafine is also available for oral administration. Terbinafine is often administered orally once a day to treat onychomycosis. Fingernail infections usually require 6 weeks of therapy, whereas toenail infections may require 12 weeks of treatment.

Naftifine and terbinafine are well tolerated and rarely cause serious adverse effects.

Other Antifungal Drugs
Flucytosine

Flucytosine is a fluorinated pyrimidine analogue that is used orally to treat severe fungal infections. The drug is accumulated by fungal cells and is converted to its active metabolite, 5-fluorouracil (5-FU), by cytosine deaminase. The metabolite is incorporated into fungal RNA, and this interferes with fungal protein synthesis (see Fig. 42-1). Unlike fungal cells, human cells lack cytosine deaminase and are unable to activate the drug.

Fungal resistance to flucytosine may result from mutations in genes encoding cytosine deaminase, cytosine permease, or enzymes that incorporate 5-FU into fungal RNA. Because drug resistance develops rapidly when flucytosine is given alone, the drug is usually administered in combination with amphotericin B. This combination produces a synergistic effect against *Candida* and *Cryptococcus* species and is effective in the treatment of pneumonia, meningitis, endocarditis, or septicemia caused by these organisms.

The adverse effects of flucytosine are usually mild. In some patients, however, hematologic toxicity and cardiopulmonary arrest have occurred.

Griseofulvin

Griseofulvin is an antibiotic derived from *Penicillium griseofulvum* (see Fig. 42-2C). The antibiotic has fungistatic activity against numerous dermatophytes, including *E. floccosum, Microsporum audouinii, M. canis, M. gypseum, T. rubrum, T. tonsurans,* and *Trichophyton verrucosum,* but it is not active against *Candida* or other fungi.

Griseofulvin is a lipophilic drug that is not very soluble in water. To enhance its dissolution in the gut, a microcrystalline form of the drug is employed in pharmaceutical preparations. Because of the drug's high lipid solubility, its absorption is increased when it is taken with a high-fat meal. The drug is deposited in keratin precursor cells of the skin, hair, and nails, where it disrupts microtubule function and inhibits the mitosis of susceptible dermatophytes. The cells are gradually exfoliated and replaced by noninfected tissue. After being metabolized in the liver, griseofulvin is excreted in the urine as inactive metabolites. Mild infections usually respond to griseofulvin therapy in 2–8 weeks, but persistent nail infections may require 3–6 months of treatment.

Griseofulvin is usually well tolerated, but it may cause dizziness, headache, insomnia, gastrointestinal bleeding, hepatitis, skin rash, or leukopenia. Griseofulvin induces the CYP3A4 isozyme of cytochrome P450 and may thereby reduce the plasma concentrations of warfarin, oral contraceptives, and barbiturates that are taken concurrently. As a result, griseofulvin may reduce the anticoagulant effect of warfarin. The clinical significance of the other drug interactions has not been established.

Ciclopirox

Ciclopirox is an *N*-hydroxy-pyridinone compound that is active against dermatophytes, *C. albicans,* and *M. furfur.* It is applied topically twice a day to treat skin infections caused by these organisms.

Tolnaftate

Tolnaftate is a nonprescription thiocarbamate drug that is used to treat tinea versicolor and mild dermatophyte infections of the skin. The drug is usually applied twice daily to the affected areas for 2–6 weeks. Like most other topical antifungal drugs, tolnaftate is not reliable for treating infections of the scalp or nail beds.

Summary of Important Points

- Polyene antibiotics and ciclopirox increase the permeability of the fungal cell membrane. Azole derivatives and allylamine drugs inhibit fungal synthesis of ergosterol.
- Flucytosine is converted to 5-fluorouracil by fungal cells and is then incorporated into fungal RNA, where it inhibits protein synthesis. Griseofulvin interferes with microtubule function and blocks mitosis.
- Amphotericin B is a polyene antibiotic that may cause renal failure and many other adverse effects. It has recently been formulated as a lipid complex that produces less toxicity.
- Amphotericin B is used to treat the most severe systemic and subcutaneous mycoses. Flucytosine and several azole derivatives (fluconazole, itraconazole, and ketoconazole) are used to treat less severe forms of these infections.
- Superficial *Candida* infections can be treated with polyene antibiotics, azole derivatives, or ciclopirox.
- Dermatophyte infections can be treated by topical or oral administration of an azole derivative or terbinafine; by oral administration of griseofulvin; or by topical administration of ciclopirox, naftifine, or tolnaftate.
- Itraconazole or terbinafine is given orally to treat onychomycosis.

Selected Readings

Bradsher, R. W. Therapy of blastomycosis. Semin Respir Infect 12:263–267, 1997.

Del Rooso, J. Q. Treatment of onychomycosis and tinea pedis with intermittent itraconazole therapy. J Am Osteopath Assoc 96:607–609, 1996.

Graybill, J. R. Itraconazole: managing mycotic complications in immunocompromised patients. Semin Oncol 25(supplement 7):58–63, 1998.

Koehler, A. P., et al. Successful treatment of disseminated coccidioidomycosis with amphotericin B lipid complex. J Infect 36:113–115, 1998.

Luke, R. G., and J. A. Boyle. Renal effects of amphotericin B lipid complex. Am J Kidney Dis 31:780–785, 1998.

Powderly, W. G., et al. A controlled trial of fluconazole or amphotericin B to prevent relapse of cryptococcal meningitis in patients with acquired immunodeficiency syndrome. N Engl J Med 326:793–798, 1992.

Rapp, R. P., et al. Amphotericin B lipid complex. Ann Pharmacother 31:1174–1186, 1997.

CHAPTER FORTY-THREE

ANTIVIRAL DRUGS

CLASSIFICATION OF ANTIVIRAL DRUGS*

DRUGS FOR HERPESVIRUS INFECTIONS
  Nucleoside analogues
  - Acyclovir, cidofovir, famciclovir, ganciclovir, penciclovir, trifluridine, and valacyclovir
  Other drugs for herpesvirus infections
  - Foscarnet

DRUGS FOR HUMAN IMMUNODEFICIENCY VIRUS INFECTION
  Nucleoside reverse transcriptase inhibitors
  - Didanosine, lamivudine, stavudine, zalcitabine, and zidovudine
  Nonnucleoside reverse transcriptase inhibitors
  - Delavirdine, efavirenz, and nevirapine
  Protease inhibitors
  - Indinavir, nelfinavir, ritonavir, and saquinavir

DRUGS FOR INFLUENZA
  - Amantadine and rimantadine

DRUGS FOR HEPATITIS
  - Interferon alfa, lamivudine, and ribavirin

DRUGS FOR OTHER VIRAL INFECTIONS
  - Interferon alfa and ribavirin

*Note that some drugs are listed more than once.

OVERVIEW

Viruses are obligate intracellular parasites that use the host cell's metabolic pathways for reproduction. This limits the number of potential sites for antiviral drug action. Furthermore, antibacterial and antifungal drugs have little or no effect on viruses. Despite these obstacles, effective antiviral compounds have been developed for the treatment of some viral infections. These include herpesvirus infections, human immunodeficiency virus (HIV) infection, influenza, and hepatitis.

Most antiviral drugs are antimetabolites of endogenous nucleosides and prevent the replication of viral nucleic acid. Other antiviral drugs inhibit the uncoating of viral nucleic acid or inhibit posttransla-

tional processing of viral proteins. Recently, scientists have used molecular modeling techniques to design a new class of drugs that act by inhibiting a protease enzyme required for maturation of the HIV virion. As knowledge about the molecular biology of viruses increases, other viral targets may be identified for future drug development.

DRUGS FOR HERPESVIRUS INFECTIONS

All herpesviruses are DNA viruses. The most common examples are **herpes simplex virus** (HSV), **varicella-zoster virus** (VZV), and **cytomegalovirus** (CMV).

HSV frequently causes **herpes genitalis** (genital herpes infection), **herpes labialis** (infection of the lips and mouth), or **herpetic keratoconjunctivitis** (infection of the cornea and conjunctiva). Less commonly, it causes **herpetic encephalitis,** a potentially fatal disease.

VZV is the cause of **chickenpox (varicella)** and **shingles (herpes zoster).** Chickenpox occurs primarily in young children. Shingles is reported more frequently in the elderly and results from activation of latent VZV in nerve root ganglia. In patients with shingles, pain and skin lesions occur in areas where the virus travels peripherally along sensory nerves to the corresponding cutaneous or mucosal surfaces. The skin lesions eventually heal but may leave residual scars. Postherpetic neuralgia is a common and disabling complication of shingles.

CMV infections in immunocompetent individuals are usually asymptomatic. Symptomatic **CMV diseases,** such as **retinitis, esophagitis,** and **colitis,** are seen most often in immunocompromised patients, including those with HIV infection or acquired immunodeficiency syndrome (AIDS).

Numerous drugs are available to treat herpesvirus infections. With the exception of foscarnet, all of the drugs are nucleoside analogues.

Nucleoside Analogues
Drug Properties

Chemistry. Most of the nucleoside analogues used to treat herpesvirus infections contain a naturally occurring purine or pyrimidine base that is coupled to a unique carbohydrate moiety (Fig. 43–1A).

Mechanisms. The nucleoside analogues are prodrugs that are phosphorylated by viral and host

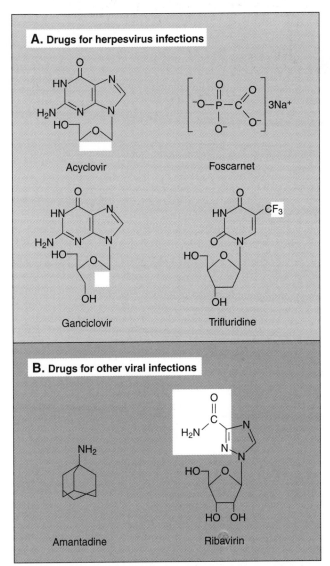

A. Drugs for herpesvirus infections

Acyclovir

Foscarnet

Ganciclovir

Trifluridine

B. Drugs for other viral infections

Amantadine

Ribavirin

FIGURE 43–1. Structures of selected drugs for herpesvirus infections (A) and other viral infections (B). Acyclovir, ganciclovir, and trifluridine are nucleoside analogues. Ribavirin, a broad-spectrum drug used in the treatment of hepatitis B, hepatitis C, and anogenital warts, is also a nucleoside analogue (a guanosine analogue). Most of these analogues contain a naturally occurring purine or pyrimidine base, which is coupled to a unique carbohydrate moiety (unshaded area). Unlike the other drugs for herpesvirus infections, foscarnet is a pyrophosphate derivative. Amantadine is a tricyclic amine compound used in the treatment of influenza.

cell kinases to form active triphosphate metabolites (Fig. 43–2). In this process, the nucleoside analogues are initially converted to monophosphate metabolites by a virus-encoded thymidine kinase. The conversion occurs only in infected host cells, thereby contributing to the selective toxicity of the analogues. Host cell kinases subsequently convert the monophosphates to active triphosphate metabolites. The active metabolites then compete with endogenous nucleoside triphosphates and competitively inhibit viral DNA polymerase. This in turn prevents the synthesis of viral DNA. Some nucleoside analogues, such as acyclovir, are incorporated into

nascent viral DNA and cause DNA chain termination because they lack the 3'-hydroxyl group required for attachment of the next nucleoside (see Fig. 43–2). Other analogues, such as ganciclovir and penciclovir, inhibit viral DNA polymerase but do not cause DNA chain termination.

Pharmacokinetics, Spectrum, and Indications. The properties and clinical uses of individual drugs for herpesvirus infections are compared in Tables 43–1 and 43–2 and discussed in greater detail below.

Viral Resistance. The incidence of resistance to the nucleoside analogues varies with the drug and viral pathogen.

Resistance of HSV and VZV to acyclovir is not common, and resistant strains are usually less infective than are sensitive strains. Furthermore, most acyclovir-resistant HSV and VZV strains are not resistant to other nucleoside analogues or to foscarnet. Most acyclovir-resistant strains have been recovered from immunocompromised patients. Loss of thymidine kinase activity is the major cause of innate and acquired resistance to acyclovir.

Resistance of CMV to ganciclovir is a more serious clinical problem than is HSV resistance, but most ganciclovir-resistant CMV strains are sensitive to cidofovir or foscarnet. Loss of a virus-specific protein kinase is the major cause of resistance to ganciclovir.

Acyclovir, Famciclovir, and Valacyclovir

Acyclovir, famciclovir, and valacyclovir are nucleoside analogues that are effective in the treatment of various HSV and VZV infections (see Table 43–2) but not in the treatment of CMV infections. All three drugs are available for oral use. In addition, acyclovir is available for intravenous and topical use.

The intravenous form of acyclovir is the most effective treatment for serious herpesvirus infections, including herpetic encephalitis and severe HSV and VZV infections in immunocompromised patients.

The topical form of acyclovir can be used to treat herpes genitalis and mild mucocutaneous infections in immunocompromised patients. In cases of herpes genitalis, however, the topical form is less effective than the oral form of acyclovir.

In its oral form, acyclovir has a relatively low bioavailability (22%). Valacyclovir, which was developed later than acyclovir, is a prodrug that is rapidly converted to acyclovir by intestinal and hepatic enzymes and is more completely absorbed than acyclovir. Because of its greater bioavailability (55%), valacyclovir requires less frequent administration than acyclovir. Famciclovir is rapidly hydrolyzed to penciclovir and has the greatest bioavailability (80%).

When acyclovir, famciclovir, or valacyclovir is given orally for the treatment of herpes genitalis, it prevents the replication of HSV and thereby reduces pain and other symptoms of acute infection. It also shortens the time to healing of lesions and reduces the amount of viral shedding. However, it does not eliminate the virus, so recurrent episodes of infection

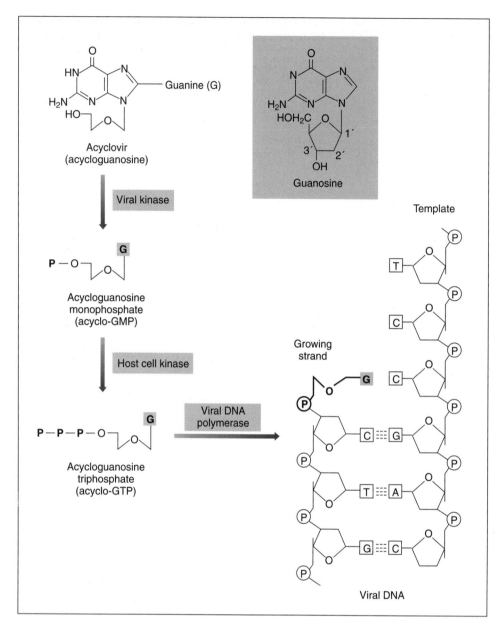

FIGURE 43–2. Mechanisms of action of nucleoside analogues used in the treatment of viral infections. Acyclovir and other nucleoside analogues are converted to active nucleoside triphosphates by viral and host cell kinases. These active nucleoside triphosphates compete with the corresponding endogenous nucleoside triphosphates and competitively inhibit viral DNA polymerase. Acyclovir and the nucleoside reverse transcriptase inhibitors (NRTIs) are incorporated into viral DNA and cause chain termination because they lack the 3′-hydroxyl group required to attach the next nucleoside. Ganciclovir and penciclovir do not cause chain termination.

are common. Shorter courses of therapy are usually sufficient for these episodes, because recurrent infections are usually milder than the initial infection. Severe herpes genitalis may require intravenous acyclovir therapy.

When acyclovir, famciclovir, or valacyclovir is given orally for the treatment of shingles, it shortens the duration of acute illness and pain and also shortens the duration of postherpetic pain. In patients with shingles, famciclovir and valacyclovir appear to be more effective than acyclovir. The newer drugs allow for less frequent administration and provide higher serum drug levels because of their greater oral bioavailability.

Acyclovir is available in an oral suspension for the treatment of children with chickenpox. The drug has a good safety record in this setting.

Acyclovir, famciclovir, and valacyclovir are well tolerated when given orally, and they do not have significant interactions with other drugs. Gastrointes-

tinal disturbances, headache, and rash are the most common side effects. Intravenous administration of acyclovir may produce phlebitis and reversible renal dysfunction.

Penciclovir

Penciclovir, the active metabolite of famciclovir, is now available in a topical cream formulation for the treatment of herpes labialis. In a study of patients with a history of frequent herpes labialis episodes, use of penciclovir was found to shorten the time to healing and the duration of pain by about a day. It also was found to decrease the duration of viral shedding.

Ganciclovir and Cidofovir

Ganciclovir and cidofovir are nucleoside analogues that are used for the prevention and treatment of CMV diseases, including retinitis, esophagitis, and colitis. Both drugs are available for intravenous use, and ganciclovir is also available for oral use. Ganciclovir is usually given initially, whereas cidofovir is generally reserved for diseases that are resistant to ganciclovir or other drugs. Ganciclovir has a relatively low oral bioavailability, so oral administration is used only for long-term suppression of CMV retinitis. Cidofovir can be given intravenously for this purpose.

Ganciclovir is about 100 times more active against CMV than is acyclovir. However, ganciclovir produces a much higher incidence of adverse effects than do acyclovir and famciclovir. The most common serious adverse effects of ganciclovir are leukopenia and thrombocytopenia. Severe myelosuppression is more likely if the drug is given concurrently with zidovudine. Other adverse effects of ganciclovir include retinal detachment, liver and renal dysfunction, rash, fever, and gastrointestinal disturbances.

TABLE 43–1.   Pharmacokinetic Properties of Antiviral Drugs*

Drug	Route of Administration	Oral Bioavailability	Elimination Half-Life (Hours)	Routes of Elimination
Drugs for herpesvirus infections				
Nucleoside analogues				
Acyclovir	Oral, IV, or topical	22%	3	Renal excretion.
Cidofovir	IV	NA	2.5	Renal excretion.
Famciclovir	Oral	80%	2	Metabolism; renal and fecal excretion.
Ganciclovir	Oral or IV	8%	4	Renal excretion.
Penciclovir	Topical	NA	NA	NA.
Trifluridine	Topical ocular	NA	NA	NA.
Valacyclovir	Oral	55%	3	Renal excretion.
Other drugs				
Foscarnet	IV	NA	5	Renal excretion.
Drugs for human immunodeficiency virus infection				
NRTIs				
Didanosine	Oral	30%	2	Metabolism; renal excretion.
Lamivudine	Oral	85%	6	Renal excretion.
Stavudine	Oral	85%	3.5	Renal excretion.
Zalcitabine	Oral	80%	2	Renal excretion.
Zidovudine	Oral or IV	65%	1	Metabolism; renal excretion.
NNRTIs				
Delavirdine	Oral	95%	7	Metabolism; renal and fecal excretion.
Efavirenz	Oral	U	U	U.
Nevirapine	Oral	92%	30	Metabolism; fecal excretion.
Protease inhibitors				
Indinavir	Oral	80%†	2	Metabolism; fecal excretion.
Nelfinavir	Oral	50%†	4.5	Metabolism; fecal excretion.
Ritonavir	Oral	80%†	4	Metabolism; fecal excretion.
Saquinavir	Oral	12%	12	Metabolism; fecal excretion.
Drugs for influenza				
Amantadine	Oral	75%	24	Renal excretion.
Rimantadine	Oral	90%	25	Metabolism; renal excretion.
Drugs for other viral infections				
Interferon alfa	Subcutaneous or IM	NA	U	Metabolism.
Lamivudine	Oral	85%	6	Renal excretion.
Ribavirin	Inhalation or IV	NA	9.5	Metabolism; renal excretion.

*Values shown are the mean of values reported in the literature. IV = intravenous; IM = intramuscular; NA = not applicable; U = unknown; NRTIs = nucleoside reverse transcriptase inhibitors; and NNRTIs = nonnucleoside reverse transcriptase inhibitors.
†Bioavailability percentages for indinavir, nelfinavir, and ritonavir are estimates based on experimental studies in animals and on plasma drug concentrations in humans.

TABLE 43–2. Clinical Uses of Drugs for Herpesvirus Infections

Drug	Herpes Genitalis	Herpes Labialis	Herpetic Keratocon-junctivitis	Herpetic Encephalitis	Chicken-pox	Shingles	Cytomegalo-virus Diseases
Acyclovir	Yes	Yes	No	Yes	Yes	Yes	No
Cidofovir	No	No	No	No	No	No	Yes*
Famciclovir	Yes	No	No	No	No	Yes	No
Foscarnet	Yes*	No	No	No	No	Yes*	Yes
Ganciclovir	No	No	No	No	No	No	Yes
Penciclovir	No	Yes	No	No	No	No	No
Trifluridine	No	No	Yes	No	No	No	No
Valacyclovir	Yes	No	No	No	No	Yes	No

*For treating patients with intolerance of or resistance to other drugs.

Cidofovir sometimes causes nephrotoxicity, neutropenia, metabolic acidosis, and other serious adverse effects. About 25% of patients have discontinued cidofovir for this reason. The drug is contraindicated in patients who are taking other nephrotoxic drugs, such as aminoglycosides or amphotericin B.

Trifluridine

Trifluridine is administered topically for the treatment of ocular herpesvirus infections. It is the most widely used nucleoside analogue in patients with herpetic keratoconjunctivitis and epithelial keratitis, and it is usually effective in treating infections that are not responsive to idoxuridine or vidarabine. The drug is generally well tolerated but may cause superficial ocular irritation and hyperemia.

Other Drugs for Herpesvirus Infections

Foscarnet is a pyrophosphate derivative (see Fig. 43–1A). It acts by blocking pyrophosphate-binding sites on viral DNA polymerase and thereby preventing attachment of nucleotide precursors to DNA. Unlike the nucleoside analogues used to treat herpesvirus infections, foscarnet does not require activation by viral or host cell kinases.

Foscarnet is active against CMV, VZV, and HSV. It must be administered intravenously and is used to treat CMV retinitis in patients with AIDS and to treat acyclovir-resistant HSV infections and shingles. Foscarnet may be combined with ganciclovir to treat infections that are resistant to either drug alone.

Adverse reactions to foscarnet include renal impairment and acute renal failure, hematologic deficiencies, cardiac arrhythmias and heart failure, seizures, and pancreatitis. Renal toxicity can be minimized by administering intravenous fluids to induce diuresis before and during foscarnet treatment.

DRUGS FOR HUMAN IMMUNODEFICIENCY VIRUS INFECTION

Remarkable advances have been made in the treatment of HIV infection and AIDS. A number of new drugs have been introduced, and the combined use of two or more drugs has been shown to markedly reduce viral loads in many HIV-positive individuals. Because many of the new drugs were introduced under the accelerated approval mechanism of the Food and Drug Administration (FDA), however, their long-term efficacy and safety have not yet been adequately studied.

Sites of Drug Action

HIV is an RNA virus that is classified as a **retrovirus.** Its replication and sites of drug action are depicted in Fig. 43–3. Once HIV enters the CD4$^+$ cell, viral RNA serves as a template to produce a complementary doubled-stranded DNA in a reaction catalyzed by **reverse transcriptase** (RNA-dependent DNA polymerase). The viral DNA then enters the host cell nucleus and is incorporated into the host genome in a reaction catalyzed by **HIV integrase.** Eventually, the viral DNA is transcribed and translated to produce large, nonfunctional polypeptides called **polyproteins.** These polyproteins are packaged into immature virions at the cell surface. As the virions are released into the plasma, an enzyme called **HIV protease** cleaves the polyproteins into smaller, functional proteins in a process called **viral maturation.**

The drugs currently available for the treatment of HIV infection act by inhibiting reverse transcriptase or by inhibiting HIV protease. Drugs that act via other mechanisms are being investigated. For example, zintevir is an investigational drug that may act by inhibiting HIV integrase, although some studies suggest that it inhibits binding or fusion of HIV to the host cell membrane.

There are two types of reverse transcriptase inhibitors: **nucleoside reverse transcriptase inhibitors** (NRTIs) and **nonnucleoside reverse transcriptase inhibitors** (NNRTIs). Small amounts of the NRTIs are converted to their active triphosphate metabolites by host cell kinases. The triphosphate metabolites compete with the corresponding endogenous nucleoside triphosphates for incorporation into viral DNA in the reaction catalyzed by reverse transcriptase. Once incorporated into DNA, the NRTIs cause chain termination in the same manner as described above for acyclovir (see Fig. 43–2). The NRTIs also inhibit host cell DNA polymerase to varying degrees,

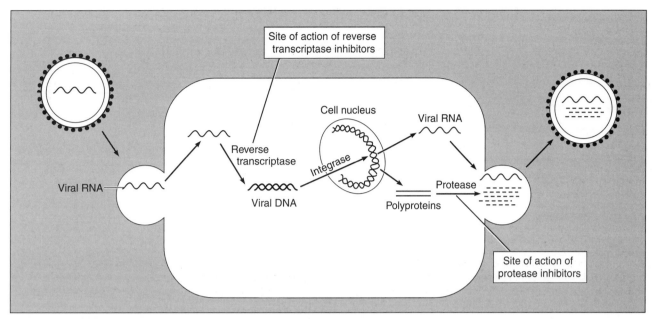

FIGURE 43–3. Sites of action of drugs for human immunodeficiency virus (HIV) infection. After the virus penetrates the host cell and becomes uncoated, the viral RNA is transcribed by reverse transcriptase to form viral DNA. Viral DNA is incorporated into the host genome in the cell nucleus by HIV integrase. The viral DNA is then transcribed to RNA. Viral RNA is incorporated into new virions and is translated to synthesize polyproteins. The polyproteins are cleaved into viral proteins by HIV protease as the new virions are released from the cell. Drugs for HIV infection inhibit reverse transcriptase or protease.

and this may account for some of their toxic effects. Unlike the NRTIs, the NNRTIs do not require phosphorylation for activity. The nonnucleoside drugs bind directly to reverse transcriptase and disrupt the catalytic site. Because they act by different mechanisms, the NRTIs and NNRTIs exhibit synergistic inhibition of HIV replication when they are given concurrently.

Nucleoside Reverse Transcriptase Inhibitors

The NRTIs were the first class of drugs developed for the treatment of HIV-positive individuals, and they are included in most HIV treatment regimens. While all NRTIs have the same basic mechanism of action, different drugs in the class serve as antimetabolites of different purine and pyrimidine bases of DNA. For this reason, an NRTI is often more effective when it is given in combination with another NRTI than when it is given alone. As shown in Table 43–3, NRTIs are often combined with one another and with NNRTIs or protease inhibitors.

Drug Properties

Chemistry. The NRTIs are synthetic derivatives of naturally occurring nucleosides (Fig. 43–4A). Didanosine is a purine base congener, whereas

---

TABLE 43–3. Drug Regimens for Treating Human Immunodeficiency Virus (HIV) Infection in Adults*

Preferred drug regimens:
- Two NRTIs (see combinations listed below) plus one protease inhibitor.
- Two NRTIs (see combinations listed below) plus one NNRTI.

Alternative drug regimens (for patients unable to take a preferred regimen):
- Two NRTIs (see combinations listed below).
- One NRTI plus one protease inhibitor.
- Two protease inhibitors alone or with either an NRTI or an NNRTI.
- One protease inhibitor plus one NRTI plus one NNRTI.

Initial NRTI combination:†	Subsequent or alternative NRTI combination:†
Zidovudine plus lamivudine	Stavudine plus didanosine
Zidovudine plus didanosine	Stavudine plus lamivudine
Stavudine plus didanosine	Zidovudine plus lamivudine
Stavudine plus lamivudine	Zidovudine plus didanosine or an NNRTI
Zidovudine plus zalcitabine	Stavudine plus lamivudine or didanosine

*NRTI = nucleoside reverse transcriptase inhibitor; and NNRTI = nonnucleoside reverse transcriptase inhibitor.
†Didanosine and zalcitabine should not be used together, because the two drugs produce similar toxicities. Zidovudine and stavudine are usually not used together, because they appear to be antagonistic.

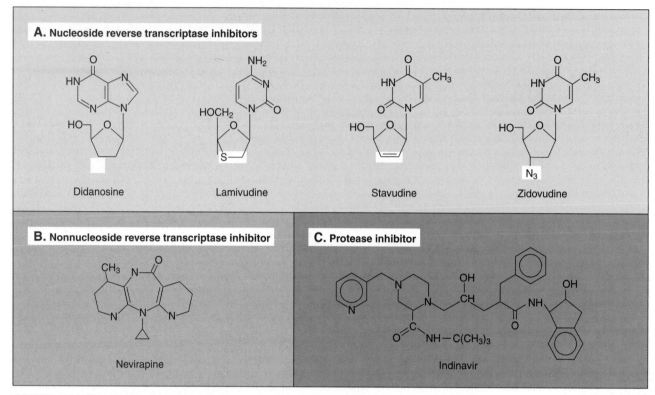

FIGURE 43-4. Structures of selected drugs for human immunodeficiency virus (HIV) infection. (A) Each nucleoside reverse transcriptase inhibitor contains a naturally occurring purine or pyrimidine base, which is coupled to a unique carbohydrate moiety (unshaded area). Didanosine is a purine base congener, whereas lamivudine, stavudine, zalcitabine, and zidovudine are pyrimidine base congeners. **(B)** Nevirapine is a tricyclic amine. **(C)** Indinavir is a pyrrolinone.

lamivudine, stavudine, zalcitabine, and zidovudine are pyrimidine base congeners.

Pharmacokinetics. All of the NRTIs can be given orally, and zidovudine can also be given intravenously. The NRTIs cross the blood-brain barrier and are distributed to the cerebrospinal fluid. The drugs are eliminated primarily by renal excretion, and renal impairment will prolong their plasma elimination half-life and may necessitate a reduction in dosage.

Spectrum and Indications. The NRTIs are the foundation of chemotherapy for HIV infection. In addition to inhibiting the replication of human and animal retroviruses, some of the NRTIs have demonstrated activity against hepatitis B virus and Epstein-Barr virus.

Viral Resistance. Resistance to NRTIs may develop during therapy and is more likely to occur in persons receiving single-drug therapy for 6 months or longer. Studies of zidovudine indicate that HIV type I (HIV-1) acquires resistance to the drug in a stepwise manner involving four or five specific mutations in the gene that encodes the reverse transcriptase enzyme. Because the virus undergoes frequent mutations, the only way to prevent resistance is to prevent HIV replication by using combination drug therapy.

Adverse Effects and Interactions. As shown in Table 43-4, the NRTIs differ in their major toxicities and in their interactions with other drugs.

Didanosine

Didanosine, or **dideoxyinosine** (ddI), is mainly used in combination with stavudine or zidovudine plus either a protease inhibitor or an NNRTI. Didanosine is not used with zalcitabine, because the two drugs produce similar toxicities, including peripheral neuropathy and pancreatitis.

Lamivudine

Lamivudine, or **3-thiacytosine** (3TC), appears to cause fewer adverse effects than do other NRTIs. Lamivudine is often used in combination with stavudine or with zidovudine. Combination therapy with these drugs produces a greater reduction in viral load than is obtained with single-drug therapy, and it also decreases the risk for emergence of drug resistance.

Stavudine

Stavudine, or **4-deoxythymidine** (d4T), is usually employed as an alternative to zidovudine in persons who cannot tolerate zidovudine or fail to respond to it. Stavudine can be combined with didanosine or lamivudine.

Zalcitabine

Zalcitabine, or **dideoxycytosine** (ddC), is less effective than zidovudine when used alone. The

Centers for Disease Control and Prevention recommends that zalcitabine be used as part of a three-drug regimen that includes zidovudine and a protease inhibitor.

Zidovudine

Zidovudine, or **azidothymidine** (AZT), was the first NRTI to be developed, and it is still the most widely used drug in this class. Zidovudine is most often combined with lamivudine or didanosine, and

it is available in a fixed-dose combination product with lamivudine. Zidovudine and stavudine are usually not used together, because they appear to be antagonistic.

Studies indicate that zidovudine treatment significantly reduces the incidence of in utero transmission of HIV from infected pregnant women to their offspring. To prevent transmission, zidovudine is administered from the 14th to the 34th week of gestation. Many authorities now recommend combination drug therapy for pregnant women with HIV infection.

TABLE 43–4. Adverse Effects and Interactions of Drugs for Human Immunodeficiency Virus (HIV) Infection*

Drug	Common Adverse Effects	Common Drug Interactions
NRTIs		
Didanosine	Gastrointestinal disturbances; pancreatitis; and peripheral neuropathy.	Didanosine decreases absorption of dapsone, delavirdine, fluoroquinolones, indinavir, itraconazole, and ketoconazole. Ganciclovir decreases excretion of didanosine and may cause toxicity.
Lamivudine	None.	Trimethoprim-sulfamethoxazole decreases renal excretion and increases serum levels of lamivudine by 30–40%.
Stavudine	Sensory neuropathy.	Dapsone, isoniazid, metronidazole, phenytoin, and vincristine may have additive neurotoxicity with stavudine.
Zalcitabine	Esophageal and oral ulcers; fever; pancreatitis; and peripheral neuropathy.	Aminoglycosides, amphotericin B, and foscarnet may reduce renal clearance of zalcitabine. Estrogens, pentamidine, sulfonamides, and other drugs that cause pancreatitis should be avoided with zalcitabine use.
Zidovudine	Anemia; fatigue; headache; hepatitis; myopathy; nausea; neutropenia; and vomiting.	Rifampin may increase metabolism and decrease the therapeutic effect of zidovudine.
NNRTIs		
Delavirdine	Rash.	Delavirdine may inhibit metabolism and increase the toxicity of astemizole, benzodiazepines, cisapride, some protease inhibitors, and rifabutin. Delavirdine and didanosine interact to decrease absorption of both drugs. Rifabutin and rifampin may induce metabolism and decrease the therapeutic effect of delavirdine.
Efavirenz	Diarrhea; dizziness; fatigue; headache; nausea; and rash.	Unknown.
Nevirapine	Fever; headache; nausea; and rash.	Nevirapine may increase metabolism and decrease the therapeutic effect of contraceptive steroids and all protease inhibitors.
Protease inhibitors		
Indinavir	Crystalluria; hemolytic anemia; hepatitis; and kidney stones (nephrolithiasis).	Indinavir may inhibit metabolism and increase the toxicity of nelfinavir and saquinavir. Delavirdine may inhibit metabolism and increase the toxicity of indinavir. Nevirapine may increase metabolism and decrease the therapeutic effect of indinavir. Didanosine decreases absorption of indinavir.
Nelfinavir	Diarrhea.	Nelfinavir may inhibit metabolism and increase the toxicity of astemizole, benzodiazepines, cisapride, indinavir, rifabutin, and saquinavir. Indinavir and ritonavir may inhibit metabolism and increase the toxicity of nelfinavir. Nevirapine may increase metabolism and decrease the therapeutic effect of nelfinavir.
Ritonavir	Asthenia; diarrhea; increased serum aminotransferase, cholesterol, and triglyceride levels; nausea; paresthesias; renal failure; and vomiting.	Ritonavir may inhibit metabolism and increase the toxicity of antiarrhythmic drugs, cisapride, nelfinavir, opioids, rifabutin, and tricyclic antidepressants. Nevirapine may increase metabolism and decrease the therapeutic effect of ritonavir.
Saquinavir	Abdominal pain; diarrhea; increased serum aminotransferase levels; and nausea.	Saquinavir may inhibit metabolism and increase the toxicity of astemizole and cisapride. Delavirdine, indinavir, and nelfinavir may inhibit metabolism and increase the toxicity of saquinavir. Nevirapine, rifabutin, and rifampin may increase metabolism and decrease the therapeutic effect of saquinavir.

*NRTIs = nucleoside reverse transcriptase inhibitors; and NNRTIs = nonnucleoside reverse transcriptase inhibitors.

Zidovudine produces bone marrow suppression and may cause anemia and neutropenia. In contrast, other NRTIs produce less bone marrow suppression but may cause pancreatitis or neuropathy.

Nonnucleoside Reverse Transcriptase Inhibitors
Drug Properties

The NNRTIs include delavirdine, nevirapine, and a newer drug called efavirenz. These drugs directly inhibit reverse transcriptase. Unlike NRTIs, they do not require metabolic activation, and they are not incorporated into viral DNA.

Pharmacokinetics. The NNRTIs are administered orally and have good oral bioavailability (see Table 43–1). They are highly lipophilic, and the concentrations that they reach in the central nervous system (CNS) are adequate for antiviral activity. The drugs are extensively metabolized before undergoing fecal and renal excretion.

Spectrum, Indications, and Viral Resistance. In vitro studies show that NNRTIs act synergistically with NRTIs and protease inhibitors against HIV. The NNRTIs are never used alone to treat patients with HIV infection, because viral resistance develops rapidly unless they are combined with other drugs. Delavirdine and nevirapine exhibit cross-resistance with each other. It is not known if they are cross-resistant with efavirenz.

Preferred and alternative treatment regimens are listed in Table 43–3. In published clinical studies, an NNRTI was often combined with zidovudine and didanosine. Results suggest that these three-drug combinations are more effective than two-drug combinations.

Adverse Effects and Interactions. NNRTIs are moderately well tolerated. Rash is the most common side effect. In patients with a mild rash, the drugs can usually be continued or restarted. However, patients should be monitored because the rash can progress to Stevens-Johnson syndrome. Drug interactions and other common adverse effects are listed in Table 43–4.

Delavirdine

Delavirdine has a shorter half-life than nevirapine and must be given more frequently.

Delavirdine inhibits the metabolism of CYP3A4, an isozyme of cytochrome P450. Concurrent use of interacting drugs (see Table 43–4) should be avoided.

Efavirenz

Efavirenz is one of the newest drugs to be approved for treatment of HIV infection. Prior to its approval by the FDA, the drug was available under a compassionate use program for patients who were intolerant of other drugs or failed to respond to them.

Efavirenz appears to be the most potent NNRTI, but its role in treating HIV-infected individuals is still under examination. Unlike other NNRTIs, efavirenz can be taken once a day.

In a phase 3 clinical trial, efavirenz was given in combination with two NRTIs (zidovudine and lamivudine).

Nevirapine

Nevirapine (see Fig. 43–4B) is usually used in combination with two NRTIs. However, when a combination of nevirapine plus an NRTI (lamivudine) and a protease inhibitor (indinavir) was used in patients with HIV infection over a 24-week period, it also demonstrated good antiviral activity.

Nevirapine has been shown to reduce maternal-fetal transmission of HIV.

In contrast to delavirdine, which inhibits cytochrome P450 isozymes, nevirapine induces cytochrome P450 and accelerates the metabolism of certain drugs (see Table 43–4).

Protease Inhibitors

Tables 43–1 and 43–4 compare information on the properties, effects, and interactions of four protease inhibitors: indinavir, nelfinavir, ritonavir, and saquinavir. Fig. 43–3 shows the site of action of these drugs.

Drug Properties

Pharmacokinetics. Protease inhibitors are given orally and are extensively metabolized by cytochrome P450 enzymes before undergoing fecal excretion. Two of the drugs, nelfinavir and ritonavir, are available in formulations for administration to pediatric patients.

Spectrum, Indications, and Viral Resistance. Protease inhibitors are active against HIV and have synergistic effects with NRTIs. The use of combinations involving protease inhibitors and either NRTIs or NNRTIs significantly reduces the viral load and slows the clinical progression of disease in patients with AIDS. Although numerous combinations have been tried (see Table 43–3), authorities now recommend combining a protease inhibitor with two NRTIs for the treatment of most HIV infections.

Viral isolates that are resistant to one protease inhibitor may be sensitive to other protease inhibitors in vitro. However, the clinical effectiveness of changing from one protease inhibitor to another after resistance has developed has not been established.

Adverse Effects and Interactions. Among the protease inhibitors, ritonavir produces the highest incidence of adverse effects, and nelfinavir appears to be the best tolerated. Protease inhibitors interact with a number of other drugs (see Table 43–4) via inhibition of cytochrome P450 enzymes. They have the greatest effect on drugs metabolized by the CYP3A4 isozyme, and they can cause a several-fold increase in the plasma concentration of these drugs.

In fact, some protease inhibitors inhibit the metabolism of other protease inhibitors, and this probably accounts for the greater oral bioavailability of saquinavir when it is administered with ritonavir. The NNRTIs also interact with protease inhibitors. Delavirdine can inhibit the metabolism and increase the toxicity of some protease inhibitors, whereas nevirapine can increase the metabolism and decrease the therapeutic effect of all of them.

Indinavir

Indinavir (see Fig. 43–4C) has demonstrated excellent clinical effectiveness in combination with lamivudine plus either zidovudine or stavudine. One study found that plasma HIV RNA levels became undetectable after 24 weeks of three-drug therapy and that the levels remained undetectable in almost 80% of patients after 100 weeks of treatment.

Indinavir is a drug that should not be taken with meals. If indinavir is combined with didanosine, the two drugs must be taken at least an hour apart because the buffering agent included in the didanosine formulation can interfere with indinavir absorption.

Nelfinavir

Nelfinavir is the newest protease inhibitor. It has been successfully employed in combination with zidovudine and lamivudine, resulting in undetectable HIV RNA levels in 80% of patients after 52 weeks of treatment. Nelfinavir should be taken with meals.

Ritonavir

Ritonavir is a potent drug with proven clinical efficacy in patients who have advanced disease, but it causes a higher incidence of adverse effects than other protease inhibitors. Adverse effects can be minimized by starting patients on lower doses and then gradually increasing the doses over 1–2 weeks. Many of the adverse gastrointestinal symptoms will subside over time with continued drug administration.

Ritonavir has a convenient twice-a-day dosing schedule and should be taken with meals.

Saquinavir

Saquinavir is usually well tolerated, but it has a lower oral bioavailability than other protease inhibitors. To enhance its absorption, saquinavir should be taken with meals that have a high fat content. The newer soft-gel capsule formulation of saquinavir has better bioavailability than the hard-gel capsule, and this may reduce the incidence of resistance and clinical failure found in early studies of the drug. The bioavailability of either formulation is markedly enhanced by taking the drug in combination with ritonavir, which inhibits CYP3A4 metabolism of saquinavir. This combination has been found to be clinically effective. Drugs that induce the CYP3A4 isozyme, such as rifabutin and rifampin, should not be used with saquinavir.

Treatment Considerations

The decision to initiate therapy for HIV infection is based on a variety of considerations, including the patient's CD4$^+$ count (expressed in terms of the number of T cells per microliter), the patient's viral load (expressed in terms of the number of HIV RNA copies per milliliter), and whether the patient has clinical symptoms of disease.

Symptomatic patients with a CD4$^+$ count under 500 are usually given drug therapy regardless of their viral load. Until recently, symptomatic patients with a CD4$^+$ count over 500 were generally given drug therapy only if their viral load exceeded 30,000. However, most authorities now recommend that treatment be started if the viral load exceeds 5000 or 10,000, despite the fact that the efficacy of treatment at this early stage has not yet been supported by clinical data.

There is no consensus about whether to treat asymptomatic patients. On the one hand, combination drug therapy is sometimes able to markedly reduce viral loads, improve CD4$^+$ counts, and prevent symptomatic illness. On the other hand, treatment is associated with drug toxicity, expense, and the potential emergence of drug resistance.

Drug regimens for treating HIV infection in adults are listed in Table 43–3. The preferred regimen for initial drug therapy consists of two NRTIs and either a protease inhibitor or an NNRTI. Before initiating treatment, the clinician should ask about other drugs that the patient is taking, since drug interactions may increase plasma drug concentrations and contribute to toxicity. To determine the response to therapy, viral loads should be measured 3–4 weeks after starting therapy and every 3–6 months thereafter. The time course of the response is highly variable. Viral suppression may take many months in patients with high viral loads.

The main reasons for changing medication after initiating therapy are treatment failure and drug toxicity. Treatment failure is indicated by a rise in the viral load to greater than 2000–5000 if previous levels were undetectable or by a rise to greater than 5000–10,000 if previous levels were lower than this. If the patient fails to respond to a drug regimen, the new regimen should include at least two new drugs. Alternative combinations of NRTIs are listed in Table 43–3. If dose-limiting or intolerable toxicity occurs, the clinician should choose alternative drugs that cause a lower incidence of the particular adverse effects experienced by the patient.

DRUGS FOR INFLUENZA

Because **influenza A virus** is one of the most common causes of infectious disease–related deaths, efforts have been made to develop methods to prevent and treat illness caused by this RNA virus. Vaccines are available for prevention, and **amantadine** and **rimantadine** are oral drugs that are currently used both to prevent and to treat influenza A.

Chemistry and Mechanisms. Amantadine (see Fig. 43–1B) and rimantadine are synthetic tricyclic amine compounds that have similar structures and act by preventing the uncoating of influenza A particles following their entry into host cells. The drugs are believed to buffer the pH of endosomes, which are membrane-bound vacuoles that surround viral particles as they enter a host cell. The buffering action prevents the acidification of the endosomes and the subsequent fusion of endosomes and viral membranes that is required for uncoating and transfer of viral nucleic acid into the cytoplasm of the host cell.

Pharmacokinetics. Amantadine and rimantadine have good oral bioavailability (see Table 43–1), and both drugs are available in liquid preparations for children. Rimantadine is less lipophilic than amantadine and does not cross the blood-brain barrier. For this reason, rimantadine is associated with fewer CNS side effects. Unlike amantadine, rimantadine is extensively metabolized to inactive compounds before undergoing renal excretion, and doses of rimantadine do not need to be adjusted in persons with renal insufficiency. The half-life of each drug is about 24 hours.

Spectrum and Indications. Amantadine and rimantadine are active against influenza A but not against influenza B. The drugs are 70–90% effective in preventing influenza if they are administered prior to exposure to the virus. They are also effective in reducing the duration and severity of influenza if they are administered within 48 hours of the onset of clinical illness.

Amantadine and rimantadine are usually administered once or twice a day for 5–7 days, but they may be given for longer periods of time during outbreaks of influenza. They are particularly useful in controlling epidemics in institutionalized elderly patients, who have a high risk of influenza-related complications and secondary infections. The drugs are also useful in the management of immunodeficient patients, who may not develop adequate immunity following influenza vaccination.

Adverse Effects. Mild CNS side effects caused by amantadine include nervousness, anxiety, insomnia, and difficulty in concentrating. In most cases, these effects diminish with continued drug administration and disappear when the drug is stopped. However, more serious CNS side effects, including hallucinations and seizures, sometimes occur in elderly patients. Rimantadine has a much lower incidence of CNS side effects and may be preferred for the treatment of patients with a higher risk of these adverse effects.

DRUGS FOR HEPATITIS

Lamivudine inhibits the replication of **hepatitis B virus** and has been approved as the first orally effective drug for patients with hepatitis B. As discussed earlier in this chapter, the drug also inhibits the replication of HIV. Unlike HIV, which is an RNA virus, hepatitis B virus is a DNA virus. Lamivudine is active against hepatitis B virus because the replication of this virus depends on reverse transcription of an intermediate RNA. Reverse transcription produces a negative-sense strand of DNA. The negative-sense DNA then serves as a template for synthesis of positive-sense DNA.

As discussed below, **ribavirin** is active against **hepatitis A and C viruses,** whereas **interferon alfa** is active against **hepatitis B and C viruses.** Hepatitis A and C viruses are both RNA viruses.

DRUGS FOR OTHER VIRAL INFECTIONS
Ribavirin

Chemistry and Mechanisms. Ribavirin is a synthetic guanosine analogue (see Fig. 43–1C) that acts by several mechanisms to inhibit the synthesis of viral nucleic acid. Ribavirin is activated by kinases that phosphorylate the drug. The active metabolites disrupt cellular purine metabolism by inhibiting inosine monophosphate dehydrogenase and thereby causing a deficiency of guanosine triphosphate. This deficiency in turn inhibits the synthesis of viral DNA and RNA. Unlike acyclovir and some reverse transcriptase inhibitors, ribavirin also inhibits the synthesis of host cell nucleic acid, and this may account for some of the toxicity of ribavirin.

Pharmacokinetics, Spectrum, and Indications. Table 43–1 outlines the pharmacokinetic properties of ribavirin.

The drug is a broad-spectrum antiviral drug that is active in vitro against a wide range of RNA and DNA viruses. These include **adenovirus, Colorado tick fever virus, Crimean-Congo hemorrhagic fever virus, Hantaan virus, hepatitis A and C viruses, herpesviruses, influenza A and B viruses, Lassa virus, measles virus, Muerto Canyon fever virus, mumps virus, respiratory syncytial virus, Rift Valley fever virus,** and **yellow fever virus.**

Although ribavirin has been successfully employed to treat infections caused by several of these viruses, the only FDA-approved indication is for the treatment of **severe respiratory syncytial virus infection.** For the treatment of neonates with this type of infection, ribavirin is administered by aerosol, using a small-particle aerosol generator. Influenza has also been treated by aerosol administration, whereas most other viral infections have been treated by intravenous administration.

Adverse Effects and Interactions. When ribavirin is given by inhalation, it can cause serious pulmonary and cardiovascular effects, including apnea, pneumothorax, worsening of respiratory status, and cardiac arrest. When the drug is given intravenously, seizures may occur. Ribavirin is teratogenic in animals, and its use is contraindicated in pregnant or lactating women. Ribavirin antagonizes the antiviral effects of zidovudine and zalcitabine, so concurrent therapy with these drugs should be avoided.

Interferon Alfa

Interferons are now available through recombinant DNA technology for the treatment of some viral infections, as well as for the treatment of neoplasms and other conditions (see Chapter 45).

Chemistry and Mechanisms. The interferons are a group of naturally occurring proteins that are produced by host cells in response to a viral infection. The interferons have multiple immunomodulating effects and antiproliferative effects, and their most important mechanisms of action in the treatment of specific disorders are uncertain. The antiviral activity of interferons results in part from induction of proteins that inhibit viral penetration or uncoating, inhibit viral peptide elongation, or degrade viral messenger RNA (mRNA).

Pharmacokinetics, Spectrum, and Indications. Interferon alfa is active against **hepatitis B and C viruses** and against some **papillomaviruses.**

Treatment with interferon produces clinical remission in some patients with **hepatitis B** or **hepatitis C.** Two forms of interferon used in treating patients with hepatitis are interferon alfa-2a and interferon alfa-2b. In patients with chronic hepatitis C, these forms of the drug appear to have similar effectiveness. The drugs are administered subcutaneously or intramuscularly three times a week for at least 12 months. In some studies, better results were obtained with 18–24 months of therapy, and combination therapy with interferon and ribavirin produced a higher response rate than therapy with either drug alone. In clinical studies of chronic hepatitis B, interferon treatment was found to result in loss of hepatitis B antigens, normalization of serum aminotransferase activity, sustained histologic improvement, and a lower risk of progression of liver disease in about one-third of the patients. However, AIDS patients with hepatitis B responded poorly to interferon treatment.

Interferon alfa is also effective in the treatment of **anogenital warts (condylomata acuminata),** which are caused by several types of papillomavirus. For this infection, the interferon is injected directly into the lesions three times a week for 3 weeks, with a repeated course of treatment after 12–16 weeks.

Adverse Effects. Interferons may cause a large number of serious and unpleasant adverse effects, including hematologic toxicity, cardiac arrhythmias, changes in blood pressure, CNS dysfunction, gastrointestinal distress, chills, fatigue, headache, and myalgia.

Summary of Important Points

- Acyclovir, famciclovir, penciclovir, and valacyclovir are nucleoside analogues used for the treatment of herpes simplex virus (HSV) and varicella-zoster virus (VZV) infections.
- Trifluridine is a nucleoside analogue used for the treatment of herpetic keratoconjunctivitis.
- Cidofovir and ganciclovir are nucleoside analogues used for the prevention and treatment of cytomegalovirus (CMV) diseases, such as retinitis, esophagitis, and colitis.
- Valacyclovir is a prodrug that is converted to acyclovir in vivo. It has better oral bioavailability than acyclovir.
- Acyclovir, ganciclovir, and penciclovir are selectively phosphorylated to their monophosphate metabolites by viral kinases, and then host cell kinases convert them to triphosphates. Other nucleoside analogues, including those for treating human immunodeficiency virus (HIV) infection, are phosphorylated only by host cell kinases.
- Acyclovir and most nucleoside reverse transcriptase inhibitors (NRTIs) cause chain termination when they are incorporated into viral DNA. Ganciclovir and penciclovir inhibit viral DNA polymerase but are not incorporated into viral DNA.
- Foscarnet is a nonnucleoside drug used to treat CMV retinitis and acyclovir-resistant HSV and VZV infections.
- NRTIs, nonnucleoside reverse transcriptase inhibitors (NNRTIs), and protease inhibitors are three classes of drugs for the treatment of HIV infection. Various combinations of these drugs act synergistically to reduce viral loads and ameliorate symptoms. The most commonly used combinations consist of two NRTIs plus either a protease inhibitor or an NNRTI.
- Frequently used NRTIs include zidovudine, which may cause anemia and neutropenia, and didanosine and zalcitabine, which may cause neuropathy and pancreatitis.
- Protease inhibitors and NNRTIs interact with a large number of drugs via inhibition or induction of cytochrome P450 isozymes.
- Amantadine and rimantadine are used in the prophylaxis and treatment of influenza. They act by preventing the uncoating of influenza A virus.
- Ribavirin is a broad-spectrum antiviral drug that is primarily used to treat respiratory syncytial virus infection in neonates.
- Interferon alfa is used to treat hepatitis B, hepatitis C, and anogenital warts. Lamivudine, an NRTI, is also used to treat hepatitis B.

Selected Readings

Carpenter, C. C., et al. Antiretroviral therapy for HIV infection in 1998: updated recommendations of the International AIDS Society—USA panel. JAMA 280:78–86, 1998.

Chesebro, M. J., and W. D. Everett. Understanding the guidelines for treating HIV disease. Am Fam Phys 57:315–322, 1998.

Deeks, S. G., et al. HIV-1 protease inhibitors. JAMA 277:145–152, 1997.

Drugs for HIV infections. Med Lett Drugs Ther 39:111–116, 1997.

Drugs for non-HIV viral infections. Med Lett Drugs Ther 39:69–76, 1997.

Erlich, K. S. Management of herpes simplex and varicella-zoster virus infections. West J Med 166:211–215, 1997.

Foudraine, N. A., et al. Improvement of chronic diarrhea in patients with advanced HIV-1 infection during potent antiretroviral therapy. AIDS 12:35–41, 1998.

Gazzard, B. G. Efavirenz in the management of HIV infection. Int J Clin Pract 53:60–64, 1999.

Guidelines for the use of antiretroviral agents in HIV-infected adults and adolescents. MMWR Morb Mortal Wkly Rep 47:43–82, 1998.

Hovanessian, H. C. New developments in the treatment of HIV disease: an overview. Ann Emerg Med 33:546–555, 1999.

Kempf, D. J., et al. The duration of viral suppression during protease inhibitor therapy for HIV-1 infection is predicted by plasma HIV-1 RNA at the nadir. AIDS 12:F9–F14, 1998.

Lo, J. C., et al. "Buffalo hump" in men with HIV-1 infection. Lancet 351:867–870, 1998.

Lucas, G. M., et al. Highly active antiretroviral therapy in a large urban clinic: risk factors for virologic failure and adverse drug reactions. Ann Intern Med 131:81–87, 1999.

McCarthy, M. Low-cost drug cuts perinatal HIV-transmission rate [news]. Lancet 354:309, 1999.

Michelet, C., et al. Safety and efficacy of ritonavir and saquinavir in combination with zidovudine and lamivudine. Clin Pharmacol Ther 65:661–671, 1999.

Moyle, G. J., et al. Antiretroviral therapy for HIV infection: a knowledge-based approach to drug selection and use. Drugs 55:383–404, 1998.

Notermans, D. W., et al. Decrease of HIV-1 RNA levels in lymphoid tissue and peripheral blood during treatment with ritonavir, lamivudine, and zidovudine. AIDS 12:167–173, 1998.

Palella, F. J., et al. Declining morbidity and mortality among patients with advanced human immunodeficiency virus infection. N Engl J Med 338:853–860, 1998.

Perry, C. M., and S. Hoble. Saquinavir soft-gel capsule formulation: a review of its use in patients with HIV infection. Drugs 55:461–486, 1998.

Sarmati, L., et al. Increase in neutralizing antibody titer against sequential autologous HIV-1 isolates after 16 weeks of saquinavir (Invirase) treatment. J Med Virol 53:313–318, 1997.

Staszewski, S., et al. Virological response to protease inhibitor therapy in an HIV clinic cohort. AIDS 13:367–373, 1999.

Valdez, H., et al. Human immunodeficiency virus 1 protease inhibitors in clinical practice: predictors of virological outcome. Arch Intern Med 159:1771–1776, 1999.

Wintermeyer, S. M., and M. C. Nahata. Rimantadine: a clinical perspective. Ann Pharmacother 29:299–310, 1995.

CHAPTER FORTY-FOUR

ANTIPARASITIC DRUGS

OVERVIEW

Endoparasitic infections are extremely common in many parts of the world, particularly in areas where the climate is warm and moist, the sanitation is poor, and insects and other vectors of disease are prevalent. In fact, billions of people in tropical and subtropical regions are infected with **protozoa** (single-cell organisms that dwell in the lumen, tissue, or blood) and **helminths** (worms, including nema-todes, trematodes, and cestodes). Factors such as immigration, an increase in the number of international travelers, and an increase in the number of individuals who have acquired immunodeficiency syndrome (AIDS) and are therefore at greater risk for opportunistic infections have all increased the probability that physicians will see endoparasitic infections that were rarely found in their usual patient population.

Since 1960, the introduction of new drugs has enabled remarkable advances in the chemotherapy of some endoparasitic infections. Albendazole and mebendazole have significantly improved the treatment of several intestinal nematode infections, while praziquantel has revolutionized the treatment of trematode and cestode infections. At the same time, metronidazole and tinidazole have provided more effective and less toxic drugs for the treatment of amebiasis, giardiasis, and trichomoniasis. Despite these advances, the drugs that are available for the treatment of filariasis, leishmaniasis, and trypanosomiasis are considered inadequate because of their toxicity, low efficacy, or need to be given parenterally for such long periods.

Unlike endoparasitic infections, **ectoparasitic infestations** are caused by organisms that live on the skin or hair shafts of patients. The most common examples are the **lice** and **mites** that cause pediculosis and scabies, respectively. Permethrin is a new drug that can be applied topically to eradicate these ectoparasites.

Table 44–1 provides information about the causes and treatment of numerous protozoal infections, helminthic infections, and ectoparasitic infestations. The antiparasitic agents that are commonly used or represent pharmacologic advances are discussed in this chapter. In some cases, an antibacterial or antifungal agent (such as tetracycline or amphotericin B) is listed as either a preferred or alternative drug, and these agents are discussed in earlier chapters. A detailed discussion of other agents listed in the table is beyond the scope of this chapter.

DRUGS FOR INFECTIONS DUE TO LUMEN- AND TISSUE-DWELLING PROTOZOA

Amebiasis, balantidiasis, cryptosporidiosis, giardiasis, and trichomoniasis are examples of infections caused by protozoan parasites that dwell in the lumen and tissues of their human hosts. Among the agents used to treat these infections are metronida-

461

TABLE 44–1. Causes and Treatment of Protozoal Infections, Helminthic Infections, and Ectoparasitic Infestations*

Condition	Most Common Pathogens	Preferred Drugs	Alternative Drugs
Infections due to lumen- and tissue-dwelling protozoa			
Amebiasis	*Entamoeba histolytica.*	Metronidazole/iodoquinol; metronidazole/ paromomycin; metronidazole/diloxanide furoate.†	Tinidazole.†
Amebic meningoencephalitis	*Naegleria fowleri.*	Amphotericin B.	None.
Balantidiasis	*Balantidium coli.*	Tetracycline.	Iodoquinol; metronidazole.
Cryptosporidiosis	*Cryptosporidium parvum.*	Paromomycin.	None.
Dientamoeba infections	*Dientamoeba fragilis.*	Iodoquinol; paromomycin.	Tetracycline.
Giardiasis	*Giardia lamblia.*	Metronidazole.	Tinidazole;† paromomycin.
Trichomoniasis	*Trichomonas vaginalis.*	Metronidazole.	Tinidazole.†
Infections due to blood- and tissue-dwelling protozoa			
African trypanosomiasis (sleeping sickness)	*Trypanosoma brucei.*	Suramin/melarsoprol;† suramin.†	Pentamidine.
American trypanosomiasis (Chagas' disease)	*Trypanosoma cruzi.*	Nifurtimox.	Benznidazole.†
Babesiosis	*Babesia* species.	Clindamycin/quinine.	None.
Leishmaniasis	*Leishmania* species.	Sodium stibogluconate.†	Amphotericin B; pentamidine; paromomycin.
Malaria	*Plasmodium* species.	See text.	See text.
Pneumocystis infections	*Pneumocystis carinii.*	Trimethoprim/ sulfamethoxazole.	Atovaquone;† pentamidine; trimetrexate/leucovorin.
Toxoplasmosis	*Toxoplasma gondii.*	Pyrimethamine/sulfadiazine; pyrimethamine/ sulfadiazine/leucovorin; spiramycin.†‡	Pyrimethamine/clindamycin; pyrimethamine/dapsone.
Infections due to nematodes			
Ascariasis	*Ascaris lumbricoides.*	Albendazole; mebendazole; pyrantel.	None.
Capillariasis	*Capillaria philippinensis.*	Mebendazole.	Albendazole.
Cutaneous larva migrans	*Ancylostoma braziliense, Ancylostoma caninum,* and *Necator americanus.*	Thiabendazole.	Ivermectin; albendazole.
Dracunculiasis (guinea worm infection)	*Dracunculus medinensis.*	Metronidazole/manual removal of worm.	Mebendazole; thiabendazole.
Enterobiasis (pinworm infection)	*Enterobius vermicularis.*	Albendazole; mebendazole; pyrantel.	None.
Filariasis	*Brugia malayi* and *Wuchereria bancrofti.*	Diethylcarbamazine.	Ivermectin.
Hookworm infection	*Ancylostoma duodenale* and *N. americanus.*	Albendazole; mebendazole; pyrantel.	None.
Loiasis	*Loa loa.*	Diethylcarbamazine.	Ivermectin.
Onchocerciasis (river blindness)	*Onchocerca volvulus.*	Ivermectin.	None.
Strongyloidiasis	*Strongyloides stercoralis.*	Ivermectin.	Thiabendazole; albendazole.
Trichinosis	*Trichinella spiralis.*	Mebendazole/ corticosteroids.	Albendazole.
Visceral larva migrans	*Toxocara* species.	Diethylcarbamazine; diethylcarbamazine/ corticosteroids for severe disease.	Albendazole; mebendazole.
Whipworm infection	*Trichuris trichiura.*	Mebendazole.	Albendazole.
Infections due to trematodes			
Chinese liver fluke infection	*Clonorchis sinensis.*	Praziquantel.	Albendazole.
Lung fluke infection	*Paragonimus westermani.*	Praziquantel.	Bithionol.†
Schistosomiasis	*Schistosoma* species.	Praziquantel.	Oxamniquine for *Schistosoma mansoni* infection.
Sheep liver fluke infection	*Fasciola hepatica.*	Bithionol.†	Triclabendazole.†

Continued

TABLE 44–1. **Causes and Treatment of Protozoal Infections, Helminthic Infections, and Ectoparasitic Infestations*** *(Continued)*

Condition	Most Common Pathogens	Preferred Drugs	Alternative Drugs
Infections due to cestodes			
Beef tapeworm infection	*Taenia saginata.*	Praziquantel.	None.
Cysticercosis	*Taenia solium* (larvae).	Albendazole; praziquantel; praziquantel/ corticosteroids.	None.
Dog tapeworm infection	*Dipylidium caninum.*	Praziquantel.	None.
Dwarf tapeworm infection	*Hymenolepis nana.*	Praziquantel.	None.
Echinococcosis	*Echinococcus granulosus.*	Albendazole/surgical drainage or resection of hydatid cyst.	Mebendazole/surgical drainage or resection of hydatid cyst.
Fish tapeworm infection	*Diphyllobothrium latum.*	Praziquantel.	None.
Pork tapeworm infection	*T. solium* (adult worms).	Praziquantel.	None.
Infestations due to ectoparasites			
Pediculosis (lice infestation)	*Pediculus humanus capitis, Pediculus humanus corporis,* and *Phthirus pubis.*	Permethrin.	Ivermectin; crotamiton.
Scabies (mite infestation)	*Sarcoptes scabiei.*	Permethrin; malathion.	Pyrethrins/piperonyl butoxide; ivermectin.

*Drugs are listed in their general order of recommended use, with the drug or drug combination used most often listed first. Drugs used in combination are separated by the symbol / , such as the combination of metronidazole and iodoquinol, which is listed as metronidazole/iodoquinol.
†In the USA, this drug is either not marketed or is only available from the Centers for Disease Control and Prevention.
‡Spiramycin is for fetal *Toxoplasma* infection.

zole, iodoquinol, paromomycin, and diloxanide furoate (see Table 44–1). In patients with amebiasis, metronidazole acts primarily as a tissue amebicide, whereas the other three drugs act as luminal amebicides.

Metronidazole

Chemistry and Pharmacokinetics. Metronidazole is a nitroimidazole compound (Fig. 44–1A). It is well absorbed from the gut and is widely distributed to tissues and fluids throughout the body, including the liver and central nervous system. The drug is extensively metabolized before undergoing renal excretion. Metronidazole is usually administered orally, although an intravenous preparation is available for use in patients with severe infections.

Spectrum and Mechanisms. Metronidazole is active against several anaerobic protozoa that commonly cause infection. These include *Entamoeba histolytica* (the agent of amebiasis); *Giardia lamblia* (giardiasis); *Trichomonas vaginalis* (trichomoniasis); and *Balantidium coli* (balantidiasis). Metronidazole is also active against anaerobic bacteria, including *Bacteroides fragilis, Clostridium difficile,* and anaerobic *Peptostreptococcus* and *Streptococcus* species.

Anaerobic protozoa have pyruvate:ferredoxin oxidoreductase, an enzyme that is not found in mammalian cells. In susceptible anaerobic protozoa, this enzyme transfers electrons to the nitro group of metronidazole to form intermediates that bind to DNA and proteins and thereby produce a cytotoxic effect.

Indications. Metronidazole is the drug of choice for **amebiasis, giardiasis,** and **trichomoniasis** and is used as an alternative drug in the treatment of **balantidiasis.**

Patients with amebiasis may suffer from intestinal infection, with or without dysentery, hepatic abscesses, or other extraintestinal manifestations of disease. Metronidazole acts primarily as a tissue amebicide and is usually given in combination with a luminal amebicide, such as iodoquinol, for the purpose of eradicating intestinal amebas.

Giardiasis causes abdominal discomfort and diarrhea in persons infected with the cyst form of *Giardia.* In the western USA, *Giardia* cysts are sometimes present in contaminated streams and ponds and are ingested by campers. The administration of metronidazole for 5 days usually cures the infection.

Trichomoniasis is a sexually transmitted disease that produces vaginitis in women but is usually asymptomatic in men. To prevent reinfection, it is important to treat patients and their sexual partners. Treatment may consist either of a single large dose of metronidazole or of smaller doses taken over a 7-day period.

Metronidazole is also used in the management of several disorders that are not caused by protozoa. For example, it is sometimes used in the management of patients with **dracunculiasis (guinea worm infection).** This infection is caused by *Dracunculus medinensis,* a nematode found in India, Pakistan, and parts of Africa. While metronidazole is not curative, it reduces inflammation and facilitates manual removal of the worm. Metronidazole is considered the drug of

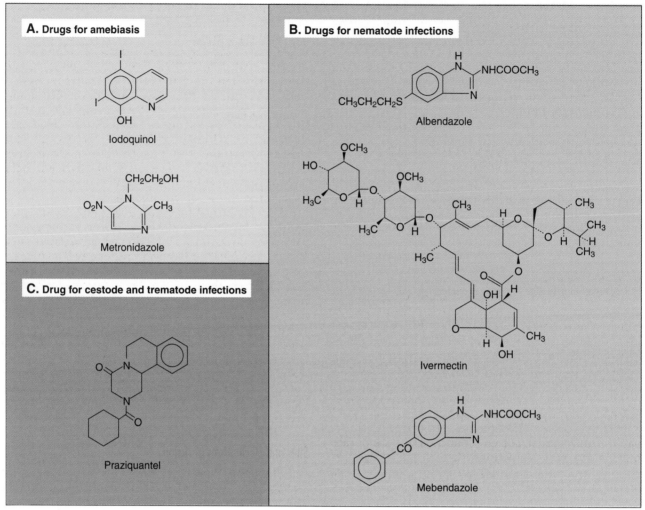

FIGURE 44–1. Structures of selected antiparasitic drugs. (A) Iodoquinol is an iodoquinoline drug, and metronidazole is a nitroimidazole compound. **(B)** Albendazole and mebendazole are benzimidazole drugs, and ivermectin is a semisynthetic derivative of an antibiotic called avermectin. **(C)** Praziquantel is an isoquinoline derivative.

choice for **enterocolitis** caused by *C. difficile,* and it is occasionally used to treat infections caused by other anaerobic bacteria. Metronidazole is available in gel or cream form for the topical treatment of **rosacea (acne rosacea),** a skin condition characterized by persistent erythema of the middle third of the face and other areas of the body.

Adverse Effects and Interactions. Metronidazole is usually well tolerated, but it causes considerable gastrointestinal discomfort in some persons. Other adverse effects include nausea, vomiting, a metallic taste, and transient leukopenia or thrombocytopenia. To reduce the gastrointestinal side effects, patients should take metronidazole with food.

Metronidazole increases the anticoagulant effect of warfarin, so the dosage of warfarin should be adjusted as necessary. Metronidazole also causes a disulfiramlike reaction with ethanol, so patients should avoid drinking alcohol while they are undergoing treatment.

Metronidazole has been shown to be mutagenic in bacteria and mammalian cell cultures. Although retrospective studies of women who took the drug during pregnancy failed to reveal an increased incidence of birth defects or cancer, it appears prudent to avoid using the drug during the first trimester of pregnancy whenever possible.

Iodoquinol, Paromomycin, and Diloxanide Furoate

Iodoquinol, paromomycin, and diloxanide furoate act as luminal amebicides but not tissue amebicides. A luminal amebicide can be used alone to treat **asymptomatic carriers of *E. histolytica,*** but it must be used in combination with a tissue amebicide to treat patients with **amebic dysentery or tissue abscesses.** The preferred combination is usually iodoquinol plus metronidazole.

Paromomycin is sometimes used to treat infections with *Cryptosporidium parvum.* **Cryptosporidiosis** usually presents as chronic diarrhea in immunocompromised persons and has been reported in up to 50% of patients with AIDS. Many methods of treatment have been tried, but none is very effective.

Paromomycin treatment has produced the greatest clinical response, but high doses of the drug must be used and long-term maintenance therapy is required to prevent relapse.

Either iodoquinol or paromomycin can be used to treat infections with *Dientamoeba fragilis,* a lumen-dwelling protozoan parasite that causes **diarrhea** and **abdominal pain.**

DRUGS FOR INFECTIONS DUE TO BLOOD- AND TISSUE-DWELLING PROTOZOA

Babesiosis, leishmaniasis, malaria, *Pneumocystis carinii* infections, toxoplasmosis, and trypanosomiasis are examples of infections caused by protozoan parasites that dwell in the blood and tissues of their human hosts.

Drugs for Malaria

Malaria is one of the most common infectious diseases in the world today and is believed to be responsible for more deaths than any other infectious disease. Four species of *Plasmodium* cause malaria: *Plasmodium falciparum, Plasmodium malariae, Plasmodium ovale,* and *Plasmodium vivax.* Most cases of malaria are due to *P. falciparum* or *P. vivax.* The disease is spread via the bites of female *Anopheles* mosquitoes and is primarily found in tropical and subtropical areas. Malaria has largely been eliminated from industrialized countries in temperate regions, so most infections that are diagnosed in people residing in the USA are infections that were acquired during travel in other countries. Neverthe-less, periodic outbreaks of mosquito-borne malaria still occur in the USA.

Malaria is transmitted when infected mosquitos inject *Plasmodium* sporozoites into the blood of the human host (Fig. 44–2). The sporozoites invade the liver, where they undergo schizogony (asexual multiplication) to form tissue schizonts. The multinucleated schizonts divide their cytoplasm to form thousands of merozoites in a process called **exoerythrocytic schizogony.** The merozoites are then released from the liver into the blood, where they infect erythrocytes and undergo **erythrocytic schizogony.** Additional merozoites are subsequently released into the blood by hemolysis.

The synchronous release of merozoites is responsible for the episodic fever observed in patients with malaria. During an infection with *P. falciparum* or *P. vivax,* the fever spikes every other day. The disease produced by *P. falciparum* (malignant tertian malaria) is more severe than that produced by *P. vivax* (benign tertian malaria), partly because *P. falciparum* causes a higher level of parasitemia and produces a persistently higher temperature during the periods between fever spikes. Whereas both *P. vivax* and *P. ovale* have a persistent exoerythrocytic stage, *P. falciparum* and *P. malariae* do not. To eradicate this persistent stage and prevent the relapse of malaria, patients infected with *P. vivax* or *P. ovale* can be treated with primaquine.

Sites and Mechanisms of Action

Fig. 44–2 shows the sites of action of drugs for malaria. As indicated above, primaquine inhibits

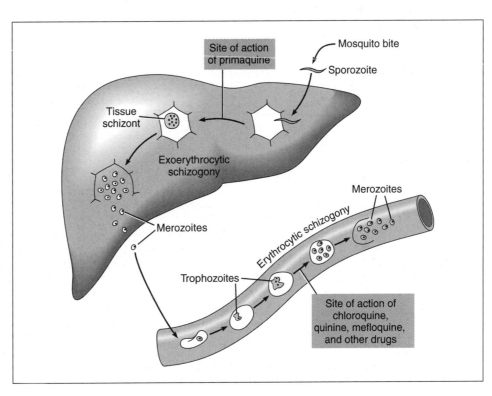

FIGURE 44–2. Sites of action of drugs for malaria. When a person is bitten by an infected mosquito, *Plasmodium* sporozoites enter the liver, form tissue schizonts, and undergo exoerythrocytic schizogony to produce merozoites. The merozoites that are released from the liver invade erythrocytes and form trophozoites that undergo erythrocytic schizogony. Some trophozoites develop into male and female gametocytes, which must subsequently pass back into a mosquito before they can develop into sporozoites and repeat the infection cycle. Primaquine blocks exoerythrocytic schizogony, while other antimalarial drugs inhibit erythrocytic schizogony.

exoerythrocytic schizogony. In contrast, all of the other antimalarial agents inhibit erythrocytic schizogony.

The mode of action of **primaquine** is uncertain, but the drug appears to act by forming quinoline-quinone intermediates that oxidize schizont membranes. These oxidizing intermediates may also be responsible for the hemolytic effect of the drug.

Chloroquine, mefloquine, quinidine, and **quinine** are believed to inhibit nucleic acid synthesis or function during erythrocytic schizogony, although the exact mechanisms of action are uncertain. Chloroquine may block the synthesis of nucleic acid, and it may also impair the ability of plasmodia to utilize hemoglobin. The selective toxicity of chloroquine may be partly explained by the drug's greater accumulation in infected erythrocytes than in uninfected cells. Quinidine and quinine appear to form a complex with plasmodial DNA, thereby preventing replication and transcription.

Sulfadoxine is a sulfonamide that acts synergistically with **pyrimethamine** to inhibit the synthesis of folic acid in plasmodia and thereby prevent the synthesis of nucleic acid. The sulfonamides inhibit dihydrofolate formation, while pyrimethamine prevents dihydrofolate reduction.

Other drugs used in the treatment of malaria include **artemether, artesunate, atovaquone,** and **proguanil.** Proguanil acts by inhibiting folate reductase, and the mechanisms of action of the other drugs are unknown.

Fig. 44–3 shows structures of selected drugs for malaria.

Chloroquine, Quinine, and Quinidine

Quinine, a drug that had been used for centuries to treat malaria, was supplanted by chloroquine after World War II. Until the 1980s, when resistance to chloroquine became widespread, chloroquine re-

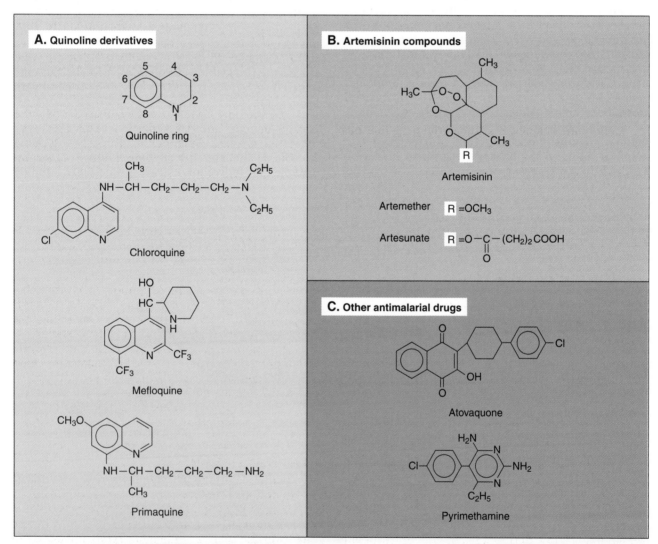

FIGURE 44–3. Structures of selected drugs for malaria. (A) Chloroquine is a 4-aminoquinoline derivative, whereas primaquine is an 8-aminoquinoline derivative. **(B)** Artemether and artesunate are derivatives of artemisinin (qinghaosu), the active ingredient of *Artemisia annua,* a plant used in traditional Chinese medicine for over 2 millennia. **(C)** Atovaquone is a naphthoquinone derivative, and pyrimethamine is a folate reductase inhibitor.

mained the drug of choice. Now that drug resistance has severely curtailed the effectiveness of chloroquine, quinine is once again being used to treat malaria in many regions of the world. In addition, other drugs have been introduced.

The only areas where most *P. falciparum* organisms are sensitive to chloroquine are the Caribbean islands, the part of Central America that is west of the Panama Canal, and parts of North Africa and the Middle East. In these chloroquine-sensitive areas, chloroquine is still the drug of choice for both the prevention and the treatment of all types of malaria, although it must be used in combination with primaquine (see below) to eradicate vivax or ovale malaria.

The most common adverse effects of chloroquine are gastrointestinal distress, nausea, and vomiting. Toxic doses may cause retinal damage and even blindness. In pregnant women, chloroquine should be used cautiously because fetal damage has been reported.

Patients with chloroquine-resistant malaria are usually treated with a combination that includes either quinine sulfate or quinidine plus either doxycycline or pyrimethamine-sulfadoxine. Alternative drugs for the treatment of chloroquine-resistant malaria are discussed in subsequent sections.

Mefloquine

Mefloquine is a newer antimalarial drug that has been used for both the prevention and the treatment of chloroquine-resistant malaria. Because cure rates with this drug have dropped from almost 100% in the 1980s to 40% by 1995, mefloquine is now primarily used for the prevention of malaria in areas where chloroquine-resistant strains are prevalent. The drug is given orally, undergoes hepatic metabolism, has a half-life of about 14 days, and is eliminated via the bile and feces.

Mefloquine may cause a severe neuropsychiatric syndrome characterized by hallucinations, anxiety, confusion, seizures, and coma. It may also cause leukopenia and thrombocytopenia.

For patients who cannot tolerate mefloquine, doxycycline (see Chapter 39) can be used for the prevention of malaria in areas where chloroquine-resistant organisms are prevalent.

Primaquine

Primaquine is an 8-aminoquinoline derivative that is active against the exoerythrocytic stage of *P. vivax* and *P. ovale.* By eradicating tissue plasmodia, it prevents the reemergence of organisms from the liver and relapse of the infection. Primaquine must be used in combination with other drugs for the treatment of infection with *P. vivax* or *P. ovale,* because primaquine is not active against the erythrocytic stage of these organisms.

Primaquine is converted to oxidizing quinoline-quinone intermediates in the body. These intermedi-

ates are believed to be responsible for the antimalarial effects and some of the toxic effects of the drug. In individuals who have hereditary glucose-6-phosphate dehydrogenase deficiency, the intermediates may oxidize erythrocyte membranes and thereby cause red cell hemolysis and hemolytic anemia. Individuals with this reaction are said to have primaquine sensitivity. A number of other drugs with oxidizing properties, including sulfonamides and sulfones, may also cause this reaction.

Pyrimethamine and Sulfadoxine

Pyrimethamine is a folate reductase inhibitor that is generally used in combination with a sulfonamide such as sulfadiazine or sulfadoxine. Pyrimethamine and sulfadiazine are used in the treatment of toxoplasmosis (a disease discussed in the next section), whereas pyrimethamine and sulfadoxine are used in the treatment of malaria.

In many parts of the world, a fixed-dose combination of pyrimethamine and sulfadoxine is available. This drug, called **pyrimethamine-sulfadoxine,** can be used in combination with quinine to treat chloroquine-resistant malaria. Although the multidrug combination is effective in some geographic areas, resistance to pyrimethamine-sulfadoxine has been reported in parts of Southeast Asia, the Amazon basin, sub-Saharan Africa, and Bangladesh.

The adverse effects of pyrimethamine-sulfadoxine include anorexia, nausea, vomiting, megaloblastic anemia, leukopenia, thrombocytopenia, hemolytic anemia, and Stevens-Johnson syndrome with epidermal necrolysis.

Proguanil and Atovaquone

Proguanil, or **chloroguanide,** is a biguanide derivative that acts as a folate reductase inhibitor. It is sometimes combined with atovaquone for the treatment of chloroquine-resistant malaria.

Atovaquone is a naphthoquinone derivative that has a high level of activity against the erythrocytic stage of all *P. falciparum* strains, including the chloroquine-resistant strains. The drug should be used in combination with doxycycline (see Chapter 39) or proguanil for the treatment of malaria, because studies indicate that a high rate of relapse occurs when atovaquone is used alone.

Atovaquone is also used in the treatment of *Pneumocystis* infections.

Artemether and Artesunate

The search for new agents to treat multidrug-resistant falciparum malaria led to the identification of artemisinin (qinghaosu) as the active ingredient of *Artemisia annua,* a plant used in traditional Chinese medicine for over 2 millennia. Two derivatives of artemisinin were subsequently found to have potent activity against the erythrocytic stages of malaria. These sesquiterpene derivatives are called artemether and artesunate, and their structures are shown in Fig. 44–3.

Artemether and artesunate have been used effectively in the treatment of over 3 million cases of falciparum malaria in Southeast Asia, and they are also being employed in sub-Saharan Africa. The drugs can be administered orally or parenterally.

Drugs for Toxoplasmosis

In immunocompetent individuals, *Toxoplasma gondii* infection is common but is rarely symptomatic. Even in cases in which it is symptomatic, treatment is not normally required.

In immunocompromised individuals and congenitally infected neonates, however, *T. gondii* can cause severe damage to many organs. For example, *T. gondii* frequently causes ocular infections and encephalitis in patients with AIDS and is the most common central nervous system disease found in these patients. *T. gondii* may cause encephalomyelitis, hydrocephaly, microcephaly, or chorioretinitis in the offspring of women who were infected for the first time during pregnancy. Women who were infected with *T. gondii* prior to pregnancy are not at risk of transmitting the infection to their offspring.

Although toxoplasmosis is usually treated with **pyrimethamine** plus **sulfadiazine,** this drug combination has some major drawbacks. First, it is not effective against *T. gondii* tissue cysts. Second, the use of pyrimethamine in combination with a sulfonamide drug sometimes induces folate deficiency and causes severe hematologic abnormalities and other adverse effects, even when the combination is given in normal doses and for short-term treatment. In patients with AIDS, high doses of pyrimethamine plus sulfadiazine are required to treat toxoplasmosis, and life-long maintenance therapy is often required to prevent reactivation of the disease. In an effort to prevent the adverse hematologic effects of pyrimethamine in these patients, **leucovorin** (folinic acid) can be added to the treatment regimen.

Unfortunately, the toxic side effects of pyrimethamine plus sulfadiazine preclude its administration in up to 40% of patients with AIDS. As an alternative, pyrimethamine can be given either with **clindamycin** or with **dapsone.**

Spiramycin is a macrolide antibiotic recommended for fetal infection resulting from acute maternal infection during pregnancy.

Drugs for *Pneumocystis carinii* Infections

Because *Pneumocystis carinii* has traditionally been classified as a protozoan parasite, it is discussed in this chapter. However, results of several studies support the argument that it is actually a fungus. In addition to causing pneumonia in premature and malnourished infants, the organism causes pneumonia and other diseases in immunocompromised persons, including those with AIDS.

The treatment of choice for *P. carinii* infections is **trimethoprim-sulfamethoxazole,** a drug combination discussed in Chapter 41. **Atovaquone** (an antimalarial agent discussed earlier in this chapter), **pentamidine,** or **trimetrexate** can be used as an alternative.

Pentamidine is given intravenously for the treatment of *P. carinii* infections, but it is administered by inhalation for the prevention of pneumonia. The adverse effects of pentamidine include hematologic toxicity, ventricular tachycardia, edema, pancreatitis, bronchospasm, and Stevens-Johnson syndrome.

Trimetrexate is a new folate reductase inhibitor that is being used to treat *P. carinii* infections in persons who are unresponsive to or intolerant of other drugs. Trimetrexate blocks the synthesis of tetrahydrofolate and thereby prevents DNA synthesis and cell division in *P. carinii* organisms. Because trimetrexate also blocks folate reductase in human cells, it must be used in combination with **leucovorin,** an active form of folic acid, in order to prevent host toxicity.

Drugs for Other Protozoal Infections

Suramin, either given alone or in combination with **melarsoprol,** is the treatment of choice for **African trypanosomiasis (sleeping sickness),** a disease caused by *Trypanosoma brucei.* Melarsoprol is indicated for use in patients with late central nervous system manifestations of the disease. These drugs must be administered intravenously and may cause serious toxicity. **Pentamidine,** a drug described earlier, is used as an alternative to suramin for African trypanosomiasis.

Nifurtimox is the drug of choice for the treatment of **American trypanosomiasis (Chagas' disease),** a disease caused by *Trypanosoma cruzi.* The effectiveness of nifurtimox is limited. However, giving interferon gamma in combination with nifurtimox appears to shorten the acute phase of the illness.

The causes and treatment of **babesiosis** and **leishmaniasis** are outlined in Table 44–1.

DRUGS FOR INFECTIONS DUE TO HELMINTHS

Helminths can be classified as **nematodes (roundworms), trematodes (flukes),** and **cestodes (tapeworms).** The most common parasites in these groups are listed in Table 44–1 and are responsible for infecting billions of people throughout the world. Effective drugs are available to treat most of the helminthic infections, but the cost of drug treatment is high. Fortunately, the World Health Organization and government agencies have sponsored mass treatment programs that appear to have had a significant impact on some helminthic infections, such as onchocerciasis (river blindness) and schistosomiasis.

Anthelmintic drugs usually act either by inhibiting mitosis in the parasite (as occurs when a benzimidazole drug is used) or by causing muscle paralysis of the parasite (as occurs when ivermectin, praziquantel, or pyrantel is used). The anthelmintic drugs kill the parasites without harming host cells, but the molecular basis for their selective toxicity is not entirely clear. In many cases, a single dose or a few doses of the drug are curative.

Drugs for Nematode Infections
Albendazole, Mebendazole, and Thiabendazole

The most commonly used **benzimidazoles** are albendazole, mebendazole, and thiabendazole.

Chemistry and Pharmacokinetics. The structures of albendazole and mebendazole are shown in Fig. 44–1B.

Albendazole has poor solubility in water. Only about 5% of an oral dose of the drug is absorbed from an empty stomach. However, absorption is markedly improved if the drug is taken with a fatty meal. Albendazole is converted to albendazole sulfoxide by first-pass hepatic metabolism, and this metabolite accounts for the systemic anthelmintic activity of the drug. Sulfoxidation of albendazole also occurs in the intestinal tract. The level of albendazole in cerebrospinal fluid is about 40% of the level in plasma.

About 10% of mebendazole is absorbed from the gut, metabolized in the liver, and excreted in the urine. In contrast to mebendazole and other benzimidazoles, thiabendazole is well absorbed from the gut, and this may partly account for its higher incidence of adverse effects. Thiabendazole is completely metabolized before undergoing renal excretion.

Mechanisms. The benzimidazoles bind to β-tubulin and thereby inhibit the polymerization of tubulin dimers and the assembly of microtubules required for mitosis and other cell functions in helminths. This action is similar to that of the vinca alkaloids, which block tubulin dimer assembly in human cells and are used to treat cancer (see Chapter 45).

Spectrum and Indications. Thiabendazole is the treatment of choice for **cutaneous larva migrans,** an infection caused when the larval forms of some nematodes burrow under the skin. The drug is added to petrolatum and applied topically for the treatment of this infection. Thiabendazole is also used as an alternative drug in the treatment of **dracunculiasis** (which is usually accompanied by a painful ulcer on the foot or leg) and **strongyloidiasis** (which is sometimes accompanied by skin manifestations similar to cutaneous larva migrans).

Albendazole and mebendazole are primarily used to treat intestinal nematode infections, including **ascariasis, capillariasis, hookworm infection, pinworm infection, trichinosis,** and **whipworm infection.** For trichinosis, the anthelmintic drug is usually given in combination with a corticosteroid, such as dexamethasone, to relieve the inflammation.

As shown in Table 44–1, albendazole is also used to treat two cestode infections: **cysticercosis** and **echinococcosis.** For echinococcosis, surgical drainage or resection is usually employed in conjunction with albendazole therapy.

Parasitic Resistance. Resistance to the benzimidazoles is now a worldwide problem in veterinary medicine, but it is not yet a significant problem in human medicine.

Adverse Effects and Contraindications. The adverse effects of thiabendazole include anorexia, nausea, vomiting, paresthesias, delirium, and hallucinations. Albendazole and mebendazole are well tolerated and produce fewer adverse effects than thiabendazole does. The most common side effects of albendazole and mebendazole are mild gastrointestinal discomfort and constipation or diarrhea. The high doses of albendazole used to treat echinococcosis may cause hepatitis or hematologic toxicity. All of the benzimidazole drugs are contraindicated during pregnancy because of their potential to inhibit mitosis and impair fetal development.

Pyrantel

Pyrantel is a pyrimidine derivative. The drug activates cholinergic nicotinic receptors in the somatic muscles of nematodes and thereby produces a depolarizing neuromuscular blockade. In contrast, pyrantel has no marked effect on neuromuscular function in mammalian species. This has led investigators to conclude that the pharmacologic properties of nicotinic receptors of nematode and mammalian species are significantly different.

Pyrantel is available as an oral suspension for administration to children and adults who have **ascariasis, hookworm infection,** or **pinworm infection.** The drug is poorly absorbed from the gut and acts primarily within the intestinal tract. It is usually well tolerated, but it may cause abdominal cramps, anorexia, diarrhea, and vomiting.

Ivermectin

Chemistry and Pharmacokinetics. Ivermectin is a semisynthetic derivative of avermectin, an antibiotic obtained from *Streptomyces avermitilis.* Ivermectin has a complex macrocytic lactone structure (see Fig. 44–1B). The drug is well absorbed from the gut, undergoes hepatic biotransformation, and is excreted in the feces. Its elimination half-life is about 25 hours.

Mechanisms. Ivermectin increases the chloride permeability of invertebrate muscle cells. This hyperpolarizes the cell membrane and causes paralysis of the pharyngeal muscles in helminths. Ivermectin is believed to activate the glutamate-gated chloride channel in invertebrate tissue, but it has no effect on chloride ion permeability in mammalian tissue.

Spectrum and Indications. Ivermectin is a broad-spectrum anthelmintic drug that is active against a wide range of nematodes. It has been used to treat a number of intestinal helminthic infections in domestic animals and pets, but it is primarily used in humans to treat **strongyloidiasis** and **onchocerciasis.** In fact, the use of ivermectin in populations susceptible to onchocerciasis has revolutionized the management of this disease. Ivermectin is active against the microfilariae (skin-dwelling, first-stage larvae) of *Onchocerca volvulus,* even at a very low dosage. When a single dose is administered once a year, it can prevent the ocular form of onchocerciasis, which is called **river blindness.** Repeated treatment is necessary because the drug is not active against the adult parasites and only prevents the maturation of filarial offspring.

Ivermectin is active against all stages of the *Loa loa* parasite and is currently used as an alternative to diethylcarbamazine for the treatment of **loiasis,** a disease that may cause both ocular and skin manifestations. Ivermectin is also active against the microfilariae of *Brugia malayi* and *Wuchereria bancrofti,* parasites that cause **lymphatic filariasis.** Studies show that low doses of the drug kill *W. bancrofti,* whereas higher doses are effective against *B. malayi.* At the present time, diethylcarbamazine is still considered the drug of choice for these infections, but recent studies suggest that combination therapy with diethylcarbamazine and ivermectin may be more effective than single-drug therapy.

Recently, ivermectin has also been employed in the treatment of ectoparasitic infestations (see Table 44–1).

Adverse Effects. Ivermectin is usually well tolerated and produces few adverse effects. Uncommonly, it causes constipation, diarrhea, dizziness, vertigo, or sedation.

Diethylcarbamazine

Diethylcarbamazine is a piperazine derivative that is administered orally and is well absorbed from the gut. The drug is partly metabolized and is primarily excreted in the urine. Although it has little activity against the larger nematodes (macrofilariae such as the pinworm, hookworm, and whipworm), it is active against several microfilariae and is considered the drug of choice for the treatment of **filariasis** and **loiasis** (diseases described above). It is also the drug of choice for the treatment of **visceral larva migrans,** an infection that is caused by *Toxocara* species and is usually characterized by eosinophilia, hepatomegaly, and pneumonitis.

Diethylcarbamazine is not active against microfilariae in vitro. Studies suggest that it acts in vivo by inhibiting prostaglandin I_2 (prostacyclin) and prostaglandin E_2 both in host endothelial cells and in filariae. These actions constrict blood vessels and increase aggregation of host granulocytes. Thus, diethylcarbamazine appears to augment the innate immune response to filarial infection.

The administration of diethylcarbamazine produces a rapid filaricidal effect, which sometimes leads to a severe host hypersensitivity response to the dying microfilariae. Otherwise, the drug is well tolerated.

Drugs for Trematode and Cestode Infections
Praziquantel

When praziquantel was introduced in the early 1970s, it revolutionized the treatment of **schistosomiasis,** a disease that can affect a wide range of organs, including the skin, liver, spleen, intestinal and urinary tracts, lungs, brain, and spinal cord. As shown in Table 44–1, it is now the drug of choice for infections caused by several other tissue flukes (trematodes) and by tapeworms (cestodes).

Chemistry and Pharmacokinetics. Praziquantel is an orally effective isoquinoline derivative that is not related to any other antiparasitic drug (see Fig. 44–1C). In patients taking praziquantel, the drug is widely distributed and enters the central nervous system. It undergoes some first-pass and systemic metabolism, and the parent drug and metabolites are excreted in the urine.

Mechanisms. Each schistosome is surrounded by a tegument. Praziquantel acts to increase the calcium permeability of the tegument and thereby cause its depolarization. When the outer bilayer of the tegument is damaged, *Schistosoma* antigens that were previously hidden from host defenses are exposed. This enables host immune cells to move in and attack the schistosomes. Thus, praziquantel acts to facilitate host immunity to these flukes. The drug's mechanism of action in other flukes and in tapeworms is unknown but is thought to be similar to that in schistosomes.

Spectrum and Indications. Praziquantel is active against most tissue flukes, including the Chinese liver fluke (*Clonorchis sinensis*), the lung fluke (*Paragonimus westermani*), and the various *Schistosoma* species that cause human infections. It is also active against the larval form of the pork tapeworm (the cause of cysticercosis) and against the adult forms of the pork, beef, fish, dog, and dwarf tapeworms.

For patients with **schistosomiasis** or **other fluke infections,** three doses of praziquantel are administered in a single day. For patients with **cysticercosis,** three doses of praziquantel are given each day for a period of 2 weeks. If manifestations of **neurocysticercosis** are present, corticosteroids are given prior to praziquantel treatment. For patients with **adult tapeworm infections,** a single dose of praziquantel is usually effective.

Parasitic Resistance. Despite intensive use of praziquantel for over 20 years, no confirmed cases of parasitic resistance to the drug have been documented.

Adverse Effects. Adverse effects are uncommon but include abdominal discomfort, dizziness, drowsiness, and headache.

Bithionol and Other Drugs

Bithionol is the drug of choice for the treatment of **sheep liver fluke infection** (*Fasciola hepatica* infection) and is an alternative drug for the treatment of **lung fluke infection** (*P. westermani* infection).

Oxamniquine is used as an alternative to praziquantel for *Schistosoma mansoni* infections, but it is not useful in treating infections caused by other *Schistosoma* species.

Niclosamide was previously used to treat most tapeworm infections, but it has now been supplanted by praziquantel.

Treatment Considerations

In Africa, Central and South America, and Asia, the use of anthelmintic drugs has evolved from the treatment of individuals to the treatment of populations. This has been possible because of the development of broad-spectrum agents that are effective in a single dose. Albendazole, mebendazole, ivermectin, and praziquantel are examples of drugs that have been successfully employed as single-dose therapy to eradicate parasites in a large population.

In most parts of the USA, pinworm infection (enterobiasis) is the most common helminthic infection. It is acquired by ingesting eggs that are initially deposited by the female parasite on the perianal skin and are then transmitted to the mouth via unwashed fingers or fingernails. Contaminated clothing or bedding may also serve as a source of infection. Pinworm infection is often spread to family members, and outbreaks among children are common in day-care settings. For this reason, family members and other close contacts of the patient should be treated at the same time. In cases of pinworm infection, a dose of albendazole, mebendazole, or pyrantel should be followed 2 weeks later by a second dose of the same drug. In cases of whipworm, hookworm, or *Ascaris* infection, a single dose of an appropriate anthelmintic drug (see Table 44–1) is usually effective.

DRUGS FOR INFESTATIONS DUE TO ECTOPARASITES

The most common ectoparasites that cause illness in humans are **lice** and **mites.** These parasites cause **pediculosis** and **scabies,** respectively.

Permethrin is the treatment of choice for both types of infestation. The drug is a synthetic pyrethrin-like compound that blocks sodium currents in the neurons of parasites and thereby causes paralysis of the organisms. For pediculosis, a liquid preparation is applied in sufficient volume to saturate the hair and scalp, and then it is rinsed off after 10 minutes. For scabies, a permethrin cream is applied to the skin from head to toe, and it is left on the skin for at least 8 hours before it is washed off. For both types of infestation, a single treatment is usually effective, but it may be repeated in 1 week if necessary. Alternative drugs are listed in Table 44–1.

Summary of Important Points

- Metronidazole is the drug of choice for treating symptomatic amebiasis, giardiasis, and trichomoniasis.
- Primaquine is the only antimalarial drug that blocks exoerythrocytic schizogony. Chloroquine and other antimalarial drugs inhibit erythrocytic schizogony.
- Many strains of *P. falciparum* have become resistant to chloroquine.
- Chloroquine is used to prevent malaria in geographic regions without chloroquine-resistant plasmodia. Mefloquine or doxycycline is used to prevent malaria in regions with chloroquine-resistant plasmodia.
- Chloroquine is used for the treatment of all types of malaria caused by chloroquine-sensitive plasmodia. In cases of vivax or ovale malaria, chloroquine is given in combination with primaquine. Primaquine is active against the persistent tissue phase of *P. vivax* and *P. ovale* and prevents relapses of malaria caused by these organisms.
- Quinine sulfate or quinidine is usually given in combination with doxycycline or pyrimethamine-sulfadoxine for the treatment of malaria caused by chloroquine-resistant plasmodia.
- Toxoplasmosis can be treated with pyrimethamine plus sulfadiazine.
- Most anthelmintic drugs act either by inhibiting mitosis in the parasite (as occurs when a benzimidazole drug is used) or by causing muscle paralysis of the parasite (as occurs when ivermectin, praziquantel, or pyrantel is used). Praziquantel appears to expose parasite antigens that were previously hidden from host cell immunity.
- Albendazole, mebendazole, or pyrantel is the drug of choice for ascariasis, hookworm infection, and pinworm infection. Mebendazole is the drug of choice for capillariasis, trichinosis, and whipworm infection. Albendazole is used for cysticercosis.
- Diethylcarbamazine is the drug of choice for several forms of lymphatic filariasis, while ivermectin is used to treat onchocerciasis (river blindness) and strongyloidiasis.
- Praziquantel is the drug of choice for all forms of schistosomiasis and for most tissue fluke infections and tapeworm infections. Bithionol is used to treat sheep liver fluke infections.
- Permethrin is the drug of choice for the treatment of pediculosis and scabies.

Selected Readings

Croft, A., and P. Garner. Mefloquine to prevent malaria: a systematic review of trials. BMJ 315:1412–1416, 1997.

Croft, S. L. The current status of antiparasite chemotherapy. Parasitology 114(supplement):S3–S15, 1997.

Drugs for parasitic infections. Med Lett Drugs Ther 40:1–12, 1998.

Lee, L. H., and M. T. Caserta. Malaria: update on treatment. Pediatr Infect Dis J 17:342–343, 1998.

Liu, L. X., and P. F. Weller. Antiparasitic drugs. N Engl J Med 334:1178–1184, 1996.

Martin, R. J., et al. Target sites of anthelmintics. Parasitology 114(supplement):S111–S124, 1997.

Wang, C. C. Validating targets for antiparasite chemotherapy. Parasitology 114(supplement):S31–S44, 1997.

CHAPTER FORTY-FIVE

ANTINEOPLASTIC AND

IMMUNOMODULATING DRUGS

CLASSIFICATION OF ANTINEOPLASTIC AND IMMUNOMODULATING DRUGS

DNA SYNTHESIS INHIBITORS
Folate antagonists
- Methotrexate and trimetrexate

Purine antagonists
- Cladribine, fludarabine, mercaptopurine, and thioguanine

Pyrimidine antagonists
- Cytarabine, floxuridine, and fluorouracil

Ribonucleotide reductase inhibitors
- Hydroxyurea

DNA ALKYLATING DRUGS
Nitrogen mustards
- Chlorambucil, cyclophosphamide, ifosfamide, mechlorethamine, and melphalan

Nitrosourea drugs
- Carmustine, lomustine, and streptozocin

Platinum compounds
- Carboplatin and cisplatin

Other DNA alkylating drugs
- Busulfan, dacarbazine, mitomycin, and procarbazine

DNA INTERCALATING DRUGS
- Bleomycin, dactinomycin, daunorubicin, doxorubicin, idarubicin, and mitoxantrone

MITOTIC INHIBITORS
- Docetaxel, paclitaxel, vinblastine, vincristine, and vinorelbine

TOPOISOMERASE INHIBITORS
- Etoposide, irinotecan, teniposide, and topotecan

IMMUNOMODULATING DRUGS
Recombinant interferons and cytokines
- Aldesleukin and interferon alfa

Monoclonal antibodies
- Abciximab, daclizumab, infliximab, muromonab-CD3, palivizumab, rituximab, and trastuzumab

Other immunomodulating drugs
- Azathioprine, cyclophosphamide, cyclosporine, levamisole, methotrexate, prednisone, tacrolimus, and thalidomide

OVERVIEW

Cancer occurs after normal cells have been transformed into **neoplastic cells** through alteration of their genetic material and the abnormal expression of certain genes. Neoplastic cells usually exhibit chromosomal abnormalities and the loss of their differentiated properties. These changes lead to uncontrolled cell division and may result in the invasion of previously unaffected organs, a process called **metastasis.**

The transformation of normal cells into neoplastic cells often involves the activation of **oncogenes** and the inhibition of **tumor suppressor genes.** Continued insights into the understanding of these events may eventually lead to the development of drugs that reverse the malignant transformation of cells or that impair the metastatic process by which neoplastic cells invade other organs. Currently, however, the drugs that are available for cancer treatment act by inhibiting the replication of neoplastic cells. Many antineoplastic drugs inhibit DNA synthesis or alter DNA structure in a manner that prevents DNA replication or transcription. A smaller number of drugs inhibit mitosis and thereby prevent the multiplication of neoplastic cells. A growing number of drugs alter immune function and increase antitumor immunity or otherwise suppress tumor cell division.

Early Detection of Cancer

Many forms of cancer do not cause symptoms or become physically detectable until there are about

10^9 tumor cells in the body, which corresponds to a solid tumor occupying about a cubic centimeter of tissue. The development of better methods for early detection of cancer has improved the treatment of patients and prolonged their survival. These methods include laboratory tests to detect **tumor cell antigens,** such as the **prostate-specific antigen** (PSA) associated with prostate cancer and the **carcinoembryonic antigen** (CEA) associated with colorectal cancer. In addition to facilitating early detection and treatment, these laboratory tests help clinicians evaluate the effectiveness of treatment.

Principles of Cancer Chemotherapy
Uses and Goals of Treatment

Antineoplastic drugs are used to treat **leukemia, lymphoma,** and **other disseminated hematologic cancers** that cannot be surgically excised. They are also used in combination with surgery or radiation therapy to treat **solid tumors.** In patients with solid tumors that can be surgically removed, chemotherapy is given to eliminate or substantially reduce potential micrometastases and thereby prevent a recurrence of the malignant growth. In patients with inoperable tumors, chemotherapy is given as palliative therapy.

The goal of cancer chemotherapy is to bring about a cure or to provide palliative therapy if the cancer cannot be cured. Palliative therapy is intended to prolong useful life and reduce incapacitating symptoms. In order for a cancer to be cured, all malignant cells must be killed or removed from the body. With some forms of cancer, the immune system may be able to remove small numbers of malignant cells after surgery, radiation therapy, or chemotherapy has eliminated the vast majority of these cells.

Treatment Regimens and Schedules

Drug regimens for cancer chemotherapy are designed to optimize the synergistic effects of drug combinations while minimizing toxicity. The regimens often employ drugs that have different toxicities and different mechanisms of action in order to maximize cytotoxic effects on tumor cells while sparing host tissue.

In the treatment of some types of cancer, specific drug regimens are used for induction of remission, consolidation therapy, and maintenance therapy. **Induction therapy,** such as that used in acute lymphocytic leukemia, seeks to produce a rapid reduction in the tumor cell burden and thereby produce a symptomatic response in the patient. **Consolidation therapy** seeks to complete or extend the initial remission, and it often uses a different combination of drugs than that used for induction. **Maintenance therapy** aims to sustain the remission as long as possible, and it may employ less frequent courses of chemotherapy and different classes of drugs than were used for induction and consolidation.

Regimens for cancer treatment are among the most complicated forms of drug therapy in use today. They often employ multiple drugs administered as **pulse therapy** (intermittent courses of therapy) rather than as **continuous therapy.** Pulse therapy allows the bone marrow to recover between treatment courses and reduces the level of hematotoxicity. The dosage rate and frequency of treatment are based on various considerations, including pharmacokinetics, tumor cell cycle kinetics, and circadian variations in host sensitivity to drugs.

Drug Characteristics

Two characteristics of antineoplastic drugs that influence the design and use of drug treatment regimens are cell cycle specificity and the log kill effect.

As shown in Fig. 45–1, the **cycle of cell replication** includes the G_1, S, G_2, and M phases. DNA is replicated during the S phase, and mitosis occurs during the M phase. Because early investigators observed no activity occurring between the S and M phases, they referred to the period before S as G_1 (gap 1) and referred to the period before M as G_2 (gap 2). Cytologists now know that cells are extremely active in their preparations for synthesis and mitosis during the G_1 and G_2 phases.

Drugs that act during a specific phase of the cell cycle are called **cell cycle–specific (CCS) drugs,** whereas drugs that are active throughout the cell cycle are called **cell cycle–nonspecific (CCNS) drugs.** CCS drugs include all DNA synthesis inhibitors and mitotic inhibitors. CCNS drugs include all DNA alkylating agents and most DNA intercalating agents.

The **log kill effect** refers to the tendency of antineoplastic drugs to kill a constant fraction of the tumor cell burden with each course of chemotherapy. If a patient had 10^{12} cancer cells when treatment was started and if each course of chemotherapy produced a 4-log kill, in theory it would take 3 courses of therapy to eliminate all of the neoplastic cells and cure the patient. However, because neoplastic cells resume growth between courses of chemotherapy, more than 3 courses would be required to eliminate all of them. Furthermore, the log kill produced by repeated courses of drug therapy may be reduced by acquired drug resistance, dose-limiting toxicity, and other factors.

Problems With Cancer Chemotherapy
Drug Resistance

Drug resistance is a major cause of cancer treatment failure. Like microbial drug resistance, tumor cell resistance may be innate or acquired. Acquired drug resistance may result from genomic mutations, such as the induction or deletion of enzymes involved in drug inactivation or drug activation, respectively. The mechanisms of tumor cell resistance are similar to those of microbial drug resistance and include decreased drug accumulation, multiplication of target enzymes, altered affinity of

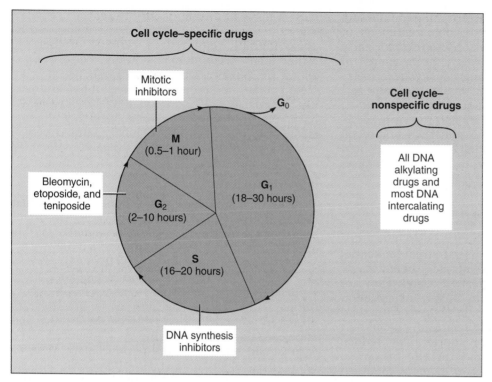

FIGURE 45–1. Cell cycle activity of antineoplastic drugs. The cycle of cell replication includes the G_1 (gap 1), S (synthesis), G_2 (gap 2), and M (mitosis) phases. Differentiated cells may enter a resting state called G_0. Cell cycle–specific drugs act primarily during the designated phase of the cycle. Cell cycle–nonspecific drugs act throughout the cell cycle.

target enzymes, loss of drug-activating enzymes, and increased function of tumor cell repair mechanisms.

P-glycoprotein transports many naturally occurring drugs out of neoplastic cells (Fig. 45–2), and its induction may lead to multidrug resistance. Because this protein is inhibited by verapamil and other calcium channel blockers, quinidine, and phenothiazines, these drugs are being studied as potential treatments to counteract tumor cell resistance. As

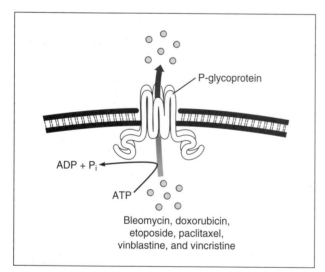

FIGURE 45–2. The P-glycoprotein mechanism of drug efflux. P-glycoprotein utilizes adenosine triphosphate to actively export bleomycin and many other naturally occurring antineoplastic drugs from the cell. Because some agents, such as verapamil, inhibit the P-glycoprotein pump and thereby allow antineoplastic drugs to stay in the cell, these agents are being studied as potential adjuncts to cancer chemotherapy. ADP = adenosine diphosphate; and ATP = adenosine triphosphate.

scientific understanding of the mechanisms of drug resistance increases, new treatments may be developed to counteract resistance.

Drug Toxicity

The most common toxicities of antineoplastic drugs (Table 45–1) result from inhibition of cell replication in the bone marrow, gastrointestinal epithelium, and hair follicles. Many antineoplastic drugs also stimulate the chemoreceptor trigger zone in the medulla and thereby elicit nausea and vomiting.

The **myelosuppression (bone marrow suppression)** produced by antineoplastic drugs often results in **leukopenia** and **thrombocytopenia,** although **anemia** may also occur. Leukopenia predisposes patients to serious infections, whereas thrombocytopenia may lead to bleeding. The onset of leukopenia is delayed because of the time required to clear circulating cells before the effect that drugs have on precursor cell maturation in the bone marrow becomes evident. With many drugs, including **methotrexate, fluorouracil,** and **cyclophosphamide,** the leukocyte count reaches its nadir in about 7 days and recovery occurs in 2–4 weeks. Nitrosourea drugs, such as **carmustine,** produce a more delayed and long-lasting suppression of leukocyte production. **Bleomycin, cisplatin,** and **vincristine** produce less myelosuppression than other antineoplastic drugs, so they are often used in combination with myelosuppressive drugs.

Although methods to prevent myelosuppression are not yet available, recombinant forms of hematopoietic growth factors, such as **epoetin alfa,**

TABLE 45–1. Major Clinical Uses and Adverse Effects of Antineoplastic Drugs*

Drug	Major Clinical Uses	Acute Toxicity	Delayed Toxicity
DNA synthesis inhibitors			
Cladribine	Hairy cell leukemia; non-Hodgkin's lymphomas.	Mild nausea and vomiting.	Myelosuppression.
Cytarabine	ANLL; non-Hodgkin's lymphomas.	Diarrhea; mild nausea and vomiting.	Hepatotoxicity; gastrointestinal and oral ulcers; myelosuppression.
Floxuridine	Renal cell carcinoma.	Diarrhea; mild nausea and vomiting.	Alopecia; gastrointestinal and oral ulcers; myelosuppression.
Fludarabine	CLL; non-Hodgkin's lymphomas.	Mild nausea and vomiting.	Myelosuppression.
Fluorouracil	Breast, colorectal, gastric, and skin cancer.	Diarrhea; mild nausea and vomiting.	Alopecia; gastrointestinal and oral ulcers; myelosuppression.
Hydroxyurea	CML; sickle cell anemia.	Mild nausea and vomiting.	Myelosuppression.
Mercaptopurine	ALL.	Usually well tolerated.	Hepatotoxicity; myelosuppression.
Methotrexate	ALL; bladder and breast cancer; non-Hodgkin's lymphomas; osteosarcoma; trophoblastic tumors.	Diarrhea; nausea.	Gastrointestinal and oral ulcers; hepatotoxicity; myelosuppression; renal toxicity.
Thioguanine	ANLL.	Usually well tolerated.	Myelosuppression.
DNA alkylating drugs			
Busulfan	CML.	Diarrhea; mild nausea and vomiting.	Myelosuppression; pulmonary fibrosis.
Carboplatin	Ovarian cancer.	Moderate nausea and vomiting.	Myelosuppression.
Carmustine	Brain tumors; malignant melanoma; multiple myeloma; non-Hodgkin's lymphomas.	Severe nausea and vomiting.	Myelosuppression; pulmonary fibrosis; renal toxicity.
Chlorambucil	CLL.	Well tolerated.	Myelosuppression; sterility.
Cisplatin	Bladder, cervical, ovarian, and testicular cancer; malignant melanoma; non–small cell lung cancer.	Acute renal failure; severe nausea and vomiting.	Mild myelosuppression; ototoxicity; renal toxicity.
Cyclophosphamide	Breast, lung, and ovarian cancer; CLL; multiple myeloma; neuroblastoma; non-Hodgkin's lymphomas; sarcoma.	Nausea; vomiting.	Alopecia; hemorrhagic cystitis; myelosuppression; pulmonary fibrosis.
Dacarbazine	Hodgkin's disease; malignant melanoma; sarcoma.	Severe nausea and vomiting.	Alopecia; myelosuppression.
Ifosfamide	Sarcoma; testicular cancer.	Nausea; vomiting.	Alopecia; hemorrhagic cystitis; myelosuppression; pulmonary fibrosis.
Lomustine	Brain tumors; non-Hodgkin's lymphomas.	Severe nausea and vomiting.	Myelosuppression; pulmonary toxicity.
Mechlorethamine	Hodgkin's disease.	Mild nausea.	Alopecia; myelosuppression.
Melphalan	Breast and ovarian cancer; multiple myeloma.	Severe nausea and vomiting.	Myelosuppression.
Mitomycin	Bladder, breast, lung, pancreatic, and stomach cancer.	Nausea; vomiting.	Alopecia; myelosuppression; pulmonary and renal toxicity; stomatitis.
Procarbazine	Hodgkin's disease.	Central nervous system depression; nausea; vomiting.	Myelosuppression; stomatitis.
Streptozocin	Carcinoid tumor; pancreatic islet cell tumor.	Severe nausea and vomiting.	Renal toxicity.
DNA intercalating drugs			
Bleomycin	Cervical, head, neck, and testicular cancer; Hodgkin's and non-Hodgkin's lymphomas; sarcoma.	Fever; mild nausea and vomiting.	Alopecia; mild myelosuppression; mucocutaneous toxicity; pneumonitis; pulmonary fibrosis.
Dactinomycin	Ewing's sarcoma; trophoblastic tumors; Wilms' tumor.	Diarrhea; nausea; vomiting.	Alopecia; myelosuppression; oral ulcers.
Daunorubicin	ALL; ANLL.	Nausea; vomiting.	Alopecia; cardiotoxicity; mucosal ulcers; myelosuppression.

Continued

TABLE 45–1.　Major Clinical Uses and Adverse Effects of Antineoplastic Drugs* (Continued)

Drug	Major Clinical Uses	Acute Toxicity	Delayed Toxicity
DNA intercalating drugs (continued)			
Doxorubicin	ALL; ANLL; bladder, breast, gastric, lung, ovarian, soft tissue, and thyroid cancer; Hodgkin's and non-Hodgkin's lymphomas; multiple myeloma; neuroblastoma; sarcoma.	Nausea; vomiting.	Alopecia; cardiotoxicity; mucosal ulcers; myelosuppression.
Idarubicin	ANLL.	Nausea; vomiting.	Alopecia; cardiotoxicity; mucosal ulcers; myelosuppression.
Mitoxantrone	ANLL.	Nausea; vomiting.	Alopecia; cardiotoxicity; mucosal ulcers; myelosuppression.
Mitotic inhibitors			
Docetaxel	Breast, ovarian, and pancreatic cancer; non–small cell lung cancer.	Usually well tolerated.	Alopecia; myelosuppression; neurotoxicity.
Paclitaxel	Breast and ovarian cancer; non–small cell lung cancer.	Usually well tolerated.	Alopecia; myelosuppression; neurotoxicity.
Vinblastine	Bladder, breast, ovarian, and testicular cancer; Hodgkin's and non-Hodgkin's lymphomas.	Nausea; vomiting.	Alopecia; myelosuppression; stomatitis.
Vincristine	ALL; Hodgkin's and non-Hodgkin's lymphomas; lung cancer; multiple myeloma; neuroblastoma; sarcoma.	Usually well tolerated.	Alopecia; mild myelosuppression; peripheral neurotoxicity.
Vinorelbine	Non–small cell lung cancer.	Nausea; vomiting.	Myelosuppression.
Topoisomerase inhibitors			
Etoposide	Non-Hodgkin's lymphomas; small cell lung cancer; testicular cancer.	Mild nausea and vomiting.	Alopecia; myelosuppression.
Irinotecan	Breast, cervical, colorectal, gastric, and lung cancer; non-Hodgkin's lymphomas.	Diarrhea; mild nausea and vomiting.	Alopecia; myelosuppression.
Teniposide	ALL.	Mild nausea and vomiting.	Alopecia; myelosuppression.
Topotecan	Glioma; lung and ovarian cancer; sarcoma.	Mild nausea and vomiting.	Alopecia; myelosuppression.
Hormones and their antagonists			
Diethylstilbestrol	Prostate cancer.	Nausea; vomiting.	Fluid retention.
Fluoxymesterone	Breast cancer.	None.	Fluid retention.
Flutamide	Prostate cancer.	Nausea; vomiting.	Impotence.
Leuprolide	Prostate cancer.	Nausea; vomiting.	Hot flashes; gynecomastia.
Prednisone	ALL; breast cancer; CLL; Hodgkin's and non-Hodgkin's lymphomas; multiple myeloma.	None.	Hyperadrenocorticism.
Tamoxifen	Breast cancer.	Nausea; vomiting.	Hot flashes; hypercalcemia.
Biologic response modifiers			
Aldesleukin	Colorectal cancer, malignant melanoma; renal cell carcinoma.	Varies with dosage and route of administration.	Fluid retention; hematologic deficiencies; hypotension; neuropsychiatric effects; renal dysfunction; skin lesions.
Interferon alfa	CML; hairy cell leukemia; Kaposi's sarcoma.	Flu-like illness.	Fatigue.
Levamisole	Colorectal cancer.	Usually well tolerated.	Granulocytopenia; mild hepatotoxicity.
Rituximab	Non-Hodgkin's lymphomas.	Chills; fever; headache; nausea.	Myelosuppression.
Trastuzumab	Breast cancer.	Chest pain; chills; dyspnea; fever; nausea; vomiting.	Unknown.

*ALL = acute lymphocytic leukemia; ANLL = acute nonlymphocytic leukemia; CLL = chronic lymphocytic leukemia; and CML = chronic myelogenous leukemia.

filgrastim, and **sargramostim,** are used to accelerate recovery from leukopenia or anemia caused by chemotherapy or bone marrow transplantation. These drugs are described more fully in Chapter 17.

The **nausea** and **vomiting** caused by antineoplastic drugs range from mild to severe. Among the antineoplastic drugs, the most emetic are **cisplatin** and **carmustine.** Fortunately, their adverse effects can be prevented or substantially reduced by pretreatment with a combination of antiemetic drugs, including serotonin antagonists such as **ondansetron,** neuroleptics such as **droperidol,** and corticosteroids such as **dexamethasone.** Another antiemetic, **metoclopramide,** is also quite useful in preventing chemotherapy-induced nausea and vomiting. The antiemetics are discussed in greater detail in Chapter 28.

Alopecia is a cosmetically distressing but less serious adverse effect of chemotherapy. It is generally reversible after treatment ends, although the hair may differ in texture and appearance from its previous condition.

Several antineoplastic drugs have characteristic organ system toxicities that appear unrelated to inhibition of cell division. For example, use of **doxorubicin** and other anthracyclines may cause **cardiotoxicity;** use of **cyclophosphamide** may cause **hemorrhagic cystitis;** use of **cisplatin** may cause **renal toxicity;** use of **bleomycin** or **busulfan** may cause **pulmonary toxicity;** and use of **vincristine, paclitaxel,** and other vinca alkaloids and taxanes may cause **neurotoxicity.**

Agents have been developed to prevent some of these organ system toxicities. For example, **dexrazoxane** was developed to prevent anthracycline-induced cardiotoxicity. Another cytoprotective drug, **mesna,** was developed to prevent cyclophosphamide-induced hemorrhagic cystitis. Cisplatin-induced renal toxicity can be partly prevented by administering fluids, along with **mannitol** and **sodium thiosulfate.** Mannitol maintains renal blood flow and tubular function, while sodium thiosulfate inactivates the drug in the kidneys. There are no specific agents to prevent pulmonary toxicity and neurotoxicity; therefore, patients at risk should be closely monitored so that treatment can be discontinued if these toxicities develop.

DNA SYNTHESIS INHIBITORS

Most of the DNA synthesis inhibitors are structural analogues of folic acid or of the purine or pyrimidine bases found in DNA. They act as antimetabolites to inhibit enzymes required for DNA base synthesis. One DNA synthesis inhibitor discussed below, hydroxyurea, is not an antimetabolite; it inhibits the conversion of ribonucleotides to deoxyribonucleotides, a process that is required for DNA synthesis. The uses, adverse effects, and chemical structures of selected DNA synthesis inhibitors are shown in Table 45–1 and Fig. 45–3.

Folate Antagonists

Methotrexate

Nearly 50 years ago, methotrexate (MTX) was used successfully to induce remission in patients with acute childhood leukemia. Today, it is the most widely used antimetabolite in cancer chemotherapy, and it is also used as an immunosuppressive drug in the treatment of rheumatoid arthritis, lupus erythematosus, and other conditions (see Chapter 30).

Chemistry and Mechanisms. The structures of MTX and folic acid are similar. However, MTX has an amino group substituted for a hydroxyl group on the pteridine ring, and it also has an additional methyl group (see Fig. 45–3A).

MTX is actively transported into mammalian cells and inhibits dihydrofolate reductase, the enzyme that normally converts dietary folate to the tetrahydrofolate form required for thymidine and purine synthesis (Fig. 45–4).

Pharmacokinetics. MTX can be administered orally or parenterally. The oral bioavailability of the drug is dose-dependent. Low doses are completely absorbed, while higher doses undergo significantly less absorption. Because MTX does not penetrate the central nervous system (CNS), it must be administered intrathecally for the prevention or treatment of CNS disease.

MTX is rapidly distributed throughout the total body water, and it is partly degraded in the intestine (by intestinal flora) and in the liver. The drug has a biphasic elimination pattern. It is primarily eliminated as the parent compound and metabolites in the urine. The terminal half-life reflects redistribution from tissues and "third space" fluids, such as ascites and pleural effusions.

Indications. The use of MTX in the treatment of choriocarcinoma, a trophoblastic tumor, was the first demonstration of curative chemotherapy. Today, MTX has a variety of uses, including the treatment of other trophoblastic tumors, bladder and breast cancer, non-Hodgkin's lymphomas, and osteosarcoma. It is especially effective for treating acute lymphocytic leukemia and for treating the meningeal metastases of a wide range of tumors.

Adverse Effects. The bone marrow and gastrointestinal mucosa are the normal tissues most sensitive to MTX toxicity. Although myelosuppression is the primary dose-limiting toxicity of the drug, severe oral ulceration (stomatitis) may also occur and necessitate dosage reduction. Administration of a fully activated form of folic acid called **leucovorin (folinic acid)** can prevent these adverse reactions, but it cannot reverse them after they have occurred. Leucovorin rescue is normally used with high doses of MTX (doses exceeding 100 mg/m^2 body surface area). Assays for MTX in plasma are readily available, and drug level monitoring provides a useful guide to the duration of leucovorin administration.

MTX may cause hepatotoxicity, especially with long-term low-dose therapy for psoriasis and rheumatoid conditions. At high doses, MTX may crystal-

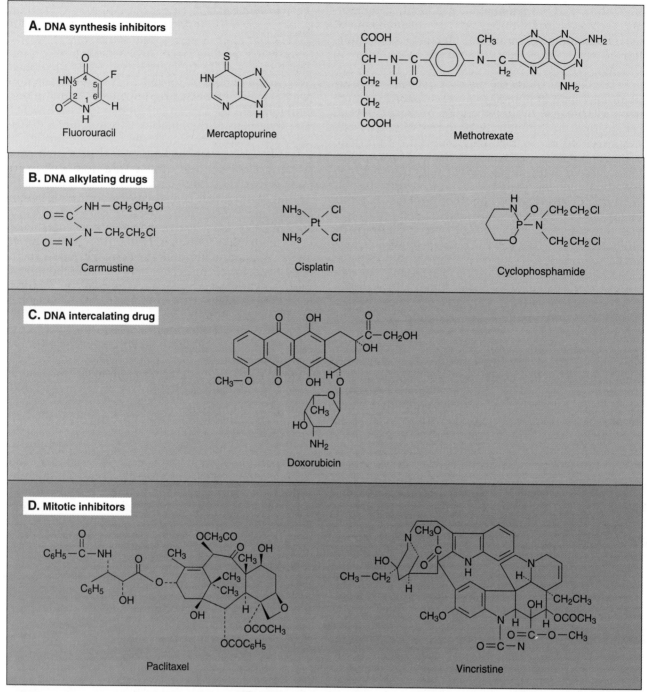

A. DNA synthesis inhibitors

Fluorouracil

Mercaptopurine

Methotrexate

B. DNA alkylating drugs

Carmustine

Cisplatin

Cyclophosphamide

C. DNA intercalating drug

Doxorubicin

D. Mitotic inhibitors

Paclitaxel

Vincristine

FIGURE 45–3. Structures of selected antineoplastic drugs. (A) DNA synthesis inhibitors include fluorouracil (5-fluorouracil), a pyrimidine antagonist; mercaptopurine, a purine antagonist; and methotrexate, a folate antagonist. **(B)** DNA alkylating drugs include carmustine, a nitrosourea drug; cisplatin, a platinum compound; and cyclophosphamide, a nitrogen mustard. **(C)** Doxorubicin is an anthracycline drug. **(D)** Paclitaxel is a taxane (taxoid), and vincristine is a vinca alkaloid.

lize in the urine and cause renal damage. To prevent renal toxicity, dosage reduction is necessary in persons with renal insufficiency.

Other Folate Antagonists

Several lipid-soluble folate antagonists that do not require active transport into cells have been developed. One of them, **trimetrexate,** is used to treat *Pneumocystis carinii* infections (see Chapter 44) and

has activity against several solid tumors. Another one, **edatrexate,** is an investigational drug for non–small cell lung cancer.

Purine Antagonists
Mercaptopurine and Thioguanine

The first purine analogue to be used in cancer chemotherapy was mercaptopurine (6-mercaptopurine, or 6-MP), a drug introduced almost 50 years ago for the treatment of acute lymphocytic leukemia. Like mercaptopurine, thioguanine (6-thioguanine, or 6-TG) is an antineoplastic agent that acts as a purine antagonist.

Chemistry and Mechanisms. Mercaptopurine and thioguanine are the thio analogues of the purine bases hypoxanthine and guanine, respectively. The drugs are believed to act similarly to inhibit purine base synthesis, although their exact mechanisms of action are still uncertain. Mercaptopurine and thioguanine inhibit several steps in the biosynthesis of purines and in purine salvage (recycling) pathways that supply purine precursors. Both drugs are activated by conversion to nucleotides through the addition of ribose phosphate. The reactions are catalyzed by hypoxanthine-guanine phosphoribosyltransferase (HGPRT), and tumor cells that delete this enzyme acquire resistance to the drugs. This probably explains why clinical cross-resistance is usually observed between mercaptopurine and thioguanine.

Pharmacokinetics. Mercaptopurine and thioguanine are given orally, and their bioavailability is variable, incomplete, and reduced by food. Both drugs are primarily eliminated by metabolism, although mercaptopurine is partly excreted unchanged in the urine after high doses. Unlike mercaptopurine, thioguanine is not metabolized by xanthine oxidase.

Indications. Mercaptopurine is used primarily for the maintenance of remission in patients with acute lymphocytic leukemia and is given in combination with MTX for this purpose. The clinical use of thioguanine is limited to maintenance of remission in patients with acute nonlymphocytic leukemia.

Adverse Effects and Interactions. Mercaptopurine and thioguanine are usually well tolerated. Myelosuppression is generally mild with mercaptopurine but may be dose-limiting with thioguanine. Long-term mercaptopurine use may cause hepatotoxicity.

To avoid toxicity, doses of mercaptopurine must be reduced by at least 50% in patients who are taking allopurinol concomitantly. Allopurinol inhibits xanthine oxidase and thereby elevates plasma levels of mercaptopurine. Allopurinol does not interact in this manner with thioguanine, since the latter is not

metabolized by xanthine oxidase. Allopurinol is often given to patients undergoing cancer chemotherapy because it inhibits the synthesis of uric acid and thereby prevents hyperuricemia and gout. Cancer chemotherapy places patients at risk for these problems because the rapid destruction of cancer cells leads to excessive purine catabolism and uric acid formation.

Fludarabine and Cladribine

Fludarabine and cladribine are both purine antagonists.

Fludarabine is a fluorinated derivative of adenine arabinoside. Adenine arabinoside is an analogue of adenosine in which the ribose moiety has been replaced with arabinose. The active triphosphate form of fludarabine blocks DNA polymerase by causing DNA chain termination. Fludarabine is a highly active agent in the treatment of chronic lymphocytic leukemia and low-grade non-Hodgkin's lymphomas.

Cladribine (2-chlorodeoxyadenosine) acts in a manner similar to fludarabine. It is primarily used for hairy cell leukemia, but it is also active against other leukemias and non-Hodgkin's lymphomas.

Pyrimidine Antagonists
Cytarabine and Fluorouracil

Chemistry and Mechanisms. Cytarabine (cytosine arabinoside, or ara-C) and fluorouracil (5-FU) are the most commonly used pyrimidine antimetabolites. Cytarabine is composed of the base cytosine and the sugar arabinose. Arabinose differs from ribose only in the position of one hydroxyl group. Fluorouracil is an analogue of thymine in which the methyl group is replaced by a fluorine atom (see Fig. 45–3A).

Cytarabine and fluorouracil are each converted to active nucleotide metabolites by tumor cell enzymes. The active metabolite of cytarabine is cytarabine triphosphate. It blocks DNA synthesis by several actions, including the inhibition of DNA polymerase and the incorporation into DNA. This incorporation causes DNA chain termination.

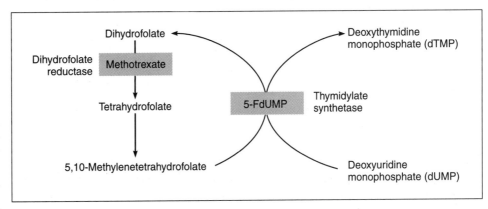

FIGURE 45–4. Inhibition of DNA synthesis by methotrexate and fluorouracil. Methotrexate inhibits dihydrofolate reductase and the conversion of dihydrofolate to tetrahydrofolate. This reduces the supply of 5,10-methylenetetrahydrofolate, the substance required for the synthesis of deoxythymidine monophosphate (dTMP). The conversion of deoxyuridine monophosphate (dUMP) to dTMP is a critical step in DNA synthesis and is catalyzed by thymidylate synthetase. This enzyme is inhibited by 5-fluorodeoxyuridine monophosphate (5-FdUMP), which is the active form of fluorouracil.

Fluorouracil has two active metabolites: 5-fluorodeoxyuridine monophosphate (5-FdUMP) and 5-fluorodeoxyuridine triphosphate (5-FdUTP). 5-FdUMP inhibits thymidylate synthetase and prevents the synthesis of thymidine, a major building block of DNA (see Fig. 45–4). 5-FdUTP is incorporated into RNA by RNA polymerase and interferes with RNA function.

Pharmacokinetics. Cytarabine can be administered intravenously or subcutaneously, and fluorouracil can be administered intravenously or topically. When the drugs are given parenterally, they are extensively metabolized before undergoing renal excretion. Cytarabine crosses the blood-brain barrier and reaches cerebrospinal fluid levels that are 40–50% of plasma levels.

Indications. Cytarabine has a narrow clinical spectrum and is primarily used in combination with daunorubicin or thioguanine for the treatment of acute nonlymphocytic leukemia. It is less frequently used to treat lymphomas.

Fluorouracil is exclusively used to treat solid tumors, especially breast, colorectal, and gastric tumors and squamous cell tumors of the head and neck. Regional delivery of the drug via the hepatic artery can produce a sustained response in patients whose colorectal cancer has metastasized to the liver. Topical application of fluorouracil is used for the treatment of actinic keratoses and noninvasive skin cancers.

Adverse Effects. Cytarabine and fluorouracil may cause nausea and vomiting, myelosuppression, and oral and gastrointestinal ulceration. Nausea and vomiting are usually mild. With fluorouracil, myelosuppression is more problematic after bolus injections, whereas mucosal damage is dose-limiting with continuous infusions. High doses of cytarabine or fluorouracil can damage the liver, heart, and other organs.

Floxuridine

Floxuridine (FUDR) is the deoxyribonucleoside derivative of fluorouracil. It acts as a pyrimidine antagonist and is used in the treatment of renal cell carcinoma.

Ribonucleotide Reductase Inhibitors

Hydroxyurea inhibits ribonucleotide reductase, the enzyme that converts ribonucleotides to deoxyribonucleotides. It thereby stops DNA synthesis and causes cells to accumulate in the S phase of the cell cycle.

Hydroxyurea is given orally and is excreted in the urine. It is primarily used to treat chronic myelogenous leukemia but is also used in the management of sickle cell anemia. In patients with the latter disease, hydroxyurea elevates the concentration of fetal hemoglobin and decreases the frequency of sickle cell crises. The dose-limiting toxicity of hydroxyurea is rapid-onset myelosuppression.

DNA ALKYLATING DRUGS

A DNA alkylating drug is an agent that cross-links DNA strands by forming covalent bonds between alkyl groups of the drug and guanine bases of DNA. The DNA alkylating drugs include nitrogen mustards, nitrosourea drugs, and several other agents. Platinum compounds, such as cisplatin, are included in this category because they also cross-link DNA.

Nitrogen Mustards

The nitrogen mustards are nitrogen analogues of the sulfur mustards that were used as chemical warfare agents in World War I. The cytotoxic effects of nitrogen mustards were discovered in the early 1940s, and the drugs were soon introduced into clinical use. They are considered the first effective antineoplastic drugs.

The nitrogen mustards are bifunctional alkylating agents that undergo spontaneous conversion to active metabolites in body fluids or are enzymatically converted to active metabolites in the liver. The strong electrophilic intermediates formed by these reactions attack the N7 nitrogen of guanine and thereby form covalent bonds with this base. Sequential attachment to two guanine residues results in cross-linking of DNA, and this prevents DNA replication and transcription (Fig. 45–5A). The alkylating drugs act throughout the cell replication cycle.

Cyclophosphamide and Ifosfamide

Chemistry and Pharmacokinetics. Cyclophosphamide and ifosfamide are prodrugs that must be converted to active metabolites by hepatic mixed-function oxidase (cytochrome P450) enzymes. The active alkylating metabolite of cyclophosphamide is thought to be phosphoramide mustard. Cyclophosphamide and ifosfamide are each partly converted to acrolein, which is probably responsible for hemorrhagic cystitis, an adverse effect that sometimes occurs with use of these drugs. Either drug can be administered intravenously, and cyclophosphamide can also be given orally. Cyclophosphamide is completely absorbed after oral administration.

Indications. Cyclophosphamide is the most widely used nitrogen mustard because of its broad spectrum of activity. It is used in the treatment of chronic lymphocytic leukemia, non-Hodgkin's lymphomas, breast and ovarian cancer, and a variety of other cancers (see Table 45–1). Because cyclophosphamide is a potent immunosuppressant, it is used in the management of rheumatoid disorders and autoimmune nephritis. It is also used in preoperative regimens for bone marrow transplantation.

Ifosfamide is primarily used to treat patients with sarcoma and patients with testicular cancer that is refractory to first-line treatments.

Adverse Effects. Adverse effects of cyclophosphamide and ifosfamide include alopecia, nausea, vomiting, myelosuppression, and hemorrhagic cystitis. Nausea and vomiting are usually mild when

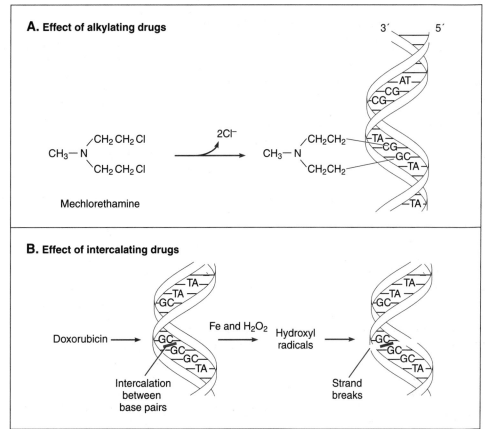

FIGURE 45–5. Mechanisms of action of DNA alkylating drugs and DNA intercalating drugs. (A) Mechlorethamine and other bifunctional alkylating drugs form electrophilic intermediates that attack the N7 nitrogen of guanine residues in DNA, thereby cross-linking DNA strands and preventing replication and transcription. (B) Doxorubicin and other anthracycline drugs intercalate between DNA base pairs. Anthracyclines are reduced to intermediates that donate electrons to oxygen to form superoxide. Superoxide then reacts with itself to make hydrogen peroxide, which is cleaved in the presence of iron to form the destructive hydroxyl radical that cleaves DNA.

cyclophosphamide is given orally, but they may be severe when it is given intravenously. The dose-limiting toxicity of cyclophosphamide is myelosuppression, whereas that of ifosfamide is usually hemorrhagic cystitis. This type of cystitis is characterized by symptoms of urinary frequency and irritation and by blood loss from the bladder. Ingestion of large amounts of fluid and the administration of **mesna,** a sulfhydryl reagent, can significantly reduce the incidence of cystitis. Mesna binds to acrolein, the toxic metabolite that causes cystitis, and converts it to an inactive substance.

Chlorambucil, Mechlorethamine, and Melphalan

Chlorambucil, mechlorethamine, and melphalan are nitrogen mustards that act via the mechanisms described earlier.

Chlorambucil is orally administered, has selective cytotoxicity for lymphocyte cell lines, and is primarily used to manage chronic lymphocytic leukemia. It is well tolerated but may cause dose-limiting myelosuppression and sterility. Long-term therapy is associated with a high incidence of secondary acute leukemia.

Mechlorethamine is a highly reactive and vesicant drug that is rapidly and spontaneously converted to its alkylating intermediate in body fluids after it is given intravenously. Mechlorethamine is a component of one of the treatment regimens for Hodgkin's disease (Table 45–2). The regimen consists

of four drugs—mechlorethamine, Oncovin (vincristine), procarbazine, and prednisone—and is called the **MOPP regimen.**

Melphalan is a nitrogen mustard that is primarily used to treat multiple myeloma (plasma cell myeloma), breast cancer, and ovarian cancer.

Nitrosourea Drugs

The nitrosourea drugs include **carmustine** (*bis*-chloroethyl nitrosourea, or BCNU), **lomustine** (CCNU), and a closely related methylnitrosourea called **streptozocin.**

Chemistry and Mechanisms. The structures of nitrosoureas are similar to those of nitrogen mustards (see Fig. 45–3B). The nitrosoureas are bifunctional alkylating drugs, and they spontaneously form active intermediates that cross-link DNA.

Pharmacokinetics. Nitrosoureas can be given orally or intravenously. They are highly lipophilic and reach cerebrospinal fluid concentrations that are about 30% of plasma concentrations. The drugs are extensively metabolized before renal excretion.

Indications. Because of their excellent CNS penetration, carmustine and lomustine have been used to treat brain tumors. Either drug can be used for lymphomas, and carmustine is also used for melanoma and multiple myeloma. Streptozocin is used only to treat carcinoid tumor and pancreatic islet cell tumor.

TABLE 45–2. Drugs or Drug Combinations Commonly Used in the Treatment of Selected Neoplastic Diseases

Disease	Treatment*
Hematologic cancers	
Acute lymphocytic leukemia (ALL)	For induction: vincristine/prednisone. For maintenance: methotrexate/mercaptopurine. For central nervous system prophylaxis: methotrexate.
Acute nonlymphocytic leukemia (ANLL)	Daunorubicin/cytarabine; cytarabine/thioguanine.
Chronic lymphocytic leukemia (CLL)	Chlorambucil; cyclophosphamide; prednisone.
Chronic myelogenous leukemia (CML)	Busulfan; hydroxyurea; interferon alfa.
Hodgkin's disease	ABVD regimen, consisting of Adriamycin (doxorubicin)/bleomycin/vinblastine/dacarbazine; MOPP regimen, consisting of mechlorethamine/Oncovin (vincristine)/procarbazine/prednisone.
Multiple myeloma	Melphalan; cyclophosphamide/prednisone.
Non-Hodgkin's lymphomas	
Histiocytic (high-grade) lymphomas	CHOP regimen, consisting of cyclophosphamide/hydroxydaunomycin (doxorubicin)/Oncovin (vincristine)/prednisone.
Nodular (low-grade) lymphomas	CVP regimen, consisting of cyclophosphamide/vincristine/prednisone.
Solid tumors	
Bladder cancer	Cisplatin; doxorubicin.
Brain tumors	Carmustine; lomustine.
Breast cancer	CMF regimen, consisting of cyclophosphamide/methotrexate/fluorouracil; CMF/prednisone; CMF/prednisone/tamoxifen or other hormones.
Bronchogenic, small cell lung cancer	Doxorubicin/cyclophosphamide/vincristine.
Choriocarcinoma	For gestational use only: methotrexate; dactinomycin.
Colorectal cancer	Fluorouracil/levamisole.
Gastric cancer	FAM regimen, consisting of fluorouracil/Adriamycin (doxorubicin)/mitomycin.
Malignant melanoma	Dacarbazine; carmustine; cisplatin.
Ovarian cancer	Cisplatin/cyclophosphamide; cisplatin/cyclophosphamide/doxorubicin; paclitaxel; docetaxel.
Renal cell carcinoma	Aldesleukin.
Sarcoma	Doxorubicin/dacarbazine.
Testicular cancer	Etoposide/bleomycin/cisplatin; vinblastine/ifosfamide/cisplatin.

*Drugs are listed in their general order of use, with the drug or drug combination used most often listed first. Drugs used in combination are separated by the symbol /, such as the combination of vincristine and prednisone, which is listed as vincristine/prednisone. For some diseases, other drugs or drug combinations are also used.

Adverse Effects. The nitrosoureas produce delayed and prolonged myelosuppression, with complete recovery taking 6–8 weeks. The thrombocytopenia caused by nitrosoureas usually occurs earlier and is more pronounced than the leukopenia produced by these drugs. Although all of the drugs cause nausea and vomiting, these effects are most pronounced with streptozocin treatment. Pulmonary damage occurs when high doses of nitrosoureas are used.

Platinum Compounds

Chemistry and Mechanisms. The drugs **cisplatin** and **carboplatin** are inorganic platinum derivatives. Cisplatin is converted to an active cytotoxic form by reacting with water to form positively charged, hydrated intermediates that react with guanine in DNA. This leads to the formation of intrastrand cross-links between neighboring guanine residues. The intrastrand links cause DNA to bend so as to distort the normal conformation of DNA and thereby impair its function. Carboplatin is believed to have a similar mechanism of action.

Indications. Cisplatin has efficacy against a wide range of neoplasms. It is given intravenously as a first-line drug for testicular, ovarian, and bladder cancer, and it is also useful in the treatment of melanoma and a number of other solid tumors.

Carboplatin has a similar spectrum of activity, but it is approved only as a second-line drug for ovarian cancer.

Adverse Effects. Cisplatin produces relatively little myelosuppression but can cause severe nausea, vomiting, and nephrotoxicity. Pretreatment with an antiemetic such as **ondansetron** will prevent or significantly reduce the severity of nausea and vomiting. The use of **mannitol** and **sodium thiosulfate** will decrease the severity of nephrotoxicity, an adverse effect associated with loss of potassium and magnesium, reduced glomerular filtration, and renal failure. Mannitol increases urine flow and may reduce binding of cisplatin to renal tubule proteins. Sodium thiosulfate accumulates in renal tubules and neutralizes the cytotoxicity of cisplatin. Renal damage caused by cisplatin is often slowly reversible.

Other DNA Alkylating Drugs
Busulfan

Busulfan is an alkyl sulfonate drug that acts as a bifunctional alkylating agent in the same manner as the nitrogen mustards act. After busulfan is administered orally, it is extensively metabolized. Its metabolites are then excreted in the urine.

Unlike other alkylating drugs, busulfan has greater activity against myeloid cells than against lymphoid cells. For this reason, it has been primarily employed in the management of chronic myelogenous leukemia.

Busulfan causes mild nausea and vomiting and produces dose-limiting myelosuppression. The most characteristic toxicity is pulmonary fibrosis ("busulfan lung"), which occurs in about 4% of patients treated on a long-term basis with the drug. Pulmonary fibrosis has its onset about 3 years after treatment begins. It is characterized by a nonproductive cough, dyspnea, and a reticular pattern on chest x-ray. No treatment has been successful, and the average survival after diagnosis is 5 months.

Dacarbazine and Procarbazine

Dacarbazine and procarbazine are atypical alkylating agents. Each drug is converted to active intermediates that can alkylate DNA, although the exact mechanisms are uncertain. Ultimately, the drugs inhibit DNA, RNA, and protein synthesis.

Dacarbazine and procarbazine are primarily used to treat Hodgkin's disease. Dacarbazine is administered intravenously and is part of the **ABVD regimen,** which consists of Adriamycin (doxorubicin), bleomycin, vinblastine, and dacarbazine. Procarbazine is given orally and is part of the **MOPP regimen,** which consists of mechlorethamine, Oncovin (vincristine), procarbazine, and prednisone. The ABVD regimen is newer than the MOPP regimen and is often used initially for the treatment of Hodgkin's disease.

Mitomycin

Mitomycin (mitomycin C) is an antineoplastic antibiotic that alkylates DNA and thereby causes strand breakage and inhibition of DNA synthesis. After the drug is administered parenterally, it is activated by hepatic reduction reactions to the active alkylating compound. Most of the drug is metabolized, but a small amount of it is excreted unchanged in the urine.

Mitomycin is primarily used in combination with vincristine as salvage therapy for breast cancer. It is also used in the treatment of non–small cell lung cancer, pancreatic and stomach tumors, and superficial transitional cell carcinomas of the bladder. Although it is administered intravenously for most types of cancer, it is administered intravesically for bladder cancer.

Mitomycin produces delayed and prolonged myelosuppression that preferentially affects platelets and leukocytes. It may also cause severe pulmonary damage and a hemolytic-uremic syndrome characterized by hemolytic anemia, renal dysfunction, and thrombocytopenia. Extravasation may result in severe necrosis.

DNA INTERCALATING DRUGS

The DNA intercalating drugs include the anthracycline drugs, bleomycin, and dactinomycin. These are some of the most widely used antitumor antibiotics. Several of the drugs have a broad spectrum of activity against hematologic cancers and solid tumors, while others have a more limited range of clinical uses.

Anthracycline Drugs
Daunorubicin, Doxorubicin, and Idarubicin

Chemistry. Daunorubicin and doxorubicin are antibiotics obtained from *Streptomyces peucetius,* and idarubicin is a semisynthetic derivative. These drugs have a four-membered anthracene ring with attached sugars (see Fig. 45–3C). Two of the four members in the ring are quinone and hydroquinone moieties that enable the compounds to accept and donate electrons and thereby promote the formation of free radicals. The anthracene ring accounts for the intense red color of the drug compounds.

Mechanisms. Several mechanisms are responsible for the cytotoxicity of the anthracycline drugs: intercalation of DNA, inhibition of topoisomerase, and formation of free radicals. The drugs bind strongly to DNA by inserting themselves between paired bases of double-stranded DNA and thereby causing deformation and uncoiling of the DNA (see Fig. 45–5B). The anthracyclines cause DNA strands to break by interfering with the action of topoisomerase II (an enzyme discussed later in this chapter) and by forming free radicals. The anthracyclines undergo reduction (addition of electrons) to form highly destructive hydroxyl radicals that produce DNA cleavage. The process appears to involve an iron-anthracycline complex that is strongly bound to DNA.

Pharmacokinetics. After intravenous administration, the anthracyclines are rapidly distributed to all body tissues except those of the CNS. They avidly bind to tissues and have large volumes of distribution and long half-lives. The drugs are extensively metabolized in the liver, and some metabolites are as pharmacologically active as the parent compounds.

Indications. Daunorubicin and idarubicin are agents used in induction and consolidation therapy for acute nonlymphocytic leukemia. Doxorubicin has a much broader spectrum of activity. It is one of the most active drugs against breast cancer, and it is also useful in the treatment of Hodgkin's disease, bladder cancer, ovarian cancer, gastric carcinoma, and other hematologic cancers and solid tumors (see Table 45–1).

Adverse Effects. Among the adverse effects of anthracyclines are myelosuppression and cardiac damage (which are dose-limiting effects), nausea and vomiting (which are dose-related and may be moderate to severe), alopecia, and mucosal ulcerations. Extravasation of the drugs during intravenous infusion may lead to severe localized tissue ulceration and necrosis. These localized reactions may progress over many weeks, and there is no effective treatment for them. Hence, exceptional care and specialized training is required for proper administration of anthracycline drugs.

The anthracyclines cause both acute and chronic cardiotoxicity. Manifestations of acute toxicity include sinus tachycardia and ventricular premature beats. These cardiac rhythm disturbances often occur during the first 24 hours and are self-limited. Chronic toxicity leads to congestive cardiomyopathy and limits the cumulative dose of anthracycline that can be given to any patient. The cardiomyopathy appears to result from iron-catalyzed formation of free radicals. Information about this process has led to the development of a cardioprotective drug called **dexrazoxane**. Dexrazoxane is a potent chelator of ferric iron, and it is believed to act by disrupting the iron-anthracycline complex and thereby preventing reactive free radical formation. Dexrazoxane is primarily given to women who have breast cancer that might benefit from continued doxorubicin therapy. Another method of preventing cardiotoxicity is to administer doxorubicin as a **liposomal complex** that is not taken up as much by cardiac tissue as is the free drug. This preparation is now approved for the treatment of Kaposi's sarcoma in patients with acquired immunodeficiency syndrome (AIDS), and it is expected to be used in the treatment of other solid tumors.

Interactions.   Drugs that increase the toxicity of doxorubicin include cyclosporine, cyclophosphamide, and mercaptopurine. Verapamil may increase the cytotoxicity of doxorubicin and other anthracycline drugs by inhibition of the P-glycoprotein that transports anthracyclines out of cells.

Mitoxantrone

Mitoxantrone is a synthetic anthracene derivative that is primarily used in combination with cytarabine for induction of remission in patients with acute nonlymphocytic leukemia. The drug is administered intravenously. Like the anthracycline antibiotics, mitoxantrone intercalates DNA and produces DNA strand breaks, but it has much less potential for free radical formation. Partly for this reason, mitoxantrone causes less cardiotoxicity, less tissue damage after extravasation, and less nausea, vomiting, mucosal ulceration, and alopecia than do doxorubicin and other anthracycline antibiotics.

Other DNA Intercalating Drugs
Bleomycin

Chemistry and Mechanisms.   Bleomycin is a mixture of two peptides obtained from *Streptomyces verticillus*. The drug has its greatest effect on neoplastic cells in the G_2 phase of the cell replication cycle. Although bleomycin intercalates DNA, the major cytotoxicity is believed to result from iron-catalyzed free radical formation and DNA strand breakage. The iron-bleomycin complex binds to DNA, which reduces molecular oxygen to oxygen free radicals that cause single strands of DNA to break.

Pharmacokinetics.   Bleomycin is administered intravenously, is widely distributed, and is primarily eliminated by renal excretion. The drug is inactivated in cells by aminohydrolase, whose low levels in skin and lung may partly account for the toxicity of bleomycin in these tissues.

Indications.   Bleomycin has a broad range of activity and is one of the most widely used antitumor antibiotics. It is useful in Hodgkin's and non-Hodgkin's lymphomas, testicular cancer, and several other solid tumors. It is particularly well known as an agent in the ABVD regimen for Hodgkin's disease (see Table 45–2).

Adverse Effects.   Bleomycin produces very little myelosuppression. For this reason, it is often combined with myelosuppressive drugs in treatment regimens. The most serious toxicities of bleomycin are pulmonary and mucocutaneous reactions. Patients taking the drug may develop pneumonitis that progresses to interstitial fibrosis, hypoxia, and death. It is therefore important to monitor patients carefully for manifestations of pulmonary toxicity, which include cough, dyspnea, rales, and pulmonary infiltrates on chest x-ray. Mucocutaneous toxicity usually presents as mild stomatitis (inflammation of the oral mucosa), skin hyperpigmentation, erythema, and edema.

Dactinomycin

Dactinomycin (actinomycin D) intercalates DNA and thereby prevents DNA transcription and messenger RNA synthesis. The drug is given intravenously, and its clinical use is limited to the treatment of trophoblastic (gestational) tumors and the treatment of pediatric tumors, such as Wilms' tumor and Ewing's sarcoma.

MITOTIC INHIBITORS

The mitotic spindle that separates the chromosomes during mitosis is made up of hollow tubules called microtubules. The microtubules are formed by the polymerization of the structural protein called tubulin. During mitosis, microtubules are continuously assembled and disassembled by means of tubulin polymerization and depolymerization. As shown in Fig. 45–6, two classes of antineoplastic drugs inhibit mitosis and cause metaphase arrest by interfering with microtubule function. The vinca alkaloids bind to tubulin and block tubulin polymerization, whereas the taxanes bind to tubulin and prevent depolymerization. By their action, the taxanes promote the formation of stable but nonfunctional microtubules. The fact that microtubules also have important roles in nerve conduction and neurotransmission may explain why use of mitotic inhibitors can cause neurotoxicity.

Vinca Alkaloids
Vincristine and Vinblastine

Chemistry and Pharmacokinetics.   Vincristine (see Fig. 45–3D) and vinblastine are natural alkaloids

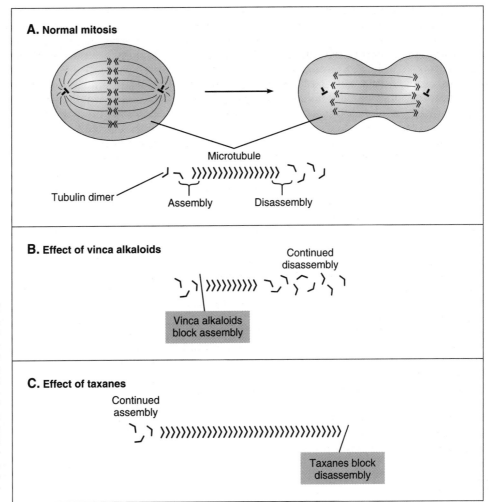

A. Normal mitosis

Microtubule

Tubulin dimer

Assembly   Disassembly

B. Effect of vinca alkaloids

Continued
disassembly

Vinca alkaloids
block assembly

C. Effect of taxanes

Continued
assembly

Taxanes block
disassembly

FIGURE 45–6. Mechanisms of action of mitotic inhibitors. **(A)** In normal mitosis, the mitotic spindle is formed by microtubules that continuously undergo assembly and disassembly as a result of tubulin polymerization and depolymerization, respectively. **(B)** Vincristine and other vinca alkaloids bind to tubulin and prevent the polymerization of tubulin dimers. **(C)** Paclitaxel and other taxanes bind to tubulin, stabilize the tubulin polymer, and thereby prevent depolymerization. Like vinca alkaloids, taxanes cause metaphase arrest.

from the periwinkle plant. Despite their structural similarity and identical mechanisms of action, the two drugs have different antitumor activities and toxicities. The oral absorption of vincristine and vinblastine is unreliable, so the drugs are administered intravenously. Neither drug enters the CNS in significant amounts. Both drugs are extensively metabolized and undergo biliary excretion.

Indications. Vincristine is often used to treat hematologic cancers, including acute lymphocytic leukemia, Hodgkin's and non-Hodgkin's lymphomas, and multiple myeloma. It also is employed in the treatment of some solid tumors, such as small cell lung cancer, neuroblastoma, and sarcoma. Vinblastine is used for lymphomas and for bladder, breast, ovarian, and testicular cancer. Vinblastine is a component of the ABVD regimen for Hodgkin's disease, while vincristine is a component of the MOPP regimen (see Table 45–2).

Adverse Effects. Vincristine produces dose-limiting neurotoxicity. It may cause a form of peripheral neuropathy that is usually distal and symmetric and affects both sensory and motor function. Suppression of deep tendon reflexes is often found and may be the earliest sign of neurotoxicity. Paresthesias of the hands and toes are also common. These

adverse effects are usually reversible and do not justify discontinuation of vincristine therapy unless they are disabling. Cranial nerve damage may cause hoarseness, facial palsies, or jaw pain, while autonomic neuropathies may cause orthostatic hypotension, abdominal pain, and constipation. In contrast to vinblastine, vincristine usually causes little myelosuppression.

The major dose-limiting toxicity of vinblastine is myelosuppression. Vinblastine usually causes little neurotoxicity.

Vinorelbine

Vinorelbine is a new semisynthetic derivative of vinblastine. It has shown good activity against non–small cell lung cancer and is being used as monotherapy for this disease.

Taxanes

Chemistry and Pharmacokinetics. The taxanes (taxoids) are plant alkaloids obtained from yew trees. In 1971, **paclitaxel** was isolated from the bark of a slow-growing Pacific yew, *Taxus brevifolia.* Because the complex ring structure of paclitaxel cannot be synthesized easily (see Fig. 45–3D) and because harvesting the bark kills the tree, efforts were made to find a more renewable source of this compound. The search resulted in the discovery of **docetaxel,** which was isolated from the needles of the European yew, *Taxus baccata.*

Paclitaxel and docetaxel are given intravenously and are eliminated via metabolism and biliary excretion.

Indications. The taxanes have good activity against several types of cancer (see Table 45–1). Paclitaxel is approved for treatment of metastatic ovarian cancer after failure of first-line drugs and for the treatment of metastatic breast cancer. Docetaxel is approved for locally advanced or metastatic breast cancer, and it is currently being evaluated for ovarian, non–small cell lung, pancreatic, and other cancers.

Adverse Effects. The major dose-limiting toxicity of taxanes is myelosuppression, particularly neutropenia. Taxanes may also cause alopecia and neurotoxicity.

TOPOISOMERASE INHIBITORS

DNA topoisomerases are enzymes that serve to maintain the normal structural topology of DNA. These enzymes relieve the torsional strain that is caused by the unwinding of DNA during the replication or transcription of DNA strands. Topoisomerases work by producing strand breaks that permit the strands to pass through the gap before the breaks are resealed. **Topoisomerase I** breaks and reseals single-stranded DNA, whereas **topoisomerase II** breaks and reseals double-stranded DNA.

Drugs that inhibit topoisomerases cause permanent strand breaks by preventing the resealing of the nicked strands of DNA. There are two groups of topoisomerase inhibitors. The podophyllotoxins inhibit topoisomerase II, whereas the camptothecin analogues inhibit topoisomerase I.

Podophyllotoxins

Chemistry and Pharmacokinetics. Podophyllin is a natural substance that is extracted from the mandrake or mayapple plant. Two semisynthetic derivatives of this substance, **etoposide** and **teniposide,** are used as antineoplastic drugs. Both drugs can be given intravenously. Although etoposide can also be given orally, its oral bioavailability varies greatly from patient to patient, so this route of administration may result in significant underdosing or overdosing. Etoposide is primarily eliminated unchanged in the urine, whereas teniposide is extensively metabolized in the liver.

Indications. Etoposide has a broad spectrum of activity against hematologic cancers and solid tumors. It is especially valuable in the treatment of testicular carcinoma, lung cancer, and non-Hodgkin's lymphomas. It also has value as a preoperative treatment for bone marrow transplantation. Because of its synergy with platinum compounds, etoposide is most frequently administered with cisplatin when it is used in combination therapy. Teniposide has a more limited spectrum of activity than does etoposide, and it is primarily used to treat acute lymphocytic leukemia.

Adverse Effects. Etoposide and teniposide are usually well tolerated, although they can produce alopecia, mild nausea and vomiting, and dose-limiting myelosuppression. They have also been associated with a low incidence of secondary nonlymphocytic leukemias.

Camptothecin Analogues

Chemistry and Pharmacokinetics. Camptothecin is an alkaloid obtained from *Camptotheca acuminata.* Although camptothecin is a potent inhibitor of topoisomerase I, it has relatively low clinical efficacy. **Irinotecan** and **topotecan** are synthetic camptothecin analogues that have greater clinical activity and less toxicity than the natural alkaloid and are given intravenously for the treatment of cancer. Irinotecan is rapidly metabolized to an active metabolite called SN-38. This metabolite has from 250-fold to 1000-fold greater antitumor activity than the parent compound. SN-38 is eliminated primarily in the bile, whereas topotecan undergoes renal excretion.

Indications. Irinotecan is approved for the treatment of colorectal cancer that has recurred or progressed following fluorouracil therapy. It is also active against lymphomas and breast, cervical, gastric, lung, and other tumors. Topotecan is active against glioma, sarcoma, and lung and ovarian tumors.

Adverse Effects. The dose-limiting toxicity of both camptothecin analogues is myelosuppression. Irinotecan produces diarrhea in a significant percentage of patients, and both drugs may cause alopecia and mild nausea and vomiting.

HORMONES AND THEIR ANTAGONISTS

Several types of hormone-dependent cancer (especially breast, prostate, and endometrial cancer) respond to treatment with their corresponding hormone antagonists. **Estrogen antagonists** are primarily used in the treatment of breast cancer, whereas **androgen antagonists** are used in the treatment of prostate cancer. **Corticosteroids** are particularly useful in treating lymphocytic leukemias and lymphomas.

The pharmacologic properties of estrogens, androgens, and their antagonists are described in Chapter 34, while those of corticosteroids are described in Chapter 33. The use of these drugs in cancer treatment is summarized below.

Hormones Used in Breast Cancer

Breast cancer is usually estrogen-dependent and can be suppressed by the administration of estrogen antagonists. **Tamoxifen** is the antagonist used most widely. This drug can be given alone to prevent breast cancer in women who have a strong family history of the disease or are otherwise highly predisposed to developing it. Tamoxifen is often employed in combination with surgery and other chemotherapeutic drugs for the treatment of breast cancer. In women over 50 years of age, adjuvant use of tamoxifen was found to reduce the annual odds of recurrence by 30%. Long-term survival appears to be greater in women receiving both cytotoxic chemotherapy and tamoxifen.

Androgens, such as **fluoxymesterone,** may also suppress the proliferation of breast cancer, but they are less effective and more toxic.

Hormones Used in Prostate Cancer

Prostate tissue is stimulated by androgens and suppressed by estrogens. For this reason, the major drugs for disseminated prostate cancer are androgen antagonists and estrogens. An androgen antagonist such as **flutamide** will block testosterone stimulation of prostate carcinoma cells. An estrogen such as **diethylstilbestrol** or a gonadotropin-releasing hormone agonist such as **leuprolide** will suppress the release of luteinizing hormone from the pituitary gland and will thereby suppress testosterone production. Estrogens also act directly to suppress prostate cancer proliferation.

Corticosteroids

Corticosteroids, such as **prednisone,** are primarily used because of their lymphocytotoxic effects in the treatment of lymphocytic leukemias, lymphomas, and multiple myeloma. Corticosteroids are relatively well tolerated and do not produce myelosuppression or other serious organ damage in most patients. For this reason, they are often combined with drugs that inhibit DNA function or mitosis in the treatment of these cancers.

IMMUNOMODULATING DRUGS

Drugs that affect the immune system are called **immunomodulators** or **biologic response modifiers.** Some of them, including recombinant interferons and cytokines, enhance antitumor immunity and are used to treat neoplastic diseases. Others act to suppress immune mechanisms and are used to treat autoimmune diseases or to prevent graft rejection following tissue transplantation. Monoclonal antibodies are immunomodulating drugs that bind to specific proteins in normal or neoplastic cells and have specific actions that have found application in a growing number of conditions, including cancers, autoimmune disorders, tissue transplantation, and infectious diseases. Based on their actions, the immunomodulating drugs can be classified as **immunostimulants** or **immunodepressants.**

Recombinant Interferons and Cytokines

Interferons are endogenous proteins that increase the activity of various cytotoxic cells in the immune system and directly inhibit the proliferation of neoplastic cells. **Interferon alfa** is an immunomodulating drug that can be administered intramuscularly, intravenously, or subcutaneously. It is used to treat Kaposi's sarcoma in patients with AIDS. In addition, it is used to treat hairy cell leukemia and chronic myelogenous leukemia and produces a clinical response in about 70% of patients with either of these diseases. In about 30% of patients with chronic myelogenous leukemia, interferon therapy causes a cytogenetic response that is characterized by loss of a chromosome called the Philadelphia chromosome.

Aldesleukin (interleukin-2, or IL-2) is a lymphokine formerly known as T cell growth factor. Aldesleukin activates IL-2 receptors and promotes B and T cell proliferation and differentiation. The antitumor effect of the drug is primarily due to increased numbers of cytotoxic T cells that can recognize and destroy tumor cells without damaging normal cells. These cytotoxic cells include natural killer cells, lymphokine-activated killer cells, and tumor-infiltrating cells.

Aldesleukin can be administered intramuscularly, intravenously, or subcutaneously. It is primarily used to treat metastatic renal cell carcinoma, but it also has activity against malignant melanoma and colorectal cancer. In about 20% of patients with renal cell carcinoma, it produces a good response, which in some cases persists for several years without further therapy.

In low doses, aldesleukin is often well tolerated and may be given as outpatient therapy. In higher doses, the drug can be quite toxic. The most common dose-limiting toxicities are hypotension, fluid retention, and renal dysfunction. Other toxicities include a broad range of hematologic deficiencies, skin lesions, and neuropsychiatric changes. The toxicities are usually reversible and can be prevented or managed by giving corticosteroids prior to aldesleukin therapy and providing vigorous supportive care. Prolonged infusions of aldesleukin appear to be less toxic than high-dose bolus injections.

Monoclonal Antibodies

Monoclonal antibodies are a new and fast-growing class of immunomodulating drugs. Table 45–3 discusses the manner in which they are assigned names and lists the clinical uses and target antigens of numerous monoclonal antibodies. **Abciximab** is discussed in Chapter 16, and **infliximab** is discussed in Chapter 28. Other monoclonal antibodies are described below.

Daclizumab is a monoclonal antibody to the high-affinity IL-2 receptor that is expressed on T cells. The antibody binds to the α subunit of the receptor, prevents IL-2 stimulation of T cell activity, and thereby reduces T cell activity against allografts. Daclizumab is used to prevent rejection of renal transplants.

Muromonab-CD3 is a monoclonal antibody to the CD3 glycoprotein that is part of the T cell antigen

TABLE 45–3. Clinical Uses and Target Antigens of Monoclonal Antibodies

Monoclonal Antibody*	Clinical Uses	Target Antigen
Abciximab	Prevent platelet aggregation and thrombosis in patients undergoing percutaneous transluminal coronary angioplasty.	Platelet glycoprotein IIb/IIIa receptors.
Daclizumab	Prevent rejection of renal transplants.	Interleukin-2 (IL-2) receptor on activated T cells.
Infliximab	Treat Crohn's disease; treat rheumatoid arthritis (investigational).	Tumor necrosis factor alpha (TNF-α).
Muromonab-CD3	Treat rejection of transplanted organs and bone marrow.	CD3 glycoprotein of the T cell antigen recognition receptor.
Palivizumab	Prevent respiratory syncytial virus (RSV) infection in infants at increased risk.	Fusion protein of RSV.
Rituximab	Treat non-Hodgkin's lymphomas.	CD20 surface antigen on non-Hodgkin's lymphoma cells.
Trastuzumab	Treat metastatic breast cancer.	Human epidermal growth factor 2 (HER2).

*Note that the names of monoclonal antibodies end in "mab" or "monab." The letters before "mab" indicate the source of the antibody: "o" for mouse, "u" for human, and "xi" for chimeric. An internal letter or syllable identifies the target of the antibody—for example, "c" for circulation (cardiovascular), "tu" for tumor, and "vi" for virus.

recognition receptor. The antibody prevents antigen access to the receptor and thereby prevents T cell activation. Muromonab-CD3 is used to treat acute allograft rejection in renal transplant patients. In addition, it is used to reverse bone marrow, cardiac, hepatic, kidney, and pancreatic transplant rejection episodes that are resistant to conventional drugs.

Palivizumab is a human monoclonal antibody to the fusion protein of respiratory syncytial virus (RSV). It is approved for prevention of RSV infection in infants with bronchopulmonary dysplasia and in premature infants whose gestational age is under 35 weeks. It is given as five monthly intramuscular doses.

Rituximab was the first monoclonal antibody approved for cancer chemotherapy. This chimeric human-murine antibody is used for treatment of relapsed or refractory B cell non-Hodgkin's lymphomas. It binds to the CD20 antigen that is found on the surface of over 90% of non-Hodgkin's lymphoma cells, as well as on normal B lymphocytes. CD20 is believed to regulate an early step in cell cycle initiation. The drug is given as an intravenous infusion.

Trastuzumab is a recombinant human monoclonal antibody to human epidermal growth factor 2 (HER2). It acts by binding to the extracellular domain of the HER2 receptor on cancer cells and thereby preventing receptor stimulation. Trastuzumab has been approved for the treatment of metastatic breast carcinoma in women who overexpress the HER2 oncogene, and it is being studied for use in combination with doxorubicin and paclitaxel. Trastuzumab is administered intravenously once a week. Its adverse effects include chills, fever, nausea, vomiting, chest pain, and dyspnea.

Microbial Products

Cyclosporine and **tacrolimus** are examples of immunomodulators that are derived from microbes. Cyclosporine is a complex fungal polypeptide, while tacrolimus is a macrolide antibiotic produced by a *Streptomyces* species. Each drug interferes with early

stages of lymphocyte proliferation by selectively blocking the production of cytokines by CD4 helper cells.

Either cyclosporine or tacrolimus can be used to prevent rejection of organ transplants and is usually given in combination with corticosteroids or other drugs. Cyclosporine can also be used to treat psoriasis and severe autoimmune diseases that are resistant to other therapeutic agents.

Cyclosporine frequently causes nephrotoxicity, hypertension, hirsutism, gingival hyperplasia, and muscle tremor. Cyclosporine is metabolized by CYP3A, a cytochrome P450 enzyme, and interacts with other drugs that inhibit or induce this enzyme. CYP3A inhibitors may increase the plasma levels and toxicity of cyclosporine, and these include erythromycin and other macrolide antibiotics, azole antifungal drugs, calcium channel blockers, and grapefruit juice. CYP3A inducers may decrease the plasma levels of cyclosporine, and these include carbamazepine, phenytoin, and rifampin.

Corticosteroids

Prednisone and other corticosteroids inhibit T cell proliferation and the expression of genes encoding various cytokines. They are used with other immunosuppressive drugs to prevent organ transplant rejection and to prevent graft-versus-host disease in patients who have undergone bone marrow transplantation. Corticosteroids are frequently employed in the treatment of various autoimmune disorders, including lupus erythematosus and rheumatoid arthritis. Their anti-inflammatory actions are also quite beneficial in these disorders (see Chapter 30).

Other Immunomodulating Drugs
Azathioprine, Cyclophosphamide, and Methotrexate

In the body, azathioprine is converted to 6-mercaptopurine. Like methotrexate, 6-mercaptopurine acts by inhibiting DNA synthesis. Cyclophosphamide acts by alkylating DNA. Because these agents prevent the proliferation of B and T lymphocytes, they are used in the prevention of organ graft rejection and in the treatment of autoimmune disorders and collagen diseases. Cyclophosphamide and methotrexate are also used in the treatment of cancer (see above).

Azathioprine is often given in combination with corticosteroids and cyclosporine or tacrolimus to patients with tissue transplants, and it is also useful in the treatment of patients with inflammatory bowel disease, rheumatoid arthritis, or lupus erythematosus. Cyclophosphamide is used primarily to treat lupus erythematosus and other autoimmune diseases and is usually given in combination with corticosteroids. Methotrexate has anti-inflammatory effects that make it especially useful in the management of rheumatoid arthritis (see Chapter 30). It is also useful in the treatment of psoriasis and severe asthma.

Levamisole

Originally used as an anthelmintic drug, levamisole was later discovered to have immunomodulating properties. The drug has complex effects that enhance T cell responses by stimulating T cell activation and proliferation. In addition to potentiating monocyte-macrophage chemotaxis and phagocytosis, it increases neutrophil mobility, adherence, and chemotaxis.

Levamisole is administered orally, and it is extensively metabolized before undergoing renal excretion. It is used in combination with fluorouracil for the treatment of colorectal cancer. In comparison with fluorouracil treatment alone, studies show that combination treatment with levamisole resulted in a 33% increase in the survival rate and a 36% decrease in the cancer recurrence rate.

Levamisole is usually well tolerated, but it causes severe granulocytopenia in up to 10% of patients. A few patients experience neurologic symptoms such as insomnia, headache, and nightmares. Mild and reversible hepatic toxicity occurs in about 40% of patients treated with the drug.

Thalidomide

Thalidomide was once banned because of its potential to cause phocomelia and other congenital malformations. It was subsequently discovered to have immunomodulating effects, and it is now being used to treat recurrent aphthous ulcers (canker sores), tuberculosis, leprosy, erythema nodosum leprosum, and the AIDS-associated wasting syndrome (cachexia).

Thalidomide appears to have both immunosuppressant and immunostimulant effects. It inhibits the production of IL-2, tumor necrosis factor alpha (TNF-α), and other cytokines. While thalidomide inhibits lymphocyte proliferation stimulated by alloantigens, some studies show that it stimulates CD8[+] cells in vitro. The mechanism of action of thalidomide in specific diseases remains to be determined.

Summary of Important Points

- Most antineoplastic drugs inhibit DNA synthesis or disrupt DNA structure and function.
- DNA synthesis inhibitors include folate antagonists (methotrexate and trimetrexate), purine antagonists (mercaptopurine, thioguanine, and others), pyrimidine antagonists (cytarabine, floxuridine, and fluorouracil), and a ribonucleotide reductase inhibitor (hydroxyurea).
- DNA alkylating drugs that cross-link DNA include nitrogen mustards (cyclophosphamide and others), nitrosoureas (carmustine and others), and miscellaneous drugs (busulfan, dacarbazine, mitomycin, and procarbazine). Platinum compounds (carboplatin and cisplatin) also cross-link DNA strands.
- DNA intercalating drugs include the anthracyclines (doxorubicin and others), bleomycin, and dactinomycin.
- Inhibitors of mitosis include vinca alkaloids (vincristine and others) and taxanes (docetaxel and paclitaxel).
- Topoisomerase inhibitors include podophyllotoxins (etoposide and teniposide) and camptothecin analogues (irinotecan and topotecan).
- Biologic response modifiers used in the treatment of cancer include interferon alfa, aldesleukin, levamisole, and two monoclonal antibodies (rituximab and trastuzumab).
- Myelosuppression is the dose-limiting toxicity of most antineoplastic drugs.
- Doxorubicin and other anthracyclines produce cardiotoxicity; cyclophosphamide causes hemorrhagic cystitis; bleomycin and busulfan produce pulmonary fibrosis; vincristine, docetaxel, and related drugs cause neurotoxicity; and cisplatin produces renal toxicity.
- Hormonal agents are used to treat some cancers, especially estrogen antagonists to treat breast cancer, androgen antagonists and estrogens to treat prostate cancer, and corticosteroids (such as prednisone) to treat lymphocytic leukemias and lymphomas.
- Immunosuppressant drugs used to prevent organ transplant rejection or to treat autoimmune diseases include monoclonal antibodies (daclizumab and muromonab-CD3), microbial products (cyclosporine and tacrolimus), corticosteroids (such as prednisone), and cytotoxic drugs (such as azathioprine).

Selected Readings

Drings, P., et al. Ifosfamide and docetaxel in non–small cell lung cancer. Semin Oncol 25:29–37, 1998.

Eisenhauer, E. A., and J. B. Vermorken. The taxoids: comparative clinical pharmacology and therapeutic potential. Drugs 55:5–30, 1998.

Ghaemmaghami, M., and J. R. Jett. New agents in the treatment of small cell lung cancer. Chest 113:86S–91S, 1998.

Glick, J. H., et al. MOPP/ABVD hybrid chemotherapy for advanced Hodgkin's disease significantly improves failure-free and overall survival: the 8-year results of the intergroup trial. J Clin Oncol 16:19–26, 1998.

Loeffler, M., et al. Meta-analysis of chemotherapy versus combined modality treatment trials in Hodgkin's disease. J Clin Oncol 16:815–817, 1998.

McNeil, C. Herceptin [trastuzumab] raises its sites beyond advanced breast cancer. J Natl Cancer Inst 90:882–883, 1998.

Nathan, F. E., and M. J. Mastrangelo. Systemic therapy in melanoma. Semin Surg Oncol 14:319–327, 1998.

Pui, C. H. Acute leukemia in children. Curr Opin Hematol 3:249–258, 1996.

Subramanian, K. N., et al. Safety, tolerance, and pharmacokinetics of a humanized monoclonal antibody to respiratory syncytial virus in premature infants and infants with bronchopulmonary dysplasia. Pediatr Infect Dis J 17:110–115, 1998.

Todeschini, G. Estimated 6-year survival of 55% in 60 consecutive adult acute lymphoblastic leukemia patients treated with an intensive phase II protocol based on a high induction dose of daunorubicin. Leukemia 12:144–149, 1998.

Uckun, F. M., et al. Biology and treatment of childhood T-lineage acute lymphoblastic leukemia. Blood 91:735–746, 1998.

INDEX

Note: Page numbers in *italics* refer to illustrations; page numbers followed by "t" refer to tables. Drug names listed in SMALL CAPITAL LETTERS are trade names (brand names). Because trade names are not discussed in the text, the index refers the reader to the listing for the generic drug name.

A

Aβ fibers, 244
Aδ fibers, 244
ABBOKINASE. See *Urokinase.*
Abciximab, 164t, 167, 487, 488t
Abdominal distention, 58
Abortion, 284, 361
Abscess, 393
Absorption, drug, 3, 9–11
ABVD regimen, 483
Acarbose, 371t, 375, 377
ACCOLATE. See *Zafirlukast.*
Accommodative esotropia, 58
ACCUPRIL. See *Quinapril.*
ACE inhibitors. See *Angiotensin-converting enzyme (ACE) inhibitors.*
Acebutolol, 80t, 83t, 84
Acetaminophen, 250, 295, 320–322
 overdose of, *321,* 322
Acetazolamide, *126,* 127t, 128t, 131
Acetohexamide, 371
Acetylation, in drug biotransformation, 15, 17, *18*
Acetylcholine, 45, *59,* 178, 179t, *180*
 ethanol inhibition of, 257
 gastric acid secretion and, 299
 inhibition of, 47–48
 properties of, 53–55
 receptors for, 47
 synthesis of, *48*
 uses of, 54–55
Acetylcholine receptor antagonists, 216t, 217t, 218
Acetylcysteine, 322
Acetylsalicylic acid. See *Aspirin.*
Acid, weak, 9, 11–12
Acinetobacter infection, 397t
Acne rosacea, 464
Acne vulgaris, 358

Acquired immunodeficiency syndrome. See *AIDS/HIV infection.*
Acromegaly, 332–333
ACTH (adrenocorticotropic hormone), 330, *331,* 332, 342
Actinomyces israelii infection, 397t
Actinomycin D, 484
ACTIVASE. See *Alteplase.*
ACULAR. See *Ketorolac.*
Acyclovir, 449–450, 451t, 452t
ADALAT. See *Nifedipine.*
Addiction, 255
Addisonian crisis, 347
Addison's disease, 346
ADENOCARD. See *Adenosine.*
Adenohypophysis, 330
 hormones of, *331,* 332–334
Adenoma, pituitary, 333, 334, 338
Adenosine, 140t, 142t, 145
Adenosine monophosphate, cyclic (cAMP), in drug-receptor interaction, 27
Adenosine receptors, 183
Adhesives, 5
Adrenal androgens, 348
 classification of, 342
Adrenal crisis, 347
Adrenal hyperplasia, congenital, 347
Adrenal insufficiency, 332, 344, 346–347
Adrenal steroids, *343,* 344–348
 classification of, 342
 inhibitors of, 342, 349
ADRENALIN. See *Epinephrine.*
Adrenergic receptor(s), 47, 68–70, 179t, 180
Adrenergic receptor agonists, 70–76
 classification of, 68
 direct-acting, 50, 68, 70–75
 for heart failure, 111, 114t, 117t, 118
 for Horner's syndrome diagnosis, 49

Adrenergic receptor agonists *(Continued)*
 indirect-acting, 50, 68, *71,* 72t, 75
 mixed-acting, 68, *71,* 72t, 75–76
β-Adrenergic receptor agonists
 classification of, 286
 for respiratory tract disorders, 286, 288t, 291, 292t
Adrenergic receptor antagonists, 50, 77–85
 classification of, 77
α- and β-Adrenergic receptor antagonists, *78,* 80t, 83t, 84–85
 classification of, 77
α-Adrenergic receptor antagonists, 77–81
 classification of, 77
 for hypertension, 79–80, *81, 82, 90,* 91t
 nonselective, 77–79, 80t
 selective, 77, *78,* 79–81, *82, 83*
β-Adrenergic receptor antagonists, *78,* 80t, 81–84
 classification of, 77
 for arrhythmias, 133
 for hypertension, 88
 for ischemic heart disease, 102
 for migraine headache, 310
 for thyroid disease, 336
 for arrhythmias, 133, 143, 144–145
 for heart failure, 120–121
 for hypertension, 81, 84, 88, *90,* 91t, 94
 for hyperthyroidism, 340
 for ischemic heart disease, 102, 103t, *104,* 108, 109t
 for migraine headache, 310, 312–313
 for thyroid disease, 340
 nonselective, 77, *78,* 80t, 81–84
 selective, 77, *78,* 80t, 84
Adrenocortical tumors, 349
Adrenocorticotropic hormone (ACTH), 330, *331,* 332, 342
Adrenogenital syndrome, 344
ADRIAMYCIN. See *Doxorubicin.*

491